# Harris' Developmental Neuropsychiatry

# Harris' Developmental Neuropsychiatry

*The Interface with Cognitive and Social Neuroscience*

Second Edition

JAMES C. HARRIS
*and*
JOSEPH T. COYLE

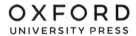

OXFORD
UNIVERSITY PRESS

# OXFORD
## UNIVERSITY PRESS

Oxford University Press is a department of the University of Oxford. It furthers
the University's objective of excellence in research, scholarship, and education
by publishing worldwide. Oxford is a registered trade mark of Oxford University
Press in the UK and certain other countries.

Published in the United States of America by Oxford University Press
198 Madison Avenue, New York, NY 10016, United States of America.

Library of Congress Cataloging-in-Publication Data
Names: Harris, James C., author. | Coyle, Joseph T., author.
Title: Harris' developmental neuropsychiatry : the interface with cognitive
and social neuroscience / James C. Harris and Joseph T. Coyle.
Other titles: Developmental neuropsychiatry
Description: Edition 2. | New York, NY : Oxford University Press, [2024] |
Preceded by Developmental neuropsychiatry / James C. Harris. New York :
Oxford University Press, 1995. |
Includes bibliographical references and index.
Identifiers: LCCN 2024020184 | ISBN 9780199928118 (paperback) |
ISBN 9780197521496 (epub) | ISBN 9780197521489 (updf) | ISBN 9780197521502 (digital online)
Subjects: MESH: Neurodevelopmental Disorders—psychology | Child |
Child Psychiatry | Child Development | Neuropsychiatry |
Cognitive Neuroscience
Classification: LCC RJ506.D47 | NLM WS 350.7 |
DDC 618.92/8—dc23/eng/20240521
LC record available at https://lccn.loc.gov/2024020184

DOI: 10.1093/med/9780199928118.001.0001

Printed by Marquis Book Printing, Canada

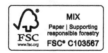

# Contents

## PART IV.   NEURODEVELOPMENTAL DISORDERS

# Foreword

This book is truly a significant contribution to the field of neuropsychiatry, but it's worthiness goes beyond the science. It is the culmination of the work of two very bright and dedicated men whose friendship and brotherly love for each other made the publication possible.

My soulmate and husband, Jim Harris, spent 5 years writing the original edition. Then in 2021 after he had spent 3 years working on this next edition, he was diagnosed with metastatic pancreatic cancer. This diagnosis was a complete surprise because he had no signs or symptoms prior to difficulty breathing 3 days prior to the diagnosis. Despite the best possible care at our academic home, Johns Hopkins, he died 6 weeks later. During all but the last 2 days of his life, he worked on the book. Unfortunately, the text was far from completed.

Our niece, Kathleen Pasko, who from the beginning was Jim's amazing assistant and organizer, edited the manuscript for grammar, punctuation, and formatting and would continue to do so. But the content was incomplete.

I knew how much this important text meant to Jim, but this was not my field, and I certainly could not complete it. So I contacted Jim's and my friend, Joe Coyle, who had advised Jim in the writing of the first edition. Despite his incredibly busy schedule and the amount of work needed, Joe undertook the completion of the text. Without Joe's input, this text would still be and probably would forever be in limbo.

The love shared by these two men for each other and for scientific excellence is the soul of this text. My hope is that the readers will feel that spirit while learning about developmental neuropsychiatry.

I also want to recognize Dr. John M. Davis for his generous contribution to this publication. His amazing friendship and support over the years means so much to Jim and me.

Catherine DeAngelis, MD, MPH

# Prologue

James (Jim) Harris, MD (1940–2021), was born in Birmingham, Alabama, but grew up in Washington, DC. He matriculated at the University of Maryland and received his Medical Degree at George Washington University School of Medicine, followed by an internship at Children's Hospital of Los Angeles. He then spent 3 years as a surgeon in the U.S. Public Health Service, serving in the Peace Corps in Thailand. After a year as a resident in pediatrics at Strong Memorial Hospital in Rochester, New York, he completed his pediatrics residency at Johns Hopkins University. He then completed a residency in child and adolescent psychiatry at Hopkins and the Kennedy Institute for the Developmentally Disabled. Rounding out his clinical training, he completed his residency in adult psychiatry at the Hopkins Phipps Clinic, receiving Board certification in pediatrics, adult, and child and adolescent psychiatry. It was during our time as residents at the Phipps Clinic that Jim and I became friends of nearly 50 years.

Among his many responsibilities at Hopkins, his most consistent identification was being the Director of Developmental Neuropsychiatry at the Kennedy Krieger Institute, a position that he held for more than 40 years. This served as his "clinical laboratory" to conceptualize the relationship between neuropsychiatry and the various behavioral manifestations of developmental disorders. With few exceptions at the time, most Divisions of Child Psychiatry were dominated by psychoanalytically trained psychiatrists with little interest in the developmentally disabled because their behavioral problems were not amenable to psychotherapy. Jim hailed from a different, empirical tradition of Leo Kanner, who first described autistic spectrum disorder (Kanner, 1943), and Leon Eisenberg, who carried out the first placebo controlled clinical trial in child psychiatry on stimulants in children with school behavioral problems (Conners et al., 1967).

At the time that Jim began to work in the Kennedy Institute, the behavioral problems of children with developmental disorders were largely ascribed to cognitive impairments and not linked to specific neuropsychopathology. Treatment was based on the Skinnerian strategies of behavioral modification as conceptualized in applied behavioral analysis wherein controlling the contingencies modified (extinguished) the offending behavior (Cataldo, 1982). Through his collaboration with Bill Nyhan on Lesch–Nyhan syndrome, which was characterized by recalcitrant self-injurious behavior, he elaborated the concept of "behavioral phenotype" and sought links between the behavior and specific brain pathology. This led, for example, to the demonstration of forebrain dysfunction of the dopamine system in the pathophysiology of self-injurious behavior in Lesch–Nyhan syndrome (Wong et al., 1996).

These observations prompted Jim to single-handedly write a textbook for Oxford University Press titled *Developmental Neuropsychiatry*. This was the first textbook to cover this topic. *Volume I: Fundamentals* reviewed the basic neuroscience advances that underpinned the relationship between the developing brain and behavioral pathology, cognitive neuroscience, and the developmental perspective that provided a new conceptual approach to these conditions. *Volume II: Assessment, Diagnosis, and Treatment of Developmental Disorders* reviewed the methods of assessment, discussed specific developmental disorders, and elaborated on the concept of behavioral phenotypes. He defined a behavioral phenotype as "a pattern of behavior that is reliably identified in groups of children with known genetic disorders and is not learned." Finally, he covered the various types of treatment. *Developmental Neuropsychiatry* was selected by Moody's as the best medical textbook published in 1996.

Since the publication of *Developmental Neuropsychiatry*, the field of developmental neuropsychiatry has changed dramatically as a consequence of seismic scientific advances. Brain imaging expanded to include magnetic resonance spectroscopy to visualize the chemical composition of the brain and functional magnetic resonance imaging to identify circuit activity related to typical and pathologic brain function. The sequencing of the human genome by 2001 transformed our ability to identify mutations and allelic variants that confer risk for developmental disorders. As the cost of sequencing the human genome fell from $100 million to less than a $1,000 per genome, genome sequencing has become routinely available for identifying genetic causes of rare developmental disorders (Bick et al., 2019). Not only has CRISPR technology made it possible to re-create in mice, rats, and even subhuman primates genetic models of developmental disorders but also it holds out the promise for potential treatments (Wong et al., 2021).

Recognizing these advances, Jim undertook in 2019 the enormous task of revising the textbook to incorporate the current state of clinical knowledge. Unfortunately, in the spring of 2021, Jim, having completed a rough draft and 70% of its fine editing, was diagnosed with pancreatic cancer, resulting in his untimely death. His wife, Catherine DeAngelis, MD, Professor of Pediatrics at Johns Hopkins, asked me to complete the final editing. Everything that is correct in this final version reflects Jim's all-encompassing knowledge of the field; any weaknesses are likely due to my oversights.

Joseph T. Coyle, MD

Eben S. Draper Professor of Psychiatry and Neuroscience (Emeritus)

Harvard Medical School and McLean Hospital

## References

Bick, D., Jones, M., Taylor, S. L., Taft, R. J., & Belmont, J. (2019). Case for genome sequencing in infants and children with rare, undiagnosed or genetic diseases. Journal of Medical Genetics, 56(12), 783–791.

Cataldo, M. F. (1982). The scientific basis for a behavioral approach to pediatrics. Pediatric Clinics of North America, 29(2), 415–423.

Conners, C. K., Eisenberg, L., & Barcai, A. (1967). Effect of dextroamphetamine on children: Studies on subjects with learning disabilities and school behavior problems. Archives of General Psychiatry, 17(4), 478–485.

Kanner, L. (1943). Autistic disorders of affective contact. Nervous Child, 2(3), 217–250.

Wong, D. F., Harris, J. C., Naidu, S., Yokoi, F., Marenco, S., Dannals, R. F., Ravert, H. T., Yaster, M., Evans, A., Rousset, O., Bryan, R. N., Gjedde, A., Kuhar, M. J., & Breese, G. R. (1996). Dopamine transporters are markedly reduced in Lesch–Nyhan disease in vivo. Proceedings of the National Academy of Sciences of the USA, 93(11), 5539–5543.

Wong, P. K., Cheah, F. C., Syafruddin, S. E., Mohtar, M. A., Azmi, N., Ng, P. Y., & Chua, E. W. (2021). CRISPR gene-editing models geared toward therapy for hereditary and developmental neurological disorders. Frontiers in Pediatrics, 9, 592571.

# Introduction

## Historical Landmarks in Developmental Neuropsychiatry

Although recognized since antiquity, explanations of the nature, causes, and treatment of intellectual and developmental disabilities have varied considerably. Historically, the earliest reference and discussion of intellectual developmental impairment may be in the Egyptian Papyrus of Thebes circa 1552 BC (Bryan, 1930). Over the intervening centuries, there has been considerable confusion about the nature and meaning of intellectual and developmental disabilities. Approaches to intervention have ranged from infanticide to exorcism and removal of evil spirits to humane education. In Greek and Roman culture, infanticide was practiced and trephining may have been used in Europe, Central, and South America as a treatment, presumably to allow such spirits to escape. Some intellectually impaired people may have become slaves and others court jesters. In the Middle Ages, demon possession continued to be suspected, but adequate care was practiced as well, for example, in the famous Hospice in Gheel, Belgium. An intellectually impaired child might also have been regarded as a changeling—an unusual child who was substituted at birth for a normal child by the fairies. In some instances, intellectually impaired people were regarded as "children of God" or harmless innocents who were allowed to wander at will. Based on this more benign view, Henry II of England promulgated legislation to provide for their protection. "Natural fools" were made wards of the king (Deitz & Repp, 1989).

Despite this early recognition and a historical distinction between neurodevelopmental disorders, intellectually impaired and those with major neurocognitive disorders (dementia), whose difficulties began later in life, an emphasis on child development and education of the intellectually impaired did not begin until the 19th century. Although the French Revolution and the American Revolution were accompanied by humane treatment and reforms in care and their aftermath saw the appearance of schools for deaf-mutes and for the blind, there was little specific study of child development. For this to occur, a new orientation toward children was required that began toward the end of the 18th century (Kanner, 1964). It was stimulated by the philosophy of Rousseau, who had emphasized the development of the child's natural, but latent, abilities through education. He viewed the child's nature as essentially good and suggested these qualities are capable of development, which was in contrast to the prevailing view that children lack innate qualities of goodness and require a rigid form of education. With a shift to considering the child's nature as essentially good, free individual expression was encouraged. The 1762 publication of *Emile* by Rousseau (1762/1911) stimulated considerable interest in Europe among educators. By emphasizing the role of the child as an active participant in learning, Rousseau's philosophy provided an orientation to the child that is an important aspect of current developmental theory.

In the 19th century, an interest in child development was further stimulated by a theory proposed to the French Academy of Sciences by Étienne Bonnet de Condillac. In his essay *Origin of Human Knowledge* and his *Treatise on the Sensations* (Crutcher, 1943), Condillac taught that "all knowledge is gained through the senses," which suggests the child's mind is a blank slate at birth. A person without language, he maintained, utilizes sight, sound, and their sensing experience of events or objects, which evoke ideas corresponding to their sensory input. He speculated that the human being first acquires the sense of smell and later acquires the other senses. Through sensory experience, intellectual abilities and knowledge of the world are established. This question of the nature of humans was the central question during the period known as the Enlightenment. Was the difference between human and animal one of kind or degree? How should wild children be classified, as human or animal? The nature of human beings and how they gain knowledge led to experiments with feral children. The most famous of these was Victor, the wild boy of Aveyron, France. Apparently, he was found in the forest living among animals. He had lacked human contact for many years and was unable to talk.

A classic study was initiated by Itard in 1800 to educate Victor (Itard, 1806). Itard was a student of Pinel, who had supervised the freeing of the insane from their chains in Paris and was the preeminent psychiatrist of that time. Despite Pinel's conclusion that Victor was intellectually impaired, Itard, following Condillac's approach, denied this. His task was to test Condillac's theory that all knowledge is acquired through the senses. Itard, under the auspices of the French Academy of Sciences, worked with Victor for 5 years. Although he made progress, Itard was not able to educate Victor successfully and finally concluded that Victor was intellectually impaired. Yet, the gains he had made with Victor were encouraging. This was the first systematic, scientific attempt to train an intellectually impaired person which demonstrated that benefits could come from education. Often neglected and an object of ridicule, it became apparent that something could be done to help an intellectually impaired person make progress. Victor's case has been reviewed in detail by Harlan Lane (1976), who suggests that Victor either had an autism spectrum disorder or was severely intellectually impaired.

Likewise, in the 19th century, the view of demon possession and the view of intellectually impaired persons as harmless innocents were replaced by early attempts to educate and house them. In 1837, Édouard Séguin, a pupil of Itard, began private instruction for intellectually impaired persons, and in 1846 he published *Idiocy and Treatment*, an approach to intervention that was the standard textbook for many years (Séguin, 1846, 1866). Itard's investigations led to the establishment of the first residential European center for young intellectually impaired people by Guggenbuhl in 1841 (Kanner, 1960). The first state school in the United States was established in Massachusetts in 1848, but it was not until 1875 that the need for care became generally recognized. Initially, the interventions were in designated educational institutions, but later it became clear that some custodial care was also needed.

During the same time period in England, J. Langdon Down described and classified syndromes in people who were intellectually impaired. He is credited with providing the first major separate classification and complete description of specific syndromes involving intellectual impairment. His general classification included congenital, accidental, and developmental categories. In 1866, Down published his observations of congenitally intellectually impaired persons in *London Hospital Reports* as "Observations on an Ethnic Classification of Idiots" (Down, 1866) and subsequently expanded them (Down, 1887). His classification was based on a then current biological theory of recapitulation: He assumed ontogeny recapitulates phylogeny. According to this theory, embryonic development in higher animals follows stages or sequences so the adult forms of lower creatures are successively passed through, one after the other, in development. Normal traits of infant life are considered more primitive but arrested, ancestral adult forms. Traits and abilities of an atypical adult were considered throwbacks or arrests in development at the level of one of the "lower races." Down included Ethiopian, Malay, Negroid, Aztec, and Mongolian as less developed forms in classifying intellectually impaired children and adults. Among these, the term "Mongolian idiot" or "mongolism" persisted for many years without reference to its racial origins. It was finally abandoned after the 21 chromosomal anomaly was demonstrated. The term "Down syndrome" is now the current usage. With Down's classification, earlier fanciful explanations were replaced by new ideas but couched in what is now an antiquated scientific theory.

Several decades later, intelligence testing was introduced. There was also an outgrowth of efforts at education of developmentally impaired persons, which led to the establishment of measures to determine intellectual ability. In France, Binet and Simon (1905, 1916) evaluated methods to deal with "backward school children" by developing a series of tests with progressively more difficult questions and subsequently arranging them by age level. In the United States, Lewis Terman (1916) standardized these tests for American children as the Stanford–Binet test. The revision of the Stanford–Binet test was published in 1916 based on assessment of 1,000 American children. Subsequently, tests were developed by Kuhlman for younger children who could not speak.

Along with intelligence, other areas of child development began to be investigated in the 19th century. In 1872, Darwin published *The Expression of the Emotions in Man and Animals*, the product of 40 years of reflection on the inheritance of behavioral patterns (Darwin, 1872/1965). Stages of development also had been considered by Darwin, and in 1877 he completed *A Biographical Sketch of an Infant* (Darwin, 1877). This study was based on notes Darwin had made on his son William's development beginning in 1839 (Bowlby, 1991). Darwin was particularly interested in behavior that occurs without being learned, such as the infant's smile. He wondered how such patterns of behavior were inherited and considered their survival value. Darwin studied emotional expression and postures as well as vocalizations. He noted how social awareness begins to focus on others and reported on the gradual differentiation of the infant cry. His studies signaled the beginning of a socioemotional approach to development.

An emphasis on child development brought to an end the view that children are miniature adults who were to be given adult responsibilities as soon as possible (Aries, 1962). In 1891, Stanley Hall began the first systematic application of the scientific method to the study of the child. Hall analyzed several thousand parent questionnaires on child development and published his results. He subsequently established the first journal of child psychology, *The Pedagogical Seminary* (Crutcher, 1943). The concept of adolescence was established as a developmental stage that follows the onset of puberty and was subsequently studied by Hall (1904).

During the same period in which an interest had emerged in child development, mental disorders in children were formally described. According to William Parry-Jones (1989), a discussion of mental disorders in children was provided by Charles West in 1852 and in 1871. William Griesinger (1867) suggested that mania and melancholia do occur in children, but hallucinations and delusions are much less common than in adults. Henry Maudsley (1867), in his *The Physiology and Pathology of the Mind*, included a chapter titled "Insanity of Early Life." After this, insanity in children gradually became differentiated from idiocy, epilepsy, and other neurological disorders. Referring to the early onset of mental disorders, Maudsley suggested that "anomalies, when rightly studied, yield rare instruction." His focus was on the chronicity of these conditions. Subsequently, Emminghaus, Moreau, and Manheimer applied adult psychiatric diagnostic terms to children (Kanner, 1959). During this period, the idea of hereditary transmission became popular, as did the view that the developing brain is vulnerable to infections, disease, head injury, frightening experiences, and bereavement (Parry-Jones, 1989). Frank Beach (1898) spoke of both organic and psychological causative factors. Puberty began to be recognized as physiologically linked to disturbance, and pubertal, or adolescent, insanity was recognized (Maudsley, 1895).

With these 19th-century origins in the education of intellectually impaired persons, the early attempts at classification, an emerging interest in socioemotional development, and the recognition of mental disorders in children, the foundation was laid for the emergence of developmental neuropsychiatry as a specialty focus in the 20th century. Moreover, during the first two decades of the 20th century, there was a dramatic change in attitude toward people with intellectual impairment. Earlier views of amorality and incorrigibility, necessitating lifelong support, were replaced by an understanding that education and community support are effective interventions.

The beginning of the 20th century saw an increased focus on behavior and on understanding juvenile delinquency. George Frederic Still (1902), in his Coulstonian lectures, described disorders of volition or moral self-control. In 1909, William Healey introduced child psychiatry into the juvenile court through the Illinois Institute of Juvenile Research. The juvenile court had previously been established in 1899 in the United States and several years earlier in Australia. Both social work assessment and psychological testing to establish the level of intelligence were introduced into the juvenile court. In 1915, Healey's book, *The Individual Delinquent*, which presented case histories of children as distinct persons, was published. That same year, the National Committee for Mental Hygiene, inspired by Clifford Beers' (1908/1981) book, *A Mind That Found Itself*, was established.

Adolph Meyer introduced objective psychology, or psychobiology, as a pragmatic approach to psychiatry early in the 20th century. The central focus of psychobiology was on the person, whose total life history must be studied along with their mental and physical capacities (Meyer, 1915; see also Lamb, 2014). A stimulus to Meyer's efforts was Emil Kraepelin's psychiatric classification, which clearly described mental disorders but did not specify treatments. According to Meyer, an emphasis on classification introduced an element of hopelessness once a diagnosis was made that little could be done to treat (Meyer, 1910). He taught that something could be done through intervention in the schools and in the social environment through interpersonal experiences that could alleviate hopelessness (Meyer, 1895). Meyer's psychobiology emphasized the contribution of life events to the development of a psychiatric disorder.

By 1920, the Commonwealth Foundation had established fellowships for psychiatrists to study difficult predelinquent and delinquent children in the schools and, through the juvenile courts, to develop sounder methods of treatment (Stevenson & Smith, 1934). In 1928, Leo Kanner, as a recipient of a Commonwealth Foundation University Fellowship, came to Johns Hopkins University to study under Adolph Meyer. In 1930, Kanner established the first child psychiatry/pediatric liaison service in a university hospital in the Johns Hopkins Harriet Lane Home. Soon afterwards, the first children's neuropsychiatric hospital opened in 1931 for the treatment of children with problems in behavior. In 1935, Kanner introduced the first English language textbook of child and adolescent psychiatry based on the first several hundred referrals seen in his pediatric consultation clinic. Many of the first cases referred to him were children who were intellectually impaired. A 1938 referral to Kanner subsequently became the first case of a new syndrome, which he described a few years later as infantile autism (Kanner, 1943). His recognition of early onset neurodevelopmental disorder in infantile autism and other disorders, which could have infantile and childhood onset, led to more careful scrutiny of early emotional development. It became apparent to Kanner that intellectually impaired persons require careful examination, have widely differing personalities, and can become emotionally disturbed.

The involvement of the parent in child development was increasingly emphasized; both parental overprotection and parental rejection were recognized. The focus on the negative aspects of the parental role in development by psychologists became so much emphasized that Kanner felt compelled to write a response, *In Defense of Mothers* (Kanner, 1941). Parents of disabled children established their own support groups to help one another cope with their child's disability. The earliest of these was the Council for the Retarded Child, which began in 1933 in Ohio, followed by the Washington Association for Retarded Children (1936) and the Welfare League for Retarded Children (1939). Once initiated, these groups eventually became nationwide organizations.

With the beginning of the eugenics movement, there was growing concern about the heredity of neurodevelopmental disorders, especially about their behavior. This led to the practice of sterilization of people with an intellectual developmental disorder. In 1927, the Supreme Court, in an 8–1 decision, upheld the legality of eugenic sterilization in the United States. In that era, the nation was caught up in a eugenics fervor. In *Buck v. Bell*, the justices allowed Virginia to sterilize Carrie Buck, a resident at the Dickensian Virginia Colony for Epileptics and Feebleminded, diagnosed (incorrectly) at the time as an imbecile. Oliver Wendell Holmes, Jr., an esteemed justice, wrote the majority decision that concluded, "Three generations of imbeciles are enough." This decision led to widespread eugenic sterilization of 70,000 American women and girls in the ensuing years (Cohen, 2016). Although by 1940, most states had abandoned practices of restricted marriage, sterilization, and institutionalization as ways to prevent future generations of intellectually impaired persons (Scheerenberger, 1983), eugenic sterilization continued into the 1960s in some states.

Moreover, during World War II, intellectually and developmentally impaired adults were designated as undesirable, as life unworthy of life; they were involuntarily euthanized (killed) in Nazi Germany. Kanner published his paper on infantile autism at a time when support for eugenic genetic engineering as a way to improve society was prevalent among scientists, so making the diagnosis of an innate neurodevelopmental condition was a serious matter. It was a time in the United States when sterilization of people with intellectual disability was legal. Moreover, in 1942, the year before Kanner's paper on infantile autism was published, Foster Kennedy, a prominent neurologist from New York, had proposed a "mercy death" for children with severe intellectual disability in an article in the *American Journal of Psychiatry* (Kennedy, 1942).

Kanner publicly opposed Kennedy in the same issue of the journal (Kanner, 1942) and offered a spirited defense for those with severe, innate developmental disorders. He insisted that all lives matter and that "we should extend the democratic ideal" to these individuals because much could be learned by studying their unique qualities.

The aftermath of World War II led an enhanced awareness of human rights, and efforts were extended to provide better treatment for intellectually impaired and mentally ill persons. With these efforts, intellectually impaired persons became a more highly visible social responsibility. The National Mental Health Act, passed in 1946, included funds for training and research for people with intellectual impairments.

With the expansion of child guidance clinics after World War II, the treatment emphasis began to focus specifically on widely recognized psychodynamic techniques. This resulted in intellectually impaired persons being increasingly excluded from guidance clinic care because there were IQ cutoff scores for this type of therapy. When new major tranquilizer medications became available, they were initially touted as effective in managing maladaptive behavior and eventually were used extensively with intellectually impaired persons. With many false starts, efforts also were made to find drugs that would cure intellectual developmental disorders.

In the 1940s and 1950s, there was new impetus to clarify the definition of intellectual developmental disorders and to develop training for specialists. In 1958, the first categorical legislation to benefit people with intellectual developmental disorders was passed (P.L. 85-926). It provided funds to universities for training professionals in care of people with intellectual developmental disorders. Social competence, in addition to cognitive level, was introduced into the classification of intellectual developmental disorders and was initially measured by Doll's Vineland Social Maturity Scale. In 1952, the American Association on Mental Deficiency formed a committee to establish a new nomenclature for people with intellectual developmental disorders. The new classification was announced in 1959 and included both adaptive and cognitive components, and it replaced the terms previously used in classification—idiot, imbecile, and moron—with the current designations of profound, severe, moderate, and mild disorders of intellectual development. In the schools, programs for people with intellectual developmental disorders were extended from serving educable (mildly impaired) to serving trainable children (moderately impaired). Difficulties with the brain-injured intellectually impaired child began to receive increasing interest during this period. Strauss and Lehtinen (1947) published *Psychopathology and Education of the Brain-Injured Child*, in which they emphasized that disturbances in perception, thinking, and emotional behavior, alone or in combination, may impede learning. Increasingly, special education programs were developed. During this era, institutions for people with intellectual developmental disorders grew in size and number. Often unable to recruit and maintain well-trained staff, these institutions frequently provided inadequate care and, in many instances, relied extensively on the use of medications for behavior management. Overcrowding, inadequate programming, high turnover rates, and inadequate community services set the stage for reform in the next decade.

In the 1960s and 1970s, stimulated by the 1962 report of the President's Panel on Mental Retardation, substantial changes in the care of developmentally disabled persons were initiated. During these years, the rights and needs of the handicapped were clearly delineated and were highlighted by President John F. Kennedy's address to the U.S. Congress (Kennedy, 1963). He announced we must act to

> bestow the full benefits of society on those who suffer from mental disabilities; to prevent the occurrence of mental illness and mental retardation wherever and whenever possible; to provide for early diagnosis and continuous and comprehensive care, in the community, for those suffering from these disorders.

The United Nations General Assembly passed the "Declaration of General and Special Rights of the Mentally Retarded," which designated that "the mentally retarded person has the same basic rights as other citizens of the same country and same age" (United Nations, 1971).

From 1950 to 1970, the number of residents in state-administered institutions increased from 125,000 to 190,000. Concern about their care led to more than 100 legal decisions that eventually resulted in the deinstitutionalization movement of the 1970s. As a result, from 1970 to 1979, the number of residents in state-administered institutions decreased by 50,000. The nation's institutional census peaked in 1967 at 194,650. By the end of fiscal year 2015, that number had declined to 21,103, a decrease of 89%.

Accompanying these reductions in institutional placement was a critical review of treatment approaches, both behavioral and pharmacological. New guidelines have been established for therapeutic interventions. The main emphasis for community and school programming has been to provide normalization for intellectually impaired persons (Wolfensberger, 1972). In 1983, Wolfensberger introduced the term *social role valorization* (SRV) to make clearer his approach to normalization. Social role valorization (SRV) emphasizes ways to make positive changes in the lives of people who are disadvantaged because of their low status in society. People who have devalued social roles are denied the benefits that society has to offer. SRV is implemented through service delivery with supports to children and adults with impairments. Wolfensberger and Thomas (2005; see also Osburn, 2006) defined SRV as

> the application of empirical knowledge to the shaping of the current or potential social roles of a party (i.e., person, group, or class)—primarily by means of enhancement of the party's competencies and image—so that these are, as much as possible, positively valued in the eyes of the perceivers.

The International Association of Social Role Valorization was established in 2013 to promote and assist organizations in implementing these concepts.

With extensive efforts at community programming, maladaptive behavior is now recognized as a major limiting factor in community placement. This recognition has led to a new emphasis on the dually diagnosed individual, the child with both a developmental disability and a mental disorder. Psychiatrists who were initially actively involved in working with intellectually and developmentally disabled children are now returning to their care with new tools and understanding based on advances in diagnosis and neurobiology, new imaging techniques, new pharmacotherapies, and a better understanding of the natural history and course of developmental disorders.

The strongest statement in regard to the right to education in the United States was the Education for All Handicapped Children Act of 1975, which mandated free and appropriate education for all intellectually impaired youngsters up to age 21 years. These guarantees were later extended to preschool children. Concurrently, new emphasis has been placed on the developmental psychopathology of attention-deficit/hyperactivity disorder, schizophrenia, Tourette's disorder, and behavioral disturbance in persons with intellectual developmental disorders. Both training and research activities have been instituted, leading to the publication of an increasing number of research articles. Journals such as the *Journal of Autism and Developmental Disorders* (Leo Kanner, founding editor), *Development and Psychopathology*, and *Developmental Medicine & Child Neurology* focus on these disorders.

Tracing the origins of a developmental perspective on childhood disorders demonstrates how attitudes toward children with developmental psychopathology have changed in the past three centuries as new knowledge has been acquired. In the chapters that follow, an integrated approach to developmental neuropsychiatric disorders is provided. The emphasis is on the child or adolescent as an experiencing person who is actively adapting to an impairment.

# References

Aries, P. (1962). *Centuries of childhood*. Jonathan Cope.

Beach, F. (1898). Insanity in children. *Journal of Mental Science, 44*, 459–474.

Beers, C. W. (1981). *A mind that found itself: An autobiography*. University of Pittsburgh Press. (Original work published 1908)

Binet, A., & Simon, T. (1905). Méthodes nouvelles pour le diagnostic du niveau intellectuel des anormaux. *L'Année Psychologique, 11*(1), 191–244.

Binet, A., & Simon, T. (1916). *The development of intelligence in children*. Williams & Wilkins.

Bowlby, J. (1991). *Charles Darwin: A new life*. Norton.

Bryan, C. (1930). *The papyrus ebers*. Appleton.

Cohen, A. S. (2016). *Imbeciles: The Supreme Court, American eugenics, and the sterilization of Carrie Buck*. Penguin.

Crutcher, R. (1943). Child psychiatry: A history of its development. *Psychiatry: Journal of the Biology and Pathology of Interpersonal Relationships, 6*(2), 191–201.

Darwin, C. (1965). *The expression of the emotions in man and animals*. University of Chicago Press. (Original work published 1872)

Darwin, C. (1877). A biographical sketch of an infant. *Mind, 2*(7), 285–294.

Deitz, D. E. D., & Repp, A. C. (1989). Mental retardation. In T. H. Ollendick & M. Hersen (Eds.), *Handbook of child psychopathology* (pp. 75–77). Plenum.

Down, J. H. L. (1866). Observations on an ethnic classification of idiots. *Clinical Lecture Reports, London Hospital Reports, 3*, 259–262.

Down, J. H. L. (1887). *On some of the mental affections of childhood and youth*. Churchill.

Griesinger, W. (1867). *Mental pathology and therapeutics*. New Sydenham Society.

Hall, S. (1904). *Adolescence*. Appleton.

Healey, W. (1915). *The individual delinquent*. Little, Brown.

Itard, J. M. G. (1806). *The wild boy of Aveyron* (G. Humphrey & M. Humphrey, Trans.). Appleton-Century-Crofts.

Kanner, L. (1941). *In defense of mothers*. Charles C Thomas.

Kanner, L. (1942). Exoneration of the feebleminded. *American Journal of Psychiatry, 99*(1), 17–22.

Kanner, L. (1943). Autistic disorders of affective contact. *Nervous Child, 2*(3), 217–250.

Kanner, L. (1959). The thirty-third Maudsley lecture: Trends in child psychiatry. *Journal of Mental Science, 105*(440), 581–593.

Kanner, L. (1960). Itard, Seguin, Howe: Three pioneers in the education of retarded children. *American Journal of Mental Deficiency, 6*, 2–10.

Kanner, L. (1964). *A history of the care and study of the mentally retarded*. Charles C Thomas.

Kennedy, F. (1942). The problem of social control of the congenital defective: Education, sterilization, euthanasia. *American Journal of Psychiatry, 99*(1), 13–16.

Kennedy, J. F. (1963). Message from the President of the United States (Document No. 58). House of Representatives, Washington, DC (88th Congress).

Lamb, S. D. (2014). *Pathologist of the mind: Adolf Meyer and the origins of American psychiatry*. Johns Hopkins University Press.

Lane, H. (1976). *The wild boy of Aveyron*. Harvard University Press.

Maudsley, H. (1867). *The physiology and pathology of the mind*. Macmillan.

Maudsley, H. (1895). *The pathology of mind: A study of its distempers, deformities and disorder*. Macmillan.

Meyer, A. (1895). *Mental abnormalities in children during primary education*. Transactions of the Illinois Society for Child Study.

Meyer, A. (1910). The dynamic interpretation of dementia praecox. *American Journal of Psychology, 21*, 385–403.

Meyer, A. (1915). Objective psychology or psychobiology: With subordination of the medically useless contrast of mental and physical. *Journal of the American Medical Association, 65*(10), 860–863.

Osburn, J. (2006). An overview of social role valorization theory. *The SRV Journal, 1*(1), 4–13.

Parry-Jones, W. L. (1989). The history of child and adolescent psychiatry: Its present day relevance. *Journal of Child Psychology and Psychiatry, 30*, 3–11.

Rousseau, J. (1911). *Emile* (B. Foxley, Trans.). Dutton. (Original work published 1762)

Scheerenberger, R. C. (1983). *A history of mental retardation*. Brookes.

Séguin, E. (1846). *Traitement moral, hygicne, et dducation des idiots et des autres enfants arricres*. Baillière.

Séguin, E. (1866). *Idiocy and its treatment by the physiological method*. William Wood.

Stevenson, G. S., & Smith, G. (1934). *Child guidance clinics: A quarter century of development*. The Commonwealth Fund.

Still, G. F. (1902). The Coulstonian lectures on some abnormal psychical conditions in children. *Lancet, 1*, 1008–1012, 1077–1082, 1163–1168.

Strauss, A. A., & Lehtinen, L. (1947). *Psychopathology and education of the brain-injured child*. Grune & Stratton.

Terman, L. M. (1916). *The measurement of intelligence*. Houghton Mifflin.

United Nations. (1971). Declaration of general and special rights of the mentally retarded.

West, C. (1852). *Lectures on the diseases of infancy and childhood*. Longman, Brown, Green & Longmans.

West, C. (1871). *On some disorders of the nervous system in childhood: Being the Lumleian Lectures delivered at the Royal College of Physicians of London in March 1871*. Longmans, Green, & Company.

Wolfensberger, W. (1972). *The principle of normalization in human services*. National Institute on Mental Retardation.

Wolfensberger, W. (1983). Social role valorization: A proposed new term for the principle of normalization. *Mental Retardation, 21*(6), 234–239.

Wolfensberger, W., & Thomas, S. (2005). *Introductory social role valorization workshop training package*. Training Institute for Human Service Planning, Leadership and Change Agentry, Syracuse University.

# PART I

# CLINICAL METHODS OF
# ASSESSMENT AND EXAMINATION
# IN DEVELOPMENTAL
# NEUROPSYCHIATRY

# 1

# Assessment, Interview, and Behavior Rating Scales

## Assessment in Developmental Neuropsychiatry

The assessment process in developmental neuropsychiatry requires a comprehensive evaluation of the individual child and their family. Three approaches are involved: (a) clinical assessment, which includes current and past family history, individual and family clinical interviews, and mental status examination of the child; (b) semistructured and structured interviews, questionnaires, behavior checklists, and rating scales; and (c) standardized tests, including psychological and neurological examinations. Background knowledge in normal child development, child psychopathology, diagnostic classification, and the specific tests used is a prerequisite. In dealing with developmental psychopathology, knowledge of the specific syndromes and their natural history is essential. The establishment of a diagnosis based on clinical assessment is complicated by difficulties in adapting the *Diagnostic and Statistical Manual of Mental Disorders*, fifth edition (DSM-5; American Psychiatric Association [APA], 2013), mental disorders classification system to children with developmental disorders and acquired neurological dysfunction. Because of the complexities of each case, familiarity with a variety of assessment approaches and instruments is important.

This chapter discusses the rationale for the clinical interview; discusses procedures involved in psychiatric interviewing; and reviews the psychiatric history, the psychiatric examination, behavior rating scales and checklists, the clinical case formulation, treatment planning, and prognosis.

## The Clinical Interview: Rationale

The interview is the main tool of investigation used with parents, other informants, and the child or adolescent. With children, adaptations of the interview process are necessary to facilitate establishing emotional contact with them. The psychiatric interview and behavioral observations that accompany it are specialized techniques. Skilled interviewing includes three main considerations (Owen et al., 2014; Russell et al., 1992; Rutter & Graham, 1968; Shaffer et al., 1999).

First, the interview is a method to acquire information. The primary goal is to establish an accurate account of the child or adolescent's behavior, emotions, and interpersonal relationships; background facts and significant life events; and obtain an understanding of their past experiences and attitudes toward others.

Both factual and emotional information is gathered during the interview process. When gathering factual information, specific questions are necessary that provide the structural component to the interview. However, the elicitation of emotional information requires an open-ended, nonstructured approach. The first goal of the interview is to establish interpersonal contact with the person to facilitate both parent and child openly discussing their difficulties. It is best to begin the interview in an unstructured way so as to elicit feelings and concerns before moving on to specific questions to establish diagnostic categories. Questions asked must be presented in a way that the patient can readily understand them and must be posed sensitively and tactfully. The aim of the interviewer is to maintain professional objectivity while establishing empathetic contact with the parent (or guardian) and child.

Second, the interview is a standard situation to assess emotions and attitudes. In working with children and adolescents, the interviewer maintains an active role from the beginning of the interview; stereotyped questions must be avoided. In whole-family interviewing, family members are engaged with one another, and interactions are promoted among them to demonstrate that everyone's communications, including those of siblings, are valued.

In the whole-family interview and in the individual interview, the interviewer must be aware of facial expressions, tone of voice, gestures, and the type of comments made. Throughout the interview process, family members and the patient will reveal a great deal about themselves as they describe their attitudes and their reactions to others. Moreover, the examiner reflects on their own reactions to the patient, and this also provides useful information in the context of the interview as a standard situation. The total interaction between the interviewer and the family member or child, then, provides an important source of information about personality and mental state. In some instances, a parent or disturbed child may elicit fear of being harmed in the interview. When this occurs, the interview may have to be terminated if the interviewer believes it cannot be conducted safely and objectively. A patient who detects fear potentially could feel more out of control and could react with aggression toward the interviewer.

Third, the interview provides an opportunity to offer support and to establish an understanding with the child and family, which may be the basis of a subsequent working relationship. The experience of being supported emotionally during the interview can become the basis of subsequent therapeutic work together. An understanding comment from the interviewer may increase confidence. Predetermined structured questioning or ill-timed interruptions can interfere with the therapeutic alliance and have the opposite effect.

In conducting the interview, the examiner should be interactive—warm, engaging, empathetic, and responsive. Nonverbal facial expression, tone of voice, and gestures can facilitate positive contact. Patients who are anxious, hostile, or suspicious may be unable to provide comprehensive factual information in their initial interview. In these instances, empathetic listening is particularly important to facilitate understanding and engagement. Because of the importance of establishing the relationship in the first interview, the examiner should not attempt to obtain information too quickly if doing so impedes this process.

In summary, the clinical interview has several aspects. It is a technique to establish an account of the present illness and to acquire information about events, experiences, and behavior. Furthermore, it provides a setting for the recording of expressed feelings, emotions, and attitudes about these events and experiences. The interview also provides an opportunity to initiate a therapeutic relationship with both the child and their family. By keeping in mind that both factual material and feelings are important, the elicitation of emotional and attitudinal information will initially be encouraged. Although specific diagnostic information is needed, the interview is approached in terms of the patient's present needs.

## The Psychiatric Interview

### Informants

Children and adolescents with developmental neuropsychiatric problems are most often referred because of parental concerns about their development, interpersonal relationships, and behavior. The assessment aims at establishing a clear account of the child or adolescent's behavior and its effects on others. Because children do not live alone and they uniformly attend school programs, their development is substantially influenced by interpersonal relationships and the attitudes of those with whom they come in contact both at home and at school. The assessment, then, involves not only the child but also the attitudes and behavior of others (parents, siblings, teachers, peers, and other significant adults) that are directed toward the child in the context of the presenting disorder. Moreover, because of limitations in the child's ability to provide a detailed account of their behavioral difficulties, informants who can describe behavior at home, at school, and in the community are essential in the assessment process. One may then compare accounts of the child's behavior in each of these settings to clarify whether the behavioral problem is situational (i.e., only occurring at home, at school, or in the community) or pervasive (i.e., occurring in all of these settings). It is not uncommon for there to be major differences in reports that come from school, home, and community.

The assessment process must take into account that children and adolescents are continually developing, so their expressed behavior and psychological symptoms must be evaluated in the context of their developmental phase. To do so, it is best to consider the child and family together as a unit. Background information about the family will assist in understanding how development has proceeded for a particular child. In addition, an understanding of the strengths and weaknesses of the family unit is essential for treatment planning. The response of parents and siblings, peers, and teachers to the child's difficulties (i.e., the impact of the behavior on others) must always be considered.

In conducting the assessment, observations of the child both alone and in their interactions with family members must be arranged. The examiner observes the child in both structured and unstructured settings. The assessment begins in the waiting area, with observations of the child with parents and/or siblings together, and continues with observations of the manner of separation when the child is taken from the family to enter the examining room. Observation in structured settings, such as neuropsychological testing, is also important.

A flexible approach is most helpful, whether the child is seen separately or as part of a family group. One approach is for the interviewer to see the child and family together to clarify the child's understanding of the reason for the consultation, to clarify if the reason for the visit was discussed between the parent and child before the visit, and to establish that interviews with both parent and child are confidential.

A complete assessment includes a phase of interviewing the whole family that allows information to be gathered about hierarchical relationships within the family, communication patterns, affective tone among family members, and alliances among them. Individual interviews are then conducted with each parent to establish their perspective on the child's difficulties. Following meeting with all family members to establish their understanding of why the child is referred, interviews with parents are conducted while the preschool or middle school child generally waits outside to be interviewed after the parents. An adolescent may be interviewed first prior to meeting with the parents.

Before leaving their parents, a child is informed about what will take place during their absence. Then the child is taken to a waiting area, where there is adequate supervision and play facilities. While waiting, the child may be given tasks to perform, such as creating a kinetic family drawing or doing other drawing tasks—for example, the "draw a person" and the "house–tree–person" tasks. Special arrangements may be necessary for preschool children who have difficulty separating from parents in an unfamiliar setting, children with intellectual developmental disorder, and brain-injured children who have severe behavioral problems.

## Interview with Parents

It is always best to see both the mother and the father together. The role of both parents in the life of the child is essential, and although the extent of involvement may differ between the parents and the child at different ages, both parents are intimately involved in the child's psychological experience whether they are physically present or not. For children with developmental disorders, involvement of both parents is of particular importance because it is not uncommon for one parent to have borne the burden of primary care, which may have precluded the other parent developing a realistic attitude and understanding of the child's abilities. Moreover, an interview with both parents together often provides an excellent opportunity to observe parental interaction and their relationship. When parents are divorced or separated and the child spends time with each of them, it may be best and more appropriate to see each parent separately.

## Information from Other Sources

Parental consent must be obtained to contact agencies, primary physicians, and other referral sources. Permission to contact the school and other agencies is essential to establish a well-rounded view of the current life situation. The teacher's account of the child's behavior at school is critical. Information about the type of classroom and the specific individualized educational program for developmentally disordered children must be reviewed as part of the assessment process. In addition, information on school attendance, particular academic strengths and weaknesses, nonacademic skills such as artistic and musical ability, behavior in the classroom and during recess, relationships with peers and with teachers, and other teacher comments are important. Moreover, behavior rating scales completed by teachers are obtained at the time of the initial assessment and on an ongoing basis. If an older adolescent or young adult is enrolled in a workshop program, then information from the job coach or supervisor will be needed.

## Developmental Aspects of Interviewing

Children are developing persons, so the diagnostic assessment must maintain a developmental perspective that considers the following: (a) Children behave differently at different ages, so knowledge of age-appropriate behavior is necessary; (b) the disorder may interfere with the normal course of development; (c) different phases of development are associated with different stresses, thus a toddler is most likely to be affected by separation experiences and a stressed adolescent may exhibit frequent mood swings; and (d) specific developmental tasks to be mastered vary with age.

The interview with the child must take into account both the child's developmental level and the child's ability to communicate. The purpose of the initial interview is to make meaningful contact with the child and establish their confidence and cooperation, to get to know the child, and to learn the child's responses to current difficulties and perception of them and also their ability to cooperate in treatment. The child may experience anxiety in encountering the interviewer, concurrently sizing up the interviewer as the interviewer makes observations and talks to the child.

When examining infants or children with severe and profound intellectual developmental disorders who have not established expressive language milestones, the initial observations must focus on social milestones. During the first year, the most important of these are the establishment of eye contact, social attachment, stranger anxiety, and the reciprocal use of language in babbling and jargon. With infants, one uses the infantile form of language called "motherese," which involves extending vowel sounds and speaking more slowly. An infant responds to the adult's mood and gestures in an active and perceptive way, which emerges from their own experience with familiar caregivers. The response to change or newness is more intense after 6 months of age when selective attachments and stranger anxiety have emerged as developmental milestones.

In examining an infant, the approach is indirect, almost casual. The interviewer should be still and quiet but close enough to observe. Initially, one makes no gesture or movement and does not use direct eye contact until the infant has looked the interviewer over from a safe and comfortable distance. In approaching an infant or a withdrawn child with intellectual developmental disorder, an outstretched hand may be offered to encourage the child to reach out. For infants and nonverbal children with intellectual developmental disorder, it is generally best for them to make the first move. In making infant observations, it is important to observe the parents' preferred holding posture and imitate it.

With toddlers and many children with intellectual developmental disorder, one should keep in mind that although they may not be speaking, their receptive language may be adequate to understand what is said about them. Because language comprehension precedes verbal expression, words they hear may be misinterpreted by them.

For children between ages 2 and 4 years who are able to talk and have a better understanding of what is said to them, the interviewer may proceed verbally and with the use of play materials. Children at this age are very literal in their understanding of the words they use and those they hear from others. Because thinking is concrete, actions may be understood in a concrete way. Descriptions to young children should avoid the use of analogies, and abstractions should be used cautiously when discussing problems with these children. Learning to speak at the child's language level will facilitate communication in future visits. In addition to literalness, children between ages 2 and 4 years may use transductive reasoning to give inanimate objects human attributes. The child may attribute feelings and motives to household objects or at least speak as if they have them. For example, a child may say a machine that has stopped has gone to sleep and may practice putting toys to sleep and waking them up. During this age period, children tend to be active and may be difficult to please or satisfy in a new office setting. Feelings such as sadness, anger, fearfulness, and jealousy are poorly modulated. Moreover, the child may have difficulty controlling anger and show unpredictability in behavior related to their emotions.

During an examination, an initial period of warming up and talking to a child about personal interests and successes may alleviate their anxiety. Younger children communicate their feelings through their behavior or through imaginary play. During play interviews, the child may show themes that reveal conflictual situations in home or in preschool settings.

By middle childhood, from age 7 years on, children are better able to express fears and feelings verbally but may be unclear about the nature of their concerns. They may ask questions in a veiled fashion, so it is essential to clarify the meaning of their questions before responding to them. A frequent and persistent question may indicate a hidden concern.

Children who are in middle childhood and adolescence may be interviewed more directly about their concerns and life experiences. For the older child, the interview is semistructured, as described in the following section.

## Interview with the Child

The child is the most important source of information and during the assessment must be seen separately unless severe separation anxiety or the extent of behavioral difficulty does not allow this. The child's view of the presenting problem should be sought out, although the quality of the child's report will vary according to developmental age. For children who are nonverbal, specific adaptations of the interview are necessary and specific devices, such as letter boards and speech aids, may be necessary to facilitate communication.

In the past, there was reluctance to use a formalized mental status examination with younger children because of concerns about the reliability of verbal information from children and a sense that the language and thought of the child are too elusive for clinical description. Concerns have been expressed regarding the child's developmental level, the age when verbal approaches could be used, and the possible transient nature of psychopathology. There have been concerns that an adult-type interview would lead to anxiety and hostility, and questions have been raised about phenomenology, psychodynamics, and their usefulness in determining etiology in younger children. Because of these considerations, interview behavior has varied, with some interviewers using direct questioning and observation and others using less formal approaches, such as play, drawings, and other imaginative methods. Yet both approaches are needed—the formal direct interview to elicit symptoms needed to make a diagnosis and the imaginal methods to establish contact and conduct treatment.

Because of past concerns about the nature of the mental status examination in the child, considerable effort has gone into improving psychiatric interviewing procedures for children and adolescents. The establishment of structured and semistructured interviews has been motivated by dissatisfaction with reliability and validity of traditional child and adolescent diagnostic procedures. The development of structured interview schedules for children followed the development of such interview schedules for adults that have been found to increase diagnostic reliability substantially; such interview schedules for children include the Child and Adolescent Psychiatric Assessment, the Kiddie Schedule for Affective Disorders and Schizophrenia, and the National Institute of Mental Health Diagnostic Interview Schedule for Children (Angold & Costello, 2000; Angold et al., 2012; Edelbrock & Bohnert, 2000; Geller et al., 2001; Hodges, Kline, et al., 1982; Hodges, McKnew, et al., 1982; Shaffer et al., 2000). Moreover, the development of a more comprehensive classification of child and adolescent disorders with more explicit diagnostic criteria has required a more standardized approach to the assessment of child and adolescent symptoms (American Psychiatric Association [APA], 2013; World Health Organization, 2019).

Face-to-face interviews are important to establish rapport with the child or adolescent, and by focusing on symptoms of concern, they help maintain the child's interest during the interview. Such interviews help clarify misunderstandings about the parents' interpretation of the child's behavior and provide an opportunity to document the context and chronicity of a child's symptoms. Although the assessment of child psychopathology requires information from parents and other informants, children are essential informants regarding their own feelings, behaviors, and social relationships. Symptom-oriented interviews are effective means for establishing diagnoses in children who may be too young to complete verbal self-reports.

The earliest structured and semistructured interviews for children are those of Lapouse and Monk (1958) and Rutter and Graham (1968). The most detailed evaluation of structured and semistructured interviewing took place in the late 1970s and 1980s. These interviews are used for both clinical and research purposes and have encountered conceptual, methodological, and technical problems in their development (Fisher et al., 2015). All of these instruments provide a list of target behaviors, symptoms, and life events that must be covered, together with guidelines for conducting the interview and recording the child or adolescent's responses. The degree of structure imposed on the interview varies from the semistructured approach, in which only general and flexible guidelines for conducting the interview and recording the information are given, to highly structured interviews that specify the exact order, wording, and coding of each item (Fisher et al., 2015). Because they can be individualized to the child and provide greater range in phrasing questions and following alternative lines of inquiry and interpreting responses, semistructured interviews are usually conducted by clinically sophisticated interviewers. Conversely, the highly structured interview, which is used most commonly in epidemiologic studies, reduces the role of clinical inference made by a more experienced examiner and can be administered by lay interviewers.

Although there are differences in the type of information gained from structured and semistructured interviews, the majority produce information about the presence, absence, severity, onset, and/or duration of specific symptoms. Some interviews produce a quantitative score regarding symptom profiles or a global index of psychopathology. Generally, assessment interview schedules are designed for parents with parallel formats for children, but some are developed specifically for children. Children can be reliable reporters especially after age 9 or 10 years. It is important to interview both child and parents. There may be differences in the child's and parents' reports of individual symptoms depending, to some extent, on whether the symptoms are externalizing or internalizing. For children with neurodevelopmental disorder, the standardized interview with the parent is used along with observation of the child.

Development of other structured interviews has led to more precise recognition of disorders, such as depression in childhood, in epidemiologic studies. However, the use of semistructured approaches to elicit the nature and extent of abnormalities of emotions, behavior, and interpersonal relationships is the most appropriate method in a clinical setting. Specific probes related to particular diagnostic criteria are incorporated into the clinical interview.

## The Psychiatric History

After establishing demographic and other background information and clarifying the reliability of the parents or other informants, the parents are asked about their specific concerns. The reason for referral is elicited, as well as a statement about the onset of the current difficulties and the family life situation at the time the difficulties began. The interviewer specifically asks about why the child is being referred at this particular time. Precipitating stressful events that may contribute to the behavioral, emotional, or interpersonal problem are reviewed, and the parents' specific concerns are addressed. Among the specific concerns to be considered are academic and school problems, antisocial behavior, emotional conflicts, regressive behavior, and interpersonal difficulties with others. The child's previous treatment should be reviewed, and the effects of the child's current behavior on family functioning should be addressed and clarified. Following these questions, a reclarification of the parents' goals in seeking help at this time is elicited.

The *family history* is reviewed, clarifying what the child's current status is in regard to stepparenting, adoption, foster care, or other family-related issues. Specific questions include the following: Who has custody of the child? Who is the child like with regard to personality and who is the child named after? The family background for both parents is obtained, including information about their own childhood, with particular emphasis on the family atmosphere in their homes as they grew up, stresses related to emotional and economic issues, and deaths or separation from close relatives. Information about the grandparents and others closely affiliated with the child is elicited, along with a developmental family history of how the parents' marriage evolved. The quality of relatedness in the current marriage, including frequency of disagreements and how disagreements are expressed, coping mechanisms, how conflict is dealt with in the family, and the relationship to the family of origin, are reviewed. The child's siblings are described in regard to age, school placement, history of significant illness, personality, and relationship to other family members.

The family history should include specific questions about developmental disorders, alcoholism, abnormal personality, suicide/homicide, mood disorders, and schizophrenia. A family history of executive dysfunction in parents and extended family members is also sought, as is parental difficulty in learning and in school achievement.

A review of *past and personal history* should include the date and place of birth, birth weight, attitude of both parents toward the pregnancy, and whether the pregnancy was planned or unplanned. If there were difficulties with the pregnancy or delivery, the emotional response of the parents to those events should be included.

*Developmental milestones* should emphasize social developmental milestones, which include eye contact, social smile, language communication, interpersonal attachment, and daily living skills. Quality of the parent–child (dyadic) relationship and the child–mother–father (triadic) relationship is discussed. Interpersonal issues that relate to feeding and illness must be considered along with the parents' attitudes toward child-rearing. Child-rearing practices and attitudes about permissiveness and limit setting are reviewed.

A *behavioral review of systems* is then carried out that includes information on temperament, early development, emotional responsiveness, antisocial behavior, attentional difficulties, self-stimulation, and play behavior.

This is followed by an *assessment of school activities*, including the age of beginning school, the current grade, schools attended, types of class placement, and emotional adjustment to beginning school. Separation problems at the time of entry into preschool or elementary school are discussed. If there were prolonged absences from school or if school years were repeated, this information along with specific difficulties in reading, writing, math, and spelling are noted. Study habits and academic goals for the child are discussed, and the child's peer relationships are clarified. If the child is teased or is a bully, this information is included, as is information about particular friendships. Attitudes toward teachers, peers, and schoolwork are obtained.

An assessment is made of the child's *awareness of sexual identity*, which includes questions regarding curiosity about their own body and about reproduction, as well as sexual interest and activities. For the adolescent, the interview includes information regarding the mastery of adolescent developmental tasks and the young person's attitude toward entry into social adolescence. One looks for mature versus pseudomature behavior and discusses attitudes toward peers, family members, and those in authority. Rebelliousness, drug-taking, periods of depression and withdrawal, and the adolescent's fantasy life are discussed with the parents. How the young person has responded to puberty, with accompanying voice changes, hair growth, and menarche, as well as masturbation and sexual concerns are discussed.

*Previous mental health history* is gathered, which includes details of any disturbances for which treatment was received and the type of treatment that was carried out. This is followed by a description of *the life situation at present*, which includes current housing; social situation; parents' work and financial circumstances; the composition of the household; the relationship with neighbors; and recent stresses, bereavement, losses, or disappointments and how both parents and child have reacted to them. A typical day in the child's life is described, which includes going to school, activities during the school day, returning home, and evening activities.

In the parent interview, questions about the child or adolescent's particular personality are addressed. This includes habitual attitudes and patterns of behavior that distinguish the child as an individual. Among the personality characteristics reviewed are attitudes toward others, including ability to trust others and to make and sustain a relationship with them. Whether the child is secure or insecure in interpersonal relationships, a leader or a follower, is established. The attitude toward interpersonal relationships—whether it is friendly, warm, and demonstrative or reserved, cold, or indifferent—is considered. Other characteristics discussed include aggressiveness, quarrelsomeness, sensitivity, and suspiciousness. The interviewer asks about the child's attitude toward themself, including self-dramatizing behavior, egocentric behavior, self-consciousness, and ambition. Moreover, attitudes of the child or adolescent to their own health and bodily functions are included in the assessment to establish whether or not the child's self-appraisal is realistic.

An *assessment of personality* also includes moral and religious attitudes, an assessment of whether the individual is easygoing or permissive, over-conscientious, perfectionistic, or conforming. Mood is considered in regard to lability and general attitude and whether the child is optimistic or pessimistic. The presence of anxiety, irritability, excessive worrying, and apathy is noted. The ability to express and control feelings of anger, sadness, pleasure, and disappointment is reviewed.

*Leisure time activities and interests*, including interest in books, pictures, music, sports, and creative activities, are noted. Determining how the child or adolescent spends leisure time is essential, including descriptions of whether the child is alone or with others during free time.

Finally, questions are asked about *daydreams, nightmares, and reactions to stress*. This involves the ability to tolerate frustration, loss, or disappointment and includes a description of circumstances that arouse anger, anxiety, or depression. Evidence of excessive use of particular psychological defenses, such as denial, rationalization, and projection, is obtained.

Because executive dysfunction interferes with adaptive behavior both at home and at school, the parent interview asks about both settings; however, teacher interviews may be necessary to cover school matters (because parents may not know). Children with executive dysfunction have difficulty regulating or organizing their behavior in relation to their schoolwork and their interpersonal activities. To clarify these problems, the history identifies the frequency and severity of target symptoms in each of these settings.

## The Psychiatric Examination (Mental State Examination)

The mental status examination must take into account the child's developmental level, along with ability and capability to engage the interviewer.

## Appearance

The first part of the interview relies on the interviewer's powers of observation. In many ways, it is the easiest part of the examination because one needs primarily to be alert and observant; however, it takes skill and experience to understand the implications of what has been observed.

The child's appearance, stature, and nutritional status are observed to determine their medical well-being. The examiner should note personal reactions to the child— that is, whether the child is personally appealing or not. Extremes in height and weight have implications metabolically and in regard to emotional development. The examiner observes whether the child is clumsy or ataxic, shows disinhibited movements, has strabismus, or shows rigid or floppy muscle tone. Skin coarseness or rash and hair abnormalities, which might suggest metabolic disorders, may be easily visible. Bruises should prompt thinking regarding child abuse, accident proneness, or clumsiness.

## Behavior Relatedness

How does the child relate to parents and to the interviewer? Does the child maintain reserve with the interviewer and only gradually warm up, or never warm up? Is the child overly friendly? Does the child make eye contact with the interviewer and show turn-taking as the dialogue progresses? Is the child sullen, angry, oppositional, reciprocal, aggressive, or totally withdrawn and preoccupied by their own thoughts and actions? The extent of relatedness varies from the child with autism spectrum disorder diagnosis who may constantly ignore others, including parents, or only make fleeting glances at them, to the shy child who may show no initial eye contact but gradually warms up over time, to the disinhibited child with Williams syndrome who hugs total strangers.

## Motor Behavior

How active and impulsive is the child? Is the child moving all over the room and getting into everything? Responding to every passing stimulus? Maintaining interest in a task or toy or losing interest quickly? Will the child pay attention and inhibit their disruptiveness when verbal limits are imposed? Does the subject squirm and fidget in the chair, stay immobile, or move normally in response to what is said to them? Does the child have nervous tics or repetitious behaviors? Are movements graceful and coordinated? Because different degrees of activity may be appropriate at different ages, a 4-year-old and a 10-year-old may show the same activity level with very different implications.

## Speech and Language

The assessment of speech and language is based not only on what is said but also on how it is said. The quality of speech gives some clues about the child's mood. Does the child speak clearly, slur words, stutter, or substitute letters (e.g., *w* for *r*)? How verbal is the child? Does the child become frustrated trying to communicate ideas, knows words but has difficulty with conceptual communication? Is the rate of speech fast or slow? Does the child whine, whisper, or shout? Does the child speak spontaneously or in monosyllabic grunts? Are the rate, rhythm, and prosody of speech appropriate? Is the volume loud or soft? Finally, can the child hear what is said and understand at a normal conversational tone? Hearing deficits for certain frequencies may make words virtually unintelligible to the listener. Alternative methods may be needed, such as communication boards for children with limited language ability; articulation problems may require an interpreter.

## Thought Process and Content

How a child thinks and what they think about can be assessed both indirectly and directly. The first part of the interview entails getting to know the child—their likes or dislikes, their friends, what they do together, what school is like, performance in school, whether they get along with parents and sibs, and their aspirations for adulthood. What are the child's preoccupations? Are there intrusive thoughts? What does the child talk about with interest and affective investment? Telling a joke or a favorite story may clarify how the child organizes their thoughts.

The second part of the interview is specifically related to why the child is being evaluated, what his parents said about coming, what the child views their problems to be, and how the child feels about the problems presented and about family relationships. In a child older than age 5 years, thought content as it relates to mood, fears, somatic problems, hallucinations, and delusions is elicited.

For adolescents, this part of the mental status examination is similar to the adult mental status examination. For adolescents, content items also focus on drug and alcohol use; difficulties with antisocial behavior; and attitudes toward dating, peers, sex, menarche, growing up, and parents.

From verbal interchanges during the interview, the interviewer assesses the coherence of the child or adolescent's thought process and whether their concerns are age, sex, and situation appropriate.

## Mood and Self-Concept (Emotional Feeling Tone and Its Outward Manifestations)

Mood and self-concept are ascertained directly and indirectly. Does the child look happy, sad, tense, or angry? Smile or seem tearful? Speak dejectedly or assertively or with excessive bravado? How does the child respond to questions about feelings, such as "When were you the most angry, happy, frightened or sad?" And what does the child do when they feel those ways? What are their specific fears and worries? Does the child like themselves, or is the child self-loathing or self-blaming? Does the child think others like them? Does the child feel picked on, and does the child "fight back"? Is the child comfortable with their gender identity? Does the child blame themself or others for their problems? Is the child overly dramatic in talking about their problems, or does the child minimize them? Is the child guarded and suspicious, irritable, or volatile? Does the child see themself as evil, bad tempered? What has the child done that the child is proud of? How does the child feel about their future? In assessing depression, the examiner focuses on loss of interest in usual activities in children who are more severely cogitatively impaired.

## Abnormal Beliefs and Interpretation of Events

Are ideas of persecution or expectation of special treatment expressed? Are there delusional beliefs? Does the child believe others can read their mind?

## Abnormal Experiences Referring to the Environment, Body, or Self

Does the child report sensory or somatic hallucinations or recurrent dreams? These areas may be addressed indirectly by asking the child if their eyes or ears ever play tricks on them, causing them to see things that others do not see or hear things others do not hear. Are there feelings of depersonalization?

## Cognition (Orientation, Memory, Attention and Concentration, and General Intelligence)

How alert is the child? Oriented to time, place, and person in an age-appropriate manner? Does the child seem to know what is happening around them, or does the child appear distracted or inattentive? How does their historical account compare to that of their parents in regard to past significant life events? Does the child know colors and body parts? Depending on the child's age, they should be able to copy the Gesell figures (circle, square, diamond, Maltese cross, and cylinder) or draw a human figure in some detail. The interviewer observes how the child draws, holds the pencil, and plans the task. How is their memory? Does the child know where they live and how they got to the place where the interview is taking place? Are there problems with attention and concentration? Can the child perform basic arithmetic (addition, subtraction, multiplication, and division)? Can the child carry out subtraction of serial 3's back from 20 and serial 7's back from 100? How is their reading comprehension? What is their level of intelligence? In play, what is their choice of toys, and how does the child approach them and use them in imaginative ways? Does the child show curiosity about how things work?

## Insight and Judgment

Does the child appreciate their role in the current difficulties and take responsibility for their behavior? What is their capacity to reflect on their behavior? Are current difficulties linked to life events or stresses?

## Behavior Rating Scales and Checklists

Behavior rating scales and checklists are commonly used in both clinical and research settings (Fisher et al., 2015). The items rated vary from highly specific behaviors to more abstract qualities of personal and social functioning. In some scales, particular constructs, such as activity level, are used; in others, broad categories of psychopathology, such as internalizing or externalizing dimensions, are included. The major rating scales utilize parents or teachers to assess the various dimensions of child psychopathology. In addition to these scales, self-reports are also available, which are completed by the child or adolescent. For children with developmental neuropsychiatric problems, the self-rating scales will often have to be read to the child because reading difficulty is commonly associated with these conditions. Reliable rating scales are based on the assumption that the parent or teacher shares a common understanding of the behavior or attribute to be rated. If the area to be rated is more abstract, a discrepancy may exist between the informant's rating and the information the therapist wishes to have rated. Raters must be able to extract information from their experiences and observations of the child that coincide with the item to be rated. Moreover, the informant and interviewer must share a common understanding about which behaviors represent the item requested on the scale. Some behaviors that may be relevant to a particular scale item might vary depending on situational or developmental issues. Finally, the raters and the interviewer must share common views about the reference points for scaling the behavior along the lines required by the particular instrument. If there are differences in understanding the base rates of the behavior, then making judgments, such as the behavior occurs "lust a little" or "very much," may be problematic.

Completion of the behavior rating scale may be affected by the educational level, intelligence, and emotional status of the informant at the time the rating is conducted, so the report may vary and not simply represent only the actual behavior of the child being rated. There also may be variability in the instrument itself in regard to how the scales are constructed, the specificity of the weighting used in questions, the time period over which ratings are made, and variations in the child's behavior from one situation to the next.

Rating scales differ from specific behavioral observations in that rating scales require the rater to make observations over longer time periods—sometimes weeks or months—and in various situations at home or in the community (e.g., in camp). Behavioral observations generally focus on highly specific time periods and very specific situations and are made during short time intervals. Consequently, ratings and direct observational measures may not be highly correlated. There are a number of reasons for this, including the fact that ratings are less clearly defined than observations, and they are more influenced by characteristics of the informant who, in research settings, tends not to be trained to the same extent as those who use direct observational methods. However, each of these approaches offers unique sources of information not attained by the other. So, although complete agreement between these two approaches is not expected, both make contributions to the assessment process.

Although there are problems inherent in the use and interpretation of rating scales, there are also advantages over other methods. Among the advantages of behavior rating scales are the following: (a) the capability of getting information from informants with many years of experience with the child in multiple settings; (b) an opportunity to collect information on behaviors that occur extremely infrequently and may be missed in short, intense observation periods; (c) the fact that they are inexpensive and efficient in regard to time needed for completion; (d) the availability of normative value when used for screening nonpsychiatric populations; (e) their availability in various forms, which allows for a variety of dimensions in child psychopathology; (f) incorporation of the views of significant people in the child's natural environment who are involved in management, care, and therapeutic interventions; (g) provision of an account for situational variation to achieve more stable ratings of the child; and (h) allowance for quantitative distinctions to be made, which are often difficult to establish using the qualitative direct observational method.

Rating scales are used in various situations, including epidemiologic research, for subgrouping of children into homogeneous clusters to determine the prognosis of clinical groups followed over longer time intervals and to allow further exploration of hypotheses related to etiology. Moreover, rating scales demonstrate sensitivity to change that may be used in treatment outcome studies for a particular condition. Some scales cover a sufficient range of child psychopathology to allow them to be used to develop a classification system for psychopathological disorders through profile analysis.

The most commonly used parent rating scales for children with learning and behavioral problems are the Conners Parent Rating Scale (Conners, 2014), the Child Behavior Checklist–Parent Form (Achenbach, 2009; Achenbach et al., 2008), and the Personality Inventory for Children (Wirt et al., 1984). Commonly used teacher rating scales include the Conners Teacher Rating Scale (Conners, 2014) and the Child Behavior Checklist–Teacher Form (Achenbach, 2009). In addition to these two teacher rating scales, there are a variety of other scales, such as the Vanderbilt ADHD Diagnostic Rating Scale (Wolraich et al., 2003). Besides individual parent and teacher ratings, other rating scales have been devised to be used by multiple informants. Moreover, rating scales are available to rate preschool behavior, affective behavior (fears and anxieties), and self-control.

## The Clinical Case Formulation

The modern case formulation builds on Adolf Meyer's psychobiological life history format that focused on an individual's response to life events and that led to George Engel's biopsychosocial model (Engel, 1977, 1980, 2009). Engel proposed that the biopsychosocial model "provides a conceptual framework and way of thinking that enables physician to act rationally . . . to become more informed and skillful in psychosocial areas" (Engel, 1980). He wrote that "our modern concept of disease includes all the parameters that bear on life itself, whether they are observable in physical, chemical, biological, genetic, morphological, psychological, interpersonal or social terms" (Engel, 1980). Its focus is on the experiencing person, their underlying neurobiology, their relationships with other people, and their environmental experience and exposures. It emphasizes that relationships are central in the provision of mental health care, utilizes self-awareness as a diagnostic and therapeutic tool, and elicits the patient's history in the context of individual life circumstances.

The clinical case formulation is a concise summary that takes into account all of the information available from the assessment process. It should begin with a brief statement of the current problem, followed by a summary of the case history and mental status examination, and conclude with a description of how the clinician understands the case from a biopsychosocial perspective (Bolton, 2015; MacNeil et al., 2012; McDougall & Reade, 1993). It is a synthesis of the assessment rather than a restatement of facts.

In DSM-5, it is not sufficient to simply check off symptoms listed to meet diagnostic criteria to make a mental disorder diagnosis. A case formulation is required in DSM-5 (APA, 2013, p. 29). The DSM-5 formulation integrates known biological, psychological, and social factors that contribute to the development of the current problem. It includes a discussion of the diagnosis and of the etiological factors and conditions that are deemed important from a review of the course of the condition. It takes into account both the patient's current life situation and background. The formulation (a) supplements the clinical diagnosis, (b) enriches the clinical database by providing a synthesis that leads to hypotheses which are testable in part by clinical observation, and (c) provides an understanding of the case that is crucial to planning treatment.

Predisposing factors, precipitating factors, perpetuating factors, and protective factors are all considered in preparing a case formulation (APA, 2013; Barker, 2004; Bolton, 2015; Flinn et al., 2015; Weerasekera, 1993; Winters et al., 2007 ). Predisposing factors are factors in the child or family that may predispose to the disorder. These include genetic and constitutional predispositions, temperament, physical abnormalities, and traumatic life events. Precipitating factors refer to experiences that may have precipitated the onset of the current problem. Precipitants interact with predisposing factors in the genesis of the disorder. Perpetuating factors are those that maintain the condition once it has become established—for example, a disruptive home environment. Finally, protective factors relate to strengths in the child and parent. Protective factors limit the severity of the disorder and assist in healthy functioning—for example, in psychological resilience.

In considering the various factors that have led to and maintain the current condition, psychodynamic issues are included in a clinical case formulation. These include three broad categories of experience: (a) key relationships, their history, and their representation in memory; (b) conflict (the type of anxiety, the coping strategy mobilized, and the solution); and (c) the experience of the self—that is, the modulation of self-concept. The method outlined below is for recording the formulation (Barker, 2004; Cameron et al., 1978; Winters et al., 2007).

## Introduction

In one or two sentences, describe the patient, the illness or problem, and why the person or family seeks assistance at this time.

## Biological Considerations

Biological considerations should be divided, when possible, into predisposing, precipitating, or perpetuating, as noted previously. If no specific neurobiological factors have been identified, this should be recorded. Neurobiological factors include genetic, medical, developmental, and temperamental factors.

## Psychological and Developmental Psychological Considerations

These might include cognitive style, self-image, and attribution of meaning to symptoms. Developmentally, it is important to list developmental tasks appropriate for the child or adolescent's age and how the disorder impacts task mastery. Age-related developmental task mastery is also considered for parents.

## Psychodynamic Issues

Key relationships, conflict, and experience of the self are included in this section. The emphasis is on psychological and/or intellectual problems within the child.

## Social Considerations

Important family and peer relationships, family diagnostic issues (e.g., mental disorders), and significant social influences on the family are discussed. One takes into account the problems of the child within the family, the problems of the child with parents and with peers, problems that occur at school, and the effects of sociocultural/religious factors on the child.

## Phenomenological

In this section of the formulation, one extracts the important findings from the mental status examination. Attempts are made to link these with underlying biological, psychodynamic, and social factors elicited in the general clinical history.

## Protective Factors

Protective factors are those that limit the disorder and facilitate adaptation and are recorded with an emphasis on the child and family strengths. These include social support and capacity for resilience.

## Hypothesis Construction

Having synthesized each of the previously mentioned areas of concern, hypotheses are generated about internal connections between psychosocial and biological events.

These associations are linked to the developmental life task important for child self-mastery at this particular age. In hypothesis construction, findings are arranged in an attempt to understand how the child and family have developed and how their current difficulties have emerged.

In summary, the clinical case formulation is not a list of difficulties but, rather, a synthesis that describes the interplay and relative importance of various issues. It should be a clearly written dynamic explanation that leads to a plan of treatment and a suggested prognosis.

---

### Example of Case Formulation

Danny is a 10-year-old boy, an only child, with a previous diagnosis of attention-deficit/hyperactivity disorder (ADHD) who is referred for escalating aggressive behavior across multiple settings. Danny's family history is notable for maternal depression but is otherwise unremarkable. Predisposing factors in his early history are notable of prematurity and postnatal anoxia, as well as placement with his grandmother at 6 months of age due to his mother's postpartum depression. Danny has a long-standing history of behavioral problems beginning in preschool, which led to a diagnosis of ADHD that has been treated with medications and behavior therapy with success. Danny can be easily reactive, although he is never aggressive. More recently, he has exhibited an onset aggression in the context of his parents' divorce and ongoing discord, his recent transfer to a new school, being bullied at school, and lack of friendships, which are all precipitation factors. Danny denies significant anxiety or depression, and hence his increased aggression has been triggered by recent stressors. Its presentation is most consistent with a diagnosis of adjustment disorder with disturbance of conduct. Danny's strengths include his above-average intelligence, solid academic performance, close relationships with his mother and grandmother, and his friendships at school.

His temperament, ADHD diagnosis, being bullied at school, and recent continuing family discord are issues that will perpetuate his behavior without focused interventions. His demonstrated strengths are his above-average intelligence, past school performance, and capacity to develop close confiding relationships with his mother and grandmother and friendships with peers at his old school. At his age, key developmental tasks are parental relationships, affect regulation when stressed, and age-appropriate peer relations with a close friend and other peers. The treatment plan needs to address the psychosocial factors that sustain his behaviors and to include focused family interventions and a review of and update to his behavioral plan and current medication. Overall, recommended treatments for his current aggression include a combination of medications, behavioral therapy, and addressing parental discord. Helping Danny find friends and recreational activities are also critical to his success; otherwise, he is at risk for continued behavioral difficulties, as well as depression and anxiety, as he embarks on adolescence.

## The Perspectives of Psychiatry Case Formulation

The perspectives of psychiatry approach to case formulation focuses on the patient's psychiatric condition from four perspectives: disease, dimensional, behavior, and life story (Peters et al., 2012). The perspectives model seeks to enhance the biopsychosocial formulation by bringing together its elements into a more integrative and rational approach to treatment planning focused on an individual patient's needs. In doing so, it considers whether the presenting psychiatric condition is best understood as a disease—for example, originating from a disorder (e.g., schizophrenia) that a person has; a dimension resulting from individual temperament and personality traits—what a person is; dysfunctional behavior (e.g., anorexia nervosa or an eating disorder)—what a person does; and life story—what a person encounters—for example, traumatic experiences such as loss of a loved one and physical or sexual abuse. The clinician considers psychiatric symptoms from all four perspectives for each person. For the DSM-5 case formulation, these perspectives can be considered within the framework of predisposing (disease, dimension, behavior, and life story), precipitating (life story), and perpetuating (disease, dimension, behavior, and life story) factors. In regard to protective factors, positive temperamental and personality traits may lead to resilience and mastery of stressful life events. Supportive family relationships may enhance resilience.

Each of these perspectives has a developmental component: Schizophrenia, for example, has a typical age of onset in late adolescence into early adulthood, temperament traits may develop into personality disorder depending on life circumstances, and behavior disorder such as anorexia nervosa typically emergences in early adolescence and psychologically reflects rejection of developmental tasks of adolescence and does not accept physical developmental changes reflecting sexual maturation. The mastery of developmental tasks in the emerging life story is linked to both emerging cognitive capacity and developmental self-emotional regulation. In regard to prognosis, mastery of age-appropriate developmental tasks is a key element.

## Neurodevelopmental Clinical Case Formulation

In case formulation of neurodevelopmental disorder cases, greater emphasis is placed on the relationship between genetic and neurological information and behavior. For example, autism spectrum disorder, ADHD, Tourette's disorder, and schizophrenia may be approached by emphasizing the importance of neurodevelopment in the formulation (Solomon et al., 2009). For known genetic syndromes, the genetic etiology, known central nervous system neuronal architectural features, and neuropsychological test findings may contribute to the understanding of presenting symptoms. This is particularly true when there is a known behavioral phenotype for the disorder. In known genetic disorders, emotional dysregulation may be linked to deficits and immaturities in inhibitory neuronal circuits that are involved in self-soothing, negative affect regulation, and overall emotional regulation (Solomon et al., 2009). Despite there being a genetic etiology, environmental, psychodynamic, and learned behavior must still be taken into account and discussed in the formulation. Finally, children with neurodevelopmental disorder diagnoses may exhibit challenging behavior, especially those who are severely cognitively impaired. In these instances, a behavior plan is prepared using behavioral analysis methodology that takes into account the developmental level of the child.

## Integrated Neuroscience Perspective on Formulation for Post-Traumatic Stress Disorder

As we learn more about developmental neuroscience, targeted case formulations may be linked to specific brain mechanisms (Ross et al., 2017). For example, advances in neuroscience help us understand fear conditioning and its relationship to dysregulated brain circuits, memory reconsolidation, epigenetics, and genetic factors in post-traumatic stress disorder (PTSD). We now know that in the process of memory reconsolidation, whenever a memory is reactivated, it becomes momentarily labile and needs to be reconsolidated, leading to its weakening or strengthening. Memory is updated and may be changed based on new experience. Thus, in PTSD, each time a traumatic experience is recalled, the individual's memory must be updated. This may be detrimental in reconsolidating cognitive distortions or may be potentially helpful because it is a new opportunity for therapy based on fear extinction. Moreover, epigenetic change may follow traumatic experiences, especially those early in life. This may have long-term effects on the regulation of the hypothalamic–pituitary–adrenal axis and limit the individual's capacity to regulate the stress response in later life. Also, genetic factors may impact post-traumatic stress responses even though they are triggered by specific experiences (Ross et al., 2017). Such advances in neuroscience make possible an integrated neuroscience informed approach to both case formulation and treatment planning.

## National Institute of Mental Health's Research Domain Criteria Applications to Case Formulation

The National Institute of Mental Health established the Research Domain Criteria research framework that focuses on higher order mental domains which represent systems of emotion, cognition, motivation, and social behavior. These domains are organized into templates to seek and validate biomarkers and endophenotypes. The domains are defined as negative valence systems, positive valence systems, cognitive systems, systems for social processes, and arousal/regulatory systems. Appraisal of these domains could potentially augment psychiatric histories, diagnosis, formulations, and treatment planning. The domains are defined as follows:

> *Negative valence systems*: This domain includes responses to acute threat, responses to potential harm, responses to sustain throughout, and responses to frustrated non-report and loss.
>
> *Positive valence systems*: This domain includes approach motivation (reward validation, effort evaluation, willingness to work, expectancy/reward prediction error,

and action selection/preference-based decision-making), initial responsiveness to reward attainment, sustained/longer term responsiveness to reward attainment, and reward learning and habit.

*Cognitive systems*: Included in this domain are attention, perception, declarative memory, language, cognitive control, and working memory.

*Systems for social processes*: This domain considers the constructs of affiliation and attachment; social communication—for example, reception of facial communication, production of facial communication, reception of non-facial communication, and production of non-facial communication; perception and understanding of the self, its constructs of agency and self-knowledge; and perception and understanding of others, including animacy perception.

*Arousal/regulatory systems*: This domain includes arousal, circadian rhythms, and sleep and wakefulness.

Systematic assessment of the domains may be utilized to establish the underpinnings of psychiatric diagnoses and to identify a problem-based focus in case formulation that incorporates these domains as elements in predisposing, precipitating, perpetuating, and protective factors (Yager & Feinstein, 2017).

## Treatment Planning

Treatment planning involves determining the appropriate intervention for both the child's and the family's problems based on the clinical formulation; this takes into account the multiple conditions that influence psychological and behavioral disturbance (Dudley et al., 2015; Winters et al., 2007).

These changes may have long-term effects on the regulation of the hypothalamic–pituitary–adrenal axis. Because of the unique presentation of symptoms that are observed in the case presentation involved for each child and family, two patients with the same DSM-5 diagnosis may require different treatment approaches. This is the case because life circumstances will vary from one child to the next, and treatment needs are influenced by the child or adolescent's developmental stage and past life experiences.

Treatment planning involves the selection of curative, corrective, ameliorative, or palliative approaches for the child or adolescent patient and their family. A properly developed formulation suggests guides for appropriate intervention. The treatment modalities chosen should be the most efficacious, the least restrictive, and the most cost-effective. Although treatment planning must take into account the problem areas identified in the clinical case formulation, it must also consider the strengths of both the child patient and the family. It addresses problems in the individual (both psychological and physical), problems in the family, problems with peers, problems at school, and problems in the sociocultural environment. Treatment goals are developed for the individual child and their family, utilizing individual psychodynamic, family systems, behavioral, pharmacological, and group treatment and environmental approaches (i.e., multimodal intervention as appropriate).

## Prognosis

Once the diagnosis has been made, the parents express their worries and ask what to expect as the child grows older. They ask the clinician to predict what outcomes to expect as the child grows older.

It was prognosis, not diagnosis, that was a main objective of ancient Hippocratic medicine. Hippocrates (2009) said,

> It appears to me the most excellent thing for the physician is to cultivate prognosis: [For in] foreseeing and foretelling, in the presence of the sick . . . he will manage the cure best who has foreseen is to have bleeding from the present state matters. And he will manage the cure best who has foreseen what is to happen from the present state of matters.

The clinical challenge is risk prediction. Increasingly, we study prediction estimates of risk to guide families in decision-making. Such clinical decisions are based on additional testing, initiating or withholding treatments, and informing families about the risk for particular outcomes. Early detection leads to early intervention with supports to improve prognosis. Increasingly in neurogenetic syndromes, developmental trajectories are better understood. We seek to understand pathways from genes to cognition and complex behaviors. Prognosis emerges from a thorough case formulation and comprehensive treatment plan.

## References

Achenbach, T. M. (2009). The Achenbach *System* of *Empirically Based Assessment* (ASEBA): Development, findings, theory, and applications. University of Vermont, Research Center for Children, Youth, & Families.

Achenbach, T. M., Becker, A., Döpfner, M., Heiervang, E., Roessner, V., Steinhausen, H. C., & Rothenberger, A. (2008). Multicultural assessment of child and adolescent psychopathology with ASEBA and SDQ instruments: Research findings, applications, and future directions. *Journal of Child Psychology and Psychiatry, 49*(3), 251–275.

American Psychiatric Association. (2013). *Diagnostic and statistical manual of mental disorders* (5th ed.). American Psychiatric Publishing.

Angold, A., & Costello, E. J. (2000). The Child and Adolescent Psychiatric Assessment (CAPA). *Journal of the American Academy of Child & Adolescent Psychiatry, 39*(1), 39–48.

Angold, A., Erkanli, A., Copeland, W., Goodman, R., Fisher, P. W., & Costello, E. J. (2012). Psychiatric diagnostic interviews for children and adolescents: A comparative study. *Journal of the American Academy of Child & Adolescent Psychiatry, 51*(5), 506–517.

Barker, P. (2004). *Basic child psychiatry* (7th ed.). Wiley.

Bolton, J. W. (2015). How to integrate biological, psychological, and sociological knowledge in psychiatric education: A case formulation seminar series. *Academic Psychiatry, 39*(6), 699–702.

Cameron, P. M., Kline, S., Korenblum, M., Seltzer, A., & Small, F. (1978). II. A method of reporting formulation. *Canadian Psychiatric Association Journal, 23*(1), 43–50.

Conners, C. K. (2014). *Conners Continuous Performance Test Third Edition*. Pearson.

Dudley, R., Ingham, B., Sowerby, K., & Freeston, M. (2015). The utility of case formulation in treatment decision making; The effect of experience and expertise. *Journal of Behavior Therapy and Experimental Psychiatry, 48*, 66–74.

Edelbrock, C., & Bohnert, A. (2000). Structured interviews for children and adolescents. In G. Goldstein & M. Hersen (Eds.), *Handbook of psychological assessment* (3rd ed., pp. 369–386). Elsevier.

Engel, G. L. (1977). The need for a new medical model: A challenge for biomedicine. *Science, 196*(4286), 129–136.

Engel, G. L. (1980). The clinical application of the biopsychosocial model. *American Journal of Psychiatry, 137*(5), 535–544.

Engel, G. L. (2009). The need for a new medical model: A challenge for biomedicine. *Holistic Medicine, 4*, 37–53.

Fisher, P. W., Chin, E. M., & Vidair, H. B. (2015). Use of structured interviews, rating scales, and observational methods in clinical settings. In A. Thapar, D. S. Pine, J. F. Leckman, S. Scott, M. J. Snowling, & E. Taylor (Eds.), *Rutter's child and adolescent psychiatry* (pp. 419–435). Wiley.

Flinn, L., Braham, L., & das Nair, R. (2015). How reliable are case formulations? A systematic literature review. *British Journal of Clinical Psychology, 54*(3), 266–290.

Geller, B., Zimerman, B., Williams, M., Bolhofner, K., Craney, J. L., DelBello, M. P., & Soutullo, C. (2001). Reliability of the Washington University in St. Louis Kiddie Schedule for Affective Disorders and Schizophrenia (WASH-U-KSADS) mania and rapid cycling sections. *Journal of the American Academy of Child & Adolescent Psychiatry, 40*(4), 450–455.

Hippocrates. (2009). *The book of prognostics*. Dodo Press.

Hodges, K., Kline, J., Stern, L., Cytryn, L., & McKnew, D. (1982). The development of a child assessment interview for research and clinical use. *Journal of Abnormal Child Psychology, 10*(2), 173–189.

Hodges, K., McKnew, D. Cytryn, L., Stern, L., & Kline, J. (1982). The Child Assessment Schedule (CAS) diagnostic interview: A report on reliability and validity. *Journal of the American Academy of Child Psychiatry, 21*(5), 468–473.

Lapouse, R., & Monk, M. A. (1958). An epidemiologic study of behavior characteristics in children. *American Journal of Public Health and the Nation's Health, 48*(9), 1134–1144.

Macneil, C. A., Hasty, M. K., Conus, P., & Berk, M. (2012). Is diagnosis enough to guide interventions in mental health? Using case formulation in clinical practice. *BMC Medicine, 10*(1), Article 111.

McDougall, G. M., & Reade, B. (1993). Teaching biopsychosocial integration and formulation. *Canadian Journal of Psychiatry, 38*(5), 359–362.

Owen, G., Wesseley, S., & Murry, R. (Eds.). (2014). *The Maudsley handbook of practical psychiatry*. Oxford University Press.

Peters, M. E., Taylor, J., Lyketsos, C. G., & Chisolm, M. S. (2012). Beyond the DSM: The perspectives of psychiatry approach to patients. *Primary Care Companion for CNS Disorders, 14*(1), 11m01233.

Ross, D. A., Arbuckle, M. R., Travis, M. J., Dwyer, J. B., van Schalkwyk, G. I., & Ressler, K. J. (2017). An integrated neuroscience perspective on formulation and treatment planning for posttraumatic stress disorder: An educational review. *JAMA Psychiatry, 74*(4), 407–415.

Russell, G. F. M., Jacoby, R., Campbell, L. B., Isaacs, A. D., Farmer, A. E., Gunn, M., Prendergast, M., Holden, N. L., & Taylor, E. (1992). *Psychiatric examination: Notes on eliciting and recording clinical information in psychiatric patients* (2nd ed.). Oxford University Press.

Rutter, M., & Graham, P. (1968). The reliability and validity of the psychiatric assessment of the child. I: Interview with the child. *British Journal of Psychiatry, 114*(510), 563–579.

Shaffer, D., Fisher, P. W., & Lucas, C. P. (1999). Respondent-based interviews. In D. Shaffer & C. P. Lucas (Eds.), *Diagnostic assessment in child and adolescent psychopathology* (pp. 3–33). Guilford.

Shaffer, D., Fisher, P., Lucas, C. P., Dulcan, M. K., & Schwab-Stone, M. E. (2000). NIMH Diagnostic Interview Schedule for Children Version IV (NIMH DISC-IV): Description, differences from previous versions, and reliability of some common diagnoses. *Journal of the American Academy of Child & Adolescent Psychiatry, 39*(1), 28–38.

Solomon, M., Hessl, D., Chiu, S., Olsen, E., & Hendren, R. L. (2009). Towards a neurodevelopmental model of clinical case formulation. *Psychiatric Clinics of North America, 32*(1), 199–211.

Weerasekera, P. (1993). Formulation: A multiperspective model. *Canadian Journal of Psychiatry*, *38*(5), 351–358.

Winters, N. C., Hanson, G., & Stoyanova, V. (2007). The case formulation in child and adolescent psychiatry. *Child and Adolescent Psychiatric Clinics*, *16*(1), 111–132.

Wirt, R. D., Lachar, D., Klinedinst, J. K., & Seat, P. D. (1984). *Multidimensional description of child personality: A manual for the Personality Inventory for Children Revised 1984*. Western Psychological Services.

Wolraich, M. L., Lambert, W., Doffing, M. A., Bickman, L., Simmons, T., & Worley, K. (2003). Psychometric properties of the Vanderbilt ADHD diagnostic parent rating scale in a referred population. *Journal of Pediatric Psychology*, *28*(8), 559–568.

World Health Organization. (2019). *The ICD-10 classifications of mental and behavioural disorder: Clinical descriptions and diagnostic guidelines*.

Yager, J., & Feinstein, R. E. (2017). Potential applications of the National Institute of Mental Health's Research Domain Criteria (RDoC) to clinical psychiatric practice: How RDoC might be used in assessment, diagnostic processes, case formulation, treatment planning, and clinical notes. *Journal of Clinical Psychiatry*, *78*(4), 423–432.

# 2

# Neuropsychological Testing

## Assessing the Mechanisms of Cognition and Complex Behavioral Functioning

Neuropsychology is the study of brain–behavior relationships. It is an applied science whose focus is on the behavioral expression of brain function (Lezak et al., 2012), whereas developmental neuropsychology is the study of how brain–behavior relationships emerge in both typical and atypical development during human development (Pennington, 2009). Developmental neuropsychological testing provides a systematic *way* to evaluate areas of dysfunction that may arise in atypical development.

Developmental neuropsychological testing is an important component of the developmental neuropsychiatric examination. The developmental neuropsychiatric assessment involves the concurrent measurement of cognitive, emotional, social, and global adaptive functioning. As part of that assessment, neuropsychological examination uses psychological tests to measure cognition and complex behavioral functioning. An appreciation of neuropsychological testing will allow the clinician to consider more carefully the relationship of brain and behavior than in the standard psychiatric mental status examination, which addresses the similar areas in less depth and less systematically.

Both clinical and developmental neuropsychological testing integrate psychiatric and psychological information on behavior and the mind with neurological information on the brain and nervous system (Denckla, 1989). Neuropsychology intersects with genetics in the broader discipline of developmental cognitive neuroscience (Johnson & de Haan, 2015).

The developmental neuropsychological assessment is similar to the clinical psychological examination in using some of the same interviews, questionnaires, and standardized tests. However, the developmental neuropsychological approach uses a different conceptual/interpretive perspective by focusing on the brain–behavior relationship. The developmental neuropsychological assessment of mental status in children is particularly important in neurodevelopmental disorders where advances in neuropsychological testing make possible the specific evaluation of functions that are not addressed in standardized intelligence, achievement, and language assessment protocols. Neuropsychological testing seeks to identify the basic processes that underlie brain growth and development to better understand, for example, psycholinguistic development, emotion regulation, and memory functions.

The tests introduced in this chapter should be particularly helpful in appreciating in greater depth mental status items that deal with cognition, speech/linguistic functions, memory, attention, executive functions (vigilance, working memory, set maintenance, planning, and inhibitory motor control), praxis (planning the sequencing of learned motor behavior), and visuomotor and visuospatial functions. In addition, the processing/production of social–emotional signals (including vocal tone, facial expression, and "body language" or gesture) can be tested.

Developmental neuropsychological tests are increasingly available to assess these and other specific capacities. Such tests will account for only a proportion of the variance in the evaluation of an individual case and must be integrated into a total clinical case formulation that addresses the multiple facets of the child's life. The linking of test findings to adaptive function is crucial because children may compensate for their brain dysfunction in a way that their overall functioning is "better than they look" on the tests applied.

This chapter provides an orientation to using developmental neuropsychological testing in assessing mental functioning. It discusses a neuropsychological model of functional domains proceeding from domain-general to domain-specific interactive specialization, introduces the construct of neuroconstructionism, reviews current issues in the application of tests and instrument development, provides a comparison of neuropsychological and clinical psychological approaches to assessment, considers the differences in brain–behavior relationships between adults and children on neuropsychological testing, reviews indications for neuropsychological testing, discusses assessment strategies for the neuropsychological capacities tested, and provides a description of the types of tests used and a rationale for their use.

## Neuropsychological Models of Functional Domains

### Domains of Function

Neuropsychologists generally consider development to be "domain-specific" and refer to domain-general and domain-specific behavior. Domain-specific regions of the brain are dynamically constructed, emerging from the interaction of genes and environment over time (interactive specialization). A domain is defined as a set of representations sustaining a particular area of knowledge (e.g., language). Traditionally, reference was made to a modular single deficit model as the accepted causal model for the neuropsychology of learning disorders. This model has been replaced by a multiple deficit etiological model. Pennington (2009) and others review the evidence that led to the abandonment of this simple model and raise important questions about the earlier use of the term innateness. It is proposed that those brain regions specialized for processing, for example, facial perception and language are not innate but, rather, become specialized as a result of cortical neuroplasticity with experience. For example, it was long proposed that language lateralization was *innately* localized in the left hemisphere of the brain rather than being the consequence of developmental processes. Elizabeth Bates and collaborators (Ballantyne et al., 2007, 2008; Bates & Dick, 2002; Bates et al., 2001; Vicari et al., 2000) provided evidence that localization is indeed the result of developmental processes. They prospectively studied infants with unilateral brain lesions. Before 6 months of age, injury to either hemisphere temporarily disrupted language development. But by ages 5–7 years, language was within normal limits for both. If language was innate to the left hemisphere, then early lesions should have had a persistent deficit and a far worse outcome than the right hemisphere group. Moreover, follow-up studies of perinatal stroke (Trauner et al., 2013) found that early language development takes a different developmental course than in typical language development. This suggests that brain reorganization results from plasticity of the developing brain (Stiles et al., 2012).

The approach to assessing clinical brain–behavioral relationships in developmental neuropsychology increasingly emphasizes these domain-general and emerging domain-specific interactive specialization of functions. Just as the quantitative genetic model does in behavioral genetics, the multiple deficit model is a multifactorial model for complex behavioral disorders. This model posits interactive risk and protective factors that might be either genetic or environmental (Pennington, 2009). These risk and protective factors mediate cognitive development and result in behavioral symptoms. No one factor is fully causative for a disorder. Thus, co-occurring conditions—for example, attention deficit disorder and learning disorder in reading—can be explained by shared etiological and cognitive risk factors. This approach supports a dimensional view that is continuous and quantitative rather than a categorical approach for diagnosis. Ultimately, each disorder has its own risk factors and others that are shared.

## Neuroconstructionism

Karmiloff-Smith challenged the earlier modular hard-wired maturational model in the ontogenesis of brain functions in her neuroconstructionism model (Karmiloff-Smith, 1998; see also Farran & Karmiloff-Smith, 2012; Mareschal et al., 2007). The neuroconstruction model, like interactional specification, emphasizes the plasticity of the developing brain and the emergence of domains that results from developmental interaction of genes, environment, and personal choice (mastery motivation).

Cortical networks are not genetically determined. A neuroconstructivist approach proposes that brain function begins in early life with biases that are relevant to the processing of certain kinds of inputs over other inputs. With experience, such processing becomes domain-specific over time through neuronal competition, with gradual specialization in location and modularization of brain function. This is accomplished through flexible, plastic, self-structuring brain systems. These are open to environmental influences at the level of gene expression, cognition, and behavior. Developmental change is the rule at each level. For example, cortical areas are more highly interconnected in the infant brain than in the adult brain. Over time, with strengthening of some connections and the pruning of others, localization and specialization of brain functions take place.

The ratio of white matter to gray matter is not static, changing as it does over developmental time. The thickness of fiber bundles in the corpus callosum between the two hemispheres is different in infancy than later in brain development. Neural processing of faces or language demonstrates that in early development, neural activity is widely distributed across cortical regions across both hemispheres. However, later in development, it is gradually fine-tuned to be more predominant in one hemisphere (Karmiloff-Smith, 2015). The neuroconstructionism model is increasingly being utilized in developmental studies. Intelligence has been examined as a developing function using this approach. A neuroconstructivist approach helps explain how intelligence may rise or fall as a result of the developing brain systems interacting with environmental factors (Rinaldi & Karmiloff-Smith, 2017). Farran and Karmiloff-Smith (2012) illustrate the neuroconstructivist approach in life span studies carried out in patients with Williams syndrome.

## Comparison of Neuropsychological and Clinical Psychological Approaches

Neuropsychological evaluation is similar to clinical psychological examination, but there are differences in conceptualization; however, some of the same goals are shared and the same testing environment is used. There are also differences in that the neuropsychologist goes into greater depth in the way tests are grouped and in how the test data are interpreted regarding brain function. Neuropsychology utilizes knowledge gained from psychological, psychiatric, and neurological research to understand brain–behavior relationships. Developmental neuropsychological testing differs from standardized clinical psychological test batteries that tend to be more general in their approach and place their primary emphasis on intelligence and personality assessments or use educational test batteries that generally include intelligence and educational assessments. Although aspects of cognitive processing may be addressed in some of these test batteries—for example, in sections of the Wechsler Intelligence Scale for Children–5 (WISC-5; Wechsler, 2014)—the focus of these tests is not primarily on establishing domains of brain function with implications for brain organization. Still, adaptations of components of these tests may be used in neuropsychological contexts.

For example, when a clinical psychologist performs a test of intelligence, the goal is to determine an individual's overall functional capacity. Instead, the neuropsychologist is specifically interested in the various psychological and neurological components that form the basis for the individual's ability or inability to perform. On these tests, general intelligence is of limited validity in children or adolescents with brain dysfunction. In such children, the summary IQ score has limited meaning when there is substantial subtest variability. The developmental neuropsychologist addresses these developmental issues by choosing tests for a particular child to individualize the assessment.

## Interpretations of Brain–Behavior Relationships in Adults and Children

Child neuropsychology differs from adult neuropsychology just as developmental psychology differs from adult psychology (Baron, 2010). The major areas of brain dysfunction responsible for neuropsychological dysfunction studied in children differ from those in adults. In developmental neuropsychology, there are two major considerations in studying impaired brain systems in children compared to adults. First, there are differences in the effects of brain injury when it occurs in the developmental period in children, in contrast to brain injury effects on the mature brain in adulthood. Second, there are differences between acquired and congenital neurodevelopmental disorders, regardless of the age when they are seen by the clinician.

The adult neuropsychological database was largely established through the evaluation of adults with known brain damage (strokes, seizures, tumors, penetrating wounds, and head trauma). These adult studies with acquired disorders have contributed substantially to our understanding of the parts or systems of the brain that are involved in a number of psychological functions. Adult neuropsychology has focused on the impact of documented focal and diffuse acquired brain lesions on behavior and findings from experimental brain lesions in animals. However, in pediatric neuropsychology, experiments in immature animals have not proven as useful because of the plasticity of the developing brain. The types of lesions seen in adults, such as strokes and penetrating wounds, occur far less commonly in children, whereas congenital malformations related to pre- and postnatal developmental insults (prematurity, intraventricular hemorrhage, and ischemia/anoxia) are more common. A majority of the neuropsychological dysfunctions of early life are not associated with known brain insults, nor are they associated with lesions demonstrable on routine neuroimaging studies. In childhood, acquired pathologies, such as trauma, tumors, and infarctions, when they do occur, may have different neuropsychological presentations when they impact an immature brain (Baron, 2018; Dennis & Levin, 2004). Unlike adult head injury, in children the injury occurs in the context of ongoing physical and cognitive development. The age of head injury and time since it occurred may be significant moderators in regard to consequences throughout the life span.

Developmental neuropsychological testing evaluates changes associated with injuries that occur during development and is used to monitor progress in rehabilitation programs. When injury does occur at any age, recovery may involve reversible changes in the affected brain regions. Recovery also may involve compensatory processes. The accomplishment of complex behavior depends on the contributions of multiple and widely distributed brain systems that may be spared following injury. Noninvolved regions may be activated and provide flexibility in task performance and lead to demonstrable resiliency in the face of focal damage when lesions occur during the developmental period. New developmental acquisitions may involve compensation by undamaged functional units that may not be available in the more mature, differentiated, and committed adult brain.

Plasticity in the immature brain is essential to recovery, and its understanding is important in rehabilitation programs. It is possible that children who sustain major lesions in one hemisphere during development may compensate by involvement of the other hemisphere. If such compensation does take place, these brain regions are not lost and may not establish their usual developmental function; in a sense, they have been crowded out. For example, large lesions of the left perisylvian cortex may be compensated by language development taking place in the right hemisphere so that potential visuospatial skill deficits may occur. Moreover, the lesion may remain silent after damage and emerge at a later time during development when that particular function is normally expected to arise. Insight, initiative, and executive functions that are expected during adolescence may be affected by brain damage earlier in life. Neuropsychological testing should examine such possibilities and clarify whether or not they do occur. Therefore, the neuropsychological study of acquired disorders in adults only indirectly serves to provide a framework to study developmental disorders. This is especially the case for most children with intellectual developmental disorder, autism spectrum disorder (ASD), attention-deficit/hyperactivity disorder (ADHD), and specific learning disabilities. In these conditions, rather than examining acquired damage, the assessment evaluates differences in the formation and integration of the brain systems themselves that arise during development. When developmental neuropsychiatric disorders are assessed, the methods used are distinct from those used in adults.

Developmental level is a key focus and impacts how the examiner engages the patient for testing, choice of instrument used, selection criteria for evaluating performance, and clinical interpretation of behavior. An emphasis is placed on integrating the patient's past history into the case formulation and conclusions. Specific recommendations are made to ensure the inclusion of individual strengths in coping at home, school, and in the community (Baron, 2010, p. 480). Developmental neuropsychological testing is increasingly available to designate patterns of performance that may be used in diagnosis, patient management, habilitation, and rehabilitation planning in developmental disorders.

Intellectual developmental disorder syndromes and other learning disorders have been recognized since the 19th century, but it is only recently that developmental neuropsychologists have emphasized them. This focus has received greater attention with the introduction of the brain imaging techniques of computed tomography (CT) in the 1970s, magnetic resonance imaging (MRI) and positron emission tomography in the 1980s, followed later by functional MRI (fMRI) and diffusion tensor imaging. Neuroimaging technology attempts to correlate specific aspects of information processing with specific brain systems. Structural imaging methods (e.g., CT and MRI) are used to link damage in particular brain regions with behavioral deficits. fMRI investigates physiological changes associated with brain activity. Links to brain structure or physiology may validate neuropsychological assumptions for the developmental disorders.

The role of genetic abnormalities in the development of various brain systems is a major area of focus in developmental neuroscience and developmental neuropsychology. In chromosomal abnormalities, in which gene defects are associated with systemic disorder, the neuropsychological investigation may be used to establish their profound effects on brain development.

In summary, neuropsychological test procedures have been used both in learning disorders of unknown etiology and in intellectual developmental disorder and neurogenetic syndromes, such as fragile X syndrome, Down syndrome, and Williams syndrome (Nussbaum et al., 2016).

## Issues in the Application of Tests and Instrument Development

Neuropsychological testing uses standardized means for clarifying deficits or impairments to identify strengths and capacities that may be used adaptively. Normative referencing is essential because capacities such as intellect, memory, and various functional domains are variable in the normal population. *Normative referencing* refers to the process of constructing norms on the typical performance of a group of individuals on a test. Tests that compare an individual's score against the scores of groups are termed *norm-referenced assessments*. Peer group normative data are required and include average levels of performance and the variability (standard deviation) of those performances on the test. An extensive number of instruments with normative data are available for use in individuals for classical psychometric and achievement testing. New data are regularly collected and critically scrutinized for interrater reliability and test–retest reliability for neuropsychological tests. Among the variables that need to be considered are gender, age, educational experience, suspected brain involvement, and sociocultural setting. In the assessment, both the effects of illness or trauma and premorbid abilities also must be considered.

Several considerations arise uniquely in developmental neuropsychological instrument development and testing (Baron, 2018). These include problems of reliability, developmental changes in cognition over time, special applications to learning disorders, appropriately designated domains for study, and concurrent testing for emotional disturbance and adaptive functioning (Denckla, 1989). These considerations are as follows:

> *Use of assessment techniques originally developed for adults*: Techniques are similar for children and adults, but the approach must be adapted for developmental level. Tests have been normed for infants, children, and adolescents and specially developed for them. Attention, language, and social deficits must be considered in test cooperation. Clinical judgment must be used when testing outside the child's age range, especially for those with neurodevelopmental disorders. Mental age must be taken into account to bring out individual strengths. An older adolescent or young adult with an intellectual developmental disorder who might typically be administered the Wechsler Adult Intelligence Scale adult intelligence test by chronological age criteria would instead appropriately be tested with the WISC-5 youth intelligence test for a better determination of their abilities.
>
> *The problem of developmental change*: A major issue is the problem of developmental change or developmental sensitivity. The child development literature documents changing skills with increasing age as the child gradually attains the mastery of complex adult skills. Existing neuropsychological measures are operationalized and adapted according to developmental level. Newer age-appropriate measures have been linked to neuropsychological theory (Pennington, 2009).
>
> *Limited behavioral repertoire and difficulty in personal engagement with the examiner in testing*: Because infants and preschool children show limited behavioral responses, observations must supplement more formal testing for the youngest children. Those with a diagnosis of moderate to severe cognitive deficits, oppositional behavior, and attentional deficit also require observation and adjustments in testing to facilitate their cooperation.

## Indications for Neuropsychological Testing

The following are indications for neuropsychological tests (Lezak et al., 2012):

> *Diagnostic evaluation of developmental disorders*: Developmental neuropsychological assessment is important in identifying domains of dysfunction that may be

related to an individual's cognitive functioning, language ability, attention, executive functioning, visual–spatial abilities, memory, motor ability, academic achievement, personality assessment, emotional and behavioral functioning, and adaptive living skills.

*Detection of conditions not demonstrated on standard diagnostic testing*: Disorders may be suspected on clinical examination that are not revealed on routine clinical psychological testing. For example, specific learning disorders that are suspected may ultimately be defined in terms of developmental neuropsychology. Moreover, mild or subtle sequelae of traumatic brain injury may not be recognized with routine testing and require neuropsychological testing.

*Monitoring the neuropsychological status of patients*: Baseline and subsequent neuropsychological testing is needed to follow up head trauma, monitor behavioral change related to drug treatment, and document any cognitive or behavioral change following other injury or toxic exposure. Baseline test data are collected at the time of presentation, and the individual's progress is followed over time. For example, the neuropsychologist might monitor changes related to drug treatment for complex partial seizures or changes following surgery for a brain tumor.

*Characterization of the cognitive capacities in planning rehabilitation programs*: Full characterization of cognitive capacities is particularly important in patients with brain injuries to determine rehabilitation needs and to help find an appropriate school setting and placement. The assessment is carried out to evaluate cognitive strengths and weaknesses. Acute epoch assessments are performed as soon as the patient is alert enough to cooperate, and chronic epoch assessments are carried out 3 or more months after the event. These assessments are used to evaluate recovery, assess therapies, and determine suitability of educational or vocational programs.

*Medicolegal situations*: Neuropsychological testing may be an important component in forensic assessment. Executive function testing, evaluation of memory, assessment for learning disorder, and overall assessment of cognitive ability may be important in establishing the individual's culpability in legal cases. Dysfunction in any of these areas may constitute a mitigating circumstance in legal cases. Brain injury and associated cognitive impairment may be grounds for a legal suit, and damages may be claimed by the family on behalf of the child. In some instances, hard neurological signs (e.g., weakness, sensory loss, and paralysis) may be absent and neuroimaging findings may be questionable following trauma. In these instances, a comprehensive neuropsychological profile assumes particular importance to clarify the nature of the injury. Neuropsychological testing may provide the objective evidence needed to support the plaintiff's claim.

*Research*: Neuropsychological testing has become an integral part of many research programs. Those test procedures linked to neuroimaging techniques are assuming increasing importance in child and adolescent neuropsychiatry. Models such as Pennington's multiple deficit model (Pennington, 2009) provide an orientation to developmental neuropsychological research that is critical for progress in this area.

## Assessment Strategies

Neuropsychological testing uses several strategies including the fixed test battery, a more flexible hypothesis-driven approach that uses tests chosen based on the particular referral question, and a combination fixed/flexible test battery approach. Tests involving the assessment of intelligence, adaptive function, and personality are used by neuropsychologists but are not a core part of the neuropsychological assessment.

Neuropsychological testing is organized to evaluate certain functional domains; the goal of testing is to evaluate these domains adequately. The tests used for these evaluations are continually being refined. Because assessment of domains of function is sought, the specific tests used will vary, so no specific core battery is recommended for developmental neuropsychological testing. Instead, commonly used tests are discussed in the text and listed in the tables. Standard texts include *A Compendium of Neuropsychological Tests* (Strauss et al., 2006), *Neuropsychological Assessment* (Lezak et al., 2012), *Buros Mental Measures Yearbook* (updated every 3 years; Carlson et al., 2017), and *Neuropsychological Evaluation of the Child* (Baron, 2018). These should be consulted for a more detailed description of tests.

## Assessment Domains/Test Results

Several stages of analysis are involved in evaluating neuropsychological test results (Denckla, 1989). At the first level of analysis, the individual's level of performance is established in a similar manner to the calculation of results that might be performed by a clinical psychologist. This aspect of the evaluation establishes whether or not a particular behavioral function is at the level expected for age. The individual level of performance is determined, and raw scores obtained from the test are converted into an age or grade equivalent, a percentile rank or a scale score, to judge whether the individual's performance is below, at, or above average.

The second stage in evaluating neuropsychological test findings is the analysis of the constituent skills that are required to perform the particular function being tested. Can the child or adolescent recognize the figure they are asked to describe, or is the child capable of writing out an answer? Because many test results require graphomotor activity, they must be interpreted according to the child's capacity to perform the function. For example, failure on a test of copying designs might be the result of faulty perception of the designs, so visual perception would need to be evaluated.

## Psychological Capacities Tested

### Cognitive/Intellectual Assessment

Intelligence tests are used by both child psychologists and child neuropsychologists. In intelligence testing, several obstacles may interfere with obtaining an accurate assessment of the child's overall functioning. To address them, it is important to make the correct choice among the available instruments for children with brain disorders.

Obstacles include the high prevalence of associated problems in attention, concentration, motivation, and behavior in children with learning disorders and intellectual developmental disorder. Available intelligence tests vary in their applicability to children with neurodevelopmental disorders. Existing medical conditions, particularly neurological disorders, may influence the assessment process. The selection of appropriate instruments can be difficult, and consideration must be given to the variety of instruments available because several tests assess similar aspects of functioning. Attention must be given to the child's reported developmental level and behavioral difficulties and the range and complexity of the child's presenting problems. The referral questions, goal of the assessment, and awareness of the limitations of existing instruments are taken into account in choosing the test instrument to be used. Table 2.1 lists some of the instruments used for cognitive and assessment and intelligence testing by both clinical and developmental neuropsychologists.

To assess the probability that an individual has a learning disorder or intellectual developmental disorder, several screening strategies have been recommended. One strategy for intellectual developmental disorder is to include a robust measure of cognitive ability, such as the WISC-5 (Wechsler, 2014). In addition, a measure of adaptive behavior is needed, as described in the next section, for the diagnosis of intellectual developmental disorder. Caution is advised when testing children who function in the severe to profound range of intellectual developmental disorder. Assessment is difficult because of the limited repertoire of behaviors in children with a mental age of less than 2 or 3 years. Their behaviors may impact the validity of the assessment results.

## Intelligence Testing

Intelligence tests were originally constructed to measure, by multiple methods, a general intelligence, or G factor, that would predict future adaptive capacity. These tests were not developed as tests of specific brain functions. Despite this, a standardized IQ test is included as part of most neuropsychological test batteries. Tests such as the WISC-5 are standardized for ages 6–16 years and have the advantage of broad-based, large-scale normative data, which make them useful for neuropsychological assessment. The IQ tests are very helpful in establishing the likelihood of success in a conventional school program.

The original WISC appeared in 1949 and has been successively revised and updated since then to the current WISC-5. Each successive edition has been renamed to account for the Flynn effect (an increase of approximately 3 IQ points per decade) to maintain the average score of 100 on the WISC-5 (Flynn, 1984, 2012; Flynn & Widaman, 2008; Trahan et al., 2014).

The WISC-5 is composed of indices and used for assessing the intelligence of children. It assesses cognitive abilities across five domains: Verbal Comprehension (i.e., Similarities and Vocabulary subtests), Visual Spatial (i.e., Block Design and Visual Puzzles subtests), Fluid Reasoning (i.e., Matrix Reasoning and Figure Weights subtests), Working Memory (i.e., Digit Span and Picture Span subtests), and Processing Speed (i.e., Coding and Symbol Search subtests). The WISC-5 is the primary measure used

**Table 2.1** Cognitive/Intellectual Assessment Measures

| Assessment Tool | Age Range |
| --- | --- |
| Bayley Scales of Infant and Toddler Development, Third Edition (Bayley-III)<br>Assesses cognitive abilities, motor, and behavioral development (e.g., attention/arousal, orientation/engagement, emotional regulation, and motor quality) in infants and preschoolers. | 1–42 months |
| Mullen Scales of Early Learning<br>Assesses cognitive abilities and motor development across five domains: Gross Motor, Visual Reception, Fine Motor, Expressive Language, and Receptive Language. | Birth to 68 months |
| Differential Ability Scales, Second Edition (DAS-II)<br>Assesses a variety of cognitive abilities, including verbal and visual working memory, immediate and delayed recall, visual recognition and matching, processing and naming speed, phonological processing, and understanding of basic number concepts. | 2:6–17:11 years |
| Wechsler Preschool and Primary Scale of Intelligence–Fourth Edition (WPPSI-IV)<br>Assesses cognitive abilities across five domains: Verbal Comprehension (i.e., Receptive Vocabulary, Information, and Similarities), Visual Spatial (i.e., Block Design and Object Assembly), Fluid Reasoning (i.e., Matrix Reasoning and Picture Concepts), Working Memory (i.e., Picture Memory and Zoo Locations), and Processing Speed (i.e., Bug Search and Cancellation). A Full Scale IQ can be calculated. | 2:6–7:7 years |
| Wechsler Intelligence Scale for Children, Fifth Edition (WISC-V)[a]<br>Assesses cognitive abilities across five domains: Verbal Comprehension (i.e., Similarities and Vocabulary subtests), Visual Spatial (i.e., Block Design and Visual Puzzles subtests), Fluid Reasoning (i.e., Matrix Reasoning and Figure Weights), Working Memory (i.e., Digit Span and Picture Span), and Processing Speed (i.e., Coding and Symbol Search). This measure is the primary measure used to determine intellectual abilities in children. | 6:0–16:11 years |
| Stanford-Binet Intelligence Scales–Fifth Edition (SB5)<br>Assesses intelligence in children and adults across five domains: Fluid Reasoning (i.e., Object Series, Matrices, Early Reasoning, Verbal Absurdities, and Verbal Analogies), Knowledge (i.e., Procedural Knowledge, Picture Absurdities, and Vocabulary), Quantitative Reasoning (i.e., Quantitative Reasoning), Visual–Spatial Processing (i.e., Form Board, Form Patterns, and Position and Direction), and Working Memory (i.e., Delayed Response, Block Span, Memory for Sentences, and Last Word). | 2:0–85+ years |
| Leiter International Performance Scale, Third Edition (Leiter-3)[b]<br>Assesses visual spatial intellectual abilities, attention, and memory across three composite domains (i.e., Nonverbal IQ, Nonverbal Memory, and Processing Speed) and five supplemental scores (i.e., Attention Sustained Errors, Attention Divided Correct, Attention Divided Incorrect, Nonverbal Stroop Congruent Incorrect, and Nonverbal Stroop Incongruent Incorrect). | 3:0–75+ years |

*(continued)*

Table 2.1 Continued

| Assessment Tool | Age Range |
|---|---|
| Comprehensive Test of Nonverbal Intelligence, Second Edition (CTONI-2)<br>Assesses cognitive abilities with minimal language and motor demands across two domains: Pictorial Scale (i.e., Pictorial Analogies, Pictorial Categories, and Pictorial Sequences subtests) and Geometric Scale (i.e., Geometric Analogies, Geometric Categories, and Geometric Sequences subtests). A Full Scale IQ can be calculated. | 6:0–89:11 years |
| Kaufman Assessment Battery for Children (K-ABC)<br>Assesses cognitive abilities across five domains: Simultaneous (i.e., Triangles, Face Recognition, Pattern Reasoning, Block Counting, Story Completion, Conceptual Thinking, Rover, and Gestalt Closure subtests), Sequential (i.e., Word Order, Number Recall, and Hand Movements subtests), Planning (i.e., Pattern Reasoning and Story Completion subtests), Learning (i.e., Atlantis, Atlantis Delayed, Rebus, and Rebus Delayed subtests), and Knowledge (i.e., Riddles, Expressive Vocabulary, and Verbal Knowledge subtests). | 2:6–12:6 years |

[a]The Wechsler Abbreviated Scale of Intelligence, Second Edition (WASI-II) is an abbreviated measure of cognitive assessment for individuals ages 6:0–90:11 years. The Wechsler Adult Intelligence Scale, Fourth Edition (WAIS-IV) is a measure of cognitive assessment for individuals ages 16–90 years.

[b]The Universal Nonverbal Intelligence Test (UNIT) is another measure of nonverbal cognitive abilities for individuals ages 5:0–17:11 years.

to determining intellectual abilities in children. The indices measure a child's ability in each of the specific cognitive domains. Five ancillary composite scores are derived from combinations of primary or primary and secondary subtests. Overall, there are 21 subtests that are used to yield 15 composite scores. Complementary subtests yield composite scores linked to cognitive abilities pertinent to identification of learning disabilities in reading and mathematics.

The Verbal Comprehension Index assesses verbal reasoning, comprehension, and verbal expression. It reflects an individual's ability to apply information that has been acquired over time. The Visual Spatial Index assesses the ability to analyze visual–spatial relationships. The Fluid Reasoning Index reflects the ability to analyze or solve problems without the benefit of prior experience or instruction. The Working Memory index assesses short-term memory. Working memory measures the individual's ability to recite or accurately rearrange information after just one exposure. Therefore, it not only reflects rote memory but also requires focused attention and concentration. The Processing Speed Index assesses an individual's ability to quickly discriminate between various shapes, and it also assesses cognitive efficiency due to the timed nature of the task.

## Issues in Intelligence Testing

### Test Interpretation in Infants and Young Children

It is not appropriate to make long-term predictions on the basis of assessments of intelligence in infancy. In addition to qualitative changes in cognitive function, there is a lack of continuity in assessed intelligence from infancy to later childhood. Behavior in very young children is less predictable because of rapid developmental spurts and lags. Children who test in the severe and profound ranges of intellectual developmental disorder will often show inadequate attention and concentration, affecting the reliability of tests. Moreover, infants who score in the severe intellectual developmental disorder range during the first years of life are likely to obtain scores in the same range during the school years. Developmental problems in testing preclude the diagnosis of intellectual developmental disorder on the basis of a single test score in infancy. Reliability problems also may interfere with adequate assessment of adaptive functioning for infants and young children.

For children older than age 2 years, there is also difficulty in interpreting psychological testing. For the younger mental ages, tests do not provide enough information to allow sufficient variability in items to clarify the degree to which a child is delayed. On a practical level, we may only be able to determine from a test that the young child is unable to succeed on tasks in a given area. An adequate test must have items that are appropriate for at least 1 year below the child's mental age; therefore, to assess a moderately intellectual developmental disabled 5-year-old child with a mental age of approximately 2½ years, an adequate testing instrument must have items at the 18-month level of functioning. Similar problems are involved in assessing variability across various domains of functioning (i.e., subtest scores) because of floor effects. In this instance, a paucity of items occurs at the child's baseline ability of several subscales within an assessment instrument. Another difficulty with early intellectual assessment instruments is their reliance on individual verbal capacities. Because of the high correlation between language functioning and intelligence, ordinarily it is true that the lower an individual's IQ, the poorer their language ability. This makes it difficult to select an appropriate intelligence test for a child with limited expressive language skills. To deal with this issue, instruments have been devised for children with severe deficits in language. They include the Leiter International Performance Scale (Roid et al., 2013) and the Comprehensive Test of Nonverbal Intelligence, Second Edition (CTONI-2; Hammill et al., 2009). However, depending on the subject, difficulties may arise in the neuropsychological interpretation of intelligence tests of this kind.

## Intelligence Testing in Neuropsychological Assessment

In general, standardized IQ tests contribute to the neuropsychological battery in that they provide an overall ability level score, provide a basis for conducting more specific neuropsychological testing, and offer extensive normative information for certain subtests that may be relevant for the neuropsychological assessment.

## Excessive Reliance on the Overall Summary Score (the Full Scale IQ) to Characterize a Patient

When there are significant differences in the domains of intellectual functions (i.e., verbal comprehension, visual–spatial abilities, fluid reasoning, working memory, and processing speed), it is best to view each domain independently instead of using the calculated Full Scale IQ number (Heffelfinger, 2014). Scores on intelligence tests are used to separate children with generalized cognitive impairment (e.g., intellectual developmental disorder) from those with isolated forms of learning disability. Definitions of learning disability are used for making placement decisions include intelligence as an indicator of learning potential. Discrepancy between cognitive ability (IQ) and academic achievement is used in diagnosing learning disabilities by examining statistical differences between intellectual measures and academic achievement measures. In addition, learning disabilities also can be diagnosed based on statistically significant weaknesses in academic abilities compared to same-age or same-grade peers. Specific learning disability criteria are listed as neurodevelopmental disorders in the fifth edition of the *Diagnostic and Statistical Manual of Mental Disorders* (DSM-5; American Psychiatric Association, 2013).

## Mood and Motivation

Mood and motivation underlie the capacity to participate fully in neuropsychological testing. Tests of attention are sensitive to disturbances in mood and motivation. The extent of motivation is evaluated through observation and in monitoring participation in the testing procedure. The ability to cooperate, sustain effort, and the extent of encouragement needed to complete a task are all observed. Motivation and task persistence overlap, so those with poor motivation may do poorly on tasks that require perseverance. Specific disturbances in motivation are referred to as apathy and may be signaled by "I don't know" responses or delays in beginning a task. Encouragement and prompting may be necessary to obtain a correct estimate of ability in the apathetic child.

## Adaptive Functioning Measurement

The primary focus of neuropsychological testing is to establish an accurate description of a child's abilities based on test results that are then used in the diagnostic and rehabilitation process. However, from these tests, little can be inferred about the child's ability to function in daily living situations at home and in new situations or in school and residential settings. Specific tests for adaptive function to assess such abilities as self-care must be utilized. These include the Adaptive Behavior Assessment System, Third Edition (ABAS-3); the Vineland Adaptive Behavior Scales, Third Edition (Vineland-3; Sparrow et al., 2016); and the Diagnostic Adaptive Behavior Scale (DABS); see Table 2.2. For example, the Vineland assesses adaptive abilities across five domains: Communication, Daily Living Skills, Socialization, Motor Skills, and Maladaptive Behavior.

## Speech and Linguistic Function

In DSM-5, language disorder, speech sound disorder, childhood-onset fluency disorder (stuttering), and social (pragmatic) communication disorder are listed. Social (pragmatic) communication disorder is a new DSM-5 disorder.

**Table 2.2**  Adaptive Functioning Assessment Measures

| Assessment Tool | Age Range |
| --- | --- |
| Adaptive Behavior Assessment System, Third Edition (ABAS-3) Assesses adaptive abilities through parent/primary caregiver (ages birth to 5 years), teacher/day care provider (ages 2–5 years), parent (ages 5–21 years), teacher (ages 5–21 years), and self (ages 16–89 years) report across 11 skill areas and three adaptive domains: Conceptual (Communication, Functional Academics/Pre-Academics, and Self Direction), Practice (Community Use, Home/School Living, Health and Safety, Self-Care, and Work), and Social (Leisure and Social). An overall score is calculated as the General Adaptive Composite. | Birth through Adulthood |
| Vineland Adaptive Behavior Scales, Third Edition (Vineland-3) Assesses adaptive abilities through clinical interval, parent/caregiver report, or teacher report across five domains: Communication (i.e., Receptive, Expressive, and Written), Daily Living Skills (i.e., Personal, Domestic, and Community), Socialization (i.e., Interpersonal Relationships, Play and Leisure, and Coping Skills), Motor Skills (i.e., Fine and Gross), and Maladaptive Behavior (i.e., Internalizing and Externalizing). | Birth through Adulthood |
| Diagnostic Adaptive Behavior Scale (DABS) Assesses adaptive abilities across three domains: Conceptual Skills (i.e., literacy; self-direction; and concepts of number, money, and time), Social Skills (i.e., interpersonal skills, social responsibility, self-esteem, gullibility, naiveté, social problem-solving, following rules, obeying laws, and avoiding being victimized), and Practical Skills (i.e., activities of daily living, occupational skills, use of money, safety, health care, travel/transportation, schedules/routines, and use of the telephone). | 4:0–21:0 years |

## Assessment of Language Structure

In linguistic theory, the major components of language or linguistic features include phonology, syntax, morphology, and semantics. The assessment of language structure includes phonological assessment (phonic and phonetic skills), lexical and semantic skills, and syntactic skills. Instruments for assessment of language structure are well characterized (Table 2.3). Assessments of language use (i.e., pragmatic language), also shown in Table 2.3, are of increasing importance but are less well characterized.

### Phonological Processing (Phonetics and Phonics)

*Phonology* refers to the sound system of language. The most important aspect of phonology is phonemes, the study of significant speech sounds. Phonemes are significant if they alter the meaning of words—for example, in the words *best* and *rest*, the "b" and "r" sounds change the meaning of the words. A second phonological category is *phonetics*, which refers to specific and discrete sounds called phonemes—for example, the "a" in *art* and the "a" in *above* sound different but do not change the meaning of words. Phonological skills are assessed in the areas of phonetics (articulation, the output side) and phonemic segmentation (recognition of phonic patterns, the input side). Phonological assessment is necessary to evaluate children with reading disorders.

Table 2.3 Language Assessment Measures

| Domain | Subdomain | Assessment Tool | Age Range |
|---|---|---|---|
| Language | Receptive Language | Peabody Picture Vocabulary Test, Fifth Edition (PPVT-5) Assesses receptive language abilities based on words in Standard American English. | 2:6–90+ years |
| | | Receptive One-Word Picture Vocabulary Tests, Fourth Edition (ROWPVT-4) Assesses one-word receptive vocabulary abilities in Standard American English. | 2:0–70+ years |
| | Expressive Language | Expressive Vocabulary Test, Second Edition (EVT-2) Assesses expressive language abilities based on words in Standard American English. | 2:6–90+ years |
| | | Expressive One-Word Picture Vocabulary Tests, Fourth Edition (EOWPVT-4) Assesses one-word expressive vocabulary abilities in Standard American English. | 2:0–70+ years |
| | Phonological Processing | Comprehensive Test of Phonological Processing–Second Edition (CTOPP-2) Assesses phonological processing abilities related to reading across five composite domains: Phonological Awareness, Phonological Memory, Rapid Symbolic Naming, Rapid Non-Symbolic Naming, and Alternate Phonological Awareness. | 4:0–24:11 years |
| | | A Developmental Neuropsychological Assessment, Second Edition (NEPSY-II) Assesses a variety of domains; subtests can be administered independently to assess specific areas. Relevant subtests for assessing language comprehension include Phonological Processing and Repetition of Nonsense Words, which assess phonemic awareness and phonological encoding and decoding. | 3:0–16:0 years |
| | | Clinical Evaluation of Language Fundamentals, Fifth Edition (CELF-5) Assesses the presence of language and communication disorders. Different subtests compose the Core Language Score dependent on age. Other composite scores include Receptive Language Index, Expressive Language Index, Language Content Index, Language Structure Index (ages 5–8 years only), and Language Memory Index (ages 9–21 years only). | 5:0–21:11 years |
| | Pragmatics | A Developmental Neuropsychological Assessment, Second Edition (NEPSY-II) Assesses a variety of domains; subtests can be administered independently to assess specific areas. Relevant subtests for assessing rapid naming include Speeded Naming, which assesses rapid semantic access to and production of names of colors, shapes, sizes, letters, or numbers. | 3:0–16:0 years |

| | | |
|---|---|---|
| | Autism Diagnostic Observation Schedule, Second Edition (ADOS-2)<br>Assesses symptoms of autism spectrum disorder across age, developmental level, and language skills. It is a semistructured, standardized assessment of communication, social interaction, play, and restricted and repetitive behaviors. | 12 months to adulthood |
| Rapid Naming/ Naming | Rapid Automatized Naming and Rapid Alternating Stimulus Tests (RAN/RAS)<br>Assesses ability to name stimulus items (e.g., letters, colors, and names) as quickly as possible without making mistakes. | 5:0–18:11 years |
| | A Developmental Neuropsychological Assessment, Second Edition (NEPSY-II)<br>Assesses a variety of domains; subtests can be administered independently to assess specific areas. Relevant subtests for assessing rapid naming include Speeded Naming, which assesses rapid semantic access to and production of names of colors, shapes, sizes, letters, or numbers. | 3:0–16:0 years |
| | Boston Naming Test, Second Edition (BNT-2)<br>Assesses visual naming ability using black-and-white drawings of common objects. | 25:0–88:0 years |
| Repetition | Wide Range Assessment of Memory and Learning, Second Edition (WRAML-2)<br>Assesses a variety of memory abilities. The relevant subtest to measure ability to repeat language is Sentence Memory, which assesses an individual's ability to repeat sentences verbatim. | 5:0–90:0 years |
| Fluency | A Developmental Neuropsychological Assessment, Second Edition (NEPSY-II)<br>Assesses a variety of domains; subtests can be administered independently to assess specific areas. Relevant subtests for assessing language comprehension include Word Generation, which assesses verbal productivity through the ability to generate words within specific semantic and initial letter categories. | 3:0–16:0 years |
| | Delis–Kaplan Executive Function System (DKEFS)<br>Assesses a variety of executive functions, including verbal fluency productivity. The relevant subtest is Verbal Fluency, which measures an individual's ability to generate words within specific initial letter and semantic categories. | 8:0–89:0 years |
| Comprehension | A Developmental Neuropsychological Assessment, Second Edition (NEPSY-II)<br>Assesses a variety of domains; subtests can be administered independently to assess specific areas. Relevant subtests for assessing language comprehension include Comprehension of Instruction, which assesses comprehension of oral instructions. | 3:0–16:0 years |

A screening of an individual's articulation can be made based on language samples that are collected as part of a language assessment battery. For example, phonemic awareness might be assessed by evaluating phonemic segmentation testing of phonological memory and assessing visual recognition of phonic patterns. Tests evaluating these areas may be used to distinguish normal readers from reading-disabled children. Core tests are shown in Table 2.3.

### Lexical and Semantic Skills (Primarily Naming and Word Retrieval)

The term *semantics* refers to the study of meaning in language. Semantics involves attaching meaning to phonological forms and prescribes the rules that determine how meaning is conveyed in sentences. Lexical and semantic skills are used in studies to compare various learning-disabled groups with controls. Semantic tests are frequently used with reading-disabled groups. Study results show that reading-disabled subjects perform at a lower level on these tests than do controls. These tests are good predictors of reading disability. Core tests shown in Table 2.3 include the Boston Naming Test, the Rapid Automatized Naming Test (picture naming), and others. The best predictions come from tests that involve visual confrontational naming. Syntax is also assessed. It refers to the arrangement of words and phrases to produce well-formed sentences in a language.

## Receptive Language

The assessment of receptive language skills involves an evaluation of the child's abilities to sustain attention to verbal stimuli; to comprehend conversation, requests, and instructions; to immediately recall verbal information; to interpret a speaker's intent within a social context; and to demonstrate sensitivity to social cues present in the social milieu.

## Pragmatic Language

Although knowledge of the rules of phonology, semantics, and syntax is very important to listeners or speakers of any language, effective language communication also requires knowledge of the pragmatic rules of language. Methods for investigating this aspect of language are not as fully developed as those for phonology, semantics, and syntax. Language-related skills thought to be processed in the right hemisphere may be important in the study of pragmatic language, particularly as it relates to social skills.

The establishment of social language use begins in early life, and some pragmatic skills are acquired during infancy before the child learns to speak. These precursors include establishing eye contact, social smiling, engaging in vocal turn-taking, and the use of anticipatory gestures.

During development, children learn the pragmatic rules that govern linguistic behavior in a social context. These rules include mastery of the following abilities:

- To express a variety of communicative intentions and use appropriate sentence structure. Examples include requesting, persuading, informing, and protesting.

- To understand and produce intentions that are directly expressed, such as "Give me something to eat," or indirectly expressed, such as "I'm hungry."
- To take turns in conversation in a reciprocal manner.
- To keep the conversational interaction going and to recognize when one's turn to speak ends.
- To change and maintain a conversational topic.
- To understand and take into consideration the social context of the conversation. In this instance, the social status of the speaker and listener must be considered, and the individual's familiarity with the listener and language conceptual skills of the conversational partner are part of pragmatic understanding. One uses an understanding of the social context to decide how to express an intention—for example, when to use colloquial language or more formal language.
- To judge the amount and type of information that the communicative partner needs to understand and then communicate to meet the partner's informational needs.
- To recognize times when a communicative breakdown has occurred and how to repair that breakdown.

Pragmatic language disorders are assessed based on these pragmatic rules. The most common examples of pragmatic failures are inappropriate interpretations of indirect communicative expressions of intent. Children with language disorders may fail to communicate intentions effectively if they do not use semantic and grammatical rules appropriately. Such children may resort to simple behavioral patterns or gestures to communicate intentions. Language-disordered children may have difficulty formulating requests and in utilizing the range of linguistic strategies and devices used by normal children. Moreover, they may fail to develop the range of communicative intentions that are expected for their age. Classically, children with autistic disorder fail to display communicative intentions and interests such as commenting on their observations and spontaneously informing others about their experiences.

In addition, the inability to maintain topics and elaborate them over time with multiple conversational turns may be apparent in language-disordered children. Abnormalities in topic maintenance are seen when children exhibit limited knowledge of the topic and show attention deficits, reticence, echolalia, or perseveration. Failure to maintain the topic may also occur because the child is unable to identify the information in the speaker's utterance that pertains to the main topic and so the child may focus on inappropriate and insignificant details of what is being said to them. Such behavior puts the burden on the conversational partner to decide how to modulate or shift the intended topic or redirect the child to the original topic that led to the exchange.

Limited topic maintenance can be characteristic of children who have difficulty with memory. These children may have problems integrating information that is presented to them and establishing its context to what was previously said. When this occurs, the main conversational points may not be understood. Moreover, a language-disordered child may have difficulty inferring the underlying message of an utterance which is presented if that message is not clearly and concretely stated. Difficulty recognizing implicit links that relate one idea to the other may make it difficult to maintain a conversational topic and lead to communication breakdown.

Finally, the ability to recognize and repair communicative breakdown may be impaired in language-disordered children. The repair, then, may be accomplished, if at all, in a simplistic manner—for example, through repetition of the original message. The basic reasons for the breakdown usually include failure to supply background information, unclear articulation, production of words in combination that leads to ambiguous messages, and failure to establish the referent pronoun.

Selected subtests from a standardized test that aims to assess the subject's ability to comprehend and use language beyond the literal level and to make inferences and understand metaphoric expressions should be conducted to provide background for evaluating pragmatic skills.

## Story Narration

Narrating a story and its analysis focus on how well the subject can produce an extended and cohesive sequence of sentences to express a meaningful story. These approaches currently have limited use clinically but may be important in the research assessment of children with developmental disorders. Narrative abilities have been assessed in children with attention-deficit disorder, learning disability, ASD, and genetic syndromes such as Down syndrome and Williams syndrome. For example, boys with ADHD produced stories that supplied less overall information and were poorly organized, less cohesive, and contained more inaccuracies (Tannock et al., 1993). Tannock et al. also found that boys with ADHD may be distinguishable from boys with learning disability. Narrative production before and after stimulant treatment for ADHD is an area of ongoing investigation.

Narrative analysis is a means to assess language in mildly to moderately language-impaired children and can be an important aspect of the assessment. Story generation and story retelling have been used to assess language in older children. Both techniques can be effective ways to measure narrative ability and may activate the cognitive organizations involved with the schema of the story. Story retelling is more clinically useful with older children in assessing their story grammar ability than is story generation (Merritt & Liles, 1989). Retold stories tend to be longer and to contain more story grammar components and more complete episodes. Because of their length, retold stories facilitate more complete assessment of impaired language use, including grammatical usage, syntax, and story cohesion. Standard story retelling/comprehension test measures based on large samples of children are not currently available. However, norms within individual groups for screening purposes are being developed. Story grammar is a specific type of narrative analysis that is characterized by a formal set of rules describing stories as being joined together in predictable ways. These rules identify patterns of temporally and causally related information. Both comprehension and production of story grammar are directed by a cognitive organization referred to as "story schema."

Story understanding requires maintaining a cognitive model that abstracts from perceptual details to describe the location, characters, actions, and causal relationships of the unfolding event. Comprehension requires activation of knowledge schemas about the expectation. In an fMRI study, regions activated included the posterior medial cortex, medial prefrontal cortex (mPFC), and superior frontal gyrus. These areas exhibited schematic event patterns that generalized across stories and subjects. Patterns activated in the mPFC, a region associated with prediction of memory for schematic knowledge, were sensitive to overall script structure (Baldassano et al., 2018).

Although stories may vary in their presentation, a well-formed narrative uses these story grammar components, either directly or inferentially, and they are both temporally and causally linked. A complete episode contains the initiating event or internal response motivating a character to formulate a goal-directed plan, an action or attempt at resolving the situation, and a direct consequence marking attainment or lack of attainment of the goal. The narrative analysis takes into account three specific elements of the story grammar: an overall description of the child's story schema in regard to frequency of the use of the story grammar components; the story hierarchy, which represents the child's use of the story grammar components in regard to their importance in communicating the narrative; and the episode complexity in regard to how the story content develops within complete or incomplete episode structures. Language-disordered children make less effective use of story grammar components and episode units when they produce narratives, and they also show poor comprehension of the causal relations linking the parts of the story.

## Attention and Executive Functioning

### Attention/Inhibition

Wakefulness and attention are essential to all other mental faculties. Neuropsychological evaluation assesses selective attention and the ability to inhibit perceptions that are irrelevant to the task demands. Attention is essential in information processing and involves basic regulatory operations of frontal lobe systems: vigilance, focusing attention, anticipating, maintaining psychological set, and exercising interference control (Noble & Kastner, 2014; Posner, 2012). Difficulty with attention may be neurocognitive or linked to anxiety and personal preoccupations.

Developmentally, problems in attention and concentration are most apparent in young children and in children who are diagnosed with intellectual developmental disorder throughout their life span. Disorders in attention are most commonly associated with sleep deprivation, post-traumatic brain injury, substance abuse, and ADHD. Children and adolescents with intellectual developmental disorder may meet diagnostic criteria for ADHD more often than mental age- or chronologically age-matched peers. The neuropsychological assessment of attention/inhibition is utilized for the assessment of children with ADHD along with the more commonly used parent and teacher behavior rating scales. Attention and executive functioning assessment measures are shown in Table 2.4.

One of the most frequently used measures of inattention and impulsivity is the Continuous Performance Test (CPT), which was originally developed as a measure of vigilance. Many versions of the CPT have been developed, but the basic methodology is the same as the original. Subjects are presented with a variety of stimuli that are displayed on a screen for a short duration, and they are instructed to respond to a

**Table 2.4** Attention and Executive Functioning Assessment Measures

| Domain | Assessment Tool | Age Range |
|---|---|---|
| Attention | Conners Continuous Performance Test, Third Edition (Conners CPT-3)<br>Assesses impulsivity and attention-related concerns across four clusters: Inattentiveness (i.e., Detectability, Omissions, Commissions, Hit Reaction Time, Hit Reaction Time Standard Deviation, and Variability), Impulsivity (i.e., Hit Reaction Time, Commissions, and Perseverations), Sustained Attention (i.e., Hit Reaction Time Block Change, Omissions by Block, and Commissions by Block), and Vigilance (i.e., Hit Reaction Time Inter-Stimulus Interval Change, Omissions by Inter-Stimulus Interval, and Commissions by Inter-Stimulus Interval), in addition to measuring response style. | 8:0+ years |
| | Conners 3rd Edition Parent, Teacher, and Self Report<br>Assesses attention-deficit/hyperactivity disorder (ADHD) and most common comorbid problems in home, social, and school settings across parent/caregiver, teacher, and youth self-reports. Content areas include inattention, hyperactivity/impulsivity, learning problems, executive functioning, defiance/aggression, and peer/family relations. DSM-5 symptom scales measured by these reports include ADHD inattentive presentation, ADHD hyperactive–impulsive presentation, conduct disorder, and oppositional defiant disorder. | 6:0–18:0 years |
| | ADHD Rating Scale–5, Home Version and School Version<br>Assesses inattentive and hyperactive–impulsive symptoms in home (completed by parent/caregiver) and school (completed by teacher) settings. There is a Spanish home version. Purchasers get permission to reproduce the forms and score sheets for repeated use. | 5:0–17:0 years |
| | Test of Everyday Attention for Children, Second Edition (TEA-Ch-2)<br>Assesses aspects of attention. In children ages 5–7 years, assesses selective and sustained attention. In children ages 8–15 years, assesses selective attention, sustained attention, and attentional switching. | 5:0–15:0 years |
| | Test of Variables of Attention, Version 9 (TOVA 9)<br>Assesses attention and inhibitory control through a 22-min-long continuous performance test. A shorter version (11 min) is administered to children ages 4–5:5 years. | 4:0–80:0 years |
| Executive Functioning | A Developmental Neuropsychological Assessment, Second Edition (NEPSY-II)<br>Assesses a variety of domains; subtests can be administered independently to assess specific areas. Relevant subtests for assessing attention and executive functioning include Animal Sorting, Auditory Attention and Response Set, Clocks, Design Fluency, Inhibition, and Statue. These subtests assess inhibition of learned and automatic responses; monitoring and self-regulation; vigilance; selective and sustained attention; the capacity to establish, maintain, and change a response set; nonverbal problem-solving; planning and organizing a complex response; and figural fluency. | 3:0–16:0 years |

**Table 2.4** Continued

| Domain | Assessment Tool | Age Range |
|--------|-----------------|-----------|
| | Wisconsin Card Sort Test (WCST)<br>Assesses ability to form abstract concepts, to shift and maintain set, and to utilize feedback. | 6.5 years through Adulthood |
| | Delis–Kaplan Executive Function System (DKEFS)<br>Assesses a variety of executive functions, including visual scanning, number sequencing, letter sequencing, number–letter switching, motor speed, verbal fluent productivity, nonverbal fluent productivity, inhibition of an overlearned response and flexibility, problem-solving, verbal and nonverbal concept formation, flexibility of thinking, deductive reasoning, planning, and metaphorical thinking. | 8 years through Adulthood |
| | Behavior Rating Inventory of Executive Function, Second Edition (BRIEF-2)<br>Assesses executive function and self-regulation through parent, teacher, and self-report. The behavioral regulation index measures inhibition and self-monitoring. The emotional regulation index measures cognitive shifting and emotional control. The cognitive regulation index measures initiation, task completion, working memory, planning/organization, task monitoring, and organization of materials. | 5:0–18:0 years |

predefined "target stimulus." A number of indices are recorded, including omission errors (failures to detect the target) and commission errors (responses to nontargeted stimuli). In addition, response times for correct detections and for various commission errors and variability may be recorded. Commonly used CPT tests, such as the Conners Continuous Performance Test, Third Edition (Conners CPT-3; Conners, 2014), and the Test of Variables of Attention (TOVA; Greenberg et al., 2017), are described in Table 2.4.

Attentional problems may interfere with the neuropsychological assessment process and make it difficult to determine if an incorrect test response reflects lack of attention or lack of knowledge. Fluctuations in attention occurring over a 45- to 90-min testing session may influence the results; moreover, reduced attention is a common sign of fatigue during testing. When demands are placed that require attention during the testing procedure, motor overflow may become apparent. Denckla (1985) developed a neurological examination to measure such subtle signs in individuals with ADHD. This is the Physical and Neurological Examination for Soft Signs (PANESS), which has been updated to evaluate the effects of gender and age on the examination (Larson et al., 2007).

## Executive Functions

The term *executive function* applies to capacities that include attending in a selective and focused manner, inhibition of off-task responding, self-monitoring, flexible concept formation, planning, judgment, and decision-making. They are linked to the frontal lobe but involve other brain regions connected to the frontal lobe (e.g., the basal ganglia).

Executive functioning refers to the individual's ability to conceptualize long-term goals, develop possible alternatives for goal attainment, choose among the alternatives in a logical manner, organize the specific steps necessary for goal attainment, and evaluate the extent to which these steps are efficient in reaching the goal. Executive function refers to the self-regulatory process whereby the individual is constantly attending, evaluating the extent to which their thoughts or actions are fitting the demands of the situation, as well as the ability to shift and self-correct when confronted with negative feedback from the situation. It is dependent not only on the individual's ability to conceptualize, organize, attend, apply rules, and reason inductively and deductively but also on the individual's capacity for selective attention and inhibition of task-irrelevant perceptions and thoughts. Development of executive functioning follows a series of developmental stages progressing from inhibition (earliest) to working memory, organizing things and spaces, planning sequences (timelines), generating strategies, and self-monitoring (Denckla, 2019).

To evaluate executive dysfunction in children, the developmental neuropsychiatric interview of the child is tailored to gather data from parents on particular behaviors that require executive function, and the child is tested directly on tests shown in Table 2.4. Because executive dysfunction interferes with adaptive behavior both at home and at school, the parent interview should cover both settings, and teacher interviews are necessary to cover school matters. Children with executive dysfunction have difficulty regulating their behavior as it pertains to their schoolwork and their interpersonal activities. To identify these adaptive problems, the clinical history clarifies the frequency and severity of target symptoms of executive dysfunction in each setting: home, school, and community. In addition, the presence of associated neurological and psychological findings that are related to executive function is assessed. The presence of executive dysfunction symptoms, how these symptoms manifest in everyday life, their developmental history in regard to time of initial symptom onset, and the presence of associated difficulties are evaluated.

## Neuropsychological Testing of Executive Function

The assessment of executive function is carried out in parallel with all of the psychoeducational and neuropsychological tests that are administered for the various cognitive content areas. Executive function status affects and impinges on content-based assessment. Executive function cannot be evaluated without the cognitive challenge of the test contents, which affect executive function processes. In assessing executive function, the examiner must focus on the processes the child follows in responding to the items presented. Because of the structured nature of the routine assessment procedure, the deficiency (an absence of expected behavior) that one seeks to demonstrate in executive function may be compensated for as the examiner, in a one-on-one situation, works to maintain the child's focused attention and helps the child organize the time for completing the test. Consequently, the "command and control" module of the neuropsychological repertoire of executive function is difficult to assess in structured one-on-one situations.

Only in more severe cases are obvious off-task behavior, inattentiveness, and disinhibition clearly enough seen in a one-on-one testing setting to diagnose executive dysfunction. Therefore, a period of unstructured observation around testing is essential when evaluating executive dysfunction. The examiner observes how the child approaches the content of the test information and makes clinical observations of older children. Qualitative data (e.g., the types of errors produced) are helpful to differentiate context-related processing problems from executive function problems. One may compare the level of performance on tasks that address similar content but place different demands for executive functional abilities.

Tasks that make demands on executive function processes are those that challenge the ability to tolerate boredom, to operate independently, and to generate active plans to solve problems. These tasks focus on the subprocesses of executive function, such as task initiation (focused attention and organized problem-solving), sustained effort, inhibition of off-task or unsuccessful behaviors, flexible shifts of attention, or the consideration of alternative strategies. Consequently, the examiner observes the child's ability to initiate the task, sustain attention to it, inhibit impulses that may interfere with task completion, and shift attention to the next task.

## Visual–Spatial and Visual–Motor Assessment

Visual–spatial and visual–motor defects may be present in children with a neurodevelopmental disorder. Visual–spatial and visual–motor assessment measures are shown in Table 2.5.

### Visuospatial Assessment

Visuospatial tests evaluate right hemispheric function, especially the right occipitoparietal and occipitotemporal regions. There are separate visual, perceptual, and memory systems in the brain for places and things. Moreover, visual item perception should not be confused with visuospatial processing. Visual item perception refers to visual recognition of a stimulus, whereas visuospatial processing addresses the relative position, the configuration, and the spatial orientation of visually presented items. These tests are sensitive to a variety of perceptual abilities. Typically, tests of visual/spatial functioning require no physical manipulation of test material or verbal labeling of responses. Although they do demand a significant contribution from the right hemisphere, they cannot strictly be dichotomized as free from left hemisphere involvement.

The examiner may have difficulty interpreting the results if verbal mediation has influenced performance on these "perceptual tests." However, by using a multiple-choice format and choosing configurational stimulus material that has been reported to be most specifically sensitive to right hemisphere damage, the examiner addresses this issue by shifting the balance toward nonverbal and motor-free visual processing.

**Table 2.5**  Visual–Spatial and Visual–Motor Assessment Measures

| Domain | Assessment Tool | Age Range |
| --- | --- | --- |
| Visual–Spatial | Beery–Buktenica Test of Visual–Motor Integration, Sixth Edition (VMI-6)<br>Assesses ability to integrate visual and motor abilities by having an individual copy increasingly complex geometric form. | 2:0 through Adulthood |
| | Hooper Visual Organization Test (VOT)<br>Assesses visual–spatial abilities by having individuals identify objects represented in line drawings as puzzle pieces. | 5+ years |
| | Judgment of Line Orientation (JLO)<br>Assesses spatial perception and orientation by having individuals identify lines of matching directions. | 7:0–through Adulthood |
| | Rey Complex Figure Test and Recognition Trial<br>Assesses visual–spatial constructional ability and visual memory by having an individual copy a complex shape and recall the shape from memory after a short and long delay. | 6:0–through Adulthood |
| Visual–Motor | Grooved Pegboard<br>Assesses eye–hand coordination, motor speed, and unilateral fine-motor dexterity. | 5:0–through Adulthood |
| | Purdue Pegboard<br>Assesses eye–hand coordination, motor speed, unilateral fine-motor dexterity, and bilateral fine-motor dexterity. | 5:0–through Adulthood |
| | Beery–Buktenica Test of Visual–Motor Integration, Sixth Edition (VMI-6)<br>Assesses motor abilities by having an individual copy increasingly complex geometric form. | 2:0 through Adulthood |
| | A Developmental Neuropsychological Assessment, Second Edition (NEPSY-II)<br>Assesses a variety of domains; subtests can be administered independently to assess specific areas. Relevant subtests for assessing motor abilities include Finger Tapping, Imitating Hand Positions, Manual Motor Sequences, and Visuomotor Precision. These subtests assess the ability to imitate hand positions, to produce repetitive and sequential finger movements and rhythmic sequential hand movements, and to use a pencil with speed and precision. | 3:0–16:0 years |
| | Physical and Neurological Examination for Soft Signs (PANESS)<br>Assesses basic motor function in children to reveal subtle motor deficits. These neurological subtle signs include overflow (also called "associated" or "extraneous") movements, involuntary movements (i.e., limb tremor, odd posturing, and choreiform), and dysrhythmia. These subtle signs can serve as markers for inefficiency in neighboring parallel brain systems important for control of cognition and behavior. | |

## Visual–Motor Functioning

Visual–motor functioning is closely related to visual item perception and visuospatial processing, but it adds a manipulation or graphomotor component to the perceptual function tasks. The Block Design and Object Assembly subtests from the WISC-5 require visual–motor ability. Visual–motor functioning is a necessary but not a suffi-cient condition for successful performance of these subtests. Visuographomotor ability requires visual processing, motor control, and possibly the mediation of selective at-tention and sequential organizing capacities. Some of the more advanced copy tasks involve preplanning; earlier simple designs may be highly overlearned.

## Memory

No standardized instrument to test orientation is available for children and adolescents. The clinical interview provides the best guide to the child or adolescent's orientation. The assessment of memory is an essential part of the clinical and neuro-psychological assessments. Memory functions (see Chapter 6) are typically assessed using measures listed in Table 2.6. These include the California Verbal Learning Test–Children's Version (CVLT-C; Delis et al., 2000); the Wide Range Assessment of Memory and Learning, Second Edition (WRAML2; Sheslow & Adams, 2003); the Rey Complex Figure Test and Recognition Trial (Meyers & Meyers, 1995); and A Developmental Neuropsychological Assessment, Second Edition (NEPSY-II; Korkman et al., 2007).

Memory disturbance may involve deficits in registration and retrieval. Considerable advances have been made in understanding memory and metamemory skills in

**Table 2.6** Memory Assessment Measures

| Assessment Tool | Age Range |
| --- | --- |
| California Verbal Learning Test–Children's Version (CVLT-C)[a]<br>Assesses verbal learning and memory using a multiple-trial list-learning process. It measures how verbal learning occurs or fails to occur over immediate recall, short-delay recall, long-delay recall, and recognition tasks. | 5:0–16:11 years |
| Wide Range Assessment of Memory and Learning, Second Edition (WRAML-2)<br>Assesses verbal memory (i.e., story memory and verbal learning) and visual memory (i.e., design memory and picture memory) with immediate recall, delay recall, and recognition subtests. | 5:0–through Adulthood |
| A Developmental Neuropsychological Assessment, Second Edition (NEPSY-II)<br>Assesses a variety of domains; subtests can be administered independently to assess specific areas. Relevant subtests for assessing memory and learning include List Memory, Memory for Designs, Memory for Faces, Memory for Names, Narrative Memory, Sentence Repetition, and Word Life Interference. These subtests assess immediate memory for sentences; narrative memory under free recall, cued recall, and recognition conditions; repetition and recall of words presented with interference; and immediate and delayed memory for abstract designs, faces, names, and lists. | 3:0–16:0 years |
| Rey Complex Figure Test and Recognition Trial<br>Assesses visual–spatial constructional ability and visual memory by having an individual copy a complex shape and recall the shape from memory after a short and long delay. | 6:0 through Adulthood |

[a]California Verbal Learning Test, Second Edition (CCVT-II) is used for individuals ages 16–89 years.

children. The examination of memory should include immediate and short-term retention, the pattern and rate of acquisition of new information, the efficacy of retrieval of remote and recently learned information, and the ability to make inferences based on memory. Each of the components should be assessed in both verbal and nonverbal modalities, using both recall and recognition techniques. Verbal and nonverbal memory can be assessed in any modality. Verbal memory is most conveniently studied utilizing tests that use auditory input and require verbal output. Verbal memory tests ordinarily present the child with a list of words or a paragraph and ask for verbal recall at a later time. These tests include measures of long-term recall and recognition and also demonstrate learning ability.

The most commonly used tests for recent memory involve selective reminding. Measures of selective reminding are available in both verbal and nonverbal areas. These techniques allow simultaneous analysis of a child's storage, retention, and retrieval abilities. Poor performance may relate to processing problems in the modality involved (e.g., language) and may not be caused by memory difficulty.

## Visual Memory

Among the nonverbal memory tasks, several instruments are available for use in school-aged children. In these tests, children are shown geometric figures and then asked to reproduce them from memory. Two commonly used tests are the Benton Visual Retention Test and the Rey–Osterrieth Complex Figure (Meyers & Meyers, 1995). For example, the complex figure test has been used to compare children with an ASD diagnosis with matched mental age and chronological age control groups. Meyers and Meyers found that the group with a diagnosis of ASD had no particular problems in copying the figure; however, they performed significantly worse in producing the figure from memory, which suggested they had difficulty storing information in a coherent way.

Severe amnesia in children is rare, although it may occur with acute encephalitis and head trauma. Problems with new learning following encephalitis and traumatic brain injury more commonly present as intellectual developmental disorder rather than as a focal deficit, although they may present as a specific learning disability.

## Academic Achievement

Evaluation of academic achievement is an essential part of the neuropsychological testing battery. Assessment is carried out for evaluation of each of the DSM-5 designated learning disorders. These include reading, written expression, and mathematics. For reading, there are specifiers for impairment in word reading accuracy, reading rate or fluency, and reading comprehension. For written expression, there are specifiers for spelling accuracy, grammar and punctuation accuracy, clarity, and organization of written expression. For mathematics, there are specifiers for number sense, memorization of arithmetic facts, accurate or fluent calculation, and accurate math reasoning. Severity is categorized as mild, moderate, or severe. Academic achievement assessment measures are shown in Table 2.7.

**Table 2.7**  Academic Achievement Assessment Measures

| Assessment Tool | Age Range |
| --- | --- |
| Kaufman Test of Educational Achievement–Third Edition (KTEA-3)<br>Assesses academic achievement in reading, mathematics, written language, and oral language across 19 subtests: Letter and Word Recognition, Nonsense Word Decoding, Reading Comprehension, Reading Vocabulary, Word Recognition Fluency, Decoding Fluency, Silent Reading Fluency, Math Concepts and Applications, Math Computation, Math Fluency, Written Expression, Spelling, Writing Fluency, Listening Comprehension, Oral Expression, Associational Fluency, Phonological Processing, Object Naming Facility, and Letter Naming Facility. There are 10 supplemental composite scores: Sound–Symbol, Decoding, Reading Fluency, Reading Understanding, Oral Language, Oral Fluency, Comprehension, Expression, Orthographic Processing, and Academic Fluency. | 4:0–25:11 years |
| Woodcock–Johnson, Fourth Edition (WJ-IV)<br>Assesses intellectual abilities, academic achievement, and oral language abilities. The Test of Achievement measures Letter Word Identification, Applied Problems, Spelling, Passage Comprehension, Calculation, Writing Samples, Word Attack, Oral Reading, Sentence Reading Fluency, Math Facts Fluency, and Sentence Writing Fluency. The Test of Cognitive Abilities measures Oral Vocabulary, Number Series, Verbal Attention, Letter-Pattern Matching, Phonological Processing, Story Recall, Visualization, General Information, Concept Formation, and Numbers Reversed. The Test of Oral Language measures Picture Vocabulary, Oral Comprehension, Segmentation, Rapid Picture Naming, Sentence Repetition, Understanding Directions, Sound Blending, Retrieval Fluency, and Sound Awareness. | Pre-kindergarten to 12th grade |
| Wechsler Individual Achievement Test, Third Edition (WIAT-III)<br>Assesses academic achievement across oral language (i.e., listening comprehension and oral expression), reading (i.e., early reading skills, word reading, pseudoword decoding, reading comprehension, and oral reading fluency), written expression (i.e., alphabet writing fluency, spelling, sentence composition, and essay composition), and mathematics (i.e., math problem-solving, numerical operations, and math fluency). | 4:0–50:11 years |
| Wide Range Achievement Test, Fifth Edition (WRAT5)<br>Assesses fundamental reading (i.e., word reading and reading comprehension), spelling, and mathematics skills in efficient completion times. | 5:0–85+ years |
| Bracken Basic Concept Scale: Expressive (BBCS:E) and Receptive (BBCS-3:R)<br>Assesses school readiness by evaluating understanding of Colors, Letters, Numbers/Counting, Sizes/Comparisons, and Shapes. | 3:0–6:11 years |
| Nelson–Denny Reading Test<br>Assesses reading abilities (i.e., Vocabulary and Comprehension) in high school and college students. | 14:0–65:0 years |
| Gray Oral Reading Test, Fifth Edition (GORT-5)<br>Assesses reading abilities by measuring Fluency (i.e., Rate, Accuracy, and Total) and Comprehension. | 6:0–23:0 years |
| Test of Written Language, Fourth Edition (TOWL-4)<br>Assesses writing abilities by measuring Vocabulary, Spelling, Punctuation, Logical Sentences, Sentence Combining, Contextual Conventions, Story Composition, Overall Writing, Contrived Writing, and Spontaneous Writing. | 9:0–17:11 years |

The Kaufman Test of Educational Achievement–Third Edition (KTEA-3; Kaufman, 2014) and the Woodcock–Johnson IV Tests of Early Cognitive and Academic Development (Schrank et al., 2015) are most commonly used to evaluate academic achievement. The Test of Written Language (TOWL; Hammill & Larsen, 2009) is used to evaluate the disorder of written expression. Among the learning disorders, written expression is often not fully appreciated by educators. When identified, it is important that the individual education program allows oral test-taking.

## Personality

The assessment of personality is an important accompaniment of neuropsychological assessment. The temperamental response style, sociability, affective status, activity level, and motivation to cooperate are not only important in the interpretation of test results but also may provide cues regarding the presence of a developmental neuropsychiatric disorder. Although the assessment of personality and temperament is of particular importance, there are a few generally accepted instruments available for children (Table 2.8). One inventory available is the Personality Inventory for Children.

Clinical inventories are available for pre-adolescents (Millon et al., 2005) and for adolescents (Millon et al., 1993). The Thematic Apperception Test is a classic test (Morgan & Murry, 1935), along with the Roberts Apperception Test (McArthur & Roberts, 2005). The Personality Inventory for Children (Lachar & Gruber, 1977) and the Minnesota Multiphasic Personality Inventory (MMPI; Ben-Porath & Tellegen, 2008 ; Butcher et al., 2001) are also available.

## Emotional and Behavior Ratings

Emotional and behavioral scales are shown in Table 2.9.

## Mood Ratings

Mood and affect may be clinically observed during the interview or may be specifically assessed using visual analog scales, which show little verbal mediation, and through self-reports, such as the Children's Depression Inventory (CDI; Kovacs, 2011) for children aged 8 years or older who can read. The Children's Depression Rating Scale–Revised, a clinician-rated instrument designed to measure the presence and severity of depression in children aged 6–12 years, may also be used. In the assessment of affect, apathy must be distinguished from depression. Moreover, the experience of emotion must be clarified because in some conditions, such as certain right hemispheric dysfunction presentations or in pseudobulbar palsy, the physical expression of affect (e.g., facial expression and voice tone) may be impaired, although inner experience may remain intact. Finally, with some frontal lobe lesions and in

**Table 2.8** Personality Assessment Measures

| Assessment Tool | Age Range |
|---|---|
| Millon Pre-Adolescent Clinical Inventory (MPACI)<br>Assesses personality characteristics through a self-report. Identifies emerging personality patterns (e.g., confident, outgoing, conforming, submissive, inhibited, unruly, and unstable), current clinical signs (e.g., anxiety/fears, attention deficits, obsessions/compulsions, conduct problems, disruptive behaviors, depressive moods, and reality distortions), and response validity. | 9:0–12:0 years |
| Millon Adolescent Clinical Inventory (MACI)[a]<br>Assesses personality characteristics to help identify early signs of Axis I and Axis II disorders in adolescents. Identifies personality patterns (e.g., introversive, inhibited, doleful, submissive, dramatizing, egotistic, unruly, forceful, conforming, oppositional, self-demeaning, and borderline tendency), expressed concerns (e.g., identify diffusion, self-devaluation, body disapproval, sexual discomfort, peer insecurity, social insensitivity, family disorder, and childhood abuse), and clinical syndromes (e.g., eating dysfunctions, substance abuse proneness, delinquent predisposition, impulsive propensity, anxious feelings, depressive affect, and suicidal tendency). | 13:0–19:0 years |
| Thematic Apperception Test (TAT)<br>Assesses an individual's perception of interpersonal relationships by creating stories based on pictures of relationships and social situations. This assessment can help identify dominant drives, emotions, conflicts, and complexities of personalities. | 5:0–79:0 years |
| Children's Apperception Test (CAT)<br>Assesses personality or aspects of emotional disturbance. Similar to the TAT but the pictures involve animals in social context in which the child identifies conflicts, identities, roles, family structures, and interpersonal interactions. | 3:0–10:0 years |
| Personality Inventory for Children, Second Edition (PIC-2)<br>Assesses a child's emotional, behavioral, social, and cognitive adjustment across different domains (e.g., cognitive impairment, impulsivity and distractibility, delinquency, family dysfunction, reality distortion, somatic concern, psychological discomfort, social withdrawal, and social skill deficits). | 5:0–19:0 years |

[a]The Minnesota Multiphasic Personality Inventory, Second Edition (MMPI-2) is used to assess personality characteristics of individuals ages 18+ years.

some metabolic encephalopathies, severe apathy may be noted in the absence of depression.

## Anxiety Ratings

Rating scales for anxiety—the Screen for Child Anxiety Related Disorders (SCARED; Birmaher et al., 1999) and the Revised Children's Manifest Anxiety Scale—are commonly used. SCARED assesses anxiety across four domains: panic/somatic, separation anxiety, generalized anxiety, and school phobia.

**Table 2.9** Emotional and Behavior Ratings Scales Measures

| Assessment Tool | Age Range |
| --- | --- |
| Children's Depression Inventory Second Edition (CDI-2)<br>Assesses cognitive, affective, and behavioral signs of depression through self-report. Identifies emotional problems and functional problems across subscales (e.g., negative mood/physical symptoms, negative self-esteem, interpersonal problems, and ineffectiveness). | 7:0–17:0 years |
| Screen for Child Anxiety Related Disorders (SCARED)<br>Assesses anxiety across four domains (e.g., panic/somatic, separation anxiety, generalized anxiety, and school phobia) across parent/caregiver and self-report. | 8:0–18 years |
| Beck Youth Inventories–Second Edition (BYI-II)<br>Assesses emotional and social functioning across five inventories: depression inventory, anxiety inventory, anger inventory, disruptive behavior inventory, and self-concept inventory. | 7:0–18:0 years |
| Revised Children's Manifest Anxiety Scale, Second Edition (RCMAS-2)<br>Assesses anxiety by measuring physiological anxiety, worry, social anxiety, defensiveness, and inconsistent responding. | 6:0–19:0 years |
| Behavior Assessment System for Children, Third Edition (BASC-3)<br>Assesses emotions and behavior of children across multiple methods. Teacher report measures Externalizing Problems (i.e., Hyperactivity, Aggression, and Conduct Problems), Internalizing Problems (i.e., Anxiety, Depression, and Somatization), School Problems (i.e., Attention Problems and Learning Problems), Behavioral Symptoms Index (i.e., Atypicality and Withdrawal), and Adaptive Skills (i.e., Adaptability, Social Skills, Leadership, Study Skills, and Functional Communication). Parent report measures Externalizing Problems (i.e., Hyperactivity, Aggression, and Conduct Problems), Internalizing Problems (i.e., Anxiety, Depression, and Somatization), Behavioral Symptoms Index (i.e., Attention Problems, Atypicality, and Withdrawal), and Adaptive Skills (i.e., Adaptability, Social Skills, Leadership, Activities of Daily Living, and Functional Communication). Self-report measures School Problems (i.e., Attitude to School, Attitude to Teachers, and Sensation Seeking), Internalizing Problems (i.e., Atypicality, Locus of Control, Social Stress, Anxiety, Depression, Sense of Inadequacy, and Somatization), Inattention/Hyperactivity (i.e., Attention Problems and Hyperactivity), and Personal Adjustment (i.e., Relations with Parents, Interpersonal Relations, Self-Esteem, and Self-Reliance). | Parent and teacher report: 2:0–21:11 years; self-report: 6:0–25:0 years |
| Child Behavior Checklist (CBCL), Teacher Report Form (TRF), and Youth Self Report (YSR)<br>Assess emotional and behavioral functioning through parent/caregiver, teacher, and self-reports. Symptoms scales include anxious/depressed, withdrawn/depressed, somatic complaints, social problems, thought problems, attention problems, rule-breaking behavior, and aggressive behavior. DSM-5-oriented scales include depressive problems, anxiety problems, somatic problems, attention-deficit/hyperactivity problems, oppositional defiant problems, and conduct problems. | CBCL and TRF, ages 1:6–5:0 years; CBCL, TRF, and YSR, ages 6:0–18:0 years |

**Table 2.9** Continued

| Assessment Tool | Age Range |
| --- | --- |
| Social Responsiveness Scale, Second Edition (SRS-2)<br>Assesses presence and severity of social impairment within the autism spectrum through parent/caregiver and teacher reports. Subscales include social awareness, social cognition, social communication, social motivation, and restricted interests/repetitive behavior. | 2:6 years to adult |
| Childhood Autism Rating Scale, Second Edition (CARS-2)<br>Assesses symptoms of autism spectrum disorder to determine symptom severity through quantifiable ratings based on direct observation. Areas assessed include relating to people, imitation, social–emotional understanding, emotional response, emotional expression and regulation of emotions, body use, object use, adaption to change, visual response, listening response, taste/smell/touch response and use, fear or nervousness, verbal communication, nonverbal communication, activity level, thinking/cognitive integration skills, level and consistency of intellectual response, and general impressions. | 2:0 years to adult |

## Social–Emotional Function Testing

Tests of social–emotional functioning are particularly important to evaluate social (pragmatic) communication disorder. Social communication is difficult to evaluate clinically because both the capacity to recognize affect and the interpretation of the context in which the affect occurs and the capacity to modulate as well as recognize affective expression are clinically important. An alternative approach in younger children and those who are severely cognitively impaired is the use of the Strange Situation Paradigm to evaluate attachment status. Moreover, studies of affect sharing in the context of joint attentional interactions in autistic and persons with intellectual developmental disorder are important. It should be borne in mind that the measurement of neuropsychological competencies is essential to joint attention. In any assessment, the clinical history will provide anecdotes that testify to social obtuseness.

## Behavioral Assessment

Rating scales for behavior include the Behavioral Assessment System for Children, the Achenbach Child Behavior Checklist (parent and teacher rating, and youth self-report), and Conner's Parent Rating Scale and and Teacher Rating Scale for children with a diagnosis of ADHD. For social deficits and ASD, the Social Responsiveness Scale, the Autism Diagnostic Interview (ADI), and the Autism Diagnostic Observation Schedule (ADOS) are standard assessment tools. The Social Responsiveness subscales include Social Awareness, Social Cognition, Social Communication, Social Motivation, and Restricted Interests/Repetitive Behavior. The ADI and ADOS are the standard evaluation measures for ASD.

## Evaluation of Test Results

### Interpretation of Test Results

The last stage in neuropsychological evaluation is the interpretation of results and establishment of the underlying neuropsychological profile based on the individual having used skills to complete the test successfully. This is an essential analysis from a neuropsychological perspective because it qualitatively assesses how an individual carries out a task and determines whether errors that emerge suggest a particular disorder. For example, errors on a memory test could be related to attentional drift, impulsivity, or poor planning. Several tests may contribute to the construct being assessed. For example, if the construct vocabulary is being evaluated, how should the interpretation about vocabulary differ when comparing the capacity to name a picture, tell about a word, or point to a word picture equivalent (Denckla, 1989). Analysis of results at these stages may be used to demonstrate whether or not a subject can perform the task and to detect patterns of response that might indicate psychological dysfunction. Findings may be used for hypotheses regarding an imbalance between brain systems that may be contributing to specific brain dysfunction. A case illustration demonstrating a neuropsychological test profile of an 8-year-old with a neurodevelopmental disorder is provided at the end of the chapter to illustrate the interpretation of results in neuropsychological testing.

## Conclusion

Differences in overall ability may be better understood by using neuropsychological testing techniques than standardized IQ tests. Some abilities are more stable in their functional organization than others. Following injury, the behavioral deficits seen in children may be similar to those that occur in adults who are injured in similar brain regions, and their recovery from injury will be incomplete. Yet, lesions involving some brain areas in children do not cause permanent deficits. These differences, according to the site and kind of lesion occurring in children, point to limitations in the functional capacity of the brain and provide evidence for reorganization of some regions, leading to limited recovery linked to some areas and better recovery when lesions occur in other areas. Neuropsychological testing assumes particular importance in developmental disorders in which deviations may occur in the development of the brain and the integration of cognitive domains.

Longitudinal studies of the neuropsychological development of both normal and developmentally disordered children may potentially help in the understanding of the consequences of the early experiences that shape the development of later child, adolescent, and adult abilities and talents. The early detection of differences among children may lead to better understanding of the roots of adult personality traits and adult psychopathologies, such as antisocial behavior, substance abuse, depressive disorder, and other illnesses. Moreover, differences in the potential to recover from acquired head injury in children and adults of different ages lead to better understanding of neural plasticity in the recovery process as the brain reorganizes following injury.

## Cognitive Neuropsychology and Cognitive Neuropsychiatry

In this chapter, the focus on cognitive neuropsychology complements psychiatric research in epidemiology and neuroscience. The neuropsychological assessment in the developmental disorders focuses on domains of brain functions and learning disorders and, following brain injury, addresses specific deficits that are gross and may be fixed. In contrast, the major mental disorders assessed in psychiatry use a different approach involving the use of observation, interaction, interview, and the use of rating scales and questionnaires, including those listed in Table 2.9. The neuropsychological approach tends to emphasize the underlying deficit or the discrepancy between an unusual ability and other deficiencies. However, major mental illnesses ordinarily present cognitively as aberrant behaviors or excessive activities, possibly as the consequence of the loss of inhibition. For example, hallucinations are not failures to perceive sensory input but, rather, represent the perception or internal generation of images that are reported in the absence of external stimulation.

The neuropsychologist ordinarily evaluates deficits but in some instances may investigate hyperfunctions (e.g., hyperlexia). Hyperfunctions have been studied in the description of hyperpallia (Yamadori et al., 1990) and in the evaluation of exceptional artistic ability in children with ASD, where highly developed access to brain modules, such as that for visual memory, has been postulated (O'Connor & Hermelin, 1987). There are also studies addressing a "hyper-connection" model of behavioral disturbance in association with temporal lobe epilepsy. Bear (1979) suggests that certain beliefs may attract strong affects due to the extent of increased linkage between cortical and limbic brain areas. He refers to this as a syndrome of sensory–limbic hyper-connection.

In the past quarter century, cognitive neuropsychiatry has emerged out of cognitive psychology and neuropsychiatry. It seeks to understand mental disorders in models linked to normal psychological functions. Moving beyond descriptive diagnoses, its aim is to find testable cognitive explanations for established psychiatric symptoms (Halligan & David, 2001). Cognitive neuropsychology and cognitive neuropsychiatry differ in that the psychiatrist tends to focus on mental disorders (syndromes) that are not psychological constructs, whereas the neuropsychologist focuses on specific impairments, such as phonological abnormalities in reading disability and impairments in semantic memory. The neuropsychologist addresses solitary disturbances of function that may emerge from a variety of pathological disorders and assume a final, common path. Neuropsychology may demonstrate a deficit but not explain the phenomenology of the disorder, such as seen in psychosis that represents anomalous functioning. A classic example from cognitive neuropsychiatry is the Capgras delusion (delusional misidentification syndrome), which is explained as an interruption in the indirect route to face recognition—that is, affective responses to familiar stimuli—localized in the dorsal route of vision from striate cortex to limbic system (Halligan & David, 2001).

For developmental neuropsychiatrists, the use of developmental testing is broader than that by general psychiatrists because the types of disorder differ. The developmental neuropsychiatrist works closely to incorporate findings from neuropsychology in their final formulation. The developmental neuropsychiatric focus on studying pathways from genes to cognition and complex behavior is akin to the cognitive neuropsychiatry model.

## Case Illustration: Neuropsychological Testing

The following case illustrates how neuropsychological tests can be used to identify developmental cognitive problems in a school-aged child. Test findings may be utilized in establishing an intervention program. In this case, the neurodevelopmental examination was carried out, and visual memory, spatial orientation, visual perception, language function and word fluency, selective attention, and executive functions were assessed.

### Statement of Concern

Consultation was requested by the patient's parents because of poor frustration tolerance, impulsivity, and boredom.

### Present Illness

This is an 8-year-old boy who, at age 4, was noted to be inattentive, demanding, and impulsive. As he has grown older, these problems have persisted. The patient has problems following routines that include dressing in the morning and completing chores. In school, he has difficulty concentrating, completing tasks, remembering what to do and when, remaining seated, and, in addition, has problems in handwriting. Although the oldest of three children, he is the most demanding of his mother's time and requires continuous redirection. In a group setting, he shows poor attention to task and is not "tuned in" to games. He is currently described as a perfectionist who becomes frustrated with his own imperfections.

### Past History

The patient is the product of a full-term pregnancy. His presentation was breach and required cesarean section. Birth weight was 8 lbs. The Apgar score at 5 minutes was 9. There was some difficulty in nursing, and poor coordination was noted in the early years of life, but no particular concerns were raised until age 4. In the preschool years, he had difficulty in coordination when riding a tricycle and problems with cutting, pasting, and color recognition milestones in kindergarten. He was also noted to have delays in articulation and to drool.

Contacts with peers have been limited, and only at age 8 did he begin to make friends. He is said to be a poor role model for his younger siblings because he becomes overly activated when stressed and is noncompliant with demands.

### Family History

The patient's mother indicates that she was easily distracted and overly talkative in school. She continues to have difficulty with organizational skills and reports problems in concentration. Because of her school-related problems, she did not go further than high school. The maternal grandfather has the diagnoses of Tourette's disorder, obsessive–compulsive disorder, and bipolar disorder. There is no history of learning or psychiatric problems on the paternal side of the family. Both parents were enuretic until elementary school.

## Interview with the Child

When interviewed, this 8-year-old acknowledged trouble concentrating, restlessness, and poor self-control. He indicated he has difficulty managing angry feelings and is periodically anxious and sad about his parents' criticism of his behavior. He does not report any abnormal mental experiences.

## Neurodevelopmental Examination

On the neurodevelopmental examination, be shows choreiform hand movements, slow finger sequencing, tremor, and developmental overflow on heel, toe, and tandem gait tasks. Drooling is noted when he is asked to move his tongue from side to side.

## Clinical Correlation

The choreiform movements and slow finger sequencing may correlate to the motor skill aspects of handwriting. His problems in motoric movement may be correlated with poor control over mental processes.

## Neuropsychological Testing

### Visual Memory

Visual memory was tested using the Benton Visual Retention Test. Scoring was at the 11th percentile, which is average for a child between 6½ and 7. Performance was poor but may potentially have been contaminated by the attentional demands needed for this visual memory task.

### Judgment of Spatial Orientation

The patient became fatigued on the Test of Spatial Orientation but was able to score in the low-average range within 1 standard deviation of the norms for age 8.

### Visual Perception

On the Facial Recognition Test, he scored in the average range for his age.

### Visuomotor Integration

On the Visual–Motor Test, he showed poor line quality, which may be linked to motor difficulties with sequencing and his tremor. Graphomotor problems were suggested by these findings. His best score was at the 7-year, 11-month level.

### Visual Memory and Planning

The Rey–Osterrieth Complex Figure was used. In copying the figure, his organizational ability was less than the 5-year level. Immediate recall was below the 6-year level, and delayed recall was average for a 6-year-old. However, his organization for delayed recall was at age level, although the copy that was made was disorganized. His difficulty in organization was attributed to problems in attention and difficulty in planning. The details of the complex figure were apparently lost due to inattention.

74

## Language

Language tests included the Clinical Evaluation of Language Fundamentals (CELF), syntax comprehension, naming pictured items, rapid automatized naming, and word fluency (animals/foods). Listening was poor, but his overall language was a strength. Sentence syntax comprehension was at the 8-year level, which was age appropriate. His best language skills were demonstrated on the Boston Naming Test, where he scored at the 12th-grade level. Word fluency was particularly good, with scoring at the 15-year level. Verbal learning was excellent, although problems in comprehension related to listening were a handicap. Scores on receptive language were discrepantly poor but were most probably linked to poor listening skills.

## Selective Attention

On the test of cancellation of targeted items, his visual search was poor. He approached the task in a disorganized and random way but was able to be successful within normal limits on two out of three challenges. When numbers were used, however, he vocalized the number he was searching for and had to be asked to stop the test after 6 minutes, yet he still made three errors. On the Test of Variables of Attention (TOVA), he was slow but was able to perform at age level on the commission and omission sections; however, his variability score was in the clinical range.

## Conclusion

The history, neurodevelopmental examination, and neuropsychological testing are consistent with a verbally gifted 8-year-old with attention deficit hyperactivity disorder who has difficulty listening and visually attending. The testing is consistent with severe organizational problems in the visual domain. Moreover, he has graphomotor problems that require compensation. The use of a computer for any extended writing that involves more than simple one-word or one-number responses is recommended.

The testing demonstrates executive function difficulties in regard to selective attention, organization, and planning. His disorganization in following through on requests and completing tasks requires a structured behavioral program at home so he can didactically be taught the organization skills he lacks. In addition to behavior management, pharmacotherapy with stimulant medication is recommended. The recommended dose is 0.3 mg/kg. After he is stabilized on this dose of medication, the TOVA should be repeated to see if his variability score is normalized. An additional test that may be performed to assess his narrative ability is the story retelling task, which should also be completed on and off medication.

## Acknowledgments

This chapter was written in consultation with Martha B. Denckla, MD, Professor of Neurology and Pediatrics Emeritus, Johns Hopkins University School of Medicine, and Director of Developmental Cognitive Neurology Emeritus, Kennedy–Krieger Institute, Baltimore, MD. Rachel Landsman, PhD, consulted on current neuropsychology tests and provided the tables.

# References

American Psychiatric Association. (2013). *Diagnostic and statistical manual of mental disorders* (5th ed.). American Psychiatric Publishing.

Baldassano, C., Hasson, U., & Norman, K. A. (2018). Representation of real-world event schemas during narrative perception. *Journal of Neuroscience, 38*(45), 9689–9699.

Ballantyne, A. O., Spilkin, A. M., Hesselink, J., & Trauner, D. A. (2008). Plasticity in the developing brain: Intellectual, language and academic functions in children with ischaemic perinatal stroke. *Brain, 131*(11), 2975–2985.

Ballantyne, A. O., Spilkin, A. M., & Trauner, D. A. (2007). Language outcome after perinatal stroke: Does side matter? *Child Neuropsychology, 13*(6), 494–509.

Baron, I. S. (2010). Maxims to a model for the practice of pediatric neuropsychology. In K. O. Yeates, M.D. Ris, H. G. Taylor, & B. F. Pennington (Eds.), *Pediatric neuropsychology: Research, theory, and practice* (2nd ed., p. 480). Guilford.

Baron, I. S. (2018). *Neuropsychological evaluation of the child: Domains, methods, & case studies* (2nd ed.). Oxford University Press.

Bates, E., & Dick, F. (2002). Language, gesture, and the developing brain. *Developmental Psychobiology, 40*(3), 293-310.

Bates, E., Reilly, J., Wulfeck, B., Dronkers, N., Opie, M., Fenson, J., Kriz, S., Jeffries, R., Miller, L., & Herbst, K. (2001). Differential effects of unilateral lesions on language production in children and adults. *Brain and Language, 79*(2), 223-265.

Bear, D. M. (1979). Temporal lobe epilepsy: A syndrome of sensory–limbic hyperconnection. *Cortex, 15*(3), 357–384.

Ben-Porath, Y. S., & Tellegen, A. (2008). *Minnesota Multiphasic Personality Inventory-2 Restructured Form.* University of Minnesota Press.

Birmaher, B., Brent, D. A., Chiappetta, L., Bridge, J., Monga, S., & Baugher, M. (1999). Psychometric properties of the Screen for Child Anxiety Related Emotional Disorders (SCARED): A replication study. *Journal of the American Academy of Child & Adolescent Psychiatry, 38*(10), 1230-1236.

Butcher, J. N., Graham, J. R., Ben-Porath, Y. S., Tellegen, A., Dahlstrom, W. G., & Kaemmer, B. K. (2001). *Minnesota Multiphasic Personality Inventory-2: Manual for administration, scoring, and interpretation.* University of Minnesota Press.

Carlson, J. F., Geisinger, K. F., & Jonson, J. L. (Eds.). (2017). *The nineteenth mental measurements yearbook.* The Buros Center for Testing.

Conners, K. C. (2014). *Conners Continuous Performance Test (Conners CPT-III) and Conners Continuous Auditory Test of Attention (Conners CATA): Technical manual.* Multi-Health Systems.

Delis, D. C., Kramer, J. H., Kaplan, E., & Ober, B. A. (2000). *California Verbal Learning Test, Second Edition.* Pearson.

Denckla, M. B. (1985). Revised Neurological Examination for Subtle Signs. *Psychopharmacology Bulletin, 21*(4), 773–779.

Denckla, M. B. (1989). Neuropsychology and its role in the diagnosis of learning disabilities. In M. B. Denckla (Ed.), *Attention deficit disorders, hyperactivity~ and learning disabilities: Current theory and practical approaches.* Ciba-Geigy.

Denckla, M. B. (2019). *Understanding learning and related disabilities.* Routledge.

Dennis, M., & Levin, H. S. (2004). New perspectives on cognitive and behavioral outcome after childhood closed head injury. *Developmental Neuropsychology, 25*(1–2), 1–3.

Farran, E. K., & Karmiloff-Smith, A. (2012). *Neurodevelopmental disorders across the lifespan: A neuroconstructionist approach.* Oxford University Press.

Flynn, J. R. (1984). The mean IQ of Americans: Massive gains 1932 to 1978. *Psychological Bulletin, 95*(1), 29–51.

Flynn, J. R. (2012). *Are we getting smarter? Rising IQ in the twenty-first century.* Cambridge University Press.

Flynn, J. R., & Widaman, K. F. (2008). The Flynn effect and the shadow of the past: Mental retardation and the indefensible and indispensable role of IQ. *International Review of Research in Mental Retardation, 35*, 121–149.

Greenberg, L. M., Holder, C., Kindschi, C. L., Swalwell, S. S., Greenberg, A., & Dupuy, T. (2017). *Test of Variables of Attention (Version 9.0)* [Computer software]. TOVA.

Halligan, P. W., & David, A. S. (2001). Cognitive neuropsychiatry: Towards a scientific psychopathology. *Nature Reviews Neuroscience, 2*(3), 209–215.

Hammill, D. D., & Larsen, S. C. (2009). *Test of written language: TOWL4.* PRO-ED.

Hammill, D. D., Pearson, N.A., & Wiederholt, J. L. (2009). *Comprehensive Test of Nonverbal Intelligence–Second Edition.* Pearson.

Heffelfinger, A. (2014). Issues in the assessment of children. In M. W. Parsons & T. E. Hammeke (Eds.), *Clinical neuropsychology: A pocket handbook for assessment* (3rd ed.). American Psychological Association.

Johnson, M. H., de Hann, M. D. H. (2015). *Developmental cognitive neuroscience* (4th ed.). Wiley.

Karmiloff-Smith, A. (1998). Development itself is the key to understanding developmental disorders. *Trends in Cognitive Sciences, 2*(10), 389–398.

Karmiloff-Smith, A. (2015). An alternative to domain-general or domain-specific frameworks for theorizing about human evolution and ontogenesis. *AIMS Neuroscience, 2*(2), 91–104.

Kaufman, A. S. (2014). *Kaufman Test of Educational Achievement–Third Edition* (KTEA-3). Pearson.

Korkman, M., Kirk, U., & Kemp, S. (2007). *NEPSY Second Edition.* Pearson.

Kovacs, M. (2011). *Children's Depression Inventory, Second Edition.* MHS Assessments.

Lachar, D., & Gruber, C. P. (1977). *Personality Inventory for Children, Second Edition.* Western Psychological Services.

Larson, J. C., Mostofsky, S. H., Goldberg, M. C., Cutting, L. E., Denckla, M. B., & Mahone, E. M. (2007). Effects of gender and age on motor exam in typically developing children. *Developmental Neuropsychology, 32*(1), 543–562.

Lezak, M. D., Howieson, D. B., Bigler, E. D., & Tranel, D. (2012). *Neuropsychological assessment* (5th ed.). Oxford University Press.

Mareschal, D., Johnson, M., Sirois, S., Spratling, M., Thomas, M., Spratling, M. W., & Westermann, G. (2007). *Neuroconstructivism: How the brain constructs cognition.* Oxford University Press.

McArthur, D. S., & Roberts, G. E. (2005). *Roberts Apperception Test for Children.* Western Psychological Services.

Merritt, D. D., & Liles, B. Z. (1989). Narrative analysis: Clinical applications of story generation and story retelling. *Journal of Speech and Hearing Disorders, 54*(3), 438–447.

Meyers, J. E., & Meyers, K. R. (1995). *Rey Complex Figure Test and Recognition Trial.* Psychological Assessment Resources.

Millon, T., Millon, C., Davis, R., & Grossman, S. (1993). *Millon Adolescent Clinical Inventory.* Pearson.

Millon, T., Tringone, R., Millon, C., & Grossman, S. (2005). *M-PACI: Millon Pre-adolescent Clinical Inventory: Manual.* Pearson.

Morgan, C. D., & Murray, H. A. (1935). A method for investigating fantasies: The Thematic Apperception Test. *Archives of Neurology & Psychiatry, 34*(2), 289–306.

Noble, A. C., & Kastner, S. (2014). *The Oxford handbook of attention.* Oxford University Press.

Nussbaum, R. L., McInnes, R. R., Willard, H. F., & Hamosh, A. (2016). Cancer genetics and genomics. In *Thompson & Thompson Genetics in Medicine* (8th ed., pp. 309–331). Elsevier.

O'Connor, N., & Hermelin, B. (1987). Visual and graphic abilities of the idiot savant artist. *Psychological Medicine, 17*(1), 79–90.

Pennington, B. F. (2009). *Diagnosing learning disorders: A neuropsychological framework.* Guilford.

Posner, M. I. (2012). *Attention in a social world.* Oxford University Press.

Rinaldi, L., & Karmiloff-Smith, A. (2017). Intelligence as a developing function: A neuroconstructivist approach. *Journal of Intelligence, 5*(2), Article 18.

Roid, G. H., Miller, L. J., Pomplun, M., & Koch, C. (2013). *Leiter International Performance Scale (Leiter-3).* Western Psychological Services.

Schrank, F. A., McGrew, K. S., Mather, N., LaForte, E. M., Wendling, B. J., & Dailey, D. (2015). *Woodcock–Johnson IV Tests of Early Cognitive and Academic Development.* Riverside.

Sheslow, D., & Adams, W. (2003). *Wide Range Assessment of Memory and Learning (WRAML2).* Pearson.

Sparrow, S. S., Cicchetti, D. V., & Saulnier, C. A. (2016). *Vineland Adaptive Behavior Scales, Third Edition (Vineland-3).* Pearson.

Stiles, J., Reilly, J. S., Levine, S. C., Trauner, D. A., & Nass, R. (2012). *Neural plasticity and cognitive development: Insights from children with perinatal brain injury.* Oxford University Press.

Strauss, E., Sherman, E., & Spreen, O. (2006). *A compendium of neuropsychological tests: Administration, norms, and commentary* (3rd ed.). Oxford University Press.

Tannock, R., Purvis, K. L., & Schachar, R. J. (1993). Narrative abilities in children with attention deficit hyperactivity disorder and normal peers. *Journal of Abnormal Child Psychology, 21*(1), 103–117.

Trahan, L. H., Stuebing, K. K., Fletcher, J. M., & Hiscock, M. (2014). The Flynn effect: A meta-analysis. *Psychological Bulletin, 140*(5), 1332–1360.

Trauner, D. A., Eshagh, K., Ballantyne, A. O., & Bates, E. (2013). Early language development after peri-natal stroke. *Brain and Language, 127*(3), 399–403.

Vicari, S., Albertoni, A., Chilosi, A. M., Cipriani, P., Cioni, G., & Bates, E. (2000). Plasticity and reorganization during language development in children with early brain injury. *Cortex, 36*(1), 31–46.

Wechsler, D. (2014). *Wechsler Intelligence Scale for Children–Fifth Edition.* Pearson.

Yamadori, A., Osumi, Y., Tabuchi, M., Mori, E., Yoshida, T., Ohkawa, S., & Yoneda, Y. (1990). Hyperlalia: A right cerebral hemisphere syndrome. *Behavioural Neurology, 3*(3), 143–151.

# PART II
# DEVELOPMENTAL COGNITIVE
# NEUROSCIENCE

# 3

# Attention

## Attention Systems

In his *Principles of Psychology*, William James (1890) suggested that attention is at the center of human performance. He wrote attention is the taking into possession of the mind, in clear and vivid form, of one out of what seem several simultaneously possible objects or trains of thought. Focalization and concentration of consciousness are of its essence.

Now, more than a century later, developments in developmental cognitive neuroscience allow the physiologic analysis of higher cognitive functions and provide a means to study attention and identify a functional anatomy of the human attentional system. The attention system is basic for the selection of information for conscious processing. Attention is the essential link between mind and brain in connecting the mental level of description (developmental cognitive science) with the anatomic level (brain neuroscience). Attention and executive functioning are emergent mental properties that result from the evolution of the human brain. Mental properties interact causally at their own higher level and may exert causal control downward. Attention allows the causal coordination of brain systems through mental states. Its study may allow us to better understand how voluntary control over autonomic systems can be accomplished. Yet it must be kept in mind that attention processes are the activities of people and not of brains. Attention to the social world is critical in child development (Posner, 2011). Multiple experimental methods have converged to allow the study of attention. These include mental chronometry, brain lesions, electrophysiology, and neuroimaging studies.

This chapter discusses definitions of attention and its characteristics; describes genes and attentional networks; reviews anatomic substrates for attention, summarizing development neuroimaging studies; considers attention and self-regulation in infancy and child development; discusses attention training in childhood; and reviews neurodevelopmental disorders characterized by attention deficits.

## Definition and Characteristics of Attention

Attention (Oyebode, 2018) is the active or passive focusing of consciousness on the external world and the inner life. Attention is active when externally focused, and it is passive when focusing on the flow of internal events. Attention may be voluntary or involuntary. It is voluntary when effort is focused on an internal or external event by choice or intention, and it is involuntary when an event or object attracts attention without deliberate conscious choice or intentional effort.

Attention is not the same as consciousness, although it depends on it, in that full attention is not possible with reduced consciousness. Yet varying degrees of attention are
possible with full consciousness. An object is held in attention voluntarily at a particular
focus and becomes the center of attention. Events outside this center, which are peripheral to awareness, may intrude and reduce the clarity of attention. Regarding thought,
active attention focuses and guides its direction. When focused, attention is used to
clarify and make thought coherent. Passive attention observes the flow of the thought
associations that pass voluntarily into awareness or consciousness.

The attention system is anatomically separate from brain systems that integrate sensory input. It is involved in decision-making that leads to choice. Attention engages a
network of anatomical regions. Each of these anatomical regions is involved in different
attentional functions. There is a discrete anatomical organization of attention systems
that is divided into three networks (Petersen & Posner, 2012): the alerting network
(brain stem arousal) linked to sustained vigilance, the orienting system involving the
parietal cortex, and the executive network involving the midfrontal/anterior cingulate
brain regions. When attention is used to focus on sensory experience, the term "orientation" is used. Orientation refers to setting attention in time and place within the realities
of one's person and situation. As an executive target detection system, attention selects
sensory input from sensory channels and working memory. Attention may be closely
bound to such memory.

The visual metaphor, the mind's eye, is useful when describing attention. Using this
visual metaphor, we see that attention may be focused or peripheral or may come onto
a central point of clarity. When one is concurrently alert and vigilant, attention may
either move easily from one object to another or become absorbed. In absorption, it
is narrowed through focus on a particular object so that other awarenesses are not recorded in memory. Attention is normally reduced with fatigue and boredom (reduction of affective interest in an object or person), during sleep, and under hypnosis.
In dreams, attention is purely passive except during the uncommon phenomenon of
lucid dreaming (Baird et al., 2019; Filevich et al., 2015). Attention is decreased in states
in which alertness or consciousness is reduced, as in epilepsy, head injury, drug- and
alcohol-induced states, increased intracranial tension, and brain stem lesions involving
the reticular formation. Attention may be enhanced by drugs such as stimulants; dissociated in hysterical states; or narrowed in mood disorders, in which it may assume the
quality of state boundness in depressive illnesses.

## Genes and Attentional Networks

The relationship of changes in brain attention network connectivity to behavior and self-
regulation from infancy into childhood and adolescence is influenced by gene expression and life experiences. Because gene expression interacts with life experience during
development, psychosocial interventions potentially may improve brain network
functioning. Each of the attentional networks has a predominant neuromodulator that
originates in subcortical regions of the brain. The alerting network neuromodulation
arises in the locus coeruleus. The orienting network neuromodulator is acetylcholine in
the basal forebrain. The neuromodulator for the executive network is dopamine from

the ventral tegmental brain region (Posner et al., 2016). Thus, dopamine activity may facilitate the efficiency of the executive network (Fossella et al., 2002). Knowledge about neuromodulators and attention networks has led to a search for candidate genes that may influence attention network efficacy. Alleles of the catechol-O-methyltransferase (*COMT*) gene, the dopamine D4 receptor gene (*DRD4*), the monoamine oxidase A (*MAOA*) gene, and other dopamine-related genes have been associated with the attention and the psychological capacity to resolve conflict; the anterior cingulate cortex is a brain network node in mediating conflict (Diamond et al., 2004).

Brain imaging studies have mapped genetic variations which are involved in executive function and brain activity are described by Fan, Fossella, et al. (2003). These authors examined genetic variation of *MAOA* and *DRD4* gene correlates with executive attention. Subjects were grouped according to whether they were homozygous/ hemizygous for the four-repeat allele of MAOA or homozygous/hemizygous or heterozygous for the three-repeat allele and their association with brain activation and conflict resolution. Similar comparisons were made for the *DRD4* gene. They studied the two genes as associated with efficient handling of conflict in reaction time experiments. A polymorphism was identified in persons with the allele that was associated with improved behavioral performance with greater activation in the anterior cingulate using the Attention Network Test (ANT). Their findings demonstrate that there are genetic differences among individuals in the efficiency of attention network function and illustrate that genes may influence attention.

A follow-up study examined the role of the *MAOA* and *DRD4* genes in the development of self-regulation during infancy and childhood (Posner et al., 2014). The study was initiated in 7-month-old infants; these children were retested and genotyped at age 2 years and tested again at age 4 years using the ANT. As infants, the orienting visual task was used to monitor orientation. Infants were monitored as they moved their head and as they moved their eyes to the location of the stimulus, with assessment of anticipatory looking and reaching toward novel objects. Infants were found to have a rudimentary attention system. Their orientation was correlated with positive affect and served as an early emotional regulatory system. At later ages, executive functioning was involved in emotion regulation.

Executive attentional activity is correlated with dopamine genes, which are important in the early development of attention networks. Polymorphic variants of the *COMT* gene (chromosome 22), previously shown to be related to executive attention in adults and older children, is also be related to attention in toddlers (Voelker et al., 2009). Haplotypes of the *COMT* gene also influence anticipatory looking at ages 18– 20 months. A 7-repeat variations of the *COMT* gene is related to parent-reported positive affect. Thus, there is a genetic link between emotion regulation and emotional reactivity in early development.

The dopamine *DRD4* gene (chromosome 11) encodes the dopamine D4 receptor, which monitors extra-synaptic dopamine concentrations in prefrontal brain regions that are involved in executive attention. The 7-repeat allele of the dopamine *DRD4* gene is associated with risk-taking behavior and attention-deficit/hyperactivity disorder (ADHD) in candidate gene studies. In a longitudinal study beginning in infancy, child–caregiver interaction was rated on a five-dimension scale of quality of parenting that included dimensions of support, autonomy, stimulation, lack of hostility, and self-confidence in their children. Parenting was rated as high quality or lower quality. For children with the 7-repeat gene variant, variations in parenting quality were demonstrated. Children with this allele and high-quality parenting showed normal levels of risk-taking behavior, whereas those with lower quality parenting demonstrated high risk-taking (Sheese et al., 2007). For children who did not have the 7-repeat polymorphism, parenting variation was correlated to impulsivity and risk-taking.

The finding that a child with the 7-repeat allele, one associated with ADHD, when paired with enriched parenting, showed less risk-taking behavior and more positive behavior is consistent with differential genetic sensitivity to the social context–environment model. The model proposes that gene variants demonstrate plasticity, making effects contingent on whether the environment is enriched or rejecting (Belsky & Pluess, 2009; Boyce, 2016). In the positive environment, the child thrives, whereas in the rejecting one, the child does more poorly than expected. Differential sensitivity to environmental context raises interesting questions regarding nature and nurture. If in evolution, genetic variants are selected that facilitate sensitivity to positive and negative nurturing, this provides important new light on the relationship of genes and environmental influences.

*Epigenetics* refers to mechanisms whereby the environment can produce long-term alterations in gene expression without altering the nucleotide sequence in the DNA. Thus, epigenetic mechanisms mediate the effects of life experience through altering gene expression. Several mechanisms mediate epigenetic effects, including histone modification, which affects chromatin structure, and cytosine methylation, which in promoter sites alters gene expression. Epigenetic changes may play a role in social adaptation. Thus, enriched social support may compensate for developmental deficits.

Alleles of the methylenetetrahydrofolate reductase (*MTHFR*) regulate the availability of the methyl donor that mediates cytosine methylation. In one study involving 7-year-old children, who were homozygous for the C allele of *MTHFR*, interaction with the *COMT* gene demonstrated greater improvement in reaction time in conflict resolution following practice on the ANT. These findings suggest that the methylation acts on or through genes that impact the executive attention network. Moreover, some participants showed initial improvement on the ANT followed by subsequent decline. The authors found that alleles of the gene encoding dopamine β-hydroxylase gene (*DBH*), the enzyme that converts dopamine to norepinephrine, were linked to decline in performance. They concluded that their findings indicate a genetic dissociation between improved attentional performance when learning and a decline with practice in performance (Voelker, Sheese, et al., 2017). Overall, they found that epigenetic mechanisms involving DNA methylation are important regulators of synaptic plasticity and "experience-dependent behavioral change" (Day et al., 2013, p. 1445). This provocative study requires replication because of its limited statistical power.

In summary, attentional research seeks to clarify how developmental change in brain connectivity is linked to behavioral markers in children at different ages (Posner et al., 2014). Allelic variants of specific genes may be associated with individual responses in studies of attention. That genes interact with the environment makes clear the importance of studying genetic variation and genetic–environment interactions regarding attention networks. A greater understanding of epigenetic mechanisms will guide interventions that influence attention and development.

## Anatomy of Attention

Developmental cognitive neuroscience studies examine the anatomic substrates for attention. The attention system is anatomically separate from interrelated systems that integrate experience with separate brain mechanisms for attention (Petersen & Posner, 2012). Both cognitive operations and neuronal activity are important. Petersen and Posner (2012) suggest several organizational principles that focus on a unified attention system to control directed mental processing, channel involuntary memory, and redirect attention back to its original target when distractions occur. Attention involves a network of anatomic regions; there is not a single system in the brain for attention, nor is attention an aspect of general brain functioning. Brain areas involved in attention carry out different functions—that is, alerting, orientation, selective detection, sustained alert and vigilance, and executive functioning. The subsystems described are shown in Figure 3.1. This figure shows the cortical areas involved in each of the three functions of attention.

## Alerting

Alertness is a prerequisite to carry out all attentional processes. Overall alertness is affected by sensory events and rhythmic variation in attention. Psychologic and

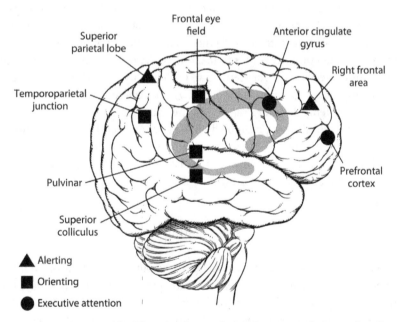

**Figure 3.1** Attention networks. The triangles, circles, and squares indicate nodes of activation of each network. Alertness is essential for other attentional operations. Alertness is influenced by sensory events and by the diurnal rhythm. The alerting system involves the right frontal area and superior parietal lobe. Orientation involves the frontal eye field, temporoparietal junction, pulvinar, and superior colliculus. Executive attention involves the anterior cingulate gyrus and prefrontal cortex.
From Posner et al. (2014); redrawn by Tim Phelps (2021).

pharmacologic studies have identified the neuromodulator norepinephrine as essential to the functioning of the alerting system (Petersen & Posner, 2012). When we attend, there is an activation of the norepinephrine system in the locus coeruleus in the brain stem to become alert. Cells in the locus coeruleus process input in two ways. One mode, referred to as tonic, is sustained and supports a tonic level of alertness over longer time intervals. The phasic mode refers to rapid change in attention; it is the basis for orienting and selective attention. Tonic, sustained, alertness predominantly involves the right cerebral hemisphere. The voluntary maintenance of sustained attention, when performing a task, involves the anterior cingulate. Conversely, rapid phasic shifts in attention focus on any incoming environmental signal. This is phasic alertness to warning information shifts, resulting in alertness and inhibition of intrinsic brain rhythms within milliseconds after awareness. We must keep in mind that the brain is continuously active. There is a default resting state when nothing is being actively processed (Raichle, 2009). Importantly, it is not alertness versus sleep that we study but, rather, alertness in the context of the brain's default state. That state is characterized by the slow oscillation between two brain networks that are within medial and lateral cortical regions of the brain. When alerted to a warning signal from the environment, the brain shifts from the resting default state to one of high alertness with increased heart rate with changes in cortical activity and increased release of norepinephrine. Such activation of the noradrenergic alerting network can be blocked by guanfacine and clonidine, drugs that reduce the release of norepinephrine (Marrocco & Davidson, 1998). Conversely, drugs that increase norepinephrine enhance danger signals to become more alert.

The norepinephrine network reaches nodes in the frontal cortex and parietal regions linked to the dorsal visual pathway and is linked to the alert attention network, whereas the orientating attention network is influenced by the neuromodulator acetylcholine. Although these mechanisms for alerting and orienting are independent, these systems work together regarding when (alerting) and where (orientating) attention is directed. Both systems allow for a rapid response to threat.

Neuroimaging studies have examined phasic and tonic alerting, finding differences in lateralization in the cerebral hemispheres. Those lateralized to the right hemisphere involve slower tonic processes, whereas those lateralized to the left hemisphere are related to higher temporal phasic alerting (Ivry & Robertson, 1998).

## Orientating

From alertness, we turn to orientation to sensory input and the study of overt and covert orientation. Overt orientating involves conscious attention and voluntary turning the eyes and body toward the source of the stimulus. Covert orientating occurs when a salient environment change causes shift in the orientation of attention. Attentive movements are coordinated early in development.

There are two brain systems that are involved in orientating to external stimuli: the dorsal and ventral attention systems. The brain region central to orientating is the superior parietal lobe. The dorsal system in parietal brain regions utilizes the frontal eye fields and intraparietal sulcus; it allows rapid control over attention (Petersen & Posner, 2012). If a target of attention is missed, attention must be refocused. The switching back process involves the temporoparietal junction. Overall, covert and overt shifts in attention involve similar brain regions. However, covert attention is separate from the motor system that involves visual saccades, although these systems interact. Finally, cholinergic systems whose source is in the basal forebrain are essential to orienting.

The ventral network is believed to be more responsive to sensory input. It is lateralized to the right hemisphere. Lesions to that brain region result in the visual neglect syndrome. The ventral network links parietal with frontal and dorsal brain regions through the temporoparietal junction. The modes of the orienting network have been studied through spatial cueing and visual search paradigms (Wright & Ward, 2008).

Sensory systems are tightly integrated to the attention orienting networks. These sensory systems are "bottom-up," involving the visual cortex and extrastriate brain regions to the temporal lobe. Ventral input is synchronized to the activity of the dorsal attention system, lending to greater attentional sensitivity (Petersen & Posner, 2012).

## Executive Control

The executive attention network is particularly important in child development. It is involved in the regulation of thought (cognitive), feelings, and actions. Basically, this third attention network is involved in executive control and executive functions. It is important in "top-down" behavioral regulation. There are two separate executive control networks for executive control (Dosenbach et al., 2008). These networks monitor conflict, engage working memory, regulate emotional states, and allow reflection to correct human error. The first executive control system is linked to the frontoparietal network; it is separate and distinct from the orienting network. The second network is the cingulo-opercular network.

In adulthood, these systems are separate, although their origin may be the same in early development. The frontoparietal system is believed to be involved in switching tasks and adjustment of attention as needed when tasks are expressed in real time. The cingulo-opercular system acts to provide a stable background for overall performance (Petersen & Posner, 2012). Lesion studies in animals and humans provide support for these two executive control systems. First, frontal midline lesions lead to a form of akinetic mutism. Although those affected with a kinetic mutism can conduct goal-oriented activities, they fail to do so. Conversely, lesions more laterally in the dorsolateral prefrontal cortex exhibit perseverations (frontoparietal symptoms) with an inability to switch from one activity to another.

Emotion regulation networks include the anterior cingulate, the frontal cortex, and the amygdala. Emotional control is linked to connectivity between the anterior cingulate and the ventral amygdala (Etkin et al., 2006). The elements of the attention networks—alerting, orienting, and executive functioning—are important in overall self-regulation. Studies using divided attention tasks such as the Stroop effect have linked these elements to specific brain regions. The Stroop effect is one of several psychological conflict tasks that assess attention shifting by introducing psychological conflict. In this task, the color on a stimulus card conflicts with color name. For example, the word "green" is presented in red ink on the card. The test measures the ability to choose the less dominant response. Similar conflict tasks on the Delis–Kaplan executive test battery assess spatial conflict and pictorial conflict. Neuroimaging studies have revealed that these conflict tasks have a common brain anatomy (Fan, Fossella, et al., 2003). For example, the Stroop effect activates areas of the cingulate gyrus that links the dorsal cingulate to cognitive tasks and the ventral cingulate for emotion-related tasks (Bush et al., 2000; Petersen & Posner, 2012). The Stroop task allows a means to understand how brain networks work in real life.

Executive function networks develop extensively from infancy into adult life. For example, anterior cingulate activation neuroimaging studies have compared infants aged 7 months with adults. Error detection is recognized at approximately age 3 years (Jones et al., 2003). In infancy, self-control systems are primarily linked to the orientation of attention (Rothbart et al., 2003). Social conflict resolution studies using parent reports have demonstrated a growing capacity for effortful control from late childhood into the adult years (Posner & Rothbart, 2007). The child's emerging attentive effortful self-control capacity associates self-regulation and executive attention. Childhood effortful control is associated with interpersonal empathy. Empathy allows the child to delay an action or impulse to avoid negative behaviors. Self-regulation is essential for child socialization.

As shown in Figure 3.2, the Attention Network Task (ANT) measures the efficiency of brain networks in children and adults by the speed of response to whether a target stimulus points left or right. Alerting cues (top left) indicate when the target will occur. Orienting cues (column 1, middle) indicate where the target will occur. Executive

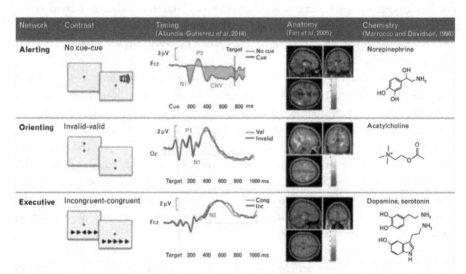

**Figure 3.2** Three attention networks measured by the Attention Network Task (ANT). This figure presents results obtained using the ANT (column 2) for alerting, orienting, and executive function networks. ANT measures the efficiency of brain networks in children and adults by the speed of responding to a target stimulus. Alerting, orienting, and executive scores from the ANT are related to the time course of brain activity measured by evoked response potentials (column 3), the anatomical location of activation of these networks in brain regions measured by fMRI (column 4), and chemical modulator pharmacological manipulations (column 5).
From Posner et al. (2016).

attention scores (column 1, bottom left) are calculated by the time to resolve conflict. In column 2, labeled Contrast, alerting cues (top left) indicate when the target will occur. Orienting cues (middle) indicate where the target will occur. Executive attention scores (bottom left) are calculated by the time to resolve conflict presented when distracting information is shown that is incongruent or congruent with the response to the stimulus. Column 3 shows alerting, orienting, and executive scores taken from the ANT related to the time course of brain activity measured by evoked response potentials. Column 4 shows the anatomical location of activation of these attention networks in brain regions measured by functional magnetic resonance imaging (fMRI), and column 5 lists chemical modulators and neurotransmitters for alerting (norepinephrine), orienting (acetylcholine), and executive control (dopamine and serotonin).

The presence of warning cues, in contrast to the absence of them (no cue), produces phasic alerting and leads to strong and fast (within a half second after presentation of the cue) neural responses involving a number of brain regions, which can be modulated by altering levels of norepinephrine in the brain. Similarly contrasting valid and invalid spatial orienting cues allows studying disengagement and switching attention from one location to another. This engages areas of the parietal and frontal cortices and is facilitated by nicotine, an agonist of the neurotransmitter acetylcholine. Finally, the presence of distracting information that is incongruent (as opposed to congruent) with the response suggested by the target produces conflict and engages executive attention. Conflict is associated with an electrophysiological response occurring as early as 200 ms following the presentation of the stimuli. This response has also been associated with activation of a number of brain regions, including the anterior cingulate and prefrontal cortices, and is modulated by levels of dopamine and serotonin in the brain.

## Attention and Self-Regulation in Infancy and Childhood

Attention develops from infancy to childhood onward in accord with the unique anatomy for each component. It develops according to connectivity in brain regions, neuromodulators, and functions (Posner et al., 2014). These functions, as they develop in infancy and childhood, are expressed in the three functional networks: alerting, orienting, and executive attention. Alerting is achieved in early development as a state of readiness to respond to environmental exposures and process them. Orienting is increasingly refined through the selection of sensory input. Executive attention monitors environmental engagement. It is involved in the mastery and resolution of conflicts between thoughts, feelings, and chosen responses.

Neuroimaging methods, fMRI, and resting-state MRI are utilized to study infants and children throughout development. At rest, brain regions in the default state remain active together. In infancy, the two attention brain networks are connected in the resting state (Gao et al., 2009). Because no task is involved in resting, connectivity can be studied in infants during this state. The connectivity networks involved are the frontoparietal brain regions related to executive attention (orienting and control) and cingulo-opercular brain regions related to executive attention networks. Moreover, brain connections change over the lifetime. During the first year of life, there is little or no connectivity between the anterior cingulate and other brain regions. Infants gradually develop longer brain connections. Infants have limited use of executive attention; they cannot regulate behavior using the executive attention network. Young children, ages 7–9 years, have shorter brain connections than adults. Such connections continue to develop into adulthood.

## Attention and Orienting in Infancy

In infancy, the alerting, orienting, and executive control systems are far less independent than in later life. At birth, sleep is predominant, with only a few hours spent in wakefulness. Alertness is stimulated by parents who arouse the infant from sleep. Arousal involves activity of the locus coeruleus. It is continually activated just as it is in later life. Endogenous alertness when waking from sleep without external stimulation also involves the locus coeruleus brain stem system (Posner et al., 2014).

Infantile alertness increases rapidly during the first 12 months of life. By 3 months of age, infants are alert most of the day. Such alertness is facilitated by stimulation from family members and daily environmental stimulation. When an alert infant moves their head and eyes to fixate on the external environment, the infant is especially attentive to the faces of caregivers (Meltzoff & Moore, 1977). Orientation is studied in infants by monitoring saccadic eye movements and examining the detection of gaze (Richards & Hunter, 1998). When the target moves, the infant's head and eyes move to refocus. Similarly, covert attention engages these same systems. The speed of reorienting improves during the first year as infants regulate their distress by orienting to sensory stimuli to maintain control of their sensory environment (Ruff & Rothbart, 2001). Caregivers redirect infant attention to facilitate the infant's regulation of their emotional state. Referred to as the *distress keeper*, such infant regulation most likely involves the amygdala system (Harman et al., 1997). The term distress keeper refers to regulation of the level of initial distress. Harman et al. (1997) found that infants could be quieted by distraction for a full minute before orientation was lost.

Importantly, it is the caregiver who facilitates infant orientation in the newborn period. However, by the fourth month, an infant has gained considerable control by alternatively disengaging their gaze from one object to directing it to another. Thus, the infant gradually gains greater control over orientation to events. As infants gain self-control, it is easier for them to be soothed by their caregivers. Later in infancy, infants begin to gain control of their behavior and their emotions. This control marks the transition from alerting and orienting to the emergence of the executive attention system.

## Development of Executive Attention in Infancy

The development of the executive attention system gradually emerges in infancy as alertness and orientation mature with increasing control of behavior and emotions. This self-control mastery is referred to as establishing effortful control (Rothbart et al., 2003; Rueda et al., 2005). Effortful control is demonstrated when a parent asks an infant to put away a toy and the infant complies. Effortful control continues to mature from 2 years onward. Before age 2 years, executive attention gradually improves with increasing duration of attention to events, positive responses to soothing, and better reorienting following distraction. For example, at approximately 7 months, detection and correction of errors are early evidence of the activity of the executive attention system. Further development of the executive functioning in the second half of the first year is illustrated by Adele Diamond's (2006) research on the A-not-B task and the reaching task. In the A-not-B task, the experimenter moves the location of a hidden object from point A to point B. The infant has previously practiced learning the location of point A and uses effortful control to now find it. In the reaching task, a conflicting route is introduced when reaching for a toy from the accustomed location. The capacity for correct response to look improves from ages 6 to 12 months. Colombo (2001) proposes that alertness, orientation to objects, and endogenous attention develop throughout the first years of life. Alerting is mature by 4 months and orienting by 6 or 7 months, whereas endogenous attention is not mastered until age 4 or 5 years.

## Attention Networks in Children

Each of the three functions of attention undergoes a long developmental process. In infancy, attention is a primarily automatic engagement. Greater voluntary control is achieved by the end of the first year of life. In the ensuing toddler and school-aged years, as the executive system gains control over attention, more goal-oriented control is achieved. At approximately age 3 years, children are better able to follow instructions and engage in research studies. Sustained attention can then be measured in tests such as the continuous performance test. The performance of young children on this test is linked to both sustained attention and their level of maturation. In one study of 3- and 4-year-olds, 30–50% of preschool children were able to complete a vigilance task. Seventy percent of 4- to 4½-year-olds and 100% of older children could do so (Levy, 1980). Developmental changes in alertness are associated with the continuing maturation of the frontal lobe of the brain.

Attention throughout childhood can be examined using a child version of the ANT (Rueda et al., 2015). The child version uses fish instead of arrows as targets. In this attention game, the goal is to feed the middle fish (the target) and make him happy by pressing a key linked to the target's direction. The ANT has been used to measure the efficiency of the targeting network. In one study, the age of participants ranged from elementary school age to adolescence. In the child, the ANT alerting shows statistically significant improvement with maturation, especially in speed of processing.

Orienting attention uses sensory input to the frontal eye fields and regions of the superior and inferior parietal pole. Connectivity between left and right parietal nodes is an important feature in orientation to visual input. Orienting speed does not show age difference in 5- and 6-year-olds, 8- to 10-year-olds, and adults for either overt or covert tasks. Voluntary orientation, disengagement, and return to the task have been studied. These tasks are dependent on cortical areas of the parietal and temporal lobes and improve with age. Endogenously adjusting attention focus is more difficult. Essentially, attention focusing and the capacity to switch attention between two different stimuli improve between ages 5, 8, and 10 years and adulthood (Posner et al., 2014). There is an age-related improvement in how quickly one can shift attention voluntarily and

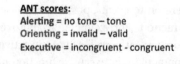

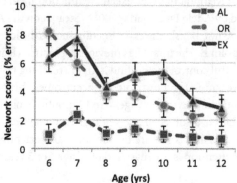

**Figure 3.3** Development of attention networks in children. This figure shows the developmental trajectory accuracy using attention network scores (calculated with percentage of errors) for children aged 6–12 years. Separate developmental trajectories are shown for each attention network. Alerting shows an earlier maturational course, whereas orienting and executive networks show a more protracted developmental trajectory in children performing the ANT. Brain evoked potential responses are measured, informing the neural mechanisms underlying them. Overall, measurement of evoked potential responses comparing adults and children indicates that children show poorer faster processing that varies according to attentional requirements.
From Pozuelos et al. (2014).

the capacity to disengage attention from an object (Brodeur & Enns, 1997). Moreover, when the orienting effect is examined by comparing reaction time to valid versus invalid cued targets, a sharpening of the development is not found until late childhood (Schul et al., 2003). Studies using the child ANT find that orienting response precision substantially improves between early and late childhood. Moreover, children between ages 6 and 12 years demonstrate interactions between alerting and orienting (Figure 3.3; Pozuelos et al., 2014).

## Executive Attention Network in Childhood

The executive attention network involves several brain regions, primarily the anterior cingulate and anterior insula (operculum) brain regions. Referred to as the cingulo-opercular network in fMRI studies, this attention network is involved in attentional performance and regulation, conflict resolution, and detection of error (Neta et al., 2017). Some parts of the executive function network are active in infancy. However, brain regions do not connect to motor control until approximately age 4 years (Posner et al., 2016). Before that, self-control is carried out primarily by use of orienting attention. One neuroimaging study of 750 subjects (aged 4–21 years) revealed that the size of the right anterior cingulate is the best predictor of capacity to resolve conflict measured by reaction time differences (Fjell et al., 2012). Imaging of white matter using diffusion tensor imaging (DTI) indicates that later in brain development, reaction time is linked to the efficiency of white matter connections. At approximately age 2 years or older, children can complete simple conflict tasks, as measured by reaction time. Awareness and self-correction of attentional errors progress between ages 2½ and 3 years, with measurably longer reaction times, suggesting children are recognizing errors. As control improves, children between ages 30 and 39 months show substantial improvement in correcting the error (Posner et al., 2014).

During the school-age years, the child version of the ANT is used to track the development of executive attention. From ages 4 to 7 years, there is substantial development of the speed of conflict resolution on the test (Rueda et al., 2005). From ages 7 to 9 years and into adolescence, there is increasing functional connectivity of the frontoparietal network involved in cognitive control (Fair et al., 2007). These findings are consistent with immaturity of frontoparietal activation in 8- to 12-year-old children on the ANT compared to adults (Konrad et al., 2005). The immaturity of frontoparietal connectivity and activation of this network most likely account for the delay in response to stimuli in young children compared to older ones. The maturation process involves long-range connectivity and focalization of effects from prefrontal sites to the midline in mature adult development. The focalization of signals in the adult compared to the child is demonstrated in neuroimaging studies. Thus, as the brain circuits that underlie executive functions become more efficient, they also become more focal (Posner et al., 2014).

In summary, throughout child development, there is substantial maturation of attention networks. The three networks mature at different rates. The ANT reveals that most of the early development of the executive network occurs before age 7 years; connectivity studies indicate increased segregation between the orienting and executive networks after age 9 years (Posner et al., 2014). Children aged 6–12 years show interaction between developing attention networks. In the adolescent years, developmental interactions between both alerting and orienting and executive attention are enhanced (Pozuelos et al., 2014).

## Attention Training in Childhood

Attention training for infants and children is an important and continuing endeavor. William James (1890) observed that infants experience the world as a "blooming, buzzing confusion" (p. 987). Thus, information must be structured for them with a clear differentiation of the learning target from background noise. For example, to do so, infant-directed speech ("motherese") exaggerates pitch and elongates words and vowel space. Such efforts carefully distinguish one phoneme from another. Brain investigations document improved attention in infants with stimulation (Wass et al., 2011). Attention training interventions seek to improve the functioning of attention networks in infants and children by practicing the use of networks. In one study, compared to a control group, infant subjects showed improvement in cognitive control in sustained attention and reduced saccadic reaction times with practice. Improvement correlated with the amount of training. Similarly, preschool children have shown enhancement of executive attention network functioning immediately after training and again after two additional months (Rueda et al., 2012). Moreover, attention training has been shown to improve children's ability to delay gratification (Murray et al., 2016). Generalization of training to daily life activities is an ongoing endeavor (Posner et al., 2016).

Mindfulness meditation attention practices can result in brain changes (Hölzel et al., 2011). The practice of mindfulness meditation has been shown to be associated with neuroplastic changes in the anterior cingulate cortex, insula, temporoparietal function, the frontal limbic network, and the default network. These studies show that mindfulness practices facilitate self-regulation. Moreover, DTI studies of adults using mindfulness training have shown specific improvements in white matter pathways around the anterior cingulate following 2 weeks of training (Tang et al., 2014). Such changes in white matter pathways may be induced by frontal theta rhythm activation during meditation practice (Voelker, Piscopo, et al., 2017). DTI studies also have shown changes in fractional anisotropy that are associated with fiber density, myelination of white matter, and efficiency of white matter in learning (speed of responses). These findings are referred to as activity-dependent myelination, a potential mechanism for new learning being associated with changes in brain connectivity (Fields, 2015). Functional anisotropy changes involve training of working memory and other tasks in adults. Similar white matter changes are reported in brain development in childhood.

## Attention Network Pathology in Neurodevelopmental Disorders

Attention deficits are commonly reported in children with intellectual developmental disorders. This has led to the belief that attention deficits are universal in these disorders. Attention deficits are most often reported when subjects, with and without an intellectual developmental disorder, matched by chronological age are compared. In such comparisons, impaired performance is expected in all aspects of functioning, including attention. However, when subjects are matched by mental age along with other developmental level measures, the percentage with impairment dropped. Those at the lower end of the normal distribution of intellectual functioning with neurodevelopmental syndromes may show attention commensurate with cognitive level.

Attention deficits reported in the literature are essentially linked to neurodevelopmental disorders. Attention deficits in children with Down syndrome, Williams–Beuren syndrome, and fragile X syndrome are reported relative to general mental age level, allowing attention deficits in specific syndromes to be compared. This approach allows comparison between syndromes to understand developmental change and stability in selective attention. The construct of visual attention is commonly studied. Several different processes are involved in visual attention, including the capacity to focus on relevant information while ignoring irrelevant information, to find new information, to compare and contrast the size of visual images, to flexibly shift cognitive strategy, to master a new task, to sustain focus on a task, and to take in new information (Iarocci et al., 2012). Despite the different mechanism involved, all these components function in a coordinated manner for information processing. Four modes of visual attention are proposed. Two of these, reflexes and habits, are unconscious; reflexes are innate, whereas habits are learned.

Developmental age-related changes are more evident in habit and conscious deliberation than in reflex action and exploration. Reflexes are stable throughout life, whereas
deliberation capacity changes most during development (Iarocci et al., 2009). The three
elements of attention as described earlier—alerting, orienting, and executive control—
have been studied with regard to reflexes and deliberation capacity. Visual reflexes
are conscious and automatically triggered by a specific environmental stimuli. Visual
orienting focuses attention to relevant objects in the environment. Orienting coordinates shifts from internal representation of an object to the object itself—for example,
scanning a crowd and unexpectedly fixating on the face of a particular person. This capacity to orient changes very little over development (Plude et al., 1994). Visual habits,
even though unconscious and automatic, are learned, whereas visual reflexes are innate.
For example, the use of arrows as directional symbols becomes so familiar that their
meaning cannot be ignored (Hommel et al., 2001). Learning to read involves repeated
rehearsal of written words until they become so familiar they can be read automatically.
Poor readers are more distracted by irrelevant words than are good readers.

Visual exploration, although controlled, is innately specified. A considerable amount
of visual processing is carried out without any specific goal. Importantly, visual attention alerts the viewer to changes in the environment. The capacity to detect changes to
the environment improves with age. This was demonstrated in a developmental study
that enrolled typically developing children and adults at ages 7, 9, 11, and 21 years.
Participants were examined using the change detection task, which is used to measure
the viewer's response to changes in the environment. Two versions of the same scene
are presented side-by-side and the subject is asked to determine what is different in the
scene. In this study, change detection improved between ages 7 and 9 years (Shore et al.,
2006). Visual deliberation involves effort with its use of executive control. Unlike exploration, deliberation is not specified innately. It involves deliberate focus on a specific
goal, orienting deliberately in response to a task, in contrast to reflexive orienting, or
deliberately switching from one visual task to another. Younger children perform more
poorly in selective attention tasks than older ones (Plude et al., 1994). In studies such as
these, developmental level and mental age must be considered as tasks become more sophisticated. However, in studying neurodevelopmental syndromes, mental age alone is
not sufficient; profiles of development are needed when making comparisons.

Attention deficits are characteristic features of neurodevelopmental disorders.
ADHD, autism spectrum disorder (ASD), schizophrenia, and a number of
neurogenetic syndromes show abnormalities in the brain's attention networks. Each of
these disorders is separately described in Part IV of this book. Studies of developmental
disorders provide a window on how disrupted attention can be studied clinically and
cognitively using systems neuroscience, cellular neuroscience, and functional genomic
approaches (Scerif & Wu, 2014). Because neurodevelopmental disorders are associated
with neurocognitive functioning in early life, they might offer a window on early developmental trajectories and changing developmental profiles over time.

Attention can be studied in neurodevelopment in both functionally defined clinical
disorders (e.g. ADHD, ASD, and schizophrenia) and genetically defined conditions (e.g.
phenylketonuria, Williams–Beuren syndrome, and fragile X syndrome). Neuroimaging
studies of clinically diagnosed ADHD demonstrate abnormalities in frontostriatal and
mesocorticolimbic brain regions. The frequency of attention deficits in neurogenetic

syndromes as well as their distinct neurocognitive profiles from infancy onwards illustrate multiple pathways to ADHD symptoms.

ADHD is a commonly occurring neurodevelopmental disorder with a prevalence of approximately 5% of children in most cultures. It is associated with poor school performance, academic underachievement, social deficits, and a greater probability of unemployment in adult life. Diagnostically in the fifth edition of the *Diagnostic and Statistical Manual of Mental Disorders* (American Psychiatric Association, 2013), the essential features of the disorder are a persistent pattern of inattention and/or hyperactivity–impulsivity that interferes with functioning in school, at home, and in the community. Core symptoms are explained based on an underlying cognitive deficit involving executive dysfunction, response inhibition, and/or motivational style. Motivational style refers to reward dysfunction, delay aversion, and difficulty in state regulation. Both executive and motivational systems are a focus of study in this disorder.

ADHD is a heterogeneous disorder. Research studies show significant large effect sizes and findings of deficits in response inhibition, vigilance, planning, and working memory. However, the extent of deficits is variable in the clinically defined disorder. ADHD is associated with both structural and functional abnormalities in brain imaging studies in right-lateralized corticostriatal networks involved in inhibitory control. fMRI neuroimaging studies show reduced activation of the inferior prefrontal cortex and caudate, in addition to frontostriatal regions.

The behavioral diagnosis may include several subtypes with different etiologies. A behavioral study of ADHD subtyped along temperamental dimensions (Karalunas et al., 2014) was conducted in pursuit of a biological basis for an ADHD subtype classification. The subtypes proposed are the surgent, irritable, and mild types. The surgent subtype has greater impulsivity than control subjects and less shyness. The irritable subtype shows higher negative affective features of temperament. The mild type showed attention deficits and more impulsiveness than a comparison group. The authors examined these subtypes using neuroimaging. They found a correlation of subtypes with attentional networks. The authors concluded that the use of temperament dimensions has clinical relevance in ADHD.

ADHD research has been extended to the examination of the default mode network (DMN). A DMN study documented that unfocused attention led to mind wandering. The DMN is active when the person is at rest. This activity is reduced when the person's attention becomes focused. In ADHD, DMN activity fails to decrease when individuals with ADHD are asked to attend to task (Sonuga-Barke & Castellanos, 2007). When children with ADHD are administered stimulant medication in DMN studies, activity is decreased with improved task engagement and reduced mind wandering (Peterson et al., 2009).

Methylphenidate, a dopamine reuptake inhibitor, is effective in reducing symptoms in the majority of cases of ADHD. Methylphenidate increases attention to a task by increasing the concentration of dopamine in the synapse. This medication facilities focused attention. Consistent with the positive response of children with ADHD to dopamine-releasing drugs, several genes implicated in dopamine transmission have been studied in ADHD using the candidate gene association method. These include the *DRD4, DRD5, DAT* (the dopamine transporter), *DBH* (dopamine β-hydroxylase), and *SNAP-25* (synapse-associated protein with a molecular weight of 25 kDa) genes, each of which had a small effect size. However, although dopamine-specific genes may increase the risk of ADHD, they may have a modulatory role rather than a causative one (Franke et al., 2009, 2010). In addition, epigenetic factors impact ADHD risk through modulating the effects of genes. Both smoking in pregnancy and low birth weight are risk factors for ADHD. Finally, a development perspective is needed to examine the stability of the ADHD diagnoses, its behavioral symptoms, and their persistence into adulthood. The majority of adults who had ADHD as children show substantial improvement and may no longer meet diagnostic criteria (Kessler et al., 2005).

Neurodevelopmental disorders such as Williams–Beuren syndrome, fragile X syndrome, and phenylketonuria are genetic disorders with early onset and high risk for inattention and hyperactivity. Study of these disorders may shed light on early predictions of attentional deficits. These genetic disorders allow further examination of the relationship of genes, brain development, and attention deficits when the genetic etiology is known. Moreover, there is the potential to examine animal models of these conditions in studying attention. Finally, development trajectories of attention and behavior can be examined from infancy onward in these rare genetic disorders (Karmiloff-Smith, 2018). The available evidence indicates that instead of a generalized deficit in attention, there are different patterns of weaknesses and strengths in attention processing among the neurogenetic syndromes reviewed here.

Children with Down syndrome (Oxelgren et al., 2017), fragile X syndrome (Grefer et al., 2016), Williams–Beuren syndrome (Leyfer et al., 2006; Rhodes et al., 2011), and early treated phenylketonuria (Antshel, 2010; Beckhauser et al., 2020) have increased rates of ADHD, with a prevalence of 34% in samples of children with Down syndrome (Oxelgren et al., 2017), 54–59 % in those with fragile X syndrome (Sullivan et al., 2006), and 65% in those with Williams–Beuren syndrome, two-thirds of whom are reported to have the inattentive type (Leyfer et al., 2006). High rates of attention deficits are reported in velocardiofacial syndrome, tuberous sclerosis complex, neurofibromatosis type 1, Turner syndrome, and other neurodevelopmental syndromes. Rates in these neurodevelopmental disorders and in phenylketonuria are far higher than those reported in population-based community studies in typically developing children, in which the rates are 3–8% (Steinhausen, 2009). Twin family and adoption studies support a genetic etiology with heritability for 60–90% (Gizer et al., 2009; Sharp et al., 2009) in non-syndromic ADHD. Impairment is noted in known developmental disorders, with impairment in orienting, vigilance, and executive control. These impairments involve neuroanatomical circuits involved in attention. Syndromic ADHD may be helpful in understanding the genetic and neural pathways underlying symptoms of ADHD, with examination of the final behavioral and cognitive phenotype characteristic of each syndrome.

Attentional impairments have been studied both within and between syndromes. The components of attention have been studied. Down syndrome is a genetic disorder caused by the presence of part or all of an extra copy of chromosome 21; it is the most common cause of intellectual developmental disorder. In Down syndrome, the first step in the attention processing, reflexive visual orienting, has been examined in comparison to typically developing children taking into account the presence or absence of distractions. Reflexive orienting was found to be intact with Down syndrome at a mental age of approximately 5 years. Voluntary (deliberate) visual orienting has been studied in children and adolescents with Down syndrome and controls matched at a mental age of 5 or 6 years. The authors found that voluntary orienting was consistent with developmental level (Goldman et al., 2005). These studies find that both reflexive visual orienting (considered innate and engaged without awareness) and voluntary visual orienting that is learned and requires visual effort are intact in Down syndrome. Despite being able to voluntarily orient, there may be difficulty in prioritizing sensory input in selecting specific locations in the environment. Other studies, however, find problems in producing or maintaining optimal vigilance and in carrying out an activity in Down syndrome. Although there may be problems with vigilance, those with Down syndrome may show better vigilance than people with other intellectual disorders of comparable mental age (Trezise et al., 2008). In Down syndrome, there are also problems in executive attention control, leading to problems in focusing attention and monitoring targets for attention (Cornish et al., 2007). When people with Down syndrome are compared to matched controls, they do show similar attention skills; however, those with Down syndrome expend greater cognitive effort in approaching tasks.

Children with Down syndrome, Williams–Beuren syndrome, and fragile X syndrome have attention deficits greater than those found in typically developing children. When the subcomponents of attention are measured in each of these syndromes, there are differences among them. Both similarities and differences characterize these neurodevelopmental syndromes. In mid- to late childhood, sustained attention is a relative strength in both Down syndrome and fragile X syndrome, and it is comparable to that of typically developing children. In contrast, with regard to inhibition, children with fragile X syndrome show greater difficulties than those with Down syndrome. Selective attention is weaker in Down syndrome than fragile X syndrome. Taken together, these results indicate different developmental trajectories of attention that are syndrome-specific, not a consequence of just having an intellectual developmental disorder. Viewed developmentally, older children with Down syndrome display poorer performance on select attention measures than typically developing children and those with fragile X syndrome. Conversely, attentional search by toddlers with fragile X shows that they display substantial preservative errors compared to other groups. Thus, perseverative errors are a marker of inhibition difficulties in fragile X syndrome. Toddlers with Down syndrome do not demonstrate this type of error. Consequently, early performance in the two syndrome groups shows difficulties that continue with their attention profiles later in childhood.

When children with Down syndrome and fragile X syndrome were compared to those with Williams-Beuren syndrome, slower attentional search differentiated the toddlers with Down syndrome when group differences in chronological age and developmental level were considered. Those with Williams–Beuren syndrome showed substantial problems differentiating targets from distractors, more so than the two other syndrome groups. Moreover, in regard to orientating, the toddlers with Williams–Beuren syndrome differed from those with fragile X syndrome in their capacity to disengage from central fixation (Cornish et al., 2007). These studies of attention in these syndromes have been extended into adulthood. Just as in infancy and childhood, the most substantial attentional problem in adults with fragile X syndrome is inhibition performance. It is significantly poorer than that of adult males with Down syndrome and mental age-matched typically developing male controls (Cornish et al., 2001).

In contrast to fragile X syndrome, inhibitory performance in Down syndrome remains relatively proficient at the functional level. Regarding selective attention, adults with fragile X syndrome show more proficient performance than adults with Down syndrome, similar to childhood measures in both syndromes. Individuals with Down syndrome do continue to improve with age in inhibition and sustained attention, whereas those with fragile X syndrome show no improvement with age on these measures (Cornish et al., 2007). Children with Down syndrome and Williams–Beuren syndrome have been compared on a test of sustained attention, the continuous performance task. This study compared sustained attention in 99 typically developing children, 25 with Williams–Beuren syndrome, and 18 with Down syndrome (Shalev et al., 2019). Rather than focus on overall differences in mean performance, the authors examined the extent that performance changed over "time on task." Children with both syndromes performed poorly compared to typically developing children. The measure of change in performance predicted teacher-rated attention deficits across all three groups. Children with Williams–Beuren syndrome showed decrements in performance over time; children with Down syndrome showed nonspecific poor performance. Thus, only children with Williams–Beuren syndrome showed decrements in performance in this study. Children with Down syndrome had a more general performance deficit; they did not show a decrement over time. These findings have practical application in education of children with Williams–Beuren syndrome because they indicate that there are benefits in giving these children frequent breaks to improve task involvement over time.

Children with Williams–Beuren syndrome (prevalence of 1 in 7,500 births) have limited attention. Deficits in control of attention are in addition to their cognitive deficits. They have a behavioral phenotype similar to typical ADHD, with high rates of inattention and hyperactivity (Cornish, Cole, et al., 2012; Rhodes et al., 2010, 2011). Fragile X syndrome (prevalence of 1 in approximately 2,400 births) is associated with significant deficits in attention and social cognition—more severe than expected for their IQ scores and developmental age (Cornish, Cole, et al., 2012; Sullivan et al., 2006). In Williams–Beuren syndrome, the dorsal stream attentional system is vulnerable to attention deficits in spatial cognition and in cognitive planning (Atkinson & Braddick, 2011). In fragile X syndrome, the fragile X mental retardation protein (FMRP) is more highly expressed in magnocellular than in parvocellular neurons in the lateral geniculate nucleus. FMRP plays a role in their hyperactivity and attention deficits (Kogan et al., 2004). This difference in protein expression affects the development and functioning of the dorsal stream in fragile X syndrome, which includes the parietal cortex (Farzin & Rivera, 2010; Kogan et al., 2004). Thus, both Williams–Beuren syndrome and fragile X syndrome have dorsal attention stream vulnerability. There are distinct molecular pathways in Williams–Beuren syndrome and fragile X syndrome that converge to the dorsal attention stream abnormalities (Walter et al., 2009). Moreover, both Williams–Beuren syndrome and fragile X syndrome have frontostriatal dysfunction. In Williams–Beuren syndrome, activity is reduced in the striatum, dorsolateral prefrontal cortex, and dorsal anterior cingulate gyrus. These brain regions are required to inhibit attention tasks such as the go–no go attentional inhibition task (Mobbs et al., 2007). These systems are also significantly less recruited to attentional responding than in typical control subjects (Hoeft et al., 2011). The previously mentioned studies were conducted with relatively high-functioning individuals with the syndrome who could complete study tasks; further study of attention is needed for genetic disorders.

In summary, across-syndrome comparisons in more cognitively impaired children show similarities and differences among neurogenetic syndromes that have attentional profiles similar to typical ADHD cases. Despite commonality in behavioral factors and dorsal attention stream vulnerability, there are differences among these syndromes. For example, toddlers and children with Williams–Beuren syndrome and fragile X syndrome differ in the way they orient their attention (Scerif & Wu, 2014). There are also different developmental trajectories of attention deficits as children with these two syndromes mature. Such changes with development indicate the importance of differentiating neurocognitive trajectories of attention deficits. How attention shapes life experiences and learning in these syndromes is an ongoing pursuit. Attention control is a developmental vulnerability across neurogenetic disorders. It interacts with learning and memory. Attention deficits in neurogenetic syndromes are discussed in more detail in Part IV. Phenylketonuria, velocardiofacial syndrome, tuberous sclerosis complex, and other genetic syndromes that have characteristic attention deficits are also discussed in Part IV.

# References

American Psychiatric Association. (2013). *Diagnostic and statistical manual of mental disorders* (5th ed.). American Psychiatric Publishing.

Antshel, K. M. (2010). ADHD, learning, and academic performance in phenylketonuria. *Molecular Genetics and Metabolism, 99*, S52–S58.

Atkinson, J., & Braddick, O. (2011). From genes to brain development to phenotypic behavior: "Dorsal-stream vulnerability" in relation to spatial cognition, attention, and planning of actions in Williams syndrome (WS) and other developmental disorders. Progress in *Brain Research, 189*, 261–283.

Baird, B., Mota-Rolim, S. A., & Dresler, M. (2019). The cognitive neuroscience of lucid dreaming. *Neuroscience and Biobehavioral Reviews, 100*, 305–323.

Beckhauser, M. T., Vieira, M. B. M., Iser, B. M., de Luca, G. R., Masruha, M. R., Lin, J., & Streck, E. L. (2020). Attention deficit disorder with hyperactivity symptoms in early-treated phenylketonuria patients. *Iranian Journal of Child Neurology, 14*(1), 93–103.

Belsky, J., & Pluess, M. (2009). Beyond diathesis stress: Differential susceptibility to environmental influences. *Psychological Bulletin, 135*(6), 885–908.

Boyce, W. T. (2016). Differential susceptibility of the developing brain to contextual adversity and stress. *Neuropsychopharmacology, 41*(1), 142–162.

Brodeur, D. A., & Enns, J. T. (1997). Covert visual orienting across the lifespan. *Canadian Journal of Experimental Psychology, 51*(1), 20–35.

Bush, G., Luu, P., & Posner, M. I. (2000). Cognitive and emotional influences in anterior cingulate cortex. *Trends in Cognitive Sciences, 4*(6), 215–222.

Colombo, J. (2001). The development of visual attention in infancy. *Annual Review of Psychology, 52*(1), 337–367.

Cornish, K., Cole, V., Longhi, E., Karmiloff-Smith, A., & Scerif, G. (2012). Does attention constrain developmental trajectories in fragile X syndrome? A 3-year prospective longitudinal study. *American Journal on Intellectual and Developmental Disabilities, 117*(2), 103–120.

Cornish, K., Munir, F., & Cross, G. (2001). Differential impact of the FMR-1 full mutation on memory and attention functioning: A neuropsychological perspective. *Journal of Cognitive Neuroscience, 13*(1), 144–150.

Cornish, K., Scerif, G., & Karmiloff-Smith, A. (2007). Tracing syndrome-specific trajectories of attention across the lifespan. *Cortex, 43*(6), 672–685.

Cornish, K., Steele, A., Rondinelli Cobra Monteiro, C., Karmiloff-Smith, A. D., & Scerif, G. (2012). Attention deficits predict phenotypic outcomes in syndrome-specific and domain-specific ways. *Frontiers in Psychology, 3*, Article 227.

Day, J. J., Childs, D., Guzman-Karlsson, M. C., Kibe, M., Moulden, J., Song, E., Tahir, A., & Sweatt, J. D. (2013). DNA methylation regulates associative reward learning. *Nature Neuroscience, 16*(10), 1445–1452.

Diamond, A. (2006). The early development of executive functions. In E. Bialystok & F. I. M. Craik (Eds.), Lifespan *cognition*: Mechanisms of *change* (pp. 70–95). Oxford University Press.

Diamond, A., Briand, L., Fossella, J., & Gehlbach, L. (2004). Genetic and neurochemical modulation of prefrontal cognitive functions in children. *American Journal of Psychiatry, 161*(1), 125–132.

Dosenbach, N. U., Fair, D. A., Cohen, A. L., Schlaggar, B. L., & Petersen, S. E. (2008). A dual-networks architecture of top-down control. *Trends in Cognitive Sciences, 12*(3), 99–105.

Etkin, A., Egner, T., Peraza, D. M., Kandel, E. R., & Hirsch, J. (2006). Resolving emotional conflict: A role for the rostral anterior cingulate cortex in modulating activity in the amygdala. *Neuron, 51*(6), 871–882.

Fair, D. A., Dosenbach, N. U., Church, J. A., Cohen, A. L., Brahmbhatt, S., Miezin, F. M., Barch, D. M., Raichle, M. E., Petersen, S. E., & Schlaggar, B. L. (2007). Development of distinct control networks through segregation and integration. *Proceedings of the National Academy of Sciences of the USA, 104*(33), 13507–13512.

Fan, J., Flombaum, J. I., McCandliss, B. D., Thomas, K. M., & Posner, M. I. (2003). Cognitive and brain consequences of conflict. *NeuroImage, 18*(1), 42–57.

Fan, J., Fossella, J., Sommer, T., Wu, Y., & Posner, M. I. (2003). Mapping the genetic variation of executive attention onto brain activity. *Proceedings of the National Academy of Sciences of the USA, 100*(12), 7406–7411.

Farzin, F., & Rivera, S. M. (2010). Dynamic object representations in infants with and without fragile X syndrome. *Frontiers in Human Neuroscience, 4*, Article 12.

Fields, R. D. (2015). A new mechanism of nervous system plasticity: Activity-dependent myelination. *Nature Reviews Neuroscience, 16*(12), 756–767.

Filevich, E., Dresler, M., Brick, T. R., & Kühn, S. (2015). Metacognitive mechanisms underlying lucid dreaming. *Journal of Neuroscience, 35*(3), 1082–1088.

Fjell, A. M., Walhovd, K. B., Brown, T. T., Kuperman, J. M., Chung, Y., Hagler, D. J., Jr., Venkatraman, V., Roddey, J. C., Erhart, M., McCabe, C., Akshoomoff, N., Amaral, D., Bloss, C., Libiger, O., Darst, B., Schork, N., Casey, B., Chang, L., Ernst, T., . . . Dale, A.; Pediatric Imaging, Neurocognition, and Genetics Study. (2012). Multimodal imaging of the self-regulating developing brain. *Proceedings of the National Academy of Sciences of the USA, 109*(48), 19620–19625.

Fossella, J., Posner, M. I., Fan, J., Swanson, J. M., & Pfaff, D. W. (2002). Attentional phenotypes for the analysis of higher mental function. *ScientificWorldJournal, 2*, 217–223.

Franke, B., Neale, B. M., & Faraone, S. V. (2009). Genome-wide association studies in ADHD. *Human Genetics, 126*(1), 13–50.

Franke, B., Vasquez, A. A., Johansson, S., Hoogman, M., Romanos, J., Boreatti-Hümmer, A., Heine, M., Jacob, C., Lesch, K.-P., Casas, M., Ribasés, M., Bosch, R., Sanchez-Mora, C., Gomez-Barros, N., Fernandez-Castillo, N., Bayes, M., Halmoy, A., Halleland, H., Landaas, E., . . . Reif, A.(2010). Multicenter analysis of the *SLC6A3/DAT1* VNTR haplotype in persistent ADHD suggests differential involvement of the gene in childhood and persistent ADHD. *Neuropsychopharmacology, 35*(3), 656–664.

Gao, W., Zhu, H., Giovanello, K. S., Smith, J. K., Shen, D., Gilmore, J. H., & Lin, W. (2009). Evidence on the emergence of the brain's default network from 2-week-old to 2-year-old healthy pediatric subjects. *Proceedings of the National Academy of Sciences of the USA, 106*(16), 6790–6795.

Gizer, I. R., Ficks, C., & Waldman, I. D. (2009). Candidate gene studies of ADHD: A meta-analytic review. *Human Genetics, 126*(1), 51–90.

Goldman, K. J., Flanagan, T., Shulman, C., Enns, J. T., & Burack, J. A. (2005). Voluntary orienting among children and adolescents with Down syndrome and MA-matched typically developing children. *American Journal on Mental Retardation, 110*(3), 157–163.

Grefer, M., Flory, K., Cornish, K., Hatton, D., & Roberts, J. (2016). The emergence and stability of attention deficit hyperactivity disorder in boys with fragile X syndrome. *Journal of Intellectual Disability Research, 60*(2), 167–178.

Harman, C., Rothbart, M. K., & Posner, M. I. (1997). Distress and attention interactions in early infancy. *Motivation and Emotion, 21*(1), 27–43.

Hoeft, F., Walter, E., Lightbody, A. A., Hazlett, H. C., Chang, C., Piven, J., & Reiss, A. L. (2011). Neuroanatomical differences in toddler boys with fragile X syndrome and idiopathic autism. *Archives of General Psychiatry, 68*(3), 295–305.

Hölzel, B. K., Lazar, S. W., Gard, T., Schuman-Olivier, Z., Vago, D. R., & Ott, U. (2011). How does mindfulness meditation work? Proposing mechanisms of action from a conceptual and neural perspective. *Perspectives on Psychological Science, 6*(6), 537–559.

Hommel, B., Pratt, J., Colzato, L., & Godijn, R. (2001). Symbolic control of visual attention. *Psychological Science, 12*(5), 360–365.

Iarocci, G., Enns, J. T., Randolph, B., & Burack, J. A. (2009). The modulation of visual orienting reflexes across the lifespan. *Developmental Science, 12*(5), 715–724.

Iarocci, G., Porporino, M., Enns, J. T., & Burack, J. A. (2012). Understanding the development of attention in persons with intellectual disability: Challenging the myths. In J. A. Burack & R. M. Hodapp (Eds.), *The Oxford handbook of intellectual disability and development* (pp. 89–96). Oxford University Press.

Ivry, R. B., & Robertson, L. C. (1998). *The two sides of perception.* MIT Press.

James, W. (1890). *Principles of psychology.* (Vol. 1). Holt.

Jones, L. B., Rothbart, M. K., & Posner, M. I. (2003). Development of executive attention in pre-school children. *Developmental Science, 6*(5), 498–504.

Karalunas, S. L., Fair, D., Musser, E. D., Aykes, K., Iyer, S. P., & Nigg, J. T. (2014). Subtyping attention-deficit/hyperactivity disorder using temperament dimensions: Toward biologically based nosologic criteria. *JAMA Psychiatry, 71*(9), 1015–1024.

Karmiloff-Smith, A. (2018). Development itself is the key to understanding developmental disorders. In A. Karmiloff-Smith, M. S. C. Thomas, & M. H. Johnson (Eds.), *Thinking developmentally from constructivism to neuroconstructivism* (pp. 97–117). Routledge.

Kessler, R. C., Adler, L. A., Barkley, R., Biederman, J., Conners, C. K., Faraone, S. V., Greenhill, L., Jaeger, S., Secnik, K., Spencer, T., Üstün, T. B., & Zaslavsky, A. (2005). Patterns and predictors of attention-deficit/hyperactivity disorder persistence into adulthood: Results from the National Comorbidity Survey Replication. *Biological Psychiatry, 57*(11), 1442–1451.

Kogan, C. S., Boutet, I., Cornish, K., Zangenehpour, S., Mullen, K. T., Holden, J. J., Der Kaloustian, V. M., Andermann, E., & Chaudhuri, A. (2004). Differential impact of the FMR1 gene on visual processing in fragile X syndrome. *Brain, 127*(3), 591–601.

Konrad, K., Neufang, S., Thiel, C. M., Specht, K., Hanisch, C., Fan, J., Herpertz-Dahlmann, B., & Fink, G. R. (2005). Development of attentional networks: An fMRI study with children and adults. *Neuroimage, 28*(2), 429–439.

Levy, F. (1980). The development of sustained attention (vigilance) and inhibition in children: Some normative data. *Journal of Child Psychology and Psychiatry, 21*(1), 77–84.

Leyfer, O. T., Woodruff-Borden, J., Klein-Tasman, B. P., Fricke, J. S., & Mervis, C. B. (2006). Prevalence of psychiatric disorders in 4 to 16-year-olds with Williams syndrome. *American Journal of Medical Genetics Part B: Neuropsychiatric Genetics, 141*(6), 615–622.

Marrocco, R. T., & Davidson, M. C. (1998). Neurochemistry of attention. In R. Parasuraman (Ed.), *The attentive brain* (pp 35–50). MIT Press.

Meltzoff, A. N., & Moore, M. K. (1977). Imitation of facial and manual gestures by human neonates. *Science, 198*(4312), 75–78.

Mobbs, D., Eckert, M. A., Mills, D., Korenberg, J., Bellugi, U., Galaburda, A. M., & Reiss, A. L. (2007). Frontostriatal dysfunction during response inhibition in Williams syndrome. *Biological Psychiatry, 62*(3), 256–261.

Murray, J., Theakston, A., & Wells, A. (2016). Can the attention training technique turn one marshmallow into two? Improving children's ability to delay gratification. *Behaviour Research and Therapy, 77*, 34–39.

Neta, M., Nelson, S. M., & Petersen, S. E. (2017). Dorsal anterior cingulate, medial superior frontal cortex, and anterior insula show performance reporting-related late task control signals. *Cerebral Cortex, 27*(3), 2154–2165.

Oxelgren, U. W., Myrelid, Å., Annerén, G., Ekstam, B., Göransson, C., Holmbom, A., Isaksson, A., Aberg, M., Gustafsson, J., & Fernell, E. (2017). Prevalence of autism and attention-deficit–hyperactivity disorder in Down syndrome: A population-based study. *Developmental Medicine & Child Neurology, 59*(3), 276–283.

Oyebode, F. (2018). *Sims' symptoms in the mind: Textbook of descriptive psychopathology.* Elsevier.

Petersen, S. E., & Posner, M. I. (2012). The attention system of the human brain: 20 years after. *Annual Review of Neuroscience, 35*, 73–89.

Peterson, B. S., Potenza, M. N., Wang, Z., Zhu, H., Martin, A., Marsh, R., Plessen, K., & Yu, S. (2009). An fMRI study of the effects of psychostimulants on default-mode processing during Stroop task performance in youths with ADHD. *American Journal of Psychiatry, 166*(11), 1286–1294.

Plude, D. J., Enns, J. T., & Brodeur, D. (1994). The development of selective attention: A life-span overview. *Acta Psychologica, 86*(2–3), 227–272.

Posner, M. I. (2011). *Attention in a social world.* Oxford University Press.

Posner, M. I., & Rothbart, M. K. (2007). Research on attention networks as a model for the integration of psychological science. *Annual Review of Psychology, 58*, 1–23.

Posner, M. I., Rothbart, M. K., & Rueda, M. R. (2014). Developing attention and self-regulation in childhood. In A. C. Nobre & S. Kastner (Eds.), *The Oxford handbook of attention* (pp. 541–571). Oxford University Press.

Posner, M. I., Rothbart, M. K., & Voelker, P. (2016). Developing brain networks of attention. *Current Opinion in Pediatrics, 28*(6), 720–724.

Pozuelos, J. P., Paz-Alonso, P. M., Castillo, A., Fuentes, L. J., & Rueda, M. R. (2014). Development of attention networks and their interactions in childhood. *Developmental Psychology, 50*(10), 2405–2415.

Raichle, M. E. (2009). A paradigm shift in functional brain imaging. *Journal of Neuroscience, 29*(41), 12729–12734.

Rhodes, S. M., Riby, D. M., Matthews, K., & Coghill, D. R. (2011). Attention-deficit/hyperactivity disorder and Williams syndrome: Shared behavioral and neuropsychological profiles. *Journal of Clinical and Experimental Neuropsychology, 33*(1), 147–156.

Rhodes, S. M., Riby, D. M., Park, J., Fraser, E., & Campbell, L. E. (2010). Executive neuropsychological functioning in individuals with Williams syndrome. *Neuropsychologia, 48*(5), 1216–1226.

Richards, J. E., & Hunter, S. K. (1998). Attention and eye movement in young infants: Neural control and development. In M. Posner (Ed.), *Cognitive neuroscience of attention* (pp. 141–172). Psychology Press.

Rothbart, M. K., Ellis, L. K., Rosario Rueda, M., & Posner, M. I. (2003). Developing mechanisms of temperamental effortful control. *Journal of Personality, 71*(6), 1113–1144.

Rueda, M. R., Checa, P., & Combita, L. M. (2012). Enhanced efficiency of the executive attention network after training in preschool children: Immediate changes and effects after two months. *Developmental Cognitive Neuroscience, 2*, S192–S204.

Rueda, M. R., Posner, M. I., & Rothbart, M. K. (2005). The development of executive attention: Contributions to the emergence of self-regulation. *Developmental Neuropsychology, 28*(2), 573–594.

Rueda, M. R., Pozuelos, J. P., & Cómbita, L. M. (2015). Cognitive neuroscience of attention from brain mechanisms to individual differences in efficiency. *AIMS Neuroscience, 2*(4), 83–202.

Ruff, H. A., & Rothbart, M. K. (2001). *Attention in early development: Themes and variations.* Oxford University Press.

Scerif, G., & Wu, R. (2014). Developmental disorders. In A. C. Nobre & S. Kastner (Eds.), *The Oxford handbook of attention* (pp. 893–925). Oxford University Press.

Schul, R., Townsend, J., & Stiles, J. (2003). The development of attentional orienting during the school-age years. *Developmental Science, 6*(3), 262–272.

Sharp, S. I., McQuillin, A., & Gurling, H. M. (2009). Genetics of attention-deficit hyperactivity disorder (ADHD). *Neuropharmacology, 57*(7–8), 590–600.

Sheese, B. E., Voelker, P. M., Rothbart, M. K., & Posner, M. I. (2007). Parenting quality interacts with genetic variation in dopamine receptor D4 to influence temperament in early childhood. *Development and Psychopathology, 19*(4), 1039–1046.

Shore, D. I., Burack, J. A., Miller, D., Joseph, S., & Enns, J. T. (2006). The development of change detection. *Developmental Science, 9*(5), 490–497.

Sonuga-Barke, E. J., & Castellanos, F. X. (2007). Spontaneous attentional fluctuations in impaired states and pathological conditions: A neurobiological hypothesis. *Neuroscience and Biobehavioral Reviews, 31*(7), 977–986.

Steinhausen, H. C. (2009). The heterogeneity of causes and courses of attention-deficit/hyperactivity disorder. *Acta Psychiatrica Scandinavica, 120*(5), 392–399.

Sullivan, K., Hatton, D., Hammer, J., Sideris, J., Hooper, S., Ornstein, P., & Bailey, D., Jr. (2006). ADHD symptoms in children with FXS. *American Journal of Medical Genetics Part A, 140*(21), 2275–2288.

Tang, Y. Y., Posner, M. I., & Rothbart, M. K. (2014). Meditation improves self-regulation over the life span. *Annals of the New York Academy of Sciences, 1307*, 104–111.

Trezise, K. L., Gray, K. M., & Sheppard, D. M. (2008). Attention and vigilance in children with Down syndrome. *Journal of Applied Research in Intellectual Disabilities, 21*(6), 502–508.

Voelker, P., Piscopo, D., Weible, A. P., Lynch, G., Rothbart, M. K., Posner, M. I., & Niell, C. M. (2017). How changes in white matter might underlie improved reaction time due to practice. *Cognitive Neuroscience, 8*(2), 112–118.

Voelker, P., Sheese, B. E., Rothbart, M. K., & Posner, M. I. (2009). Variations in catechol-*O*-methyltransferase gene interact with parenting to influence attention in early development. *Neuroscience, 164*(1), 121–130.

Voelker, P., Sheese, B. E., Rothbart, M. K., & Posner, M. I. (2017). Methylation polymorphism influences practice effects in children during attention tasks. *Cognitive Neuroscience, 8*(2), 72–84.

Walter, E., Mazaika, P. K., & Reiss, A. L. (2009). Insights into brain development from neurogenetic syndromes: Evidence from fragile X syndrome, Williams syndrome, Turner syndrome and velocardiofacial syndrome. *Neuroscience, 164*(1), 257–271.

Wass, S., Porayska-Pomsta, K., & Johnson, M. H. (2011). Training attentional control in infancy. *Current Biology, 21*(18), 1543–1547.

Wright, R. D., & Ward, L. M. (2008). *Orientation of attention.* Oxford University Press.

# 4

# Emotion

Emotions are essential to evolutionary adaptation and survival. In his classic book, *The Expression of the Emotions in Man and Animals*, Darwin (1872/2009) emphasized that natural selection focuses on both the evolution of physical structure and the domain of the mind and behavior of the emotions. He found that specific emotions have similar expression in people throughout the world. This includes remote areas where an opportunity to learn emotional expression through cultural transmission was highly unlikely. Darwin found that specific emotions find similar expression across species, indicating phylogenetic conservation. Early experimental brain research in the late 19th century sought to link emotion to the brain. If indeed emotional circuits in the brain are conserved, emotion could be explored in both animal models and human development (LeDoux & Damasio, 2013). Modern affective neuroscience examines our current understanding of emotion and the brain.

This chapter reviews definitions of emotion and related terms, historical issues in the study of emotion, the development of the primary emotions, the emergence of self-conscious emotions, the relationship of emotion and cognition (attention, memory, and decisions), and the affective neuroscience of emotion and feelings in the conscious expression of emotion (Adolphs, 2017).

## Definitions

Emotional states have been categorized according to type, intensity, and duration. Six main groups of emotions are expressed in the face: joy, surprise, fear, sadness, anger, and disgust/contempt (Ekman, 1999; Gazzaniga et al., 2019). A seventh emotion, interest, has been described (Izard, 1991). These emotions may be communicated by body postures and through facial expressions, gestures, tone of voice, and general appearance. Emotion is assessed empathetically, so if someone is friendly and cheerful on greeting, then the feeling of cheerfulness may be experienced by the recipient. One literally puts oneself in the place of another through empathy. *Emotion* is the term generally used to describe physiological and psychosomatic concomitants of mood (Oyebode, 2018). Emotion should not be confused with feeling and affect—each word has a specific meaning. Emotion refers to a state of the self, whereas the word "feeling" is more often used to describe conscious experiences of both emotions and sensations. Jaspers (1959/1963) contrasted conscious feelings associated with emotions, such as sadness and joy, with the more global, vital feelings, where an emotion is described subjectively as encompassing the whole organism. An emotional state may also be designated according to its biological purpose and, in this context, would be described as an instinct.

*Mood* is a pervasive and sustained emotional state or frame of mind that, when intense, colors a person's perception of the world (American Psychiatric Association [APA], 2013; Jaspers, 1959/1963). Moreover, a mood is a prolonged state and shows considerable variation. Mood is typically used to describe one's psychological state in relation to the environment. Feeling is the term used to describe a positive or negative reaction to an experience. *Feeling* refers to both the active experience of sensation (e.g., touch) and the subjective experience of emotion. *Affect* in psychiatry refers to the expression of emotion. Whereas feeling is an individual unique emotional response, affect describes a momentary and complex emotional arousal. Affects are processes of considerable intensity. Affect describes a pattern of observable behaviors that express subjectively experienced feeling states based on emotions such as sadness, elation, and anger. Affect fluctuates and is variable over time in response to changes in emotional state, in contrast to mood, which is pervasive and sustained over time. Therefore, there is a range of affect that may be described as labile, restricted, constricted, inappropriate, blunted, or flat (APA, 2013). Normal affective expression is indicated through variability in facial expression, voice tone, and expressive hand and body movements. When labeled, there is variability in affect with abrupt, repeated, and rapid shifts in affective expression. When restricted or constricted, there is reduction in the range and intensity of emotions expressed. Where inappropriate, there is discordance between affect expression and ideation on speech content. When blended, there is substantial reduction of emotion, sensitivity, and expression. When flat, there is an absence or near absence of affective expression (APA, 2013), with unchanging facial expressions, decreased spontaneity, and lack of vocal inflection.

In affective disorders, typically the primary focus is on mood. In sadness, there are expressions of gloom, despondency, despair, or helplessness. The actual experience by the person is qualitatively distinct from normal sadness and more like physical pain; sometimes it is described as a sense of painful abject emptiness. Similarly, there may be exacerbation of joy that progresses to mania, ecstasy, and intensification of fear, anger, and surprise.

In *General Psychopathology*, Jaspers (1959/1963) concentrated on three aspects of mood and affect: the involvement of the self, the contrast of opposites, and the object toward which the response was directed. Regarding the self, feelings are experienced by the self, but empathy may be directed toward others. The judgment that another person is sad or happy based on a facial expression or that a picture looks sad results from the response it evokes in the observer. On the other hand, the intensity of affect also is experienced in polar opposites. Visual analog scales of mood confirm this in their request for self-report rating of changes in mood. Furthermore, feelings may be directed toward an object (e.g., fear of a dog) or may have no object, as in the case of anxiety.

## History

An important contribution to the study of emotions in the 19th century was Charles Darwin's *The Expression of the Emotions in Man and Animals,* published in 1872 (Darwin, 1872/1965). He emphasized that there are specific fundamental emotions, which are expressed in overt behavior. Subsequently, in 1884, William James suggested that the outward signs of emotions, such as facial expressions or bodily responses, are not the result of prior emotional signals but, rather, that "our feeling of the bodily changes as they occur is the emotion." A similar point was made by C. G. Lange in 1885; this position is known as the James–Lange theory of emotion (i.e., an external event perceived by an individual produces a bodily response, and it is the perception of these bodily events that constitutes the emotional experience). The implication is that a specific emotional experience is produced by a specific and unique set of bodily and visceral responses. In the 1920s, W. B. Cannon (1927, 1929) published a critique of the James–Lange theory. He suggested that emotional behavior was still present when internal organs were surgically or accidentally disconnected from the central nervous system, so emotions did not differ in important ways in the associated visceral response. He noted that autonomic responses are slow and emotional experience occurs quickly. The two theorists leave us with this question: Is emotion experienced because we perceive our bodies in a particular way, or are there specific emotional neural systems in the brain that respond to environmental events? As Gregory and Zangwill (1987) ask, Do we grieve because we cry, or do we cry because we grieve?

Historically, this debate on the emotions went into decline when behavioralism was the primary paradigm in psychology. With the behavioral focus on objective and observable data, less emphasis was placed on the study of emotion. However, with the emergence of developmental cognitive psychology, cognitive aspects of emotion were fully addressed. The cognitive view is that novelty, discrepancy, and interruption of our perceived cognitive sets lead to visceral responses, which cognitively are interpreted and experienced as sadness, fear, joy, and other feelings. With the establishment of a cognitive approach to emotion, developmental cognitive neuroscience is free to study the brain mechanisms linked to emotion.

## Theories of Emotion Generation

The response to emotional experience is an adaptive one with three components: the physiologic reaction (e.g., increased heart rate), the behavioral reaction (e.g., fight or flight), and subjective feeling (e.g., fear). Theories of emotion generation seek to understand these three responses regarding the timing of the three components and whether cognition is involved (Gazzaniga et al., 2019). Because research scientists disagree on how emotions are generated and also the role that cognition plays or does not play in generating or processing emotions, several theories have been proposed to understand emotion generation (Gazzaniga et al., 2019). Those discussed here are the Cannon–Bard theory, the appraisal theory, the Singer–Scharter theory, LeDoux's fast and slow road to emotion, the evolutionary perspective, Porges' polyvagal model, Panksepp's hierarchal processing theory of emotion, and Anderson and Adolphs' view that emotions are central caused states.

Cannon and Bard (1927) proposed that emotions and their underlying physiology are experienced simultaneously and that emotional experiences are the result of neural activity in brain circuits. Consequently, when sensory stimuli are transmitted through the brain to the thalamus, the thalamus conveys them simultaneously to the neocortex and hypothalamus. The thalamic–sensory inputs are conveyed to the hypothalamus;

the cortex that receives the physiologic response evaluates their significance and generates the emotional feeling. The Cannon–Bard theory suggests that emotional experiences are created via parallel processing involving the hypothalamus and cerebral cortex. The information transmitted to the cortex determines the quality of emotional experience.

The appraisal theory (Lazarus, 1991) focuses on cognition as the first step. Thus, emotions are a response to cognitive appraisal of harm or risk. We first appraise the significance of the stimulus that alerts us to danger. In this model, cognitive appraisal comes first before emotional response or feeling. Such appraisal may be automatic and out of conscious awareness. For example, a person sees a bear, automatically senses danger, becomes aware of fear, and runs.

The next approach is the cognitive arousal theory (Schachter & Singer, 1962), which states that the body's reaction is the emotion. Schachter and Singer propose that emotional experiences occur when the brain becomes aware that the body is in the state of heightened physiologic arousal. In this theory, stimuli from the environment are conveyed to the brain, where they initiate emotionally ambiguous peripheral emotional responses, especially in the autonomic nervous system and neurohormonal systems. Nonspecific arousal is transmitted to the brain, which elicits an evaluation process. The brain interprets emotionally ambiguous states from situational cues from both the physical environment and the social environment. Earlier, William James had proposed that the physiologic feedback from the periphery determines the nature of emotional experience. However, Cannon and Bard had successfully argued that peripheral autonomic feedback was not sufficiently specific to determine the nature of experience because there were too many inputs to have a specific pattern of each one. The Singer–Schachter cognitive arousal theory solution was to add cognition in the chain between nonspecific arousal and experience. It posits that emotional arousal is followed by identifying the emotion. Joseph LeDoux (2012) has proposed instead that there are two emotion systems that act in parallel. He refers to them as fast and slow. The fast system directly engages the amygdala and bypasses the cortex. This system is an evolutionary neural system geared to produce a rapid response to danger. LeDoux's vision of earlier theories draws attention to a critical subcortical brain region, the amygdala, that is involved in receiving sensory input. The amygdala projects to structures in the hypothalamus and brain stem that regulate the autonomic expression of fear throughout the brain. In this model, transmission from the amygdala to the brain stem and cortex underlies emotion generation (Gazzaniga et al., 2019; LeDoux, 2012). This neuronal system is an experience expectant neuronal system that arose early in evolution to enhance survival when there is danger (Greenough et al., 1987). The slow system that involves cognition is more accurate but slower. This second system, involving cognition, generates conscious feelings of emotion. Conscious feelings emerge with experience during development as children learn to find words for various forms of emotional arousal—that is, feelings—and find words for fear, sadness, joy, and anger to identify patterns of emotional arousal. Consequently, words such as fear become linked to subjective feelings. LeDoux refers to those brain circuits that respond to threat as defensive and to responsive behavior as defensive behavior (LeDoux, 2014). This model is further refined in regard to appraisal of threat in Porges' neuroception, polyvagal model that focuses on the evolution of the automatic nervous system (Porges, 2001, 2004).

## Porges' Polyvagal Model

The evolution of the automatic nervous system provides a means to interpret the adaptive significance of physiologic emotional arousal that underlies social behavior. The polyvagal model accounts for neural regulation of the automatic nervous system. There are three evolving stages of response to threat. The first response, and most primitive, is social withdrawal with immobilization. If the threat is severe, feigning immobilization involves faking death in animals and psychological dissociation in traumatized humans. The second response to threat is fight or flight as defined by Cannon and Bard. The third response to threat is an adaptive response of social engagement when cognitive appraisal puts the threat in context and finds a way to assertively respond to the threat (Porges, 2001, 2004).

## Panksepp's Hierarchal Processing Theory of Emotion

Panksepp proposes that there is a hierarchal emotion control system (Panksepp & Biven, 2012; see also Gazzaniga et al., 2019). Thus, depending on the emotion, processing proceeds in one of three ways. Basic emotions, such as fear conditioning (Davis et al., 2010; LeDoux, 2014), arise from evolutionary evolved core neural networks in the subcortical brain. Subsequently, there is emotional learning elaborated by cognition. This involves the integration of limbic and paralimbic structures with the neocortex (Panksepp & Biven, 2012). Panksepp describes seven basic emotional systems across all mammalian species. When they are disrupted, the result is an emotional disorder. These emotional systems are (a) seeking (how the brain generates expectant or euphoric responses), (b) rage (aggressive responses), (c) fear (how the brain responds to physical danger), (d) lust (primitive sexual arousal), (e) care (nurturance), (f) panic/sadness and play (positive, rough and tumble interaction often accompanied in humans by "play face" to alert there is no danger), and (g) self (how emotions are elaborated in the brain to maintain self-esteem).

## Anderson and Adolphs' Emotions

Anderson and Adolphs (2014) offer a framework for studying emotion across species. They propose that emotional behaviors are a class of behaviors that evolved to express internal emotional states. These emotional states have adaptive features that apply to human emotions, such as fear and anger, and across phylogeny, and they can be modeled in organizations that are evolutionarily different from humans. They propose that emotional stimulus, such as danger, activates a central nervous system state. That activated state simultaneously activates multiple systems, resulting in separate responses. These include physiological response, feelings, cognitive changes, and behavior. This approach leads to a revised approach to operationalizing emotion within psychiatry and psychology. These authors view emotions in humans and animals fundamentally as biological phenomena. Because emotions are ubiquitous across species and evolved through processes of natural selection, studies in both animals and humans are needed.

Their focus is on the emotional state rather than the conscious experience of emotion. This approach, they propose, is compatible with manipulation by the methods of neuroscience (Adolphs & Anderson, 2018).

## Evolutionary Approaches to Emotion

In preparation for writing *The Expression of the Emotions in Man and Animals* (Darwin, 1872/1965), Darwin carefully read psychiatrist Henry Maudsley's 1870 Gulstonian lectures, *Body and Mind: Their Connection and Mutual Influence* (Maudsley, 1870). Darwin noted that pain and suffering of any kind, if long continued, cause depression and lessen the power of action. His biological approach focuses on six emotional states: happiness, sadness, fear, anger, surprise, and disgust. It includes illustrations from both nonhuman primates and men. He also referred to low spirits (anxiety, grief, and despair) and high spirits (joy, love, and devotion).

Darwin's (1872/1965) book emphasizes the evolution of emotional expression. Human faces were drawn from asylums, including the Salpêtrière in Paris and the West Riding Pauper Lunatic Asylum in Wakefield, UK. Darwin emphasizes the importance of emotional communication to facilitate psychological development and consulted with leading psychiatrists. Darwin's book on the expression of emotions has remained continuously in print. Its impact was highlighted by the New York Academy of Sciences in its retrospective on Darwin's *The Expression of the Emotions in Man and Animals* featuring more than 30 papers (Ekman, 2003).

## The Limbic System and the Emotional Brain

The proposal that neural networks of cognition and emotion are distinct in the brain was presented by James Papez in his 1937 paper, "A Proposed Mechanism of Emotion." In 1878, Paul Broca introduced the term *limbic lobe* (Latin *limbus* meaning rim) for structures that surrounded the brain stem (Pessoa & Hof, 2015). Papez proposed that emotional experience is based on connections linking the hypothalamus, anterior thalamus, cingulate gyrus, and hippocampus. Paul McLean, later chief of the National Institute of Mental Health (NIMH) Laboratory for Brain Evolution and Behavior, amplified and reconceptualized Papez's proposal in his description of the limbic system, which detailed the brain circuits involved with the processing of emotion. He viewed the limbic system as a circuit consisting of the limbic lobe and its major connections in the forebrain—the hypothalamus, amygdala, and septum—along with other portions of the orbital frontal cortex, as shown in Figure 4.1.

MacLean's identification of the limbic system as the emotional brain continues to influence those who seek to understand the evolution of emotions (Panksepp & Biven, 2012). MacLean's interest in subjective experience stemmed from his work with patients with psychomotor epilepsy because their symptoms include emotional feelings and somatic symptoms (MacLean, 1949). MacLean wrote that emotional feelings elude "the group of intellect" (p. 348) because their origins are in evolutionary primitive structures, thus preventing their verbal communication of them to others. Essentially,

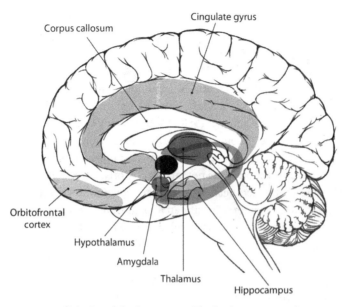

**Figure 4.1**  Anatomy of MacLean's limbic system. The limbic system, whose primary structures are identified here, contains complex neural circuits that Paul MacLean posited were involved in the processing of emotion.

FromGazzaniga, Ivry and Mangun (2019); redrawn by Tim Phelps (2021).

"this underlying biology provides a clue to understanding the difference between what we feel and what we know" (Newman & Harris, 2009, p. 3). His research on the limbic system led to the creation of the NIMH section on Limbic Integration and Behavior and subsequently to the NIMH Laboratory of Brain Evolution and Behavior. At the laboratory, MacLean traced the evolution of the brain from reptiles to mammals. Later, he reconceptualized the limbic system as the paleomammalian brain. He determined that the reptilian brain was the forerunner to the striate pallidal complex of mammals. This research led him to propose a triune brain as evolution progresses from proto-reptilian formation to the paleomammalian brain (limbic complex) to the neomammalian brain. In human evolution, these three evolutionary steps led to the integrated human brain. The matrix of the brain stem evolved from the reptilian brain and includes the reticular system, midbrain, and basal ganglia. Early mammalian structures above them include the oldest parts of the cerebral cortex, and related brain stem nuclei (limbic brain) appeared last in evolution as the elaborated cerebral cortex. The cerebral cortex and its associated nuclei of the brain stem form the most recent evolutionary advance. Metaphorically, the cerebral cortex, with its regulatory functions, serves as the "thinking cap of the brain."

Seeking to understand the evolution of social behavior, MacLean focused on the evolution of the mammalian brain and its role in family life. He found evidence that the thalamocingulate division of the limbic system was found only in mammals. He proposed that the thalamocingulate brain region mediated and facilitated maternal care, audiovisual mother–infant communication (the isolation or separation call that alerted the mother to the infant's location), nursing, and play behavior (MacLean,

1985). As evidence of the distinctness of the paleomammalian (limbic) brain function, MacLean and colleagues demonstrated that hamsters whose neocortex was removed at birth (sparing the limbic cortex) continued to play when young and provided maternal care as adults (Murphy et al., 1981). However, if the limbic cortex was injured, play was disrupted. Subsequently, MacLean and Newman demonstrated that lesions placed in the midline frontolimbic cortex in adult squirrel monkeys largely eliminated adult isolation call (LeDeux, 2012; MacLean, 1988). In the ensuing years, there has been refinement in MacLean's limbic system model. Several brain stem nuclei connected to the hypothalamus are not part of the limbic system, and other brain stem nuclei that are involved in automatic reactions were not included. Moreover, some classic limbic areas, such as the hippocampus, have been shown to have nonemotional function. The hippocampus is important for memory. Specific areas of the limbic system contribute to some emotional functions; however, the originally proposed limbic system suggested an integrated system for the mediation of emotion. Still, despite these refinements, the hippocampus does play a role in emotional learning. The model that MacLean proposed continues to be examined with more refined neurobiological methods. MacLean's views that emotional responses are necessary for survival and involve primitive neural circuits that are conserved in evolution continue to stimulate research.

That cognitive processes and emotional states function relatively independently of one another is supported by all of the theories proposed for emotional brain functioning (LeDoux & Damasio, 2013). As an evolutionary neurobiologist, Paul MacLean was interested not only in emotion and the brain but also in the behaviors that were linked to the emotional brain. More broadly, he wrote about evolutionary steps toward sociability in the transition from reptiles to mammals and humans. In a journal article, MacLean (1985) emphasized the importance of the paleomammalian brain (limbic system) in the evolution of mammals. He emphasized the functions of this part of the brain in the evolution of the family. Family life begins with mother–infant attachment signaled by the emergence of the separation call that alerts the mother to the location of the separated infant. As mammals evolved, infant vocalization elicited the release of oxytocin from the breast, which facilitated the milk letdown reflex and led to enhanced maternal social engagement with the infant. Safe and secure, the infant could enhance its repertoire of behavior to learn through play and master environmental challenges.

The inability to detect differences in patterns of autonomic effects specific to the different emotions despite evidence for differentiation of emotions at a subjective level has created difficulties for emotion theory. Because we feel distinct emotions in the absence of objective evidence for autonomic differentiation, emotions must involve the integration of separate response components. Among these are autonomic activity and the cognition of external events plus patterned feedback from motor systems, such as the face. The cognitive arousal hypothesis addresses these complications by stating that emotional experience is generated through the integration of a generalized state of autonomic arousal with cognitions specific for each of the emotions. Undifferentiated autonomic arousal is necessary to create the subjective experience of emotion, but a specific situation is necessary to generate the qualitative emotion, such as fear, anger, or sadness. Cognition is not a stimulus to emotional reactions, but it is the mental event that is the equivalent to the quality of the emotion. Subjective feelings, then, are critical markers for emotion, whereas expressive behaviors are used as the indicators. This approach has allowed the exploration of social and cognitive factors that are responsible for emotional experiences. Using this framework, the social context for the resolution of ambiguous emotional states is considered. Still, this model has difficulty in at least four areas. First, autonomic participation may not be necessary for emotional experience and behavior. Second, this model indicates that socialization history may be essential to create the cognitions that are required for emotional feelings. Yet, the similarity of emotional expressions and judgments across widely separate cultures is inconsistent with the socialization hypothesis based on a history of certain social experiences. There is little reason to identify the quality of emotion with cognition because the two seem different and the organization of the nervous system suggests that these two sets of events are the product of separable processing mechanisms. Third, this model fails to account for the role of the social environment in shaping individual emotional experience. Fourth, it fails to address the internal organizing functions of emotion. On the other hand, William James suggested that both autonomic feedback and feedback that occurred during the behavior itself involving the somatic muscles contribute to emotional experience. James' focus on somatic experience is considered somewhat differently in the third approach, the *facial feedback theory*. In facial feedback theory, emotional feelings result when the state of the facial muscles during emotional experiences is communicated to the brain (Izard, 1977). This approach contrasts with the cognitive arousal theory, in which the brain interprets nonspecific peripheral feedback based on external events in the environment—that is, the interpretation of feedback to the brain from the face, which is specific to the emotion expressed. It is the condition which determines the emotion that can be experienced.

Each of these first three theories requires that some form of emotional coding take place before emotional experience is generated. In the central theories, subcortical brain areas must identify the exact emotional implications of the stimulus. The cortex then produces an emotional experience appropriate to that stimulus. In the cognitive arousal theory, the brain must distinguish between emotional and nonemotional situations and generate responses. In facial feedback theory, the brain determines the emotional significance of the stimulus so that the facial muscles can be appropriately contracted and provide emotionally specific feedback. Although these approached compete with one another and are considered to be separate theories, it may be that each approach is useful in explaining various types of emotional experiences. All three of these approaches are in agreement that emotional processing precedes conscious emotional experience. Emotional processing occurs out of awareness and is not conscious. The results of nonconscious processing may be experienced as conscious content, but the processes themselves remain inaccessible. Zajonc (1980) showed that affective reactions (preference formation) may take place prior to, and independent of, conscious recognition of an environmental stimulus. The computation of the affective experience stimuli is not consciously processed in Zajonc's experiments. This indicates that the brain can compute the emotional significance of the stimulus independent of the mechanism for recognizing what that stimulus is. As a result of these experiments demonstrating nonconscious computation of behavioral and autonomic expression of emotion, the role of consciousness in the initial generation of emotion may no longer be viewed as an essential element.

The fourth approach to understanding emotion is referred to as the *perceptual–motor model*. This model focuses on understanding how emotions are constructed and the changes in emotional constructive processes over the life span. The perceptual–motor model suggests that there is a core set of emotional reactions that are present at birth and that these core reactions are elaborated during development. This model differs from the other models presented in that increased emphasis is given to the components of cognitive and expressive motor processes that generate emotions. By looking at the components of emotional reactions, we recognize that the terms "emotion" and "cognition" both stand for complex sets of partially independent processes that are integrated in the generation of emotional or cognitive reactions. In addition, emotion is a process that organizes the components that are involved in affecting behavior.

The major challenge to emotion processing theory is to specify the factors responsible for the organization of emotion. There are three components for emotional processing that must be considered: cognitive–expressive components, action systems, and somatic receptor systems. The cognitive–expressive components are sensitive to interpersonal expressive cues (e.g., facial or vocal cues) and generate parallel reactions in response to these cues. Leventhal (1991) suggests that some expressive components are closed units such as phonetic modules, which are used for the perception and production of phonetic units in speech. Although these modules may be unique to emotional reactions, others may also be components of the cognitive system.

Action systems organize general approach and avoidance behavior, and therefore they function at a higher level than the expressive components and may include more than one expressive module. These action systems may respond to a wide array of stimuli and produce a broad range of behaviors. Various memory structures may be assessed by each action system as it guides approach or avoidance.

Somatic receptor systems may integrate both expressive components and action systems with the organism's physiologic systems. These systems are integrated through hormones that are manufactured in various parts of the body, and they communicate and integrate specific functions by acting upon receptor sites or target cells. These systems integrate the brain—that is, cognitive–expressive components and action systems—with widely separate physiologic processes.

## Cognition and Emotion

Attention, memory, and decision-making are influenced by emotion. Emotional states motivate action, and they indicate what is potentially relevant and important. There is an ongoing interaction between psychological and biological processes that are involved in constructing both cognitive and emotional reactions. To consider the interaction of emotion and cognition, it is critical to take into account what level of cognitive and emotional activity is involved in the interaction. For example, to evaluate the impact of emotional states and cognitive activity, it is important to clarify whether the focus is on preattentive cognitive processes, attentional processes, or consciously generated cognitive activity. Emotions, such as joy, fear, and sadness, may have an impact on initial learning. For example, a frightened person might be more attentive to and better retain frightening memory content.

## Emotion and Memory

The relationship between emotion and memory is particularly important. Emotional arousal may facilitate the remembrance of events that occurred during a similarly aroused state. Emotional events impact encoding, stabilization and storage, and retrieval of memories. They may determine what comes into memory to be encoded; enhance consolidation and memory storage, making forgetting less likely; and enhance the judgment of the importance of memories that are retrieved. Memories stored with heightened arousal are most likely to convince the person of their accuracy; however, by being focused on specific aspects of the experience, such memory may be less accurate regarding the total event. Events occurring during intense emotional arousal seem to be preserved in memory with special accuracy and clarity. The memory of intense experiences has been referred to as the "flash bulb" memory hypothesis (Sharot et al., 2004). Memories of real-life arousing events heighten the feeling of remembering without necessarily enhancing the accuracy of such memories. Enhancement of these heightened arousal memories involves activation of the amygdala, whereas nonarousing detailed knowledge of knowing is required to activate the parahippocampal gyrus. Thus, independent neural systems are involved for highly arousing perceptually salient events that subsequently are more remembered with a subjective sense of accuracy than neutral memories for knowing details that are not accompanied by heightened arousal. Moreover, all details are recalled if there is neutral affect, and with heightened arousal, fewer details are remembered with great confidence. Finally, emotions influence cognitive decision-making. Recalling information that is relevant to future planning is personalized, and its emotional value of the information to the person is assigned at memory storage. Cognitive appraisal of the relevance of emotionally arousing events can decrease or increase emotional brain responsiveness and how memories are stored.

In the psychodynamic concept of repression (Freud, 1964), the recall of events that are associated with the arousal of emotion may produce anxiety. To defend against anxiety, the memory of events in Freud's model may be prevented from reaching conscious awareness. The mental mechanism of repression has been studied in the experimental literature in the context of perceptual defenses and subliminal processing of experiences (Erdelyi, 1985).

In addition to facilitating and inhibiting the memory of events, emotion itself may be directly remembered (i.e., emotional experiences may be directly experienced without conscious recall). This was demonstrated in a classic case by Claparede (1951). He was evaluating a brain-damaged patient with a profound memory disturbance who lacked conscious recall of experiences that had occurred only moments before the trauma. On one occasion, the examiner stuck the patient with a pin during the interview. She was asked what had just happened to her; she had no conscious memory of the event. However, in the future, she refused to shake the hand of the examiner. This suggests that the emotional memory of the unpleasant experience (painful pinprick) permitted the patient to respond appropriately by storing information that allowed her to avoid future hand contact with the examiner. Stored memory was apparently undisturbed despite the brain damage, which impaired her ability to recall the details of experience. This early experiment is significant in suggesting that brain circuits used for nondeclarative (procedural) memories may differ from those used for conscious explicit memories. Memories may represent the storage of emotionally significant experiences in the nervous system, which may influence future information processing even though these event memories are out of awareness. In this context, emotion is treated as a memory process in itself rather than one that influences memory through inhibition and facilitation.

## Neuroscience and Emotion

The amygdala's major role is emotion processing. Extensive studies have been conducted regarding its role in emotion, particularly regarding the physiology of fear. The amygdala is a small structure in the temporal lobes adjacent to the anterior hippocampus that has been identified as the source of the brain's emotional network. Early studies of Kluver and Bucy (1937) showed that damage to the temporal lobes in monkeys leads to emotional disturbance. Subsequently, it was demonstrated that damage to the amygdala alone will produce the same behavior. In the Kluver–Bucy studies, lesioned monkeys lost fear of previously frightening stimuli, attempted to copulate with members of the same sex, and tried to eat inappropriate objects. Much of this syndrome can be understood as a disconnection of the sensory and the affective or motivational properties of incoming stimuli. Although visual stimuli are perceived as visual objects, the response to them is no longer socially appropriate. The amygdala has been shown to be an essential component of the brain's emotional system and is consistently implicated in emotional processing.

The amygdala's role in emotional processing is the consequence of its anatomic connectivity. Each of the bilateral amygdalae in primates is made up of nuclei grouped into three main amygdaloid complexes. The amygdalae receive input from sensory processing areas in the neocortex and thalamus. The amygdalae project to brain stem regions that control autonomic responses, hormonal responses, and behavior. Because of this extensive connectivity, the amygdalae can transform sensory stimuli into emotional signals. Through the amygdala, sensory processing essentially becomes emotional processing. The amygdalae can both initiate and control emotional responses. With a better understanding of the functional organization of the amygdala, its role in emotion is becoming increasingly clarified (LeDoux, 2012). There are 13 nuclei of the amygdala grouped into three complexes. Each has its own unique set of afferent and efferent connections (Lang & Davis, 2006). The role of the amygdala in fear and anxiety is summarized by Davis (1992), and its connectivity is illustrated by Lang and Davis (2006).

As shown in Figure 4.2, the largest region of the amygdala is the basolateral nuclear complex, made up of lateral and basal nuclei and accessory nuclei. Of these, the lateral nucleus receives sensory inputs. Connections from this nucleus to the basal nucleus and on to the ventral striation are involved in response to threat (i.e., avoidance or escape). The centromedial complex is made up of the medial nucleus and central nucleus. Here, information forwarded from the basal nucleus leads to a response. The response involves the brain stem regions that control emotional defensive behaviors along with linked automatic and endocrine responses. Among the amygdala complexes, the

**INPUTS**

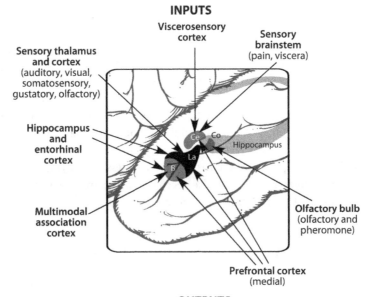

**OUTPUTS**

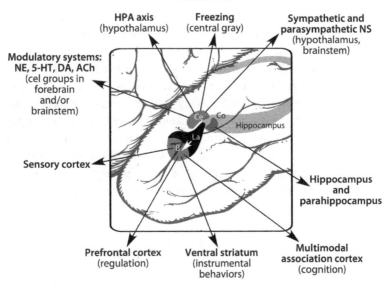

**Figure 4.2** Schematic diagram of direct connections in the amygdala. The amygdala lies deep within the medial temporal lobe adjacent to the hippocampus, as shown in Figure 4.1. The lateral nucleus is the major site receiving sensory inputs, whereas the central nucleus is the major output region for the expression of innate emotional responses and the physiological responses associated with them. Outputs to and from the lateral (La), basal (B), centromedial (Ce), and cortical (Co) nuclei of the amygdala are shown. The basal nucleus connects with striatal areas involved in the control of goal-directed behaviors. 5-HT, 5-hydroxytryptamine (serotonin); Ach, acetylcholine; DA, dopamine; NE, norcpinephrine; NS, nervous system.

FromGazzaniga, Ivry and Mangun (2019); redrawn by Tim Phelps (2021).

smallest is the cortical nucleus, whose primary input is from the olfactory bulb and olfactory complex. Its output is to the medial nucleus, and it is linked directly to the hippocampus and parahippocampal gyrus. In emotionally arousing situations, this system may modulate memory formation. With these extensive connections, the amygdala is the forebrain's most connected structure, suggesting its importance in attention, memory, and learning when responding to emotionally salient stimuli. Thus, the amygdala is important in recognizing a stimulus, its salience, and the response to it. This is pertinent in detecting danger and its avoidance. The amygdala contains receptors for the neurotransmitters glutamate, serotonin, dopamine, norepinephrine, and acetylcholine and for the peptides oxytocin, opioids, vasopressin, corticotropin-releasing factor, and neuropeptide Y. There are also receptors in the amygdala for hormones, glucocorticoids, and estrogen (Gazzaniga et al., 2019).

## Amygdala and Conditioned Fear

The amygdala has a crucial role in the expression of conditioned fear. Conditioned fear occurs when an initially neutral environmental stimulus is repeatedly paired with an aversive stimulus. Davis (1992) describes the amygdala and its efferent projections as presenting a central fear system that is involved in the expression and acquisition of conditioned fear.

As shown in Figure 4.3, there are direct connections between the central nucleus of the amygdala and hypothalamic and brain stem target areas that may be involved in the elicitation of fear and anxiety. Davis (1992) demonstrates that stimulation of efferent fibers from the amygdala to various anatomic targets leads to sympathetic activation, parasympathetic activation, increased respiration, activation of catecholamines, increased reflexes, cessation of a behavior, open-mouth movements, and adrenocorticotropic hormone release. The behaviors associated with amygdaloid stimulation include the various symptoms of fear and anxiety, such as tachycardia, respiratory distress,

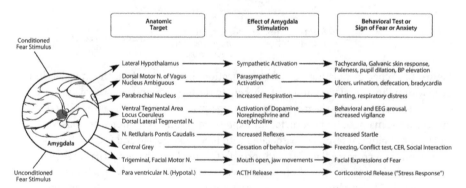

**Figure 4.3** Direct connections to hypothalamus and brain stem. Schematic diagram showing direct connections between the central nucleus of the amygdala and a variety of hypothalamic and brain stem target areas that may be involved in different animal tests of fear and anxiety. ACTH, adrenocorticotropic hormone; BP, blood pressure.
From Davis (1992); redrawn by Tim Phelps (2021).

increased startle, facial expressions of fear, and the stress response. Various sensory projections terminate in the lateral amygdaloid nucleus to produce these effects. These projections originate in the areas of the cortex and thalamus that process sensory input.

Fear conditioning is thought to occur via emotional learning processes involving thalamic–amygdala projections. Through this subcortical pathway, inputs from the thalamus to the amygdala lead to activation either before or simultaneously with the arrival of input at the cortical level. This subcortical system may play an important role in preconscious and precognitive emotional processing. Because these connections are direct, they may allow primitive sensory representations to activate quickly in emotional situations. These direct connections are reminiscent of the classic theories of Cannon and Bard (Cannon, 1929) and Papez (1937). These authors emphasized the importance of subcortical sensory transmission in the experience and expression of emotion.

## Amygdala and Social Cognition

The human amygdala is essential in the processing of emotion and socially salient stimuli. In addition to its role in conditional fear, the amygdala plays a major role in the recognition of facial emotions responding to the emotional expression of faces. Thus, it is important in social cognition (Adolphs, 2010). Emotional states have evolved to allow us to meet environmental challenges in a context-sensitive manner that allows flexibility in responding to relevant challenges rather than reflexive responses to danger. Context-sensitive responding is informed by the recognition and learning of recurring themes. Although some stimuli induce emotions, the emotional significance of the majority of emotions is learned (Adolphs, 2017).

Emotion states can be studied separately from conceptual knowledge. Emotional states have benefited from the study of patient S.M., who has a rare autosomal recessive genetic disorder, Urbach–Wiethe disease. In this disease, typically with onset at approximately 10 years of age, the amygdalae in both cerebral hemispheres are nearly destroyed by calcium depositions, although the hippocampus and neocortex are unaffected. Just as science has benefited from the study of the removal of the hippocampus bilaterally in patient H.M, S.M. allows us to study the bilateral loss of the amygdala. S.M., studied by Adolphs (2017), does not experience fear in herself nor can she produce a facial expression of fear when asked to do so. She is unable to recognize fear in other's facial expressions and does not recognize multiple emotions in a single facial expression. She does not avoid threatening situations or show automatic responses related to fear. Yet she has no difficulty in recognizing the faces of familiar people from their photographs. She can laugh; she can cry; she endorses feelings of sadness, happiness, and other emotions. She does not show learning based on unconditional fear in Pavlovian fear conditioning on standardized tests. She has normal intelligence, perception, and motor ability. She can recognize and draw expressions of sadness, happiness, anger, disgust, and surprise, but not fear. Such findings further specify the effects of damage to the amygdala and highlight its role in the recognition of facial expressions of emotion. They indicate that the amygdala does participate in the perception of social signals and offers an additional link of brain systems involving the amygdala to social cognition.

Allman and Brothers (1994) suggest that the role of the amygdala in detecting both directions of gaze and facial expressions of emotion indicates a role for the amygdala in those brain mechanisms that represent the intentions and dispositions of others. They suggest additional studies on the role of the amygdala in the interpretation of social touch and voice intonation should be performed. Brain systems linking the orbital frontal cortex and amygdala have been proposed to participate in social decision-making by correlating somatic states with behavioral situations. Neuroimaging studies find significant activation of the amygdala to fear faces in typical subjects (Morris et al., 1996). Single neurons in the human amygdala have been shown to selectively encode whole faces (Rutishauser et at., 2011).

Individuals with autism spectrum disorder (ASD) have abnormal face processing, which has been linked to the amygdala. When data were recorded from two neurosurgical cases with ASD, the subjects focused far more on the mouth than the eyes of the examiner (Rutishauser et al., 2013). The investigators found single-neuron correlates to atypical face processing. Another neuroimaging study found amygdala activity was enhanced for fear faces when the person's visual facial focus moved from the mouth to the eyes (Gamer & Büchel, 2009). Finally, oxytocin modulates amygdala reactivity to fearful eye expression, consistent with nonconscious processing. These findings provide further confirmation that the amygdala is attuned to threat signals from the eye in a social context. Typically, eyes are the facial feature that is first attended to when looking at faces. Oxytocin, the social bonding hormone, attenuated the amygdala reactivity to fearful eyes. This dampening effect may reflect reduced preconscious vigilance for facial threat when oxytocin is administered (Kanat et al., 2015).

In another study, investigators examined neurons in the human amygdala selective to perceived emotions (Wang et al., 2014). They found that the amygdala specifically encodes the subject's judgment of emotions expressed in faces, but not their perceptual judgment. The investigators recorded from 210 single neurons in the amygdala in neurosurgical cases with implanted depth electrodes. Subjects were asked to discriminate fearful and happy faces by a button press. Neurons were identified that distinguished fearful versus happy faces. Hippocampal neurons, unlike amygdala neurons, were found to encode emotions but not subjective judgment of them. The authors concluded that sensory information about faces is integrated in the amygdala and conveyed to the neocortex with reward value in a social context. This may involve connections located in the basal ganglia and prefrontal cortex and underlie subjective social judgment about facial emotions regarding approachability and trustworthiness. Although the amygdala is involved in distinguishing the relevance of facial expressions, fear conditioning, and social responsiveness, it is not the only brain region required for emotions.

Another region of importance in the study of emotions is the insular cortex. The insular cortex has reciprocal connections with the amygdala as well as the medial prefrontal cortex and anterior cingulate gyrus. Its reciprocal connectivity extends to frontal, parietal, and temporal cortical areas. All of these areas are involved with attention, memory, and cognition (Gazzaniga et al., 2019, p. 464). Importantly, the perception of bodily states (interoception) correlates with the insula activity (Garfinkel & Critchley, 2013; Terasawa et al., 2013). The anterior insula cortex supports conscious appraisal of subjective bodily and emotional states. The anterior insula cortex is involved in the appraisal of emotions and body physiology. The anterior insula cortex mediates the relations of bodily sensibility and social fear, thus increasing emotional awareness and influencing social interaction. Interoception refers to our sensitivity to stimuli within the body. Viscerosensory nerves from the afferent limb of automatic nervous reflexes are involved in automatic nervous system regulation; the efferent myelinated vagus nerve facilitates social engagement (Porges, 2001). Thus, interoception encompasses conscious visceromotor activity. Therefore, "internal physiologic and subjective emotional states are interdependent"; they are being studied as brain mechanisms that underlie the generation of emotion (Garfinkel & Critchley, 2013, p. 231). Overall, the anterior insula is believed to integrate all of the visceral and somatic input, allowing it to represent the body in the mind. Other studies (Gu et al., 2013) propose that the anterior insular cortex also works in consort with the anterior cingulate gyrus when experiencing emotional feelings. The posterior insular may be activated when there are feelings of sexual desire (Cacioppo et al., 2012). The insula apparently is the place in the brain where cognitive and emotional information becomes integrated. In summary, the insula is involved in integrating affective and cognitive information, whereas the amygdala's role is more selectively involved in affective arousal, particularly for negative environmental input.

Disgust is the emotion specifically linked to the insula; it is linked to the insula's role in the perception of bodily states. Machine learning technologies are consistent with brain representations of emotions as discrete categories. The brain fluctuates among multiple distinct emotional states at rest (Kragel et al., 2016).

## Brain Regions Involved in Happiness

Finding brain regions involved in happiness is complex. Defining happiness based on a person looking at smiling faces or watching films that amuse has proven unreliable. One study contrasted happiness and sadness in subjects conducting a cognitive task (Habel et al., 2005). The authors found that happiness and sadness involved activations of similar brain regions. With happiness, the greater activation was found in the right dorsolateral prefrontal cortex, left medial and posterior cingulate gyrus, and right inferior temporal gyrus. In sadness, the greater activation was in the transverse temporal gyrus and bilaterally in the ventrolateral prefrontal cortex, the left anterior cingulate cortex, and superior temporal gyrus. The networks are sufficiently similar that the authors concluded that positive and negative moods have similar but distinct involvement of a common network. Other authors (Sato et al., 2015) used structural magnetic resonance imaging (MRI) to correlate self-reported subjective happiness from research participants. They proposed that happiness involves the feeling of pleasure (satisfaction in life) and includes both emotional and cognitive components. Focusing on the precuneus, a brain region linked to self-consciousness, they found that it is involved in processing information regarding self-awareness and positive emotions. Participants were specifically asked to rate subjective happiness—that is, the intensity of positive and negative emotional experiences—and also describe their purpose in life. The authors found a positive relationship between subjective happiness and gray matter volume in the precuneus. Subjective happiness was found to be associated with more pleasure than displeasure, as well as positive cognitive appraisal of purpose in life.

Sato et al. (2015) proposed that their findings are consistent with meta-analyses of functional imaging data linking subjective happiness to areas of the brain that include the anterior cingulate gyrus, medial parietal cortex, posterior cingulate gyrus, precuneus, and amygdala (Zhang & Chiang-shan, 2012). Previous functional MRI (fMRI) studies had shown that states of happiness are associated with medial parietal cortex, the site of the precuneus. Moreover, the precuneus is involved in self-reference and integration of current experience with past memory and future plans (Lou et al., 2004). A study that focused on eudaimonic well-being (self-acceptance and purpose in life), not specifically on happiness, found an association with insular cortical volume (G. Lewis et al., 2014).

Sigmund Freud's model focused on the pleasure principle, equating it with happiness. Others have proposed that happiness is linked to achievement. Csikzentmihalyi (1990) proposed that happiness accompanies complete absorption in one's vocation; he proposed that bodily pleasure (e.g., eating and sexual satisfaction) while fully cognitively engaged results in the mental state of "flow." Flow, he noted, is the optimal experience of complete self-absorption in any activity—for example, sports, mastery solving math problems, dance, etc.—that enhances self-esteem. It engages those brain systems involved in pleasure, reward, and cognitive motivation. Neuroimaging and structural MRI studies, depending on how happiness is defined, emphasize subjective awareness of emotional state and heightened consciousness.

## Brain Regions and Love

Unlike the other emotions, there is not a distinguishing facial expression for love. Rather than facial expression per se, love is elicited by recalling the name of a loved one. The feeling of love has been examined in neuroimaging studies utilizing self-report rating scales. One example is the Passionate Love Scale (Gazzaniga et al., 2019). Feelings of love activate subcortical reward, emotional, motivational, and cognitive systems. These systems include the insula, caudate, putamen, anterior cingulate gyrus, bilateral posterior hippocampal, left inferior frontal gyrus, left middle temporal gyrus, and parietal lobe. Such brain activation indicates that love is a complex emotion, not a simple basic one; it involves multiple regions of the brain. Although no amygdala activation is reported for love, amygdala activation is found for lust.

Brain regions that have been studied for love with fMRI include those involving passionate love, maternal love, and unconditional love. These various forms of love activate different networks. Passionate love is mediated by a network in the subcortical region linked to cognitive areas representing attention and self-representation. The maternal love circuit overlaps with the area activated in passionate love but has its own neural circuit signature. The circuit involves the subcortical periaqueductal (central) gray matter, a brain activation region distinctive for maternal love (Ortigue et al., 2010). Love involves emotion, reward, social cognition, self-representation, and attention. Essentially, it "appears to light up much of the brain" (Gazzaniga et al., 2019, p. 468), but fMRI was not needed to prove that! Paul MacLean (1985) wrote that the evolution of the brain in humans allows us to "look with feeling"—that is, to experience empathy and love with others. Neuroimaging studies of love demonstrate this evolutionary advance. When we experience love, we integrate the whole brain.

## Development of Emotions and Feelings in Children

Infants begin signaling their emotional state from birth onwards. The earliest distinction is between positive and negative affect by expressing pleasure (smile) or displeasure (crying). Basic emotional expressions that are recognized in the first weeks of life include interest, happiness, sadness, surprise, fear, and anger; these become functional over the first 2 years of life. Infants aged 2–8 months show more interest in a live human face than a mannequin and more attention to a mannequin than a face-like object with scrambled features (Izard, 2007). Even earlier, infants on first feeding will smile when given a sweet liquid and express distress by pursing their lips, and sometimes crying, at a bitter taste. At age 4 months, anger is expressed when goals are blocked. Anger and sadness can be distinguished using measures of hypothalamic–pituitary–adrenal and automatic activity (M. Lewis et al., 2006). In addition, 4- and 5-month-old infants show anger expressions but not sadness to loss of contingent stimulation.

The capacity for emotional expression and emotion recognition arise concurrently. Emotion perception involves one's feelings and actions, as does emotional expression (Izard, 2007). At age 4 months, infants show different affective responses to the basic emotions of sadness, anger, and fear. Fear responses increase after 7 age months. At this age, infants become more fearful and wary of strangers; there is increased sadness with separation from a familiar caregiver (Smith et al., 2015). These responses are illustrated in Mary Ainsworth's "strange situation" paradigm when, depending on attachment status, intense happiness, as well as intense anger, may be shown when reunited with the parent. Moreover, anger and pain are differentiated after age 7 months. When 2- to 8-month-olds were given routine inoculations, the younger children showed broad generalized distress, whereas the older ones showed distinct anger (brows compressed together, eyelids tensed, and mouth squared).

## Recognizing Emotions in Others

Although children do not innately understand facial expressions showing discrete emotions, they do mimic them. When mothers were asked to change facial expression and tone of voice to signal different emotions, their babies showed differential responses. When mothers of 10-week-old infants appeared happy, so did their babies; if mothers appeared angry, the babies mimicked that emotion. When mothers expressed a sad face, infants became distressed and withdrawn but did not show a clearly sad face (Haviland & Lelwica, 1987). A 9-month-old infant's sadness expressions did increase when the mother showed a sad expression while the child played, and play behavior decreased, as did earlier expression of joy in play (Termine & Izard, 1988). The results of these infant studies are consistent with the universality of a limited set of basic emotions linked to the brain stem and amygdala (Adolphs, 2006).

Darwin (1877) provided an early description of emotional development based on his detailed observations of one of his children. Darwin wrote about the development of anger in his son:

> On his eighth day he frowned and wrinkled the skin around his eye before a crying fit, but this may have been pain, not anger. When nearly 4 months, there was no doubt from the manner in which blood gushed into his whole face and scalp, that he got into a violent passion. When he was 7 months, he screamed in rage when a lemon slipped away and he could not seize it with his hands. When 11 months old, if a wrong plaything was given to him, he would punch it away and beat it. I presumed that the beating was an instinctive sign of anger like the snapping of the jaws of a young crocodile just out of the egg; and not that he imagined he could hurt a plaything.

Here, Darwin proposes that emotional displays are instinctive. Current research supports the universality of basic emotions. Still, unlike Darwin, current findings do not always consider individual differences in emotion expression and emotion recognition. However, evidence from meta-analytic studies is supportive of the view that basic emotions are "natural kinds" (Izard, 2007, p. 262). Moreover, elicitation of a basic emotion requires an appropriate stimulus such as a mother's smile to elicit joy.

Finally, a basic emotion also has a feeling component linked to an associated neurobiological process. Such feelings emerge from sensory systems that alert the person to what is happening around them. Such feeling states derive from subcortical neural systems in the upper brain stem and have specific properties of motivation (Panksepp, 2005).

There is evidence that preverbal toddlers can use manual gestures to convey emotions (Vallotton, 2008). For example, 11-month-old Cathy, when seeing a stuffed toy spider, hit her chest and looked at her caregivers, who said "fear" and Cathy nodded in agreement. Infants begin to use words at approximately age 13 months, and at approximately age 20 months they begin using emotion words (Bretherton et al., 1986). In the following months, children use emotion words in spontaneous conversation. At first, they refer to their own emotions, but at approximately age 24 months, they refer to the emotions of others. A 2-year-old child's attribution of emotion is not entirely triggered by recognizing another person's human facial expressions. An infant may attribute feelings to stuffed animals and dolls. Moreover, when 2-year-olds do talk about emotional states, such as feeling good, there is no obvious associated facial signature. Young children refer to a few basic positive emotions (happy or good) and negative emotions (angry or mad, scared or afraid, and crying or sad). However, they are not necessarily engaged in self-conscious reporting of emotions. Gradually between ages 2 and 4 years, preschool children refer to past, future, and recurrent feelings. By age 3 years, children's spontaneous conversations indicate that they understand that emotions are internal feelings (Rosnay et al., 2008) which are different from causes and consequences. Also by age 3 years, children can name and provide a cause for some emotions and label happy, sad, and angry expressions. Thus, by age 3 years, language and cognition have sufficiently advanced to allow children to differentiate emotions and begin to link them (Widon, 2016). Increasingly, language allows children to not only put their feelings into words but also, in conversation, revisit past emotions and come to realize that past emotions are reactivated when given reminders. Increasingly, too, they can talk about future emotions. In time, they can describe situations for specific emotions. Thus, when interviewed, they can describe situations that elicit various emotions. They can tell when they are happy, sad, angry, or afraid. They, too, appreciate that the same situation can elicit different emotions depending on context (Rosnay et al., 2008).

How do children with developmental neuropsychiatric disorders differ from typically developing children in emotional development? Social awareness and level of cognitive functioning are important factors. For example, children diagnosed with ASD, both those with higher and those with lower cognitive capacity, are good at remembering recurrent sequences of events, but changes in those routines will induce panic in these children. Such perseverance of sameness is a clinical feature emphasized by Leo Kanner and included in the current DSM-5 ASD criteria.

Script-based situation-sensitive, concrete memory may help typically developing children in understanding emotions. They may understand that situations such as giving gifts at birthday parties make people happy, whereas other situations in which their demands are not met make people unhappy. Children with ASD can appropriately match the facial expressions that go with depictions of emotionally charged situations. They can select a sad face for a picture showing a child looking at a broken toy and choose an angry face for a picture of two children fighting. However, on these tasks, they perform poorly compared to a typically developing control group of children (Baron-Cohen, 1991). However, children with ASD do not appreciate what causes emotions, unlike neurotypically developing children, who do realize that is not the concrete situations by themselves that cause emotions. Rather, it is the way the situation is appraised that causes emotions. Unlike typically developing children, children with ASD generally lack a theory of mind—that is, they do not understand that others have beliefs, desires, intentions, and perspectives that are different from their own. Typically developing children, at ages 5 and 6 years, begin to understand the impact of beliefs on emotion. Essentially, all 5-year-olds can understand a story character's mistaken expectation. It is only at age 6 years that the majority of children can make correct attributions of surprise consistent with a character's misplaced expectation about what is going to happen. In one study, younger children's beliefs about the Red Riding Hood story were examined. Although most children realized that she did not know the wolf was waiting for her at her grandmother's cottage, they still claimed she was afraid before even seeing the wolf. When asked how she would feel when leaving home, their incorrect attribution of fear was increased the closer she was to the cottage. At each point of the journey, the children were aware that she did not know anything about the wolf, but they still insisted she was afraid (Ronfard & Harris, 2014). Older children did not have such beliefs. Developmentally, children learn that the same situation can elicit different emotions depending on the particular beliefs and desires they hold. Young children find it difficult to understand that a belief-based appraisal of an upcoming situation, accurate or not, determines how a person feels rather than the situation itself.

## Self-Conscious Emotions

The consciousness of self develops in the second year of life and is demonstrated in self-referential behaviors. For example, touching one's own nose when looking in a mirror is a form of self-reference, as are the use of pronouns "me" and "mine" and knowing when one is pretending. The emergence of self-consciousness has a profound effect on emotional life, and in later childhood and adolescence self-conscious emotions are refined. These include embarrassment, empathy, envy, pride, guilt, shame, and hubris. The measurement of these complex emotions includes not only facial expression but also vocalization and bodily behavior. These emotions are not understood until the child has sufficient consciousness of self. The sense of self emerges in development through an infant or toddler's intentional actions in social exchange with caregivers. The establishment of a sense of self is essential for the appearance of self-conscious emotions. These new emotions are developmentally complex and generally require maturation. Components of emotion increasingly maintain their original integrity, even though they may be incorporated into new organizational structures. The type of interpersonal experience may lead to variation in the organization of emotions. Cultural influences may be important too, for example, in the expression and channeling of emotions. Although basic emotions may be innate, the emotional schema involved in expression may be reorganized while retaining the basic biologic substrate. Consequently, if emotional experience is inhibited in early life, then new conditions may need to be simulated in therapy situations for the full expression of that neglected emotion.

During development, emotions show multiple component constructions at various levels, which may have a degree of functional independence. Socialization of the child may link components in typical or unexpected ways, so the expected organization may not always occur. Cognitive components, especially those associated with the sense of self, are important in the expression of emotion and its elaboration. The components represented in emotion are active processing units that use emotional schemata which may be based on basic emotions. These schemas are needed to clarify components of emotional experience, such as perceptual memory for faces, things, and places, and the differentiation between volitional and spontaneous emotional–motor behavior.

Emotional schema may reflect the operation of basic emotion components along with reciprocal interaction between emotion and consciousness. These processes, evolved throughout evolution, have underlying endocrine and somatic receptor systems. Both evolutionary development and individual development have resulted in perceptual–cognitive and motor systems that may more effectively execute this sense. Through the study of emotion, we come to understand the unity of "the mind in the body" and "the body in the mind."

Basic emotions, as discussed previously, involve bodily activity. The capacity for emotionally expressive behavior emerges in evolutionary adaptive neurobiological systems. As self-consciousness and language develop, children label basic emotions as feelings and put feelings with words. Putting feeling into words is an essential element in psychotherapy and beneficial in coping with negative experiences (Lieberman et al., 2007).

Neuroimaging studies establish the neurobiological processes that are involved in putting feelings into words to cope with negative emotions. Linguistic processing, affect labeling, results in a reduction in amygdala activity compared to perceptual processing of emotional aspects of the same image presented. Moreover, during linguistic processing, there is greater activity than during nonlinguistic processing of emotion in the right ventrolateral prefrontal cortex (rVLPFC). This results in "top-down" inhibition. The extent of rVLPFC activity is also inversely correlated with the extent of amygdala activity when labeling affect. Thus, putting feelings into words may reduce amygdala responsiveness and potentially reduce emotional distress. Moreover, the rVLPFC in this study was the only brain region specifically involved in disrupting the response of the amygdala to emotionally evocative images. The medial prefrontal cortex was found to mediate the interaction of the rVLPFC and activity in the amygdala. The medial prefrontal cortex projections to the amygdala are dense in both rats and humans. The coupling of amygdala–prefrontal regions has been shown to depend on correlations with genetic variation of the serotonin transporter (Heinz et al., 2005). The connection between the rVLPFC and medial prefrontal cortex is a mechanism whereby language and potentially other symbolic processes impact a basic limbic brain control system, leading to therapeutic benefit.

## Neuroscience and Emotion Understanding

When socially engaged with others, we infer what others may be feeling and why they feel as they do. To do so quickly, we recognize and cognitively orient to emotionally salient cues; classify other emotions into categories we know; and, utilizing theory of mind, gauge what caused the other person's emotion, actions they may be planning, and how to respond. Functional neuroscience imaging studies have examined cognitive processes and brain regions that enable our capacity for emotional understanding of others (Spunt & Adolphs, 2019). Such emotional understanding involves detecting cues, inferring emotional categories, and attributing causes for the emotion elicited in others. Figure 4.4 illustrates the network of brain structures, with the dorsomedial prefrontal cortex the most prominent among them, in inferring emotions in others and their causes.

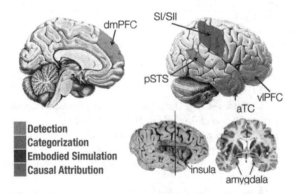

**Figure 4.4** Brain structures implicated in understanding the emotions of others. The figure shows brain structures that are proposed as implicated in our emotional understanding of others. The functional brain components are for detection of emotion, categorization, embodied simulation, and casual attribution. Each brain structure is color-coded by functional component. The most prominent regions, not all, are shown. aTC, anterior temporal cortex; dmPFC, dorsomedial prefrontal cortex; pSTS, posterior superior temporal sulcus; SI/SII, human somatosensory cortices; vlPFC, ventrolateral prefrontal cortex.
From Spunt and Adolphs (2019).

This proposal hypothesizes that we vicariously experience feelings of others in ourselves and simulate another bodily state by representing that state in somatosensory-related brain regions ($S_1$, $S_2$, and insula) in our own brain (Goldman & Sripada, 2005). This view is supported by the fact that the somatosensory-related cortices (especially in the right hemisphere) block people's ability to recognize facial emotion (Adolphs et al., 2000).

In summary, knowledge about the evolution of basic emotions, the establishment of emotional schemas, and affect labeling provide fundamental information needed to advance treatment for typically developing children and those with developmental neuropsychiatric disorders.

# References

Adolphs, R. (2006). Perception and emotion: How we recognize facial expressions. *Current Directions in Psychological Science, 15*(5), 222–226.

Adolphs, R. (2010). What does the amygdala contribute to social cognition? *Annals of the New York Academy of Sciences, 1191*(1), 42–61.

Adolphs, R. (2017). How should neuroscience study emotions? By distinguishing emotion states, concepts, and experiences. *Social Cognitive and Affective Neuroscience, 12*(1), 24–31.

Adolphs, R., & Anderson, D. J. (2018). *The neuroscience of emotion: A new synthesis.* Princeton University Press.

Adolphs, R., Damasio, H., Tranel, D., Cooper, G., & Damasio, A. R. (2000). A role for somatosensory cortices in the visual recognition of emotion as revealed by three-dimensional lesion mapping. *Journal of Neuroscience, 20*(7), 2683–2690.

Allman, J., & Brothers, L. (1994). Faces, fear, and the amygdala. *Nature, 372*, 613–614.

American Psychiatric Association. (2013). *Diagnostic and statistical manual of mental disorders* (5th ed.). American Psychiatric Publishing.

Anderson, D. J., & Adolphs, R. (2014). A framework for studying emotions across species. *Cell, 157*(1), 187–200.

Baron-Cohen, S. (1991). Do people with autism understand what causes emotion? *Child Development, 62*(2), 385–395.

Bretherton, I., Fritz, J., Zahn-Waxler, C., & Ridgeway, D. (1986). Learning to talk about emotions: A functionalist perspective. *Child Development, 57*(3),529–548.

Cacioppo, S., Bianchi-Demicheli, F., Frum, C., Pfaus, J. G., & Lewis, J. W. (2012). The common neural bases between sexual desire and love: A multilevel kernel density fMRI analysis. *Journal of Sexual Medicine, 9*(4), 1048–1054.

Cannon, W. B. (1927). The James–Lange theory of emotions: A critical examination and an alternative theory. *American Journal of Psychology, 39*(1–4), 106–124.

Cannon, W. B. (1929). *Bodily changes in pain, hunger, fear and rage.* Appleton.

Claparede, E. (1951). Recognition and "me'ness." In D. Rapaport (Ed.), *Organization and pathology of thought* (pp. 58–75). Columbia University Press. (Reprinted from Archives de Psychologies, 1911, 79–90)

Csikzentmihalyi, M. (1990). *Flow: The psychology of optimal experience.* Harper & Row.

Darwin, C. (1877). A biographical sketch of an infant. *Mind, 2*(7), 285–294.

Darwin, C. (1965). *The expression of the emotions in man and animals* (Vol. 526). University of Chicago Press. (Original work published 1872).

Darwin, C. (2009). *The expression of the emotions in man and animals, anniversary edition* (4th ed.). Oxford University Press. (Original work published 1872)

Davis, M. (1992). The role of the amygdala in fear and anxiety. *Annual Review of Neuroscience, 15*(1), 353–375.

Davis, M., Walker, D. L., Miles, L., & Grillon, C. (2010). Phasic vs. sustained fear in rats and humans: Role of the extended amygdala in fear vs. anxiety. *Neuropsychopharmacology, 35*(1), 105–135.

Ekman, P. (1999). Basic emotions. In T. Dalgleish &M. Power (Eds.), *Handbook of cognition and emotion* (pp. 45–60). Wiley.

Ekman, P. (2003). Emotions inside out: 130 years after Darwin's "The Expression of the Emotions in Man and Animal." Proceedings of a conference. November 16–17, 2002, New York City, New York, USA. *Annals of the New York Academy of Sciences, 1000,* 1–404.

Erdelyi, M. H. (1985). *Psychoanalysis: Freud's cognitive psychology.* Freeman/Times Books/ Henry Holt.

Freud, S. (1964). *The standard edition of the complete psychological works of Sigmund Freud* (J. E. Strachey, Trans.). Hogarth.

Gamer, M., & Büchel, C. (2009). Amygdala activation predicts gaze toward fearful eyes. *Journal of Neuroscience, 29*(28), 9123–9126.

Garfinkel, S. N., & Critchley, H. D. (2013). Interoception, emotion and brain: New insights link internal physiology to social behaviour. Commentary on: "Anterior insular cortex mediates bodily sensibility and social anxiety" by Terasawa et al. (2012). *Social Cognitive and Affective Neuroscience, 8*(3), 231–234.

Gazzaniga, M. S., Ivry, R. B., & Mangun, G. R. (2019). *Cognitive neuroscience: The biology of the mind* (5th ed.). Norton.

Goldman, A. I., & Sripada, C. S. (2005). Simulationist models of face-based emotion recognition. *Cognition, 94*(3), 193–213.

Greenough, W. T., Black, J. E., & Wallace, C. S. (1987). Experience and brain development. *Child Development, 58*(3), 539–559.

Gregory, R. L., & Zangwill, O. L. (1987). *The Oxford companion to the mind.* Oxford University Press.

Gu, X., Hof, P. R., Friston, K. J., & Fan, J. (2013). Anterior insular cortex and emotional awareness. *Journal of Comparative Neurology, 521*(15), 3371–3388.

Habel, U., Klein, M., Kellermann, T., Shah, N. J., & Schneider, F. (2005). Same or different? Neural correlates of happy and sad mood in healthy males. *NeuroImage, 26*(1), 206–214.

Haviland, J. M., & Lelwica, M. (1987). The induced affect response: 10-week-old infants' responses to three emotion expressions. *Developmental Psychology, 23*(1), 97–104.

Heinz, A., Braus, D. F., Smolka, M. N., Wrase, J., Puls, I., Hermann, D., Klein, S., Grusser, S., Flor, H., Schumann, G., Mann, K., & Buchel, C. (2005). Amygdala–prefrontal coupling depends on a genetic variation of the serotonin transporter. *Nature Neuroscience, 8*(1), 20–21.

Izard, C. E. (1977). *Human emotions.* Plenum.

Izard, C. E. (1991). *The psychology of emotions.* Plenum.

Izard, C. E. (2007). Basic emotions, natural kinds, emotion schemas, and a new paradigm. *Perspectives on Psychological Science, 2*(3), 260–280.

Jaspers, K. (1963). *General psychopathology* (J. Hoenig & M. W. Hamilton, Trans.). Manchester University Press. (Original work published 1959)

Kanat, M., Heinrichs, M., Mader, I., Van Elst, L. T., & Domes, G. (2015). Oxytocin modulates amygdala reactivity to masked fearful eyes. *Neuropsychopharmacology, 40*(11), 2632–2638.

Kluver, H., & Bucy, P. C. (1937). "Psychic blindness" and other symptoms following bilateral temporal lobectomy in rhesus monkeys. *American Journal of Physiology, 119,* 352–353.

Kragel, P. A., Knodt, A. R., Hariri, A. R., & LaBar, K. S. (2016). Decoding spontaneous emotional states in the human brain. *PLoS Biology, 14*(9), e2000106.

Lang, P. J., & Davis, M. (2006). Emotion, motivation, and the brain: Reflex foundations in animal and human research. *Progress in Brain Research, 156,* 3–29.

Lazarus, R. S. (1991). *Emotion and adaptation.* Oxford University Press.

LeDoux, J. (2012). Rethinking the emotional brain. *Neuron, 73,* 653–676.

LeDoux, J. E. (2012). Evolution of human emotion: A view through fear. Progress in Brain Research, *195,* 431–442.

LeDoux, J. E. (2014). Comment: What's basic about the brain mechanisms of emotion? *Emotion Review, 6*(4), 318–320.

LeDoux, J. E., & Damasio, A. R. (2013). Emotions and feelings. In E. R. Kandel, J. H. Schwartz, T. M. Jessell, S. A. Siegelbaum, A. J. Hudspeth, & S. Mack (Eds.), Principles of neural science (5th ed., pp. 1079–1094). McGraw-Hill.

Leventhal, H. (1991). Emotion: Prospects for conceptual and empirical development. In R. G. Lister & H. J. Weingartner (Eds.), *Perspectives on cognitive neuroscience* (pp. 325–348). Oxford University Press.

Lewis, G. J., Kanai, R., Rees, G., & Bates, T. C. (2014). Neural correlates of the "good life": Eudaimonic well-being is associated with insular cortex volume. *Social Cognitive and Affective Neuroscience, 9*(5), 615–618.

Lewis, M., Ramsay, D. S., & Sullivan, M. W. (2006). The relation of ANS and HPA activation to infant anger and sadness response to goal blockage. *Developmental Psychobiology, 48*(5), 397–405.

Lieberman, M. D., Eisenberger, N. I., Crockett, M. J., Tom, S. M., Pfeifer, J. H., & Way, B. M. (2007). Putting feelings into words. *Psychological Science, 18*(5), 421–428.

Lou, H. C., Luber, B., Crupain, M., Keenan, J. P., Nowak, M., Kjaer, T. W., Sackeim, H. A., & Lisanby, S. H. (2004). Parietal cortex and representation of the mental self. *Proceedings of the National Academy of Sciences of the USA, 101*(17), 6827–6832.

MacLean, P. D. (1949). Psychosomatic disease and the "visceral brain": Recent developments bearing on the Papez theory of emotion. *Psychosomatic Medicine, 11*(6), 338–353.

MacLean, P. D. (1985). Brain evolution relating to family, play, and the separation call. *Archives of General Psychiatry, 42*(4), 405–417.

MacLean, P. D. (1988). Evolution of audiovocal communication as reflected by the therapsid-mammalian transition and the limbic thalamocingulate division. In J. D. Newman (Ed.), *The physiological control of mammalian vocalization* (pp. 185–201). Springer.

Maudsley, H. (1870). *Body and mind: Their connection and mutual influence.* Macmillan and Company, London.

Morris, J. S., Frith, C. D., Perrett, D. I., Rowland, D., Young, A. W., Calder, A. J., & Dolan, R. J. (1996). A differential neural response in the human amygdala to fearful and happy facial expressions. *Nature, 383*(6603), 812–815.

Murphy, M. R., MacLean, P. D., & Hamilton, S. C. (1981). Species-typical behavior of hamsters deprived from birth of the neocortex. *Science, 213*(4506), 459–461.

Newman, J. D., & Harris, J. C. (2009). The scientific contributions of Paul D. MacLean (1913–2007). *Journal of Nervous and Mental Disease, 197*(1), 3–5.

Ortigue, S., Bianchi-Demicheli, F., Patel, N., Frum, C., & Lewis, J. W. (2010). Neuroimaging of love: fMRI meta-analysis evidence toward new perspectives in sexual medicine. *Journal of Sexual Medicine, 7*(11), 3541–3552.

Oyebode, F. (2018). Sims' symptoms in the mind: Textbook of descriptive psychopathology. Elsevier.

Panksepp, J. (2005). On the embodied neural nature of core emotional affects. *Journal of Consciousness Studies, 12*(8–9), 158–184.

Panksepp, J., & Biven, L. (2012). *The archaeology of mind: Neuroevolutionary origins of human emotions.* Norton.

Papez, J. W. (1937). A proposed mechanism of emotion. *Archives of Neurology & Psychiatry, 38*(4), 725–743.

Pessoa, L., & Hof, P. R. (2015). From Paul Broca's great limbic lobe to the limbic system. *Journal of Comparative Neurology, 523*(17), 2495–2500.

Porges, S. W. (2001). The polyvagal theory: Phylogenetic substrates of a social nervous system. *International Journal of Psychophysiology, 42*(2), 123–146.

Porges, S. W. (2004). Neuroception: A subconscious system for detecting threats and safety. *Zero to Three, 24*(5), 19–24.

Ronfard, S., & Harris, P. L. (2014). When will Little Red Riding Hood become scared? Children's attribution of mental states to a story character. *Developmental Psychology, 50*(1), 283–292.

Rosnay, M. D., Harris, P. L., & Pons, F. (2008). Emotional understanding and developmental psychopathology in young children. In L. Feldman Barrett, M. Lewis, & J. Haviland Jones (Eds.,), *Handbook of emotions* (4th ed., pp. 343–386). Guilford.

Rutishauser, U., Tudusciuc, O., Neumann, D., Mamelak, A. N., Heller, A. C., Ross, I. B., Philpot, L., Sutherling, W., & Adolphs, R. (2011). Single-unit responses selective for whole faces in the human amygdala. *Current Biology*, *21*(19), 1654–1660.

Rutishauser, U., Tudusciuc, O., Wang, S., Mamelak, A. N., Ross, I. B., & Adolphs, R. (2013). Single-neuron correlates of atypical face processing in autism. *Neuron*, *80*(4), 887–899.

Sato, W., Kochiyama, T., Uono, S., Kubota, Y., Sawada, R., Yoshimura, S., & Toichi, M. (2015). The structural neural substrate of subjective happiness. *Scientific Reports*, *5*, 16891.

Schachter, S., & Singer, I. E. (1962). Cognitive, social, and physiological determinants of emotional state. *Psychological Review*, *69*, 379–399.

Sharot, T., Delgado, M. R., & Phelps, E. A. (2004). How emotion enhances the feeling of remembering. *Nature Neuroscience*, *7*(12), 1376–1380.

Smith, P. K., Cowie, H., & Blades, M. (2015). *Understanding children's development*. Wiley.

Spunt, R. P., & Adolphs, R. (2019). The neuroscience of understanding the emotions of others. *Neuroscience Letters*, *693*, 44–48.

Terasawa, Y., Shibata, M., Moriguchi, Y., & Umeda, S. (2013). Anterior insular cortex mediates bodily sensibility and social anxiety. *Social Cognitive and Affective Neuroscience*, *8*(3), 259–266.

Termine, N. T., & Izard, C. E. (1988). Infants' responses to their mothers' expressions of joy and sadness. *Developmental Psychology*, *24*(2), 223–229.

Vallotton, C. D. (2008). Signs of emotion: What can preverbal children "say" about internal states? *Infant Mental Health Journal*, *29*(3), 234–258.

Van Rosmalen, L., Van der Veer, R., & Van der Horst, F. (2015). Ainsworth's strange situation procedure: The origin of an instrument. *Journal of the History of the Behavioral Sciences*, *51*(3), 261–284.

Wang, S., Tudusciuc, O., Mamelak, A. N., Ross, I. B., Adolphs, R., & Rutishauser, U. (2014). Neurons in the human amygdala selective for perceived emotion. *Proceedings of the National Academy of Sciences of the USA*, *111*(30), E3110–E3119.

Zajonc, R. B. (1980). Feeling and thinking: Preferences need no inferences. *American Psychologist*, *35*(2), 151–175.

Zhang, S., & Chiang-shan, R. L. (2012). Functional connectivity mapping of the human precuneus by resting state fMRI. *NeuroImage*, *59*(4), 3548–3562.

# 5

# Language

> Nevertheless, the difference in mind between man and the higher animals,
> great as it is, is certainly one of degree and not of kind. If it be maintained
> that certain powers, such as self-consciousness, abstraction, etc., are pe-
> culiar to man, it may well be that these are the incidental results of other
> highly advanced intellectual faculties; and these again are mainly the result
> of the continued use of a highly developed language.
>
> —Charles Darwin, *The Descent of Man* (1871)

The emergence of language in human evolution is an issue of continuing interest to
cognitive neuroscientists. The establishment of language is crucial in distinguishing
humans from other species. But is its structure different in kind, resulting from genetic
changes that produce unique neural circuits specific to humans, or is it different in degree, evolving from phylogenetically older structures, as Darwin might suggest? To
address these questions, this chapter focuses on the developmental cognitive neuroscience of language (Bickerton, 1990).

Language development has been investigated throughout recorded history. Research
methods now ask about how language is acquired. Is it that language is an innate system
with specialized language centers in the brain, one that involves the reconfiguration
of mental and neural systems that are present in other species and continue to serve a
nonlinguistic function in our own species? Or, is it an emergent function that results
from competition between lexical items, phonological forms, and syntactic patterning?
If so, are there specialized linguistic centers in the brain?

This chapter reviews current issues in language development regarding these two
perspectives. It reviews the anatomy of language, discusses simulated language learning
in neural networks, considers event-related potential studies that relate to language development, and emphasizes special issues in language development. Special issues relate
to children with focal brain injury, specific language impairments, and deafness; children with genetic disorders involving language; and children who have been linguistically deprived.

## History

Without special training or carefully sequenced linguistic training, children typically
acquire natural language. The extent of language development is related to overall cognitive ability. Still, children with intellectual developmental disorders acquire language
without special training just as typically developing children do, although later. The

emergence of language is universal in children, but it does not necessarily depend on specialized language domains (Bates, 1992).

The earliest known language experiment took place in the late 7th century BC (Rymer, 1993) when Psamtik I, the first of the Saite kings of Egypt, asked, "What might be the original language of the world?" Living in a country with multiple cultures resulting from immigration, he decided to explore which language a child would speak spontaneously if deprived of early language experience. According to the Greek story, as given in Herodotus, two infants were taken from their mothers at Psamtik I's request. They were placed in isolation in a shepherd's hut, and the shepherd was told not to speak with them. They were thus reared in silence on a diet of goat's milk. Two years later, when the shepherd returned to the hut, the children went to him and spoke their first utterance. The word they spoke, *bekos*, was the word for bread in the language of the Phrygians. The ruler then stated that this was the protolanguage and established himself as perhaps the first linguistic researcher.

Psamtik I is remembered now not only for his innovation but also for scientific errors; it is unclear, for example, whether the children simply preferred the bread of this particular Phrygian culture and had not had a natural grasp of other words. However, the question that he raised in regard to spontaneous innate language production persists, and understanding language development continues to be a challenge for developmentalists.

Although children are not denied language exposure or experience for the sake of science, much of our understanding of the acquisition of language comes from extreme examples of children who have been raised in the wild, called *feral* children, without language exposure, such as the wild boy of Aveyron (H. Lane, 1977). More recently, it comes from the case of Genie (Curtiss, 1977). In other instances, children who have been abused or neglected and whose family histories replicate the isolation prescribed by the ancient Egyptian ruler are studied. Following Psamtik, a Greek philosopher, Epicurus, believed that language was a product of nature—a biological function like vision or digestion—and not the product of intellect or a specially created ability. However, later philosophers, such as Leibnitz in the 17th century, suggested that language ability was a special gift and that its form of expression was determined by natural instinct.

It was not until the 1950s when Noam Chomsky published *Syntactic Structures* (1957) that the study of language acquisition assumed scientific prominence. Previously, research focus had been on vocabulary; Chomsky changed the focus to syntax. The syntactic argument was that the grammars of different languages used the same principles. Because of this striking uniformity between languages in syntax in different cultures, Chomsky suggested that language was specific to the human species and that the rules of language are ingrained on a level "more basic than thought." This view, that of the nativist or innatist school, suggests that language develops spontaneously. However, Chomsky's approach is questioned by environmentalists (or empiricists), who propose that children learn language through interactions, primarily from interactions with their parents and particularly with their parents' speech, and that multiple brain regions are involved.

The extent to which language is innate has been the subject of debate following Chomsky's (1957) proposal that a special and separate mental organ is responsible for language. If he is correct, mental structures that support language are modular and discontinuous from other perceptual and cognitive systems. Furthermore, it suggests that the brain of a newborn child contains neuronal structures that are destined to mediate language and only language. This view is contrasted with an approach in which language is viewed as requiring the reconfiguration of mental and neuronal systems that persist from other species and develop evolutionarily, much as Darwin might have suggested. Such systems would continue to serve some nonlinguistic functions as well.

Current studies support the view that language development does appear to occur as a result of a mix of neuronal systems and includes other cognitive and perceptual functions. Linguistic theory focuses on understanding this acquisitional process. What the child brings to the language learning task is generally referred to as the *language acquisition device*. The input from parents and others is referred to as *primary linguistic data*.

## The Anatomy of Language

As Darwin proposed, there is no animal homolog for human language. Both auditory and visual sensory and perceptual systems are essential in the comprehension of language. Brain regions that make key contributions to language include the cortical (premotor cortex, motor cortex, and supplementary cortex) and subcortical (thalamus, basal ganglia, and cerebellum) brain regions. Typically, most language processing is lateralized to the left hemisphere regions that surround the sylvian fissure (Gazzaniga et al., 2019). Left hemispheric language areas include Wernicke's area (primarily located in the posterior superior temporal gyrus, parts of the anterior and lateral cortex, and the inferior parietal lobe) and Broca's area (inferior frontal cortex and the insular cortex). These regions and the white matter tracts that connect them make up the left perisylvian language network (Hagoort, 2013). Although the majority of language processing typically takes place in the left hemisphere, the right hemisphere is also involved. The right superior temporal sulcus is involved in language prosody—that is, processing the rhythms of language. Prosodic expression is an ongoing area of research in autism spectrum disorder (McCann & Peppé, 2003). The right prefrontal cortex, middle temporal gyrus, and posterior cingulate brain regions are activated for metaphorical meaning in sentences. Cortical mapping using direct cortical mapping conducted during awake surgery reveals that the anatomical localization for language varies across patients, confirming that language cannot be reliably localized based on specific anatomical regions alone. In one study, carried out in 117 patients, the frontal cortex and the posterior temporal cortex, as expected, were identified in most, but in others only identified in frontal or temporal areas (Ojemann et al., 1989). Thus, some cases had classical regions disrupted, whereas others did not. Cortical mapping of language areas is essential in neurosurgical procedures to preserve language, particularly for epilepsy surgery in children and adults (Gonen et al., 2017).

A development approach is needed to understand anatomical language mapping in the brain. Importantly, studies of the impact of early unilateral brain damage in the developing brain have been conducted. In one study, children were examined who had perinatal left hemisphere or perinatal right hemispheric stroke ($n = 71$). They were compared to typically developing children ($n = 126$) with typical language development.

At 12 months of age, there were no differences in words understood, phrases understood, or words produced, despite perinatal strokes. At 24 months, both lesion groups scored lower than typically developing children in word production, irregular words, or sentence length but did not differ from one another regarding the side of the stroke—left side versus right side. Although expressive vocabulary did not progress as expected, here, too, there were no differences in regard to lesion side. Still, gesture and word production were dissociated in the left hemisphere group (Trauner et al., 2013). Consistent with earlier studies, language development proceeds following stroke because of plasticity of the developing brain (Bates & Roe, 2001). A decade or two after experiencing perinatal stroke damage to the left hemisphere (typically the language side of the brain), affected adolescents and adults were evaluated. In this study, 12 people aged 12–25 years with left brain perinatal stroke were found to have language function for both language comprehension and production in the "normal" range but used the right hemisphere of the brain. Neuroimaging studies in these individuals showed essentially an exact opposite language region from the typical left normal language area. The right hemisphere region of the brain had the damaged part, in this instance producing a mirror-image language area (Newport et al., 2017).

The child development to lesion approach must be contrasted with the adult lesion approach. The language area in adults is the product of language development. Language learning emerges outside the typical regional area biased for language acquisition. When the typical language region is damaged, parts of the brain in the right hemisphere emerge and function as language-learning areas. Our understanding is that early in life, right hemispheric homotopic regions are heavily involved in language processing even in the healthy brain. This may be the basis for the enhancement of these right hemisphere regions' involvement in language processing when there is early brain injury (Newport et al., 2017). This reorganization takes place between birth and age 5 years, when children struggle to meet the challenges associated with language and communication learning. Neuroimaging studies show that up to approximately age 4 years, children can process language in both sides of the brain. After that time, language functions split, with the left side of the brain processing sentences and the right side of the brain processing emotion in language.

Neuroimaging studies of language networks using resting-state functional magnetic resonance imaging (fMRI) and the white matter tracks are revealing. Imaging resting fMRI in children with perinatal stroke indicates that the language networks have altered connectivity in both hemispheres. Language networks are not present at birth and develop throughout the childhood years. Dorsal and ventral white matter structural networks have been identified. The dorsal language pathway involves the arcuate and superior longitudinal fascicles. The ventral portion involves the uncinate fascicular and/or extreme capsule. Long-range intrahemispheric language connections between the inferior frontal gyrus and posterior superior temporal areas are not fully developed in typically developing 6-year-old children, consistent with such plasticity. Functional connectivity of language networks is altered in children with perinatal stroke (Newport, 2017). Children with left hemisphere stroke have comparable functional connectivity between language areas of the left and right hemispheres compared to typically developing children. This suggests that these children retain prelanguage bi-hemispheric potential and/or develop right lateralization to compensate for left hemispheric damage.

The results of the study by Newport (2017) are in accord with other evidence that supports compensatory developmental plasticity after early injury (Carlson et al., 2019).

## The Evolution of Language

Humans have a biological predisposition to language, although its evolutionary origins are not known. At issue is the question of whether or not language can be explained in terms of natural selection (Chomsky, 2006, 2017; Pinker & Bloom, 1990). Did language emerge based on an underlying cognitive mechanism specific to language or as a consequence of social behavior? Sterelny (2012) proposes that the origin of language begins with gestured communication leading to enhancement of social communication following incremental language emergence. This proposal is for gestures as the origin, not an evolutionary expansion of vocalization from great apes. Studies of vervet monkey communication in Amboseli National Park in Kenya have found that vervet monkeys give acoustically different alarm calls for different predators (Seyfarth et al., 1980). Eagle alarm calls warn for birds that may attack. Leopard calls warn of approaching terrestrial predators; monkeys will scamper and climb trees in response. For snakes, the monkeys are alerted to stand up and look around. Alerting vocalization is rare when alone and more likely to occur with kin than with non-kin, so their warning calls are not automatic. Vervet monkeys do not demonstrate theory of mind and thus do not attribute mental states to others, and although their behavior may affect others, the outcome is not cognitively intentional (Seyfarth & Cheney, 2003). However, further examination of context (specificity of alarm calls and aggressive calls) in vervet monkeys finds that when aggressive context is also taken into account, both cognitive appraisal of the situation and internal state make contributions to variations in call usage. However, the semantic properties of vervet vocalized alarm calls do not resemble human words. Such acoustic calls, vocalizations, in nonhuman primates are largely innate (Price et al., 2015). Because vocalization communication is not symbolic, it differs from human language.

If not derived from nonhuman primate vocalization, might human language evolve from manual gestures? If so, has generative language evolved from evolutionarily early human, *Homo habilis*, gesture usage rather than monkey vocalization leading to verbal language in the emergence of human, *Homo sapiens* (Corballis, 2017)? If so, language evolved out of gesture and mime with gradual conventionalization of gestural symbols. The emphasis here is on the function of language as primarily a system of communication more so than a system of thought—one in which culture may play a role in the evolutionary steps toward communicative language in humans.

The role of gesture is borne out in great apes, where gestures are more essential to communication than vocalization (Gazzaniga et al., 2019). In great apes, vocal calls are inflexible and tend to be automatically linked to an emotional state and produced in response to environmental stimuli, whereas there is flexibility in gestures. Unlike alarm vocalizations, gestures are used in social grooming and in play; some may be learned by chimpanzees, gorillas, and bonobos. Moreover, unlike vocalization, gestures are linked to attention from the communicating conspecifics. Thus, primate gestures are more akin to human language than are vocalizations. Great apes have cortical control over both hands and fingers. Although efforts to teach nonhuman primates to speak have been unsuccessful, there are notable examples of manual social communication. A chimpanzee, Washoe, learned approximately 350 signs. A bonobo, Kanzi, learned to point to abstract symbols on a keyboard and has used that information to communicate near the level of a 2-year-old child (Savage-Rumbaugh et al., 1993; Savage-Rumbaugh & Lewin, 1994). Kanzi also exhibits protosyntax. He understands word order and knows the difference between "make do" and "snake bite the doggie."

Others propose that language arose from a combination of gestures and facial movements. The left hemisphere controls motoric hand movements in humans and great apes. Still, although there is considerable support for the role of gesturing in the evolution of human language, this proposal is not fully accepted. An anthropologist has proposed that gestural and oral communication could have evolved in parallel or that brain oral–aural and kinesthetic modulates evolved together (Kendon, 2017). Kendon points to the close coordination of babbling and hand movements in human infants (Trevarthen, 1979) and to babbling in the manual mode in deaf children who do not speak but make hand gestures at the age children begin to babble (Petitto & Marentette, 1991). Most declarative pointing to objects by children is accompanied by vocalization. A speaker commonly gestures when speaking, facilitating the gesture being fully understood. Although the issue is not resolved, neurologically hand and mouth are closely related brain systems. The largest relevant brain difference between human and non-human primates is the left perisylvian area, a brain region that involves left hemispheric representation of linguistic information. In the temporal lobe, there is increased connectivity with left perisylvian brain regions. The most substantial evolutionary brain changes in brain development are in the overall size and function of the left temporal cortex, which is densely interconnected with the inferior frontal and inferior parietal cortex (Gazzaniga et al., 2019).

The left hemisphere is dominant for communication in both humans and the chimpanzee. In human emotional expression, the right side of the mouth opens first and wider than the left. The left side of the mouth opens first for emotional expression. Studies indicate that left hemisphere voluntary control of hand gestures as well as vocalization might have evolved in an integrative manner. Neuroimaging methods have contributed to our understanding of the evolution of the left perisylvian language system. Dorsal and ventral language pathways in humans interconnect the temporal lobe to the inferior frontal and parietal cortex. A diffusion tensor imaging (DTI) and MRI study conducted in humans, chimpanzees, and rhesus macaque monkeys linked the arcuate fasciculus, a white matter tract important in human language (Rilling et al., 2008). This study revealed a prominent temporal lobe projection of the human arcuate fasciculus. The arcuate fasciculus is much smaller or absent in chimpanzees and rhesus macaques. It is proposed that this human track specialization is relevant in the evolution of language. The identification of this subprojection interconnecting brain areas is informative regarding the complexity of human language. Regions of the temporal lobe are key in the representation of words, their meanings, and conceptualization. These neuroimaging findings are consistent with there being remarkable changes in brain connectivity in cortical areas that are the product of human language evolution.

In summary, striking evolutionary changes in the size and functioning of the temporal cortex and its interconnectedness with the inferior frontal and inferior parietal cortex are proposed to be essential to the evolution of human language.

## Gene Mutation in the Evolution of Speech and Language

A gene mutation in the Forkhead box protein P2 (FoxP2), one gene that is involved in language production, results in a severe speech and language disorder that is inherited as autosomal dominant, affecting multiple family members (Hurst et al., 1990). This mutation has been studied extensively as potentially linked in evolution to the emergence of human speech and language (Enard et al., 2002) because language development was essential in human evolution in facilitating social organization. Language is important in the exchange of information between people. It is important for the emergence of abstraction and symbolic thought. However, extensive genomic study of FOXP2 among diverse human populations has refuted the proposal of this single gene's role in human language evolution (Atkinson et al., 2018). Neanderthals carried the same mutation, and Atkinson et al. did not find evidence of changes in the gene in *H. sapiens* evolution.

Despite there being no recent evolutionary change in the FOXP2 gene, this gene is involved in human language in birdsong (mimicry in birds) and echolocation in bats. A 1990 study of profound language disorder in the "KE" family revealed half of the family members were affected over three generations (Hurst et al., 1990). These family members have been diagnosed with developmental verbal dyspraxia. Their linguistic deficits include impaired grammar, difficulty with the morphology of words, and inability to repeat heard words. The disorder involves translocation of the 7q31.2 region of the FOXP2 gene. In humans, loss of one copy of the FOXP2 gene (haploinsufficiency) results in abnormal brain development. The FOXP2 gene is involved in synaptic plasticity, making it important in learning and memory. In addition to the KE family, FOXP2 variants have been identified in 14 individuals in three other families (Reuter et al., 2017). FOXP2 has also been implicated in attention-deficit/hyperactivity disorder (Demontis et al., 2019).

Brain imaging studies have been carried out seeking the neuronal basis of language deficits in the KE family. Structural and functional MRI studies demonstrated bilateral abnormalities in motor-related regions of the brain. Family members with the mutation have an oral–facial movement disorder. The behavioral phenotype associated with the FOXP2 mutation in the KE family affects expression and articulation of language rather than language comprehension; family members have no hearing or neurological diagnoses. This is a severe speech disorder that affects both phonology and grammar. Compared to a typically developing control group, on examination of word and nonword repetition and oral praxis, MRI studies of affected family members showed a 25% bilateral reduction in the volume of the caudate nucleus; reduction in gray matter density in the inferior frontal gyrus (Broca's area); and reduction in precentral gyrus, frontal pole, and cerebellum. However, there were elevated levels of gray matter density in the superior temporal gyrus (Wernicke's area), angular gyrus, and putamen (Gazzaniga et al., 2019; Vargha-Khadem et al., 2005). The extent of caudate volume reduction was correlated with performance on a test of oral praxis, a test of non-word repetition, and performance on the coding subtest of the Wechsler Adult Intelligence Scale.

The fMRI studies used two protocols. One involved silent verb generation and word repetition, and the other used spoken verb generation and word repetition. The fMRI studies found that affected family members have a more posterior and more extensively bilateral activation on all tasks. Considering both structural and functional

MRI results, the affected family members had less activation of Broca's areas and its right hemispheric homolog out of the putamen. Thus, brain-affected individuals, perhaps as a means of compensation, showed overactivation in nonlanguage brain areas involving postcentral, posterior, and parietal regions. Overall, these neuroimaging findings suggest that FOXP2 may have an important role in the development of putative frontostriatal and frontocerebellar networks. These networks are involved in learning, planning, and executive function of oral–facial and speech motor sequencing (Vargha-Khadem et al., 2005). Bringing together the neurophenotype of the KE family with the neural expression of FOXP2, the proposed circuit helps clarify how the KE family's mutation has led to orofacial and verbal dyspraxia in affected family members.

## Fundamentals of Language

Human language can be spoken, gestured, or written. Because it derives from the capacities of the brain, it is referred to as a natural language. There are language vocabulary, grammar, and syntactical rules. Language allows us to communicate both concrete and abstract ideas and to converse about the past, present, and future (Gazzaniga et al., 2019). What is involved to allow such communication to occur? As discussed in Chapter 17, words have meaning and a sound base that is a phonological form. Words also have a visual form referred to as orthographic form. We store representations of words and their associated concepts in the brain. Such word (lexical) representation constitutes a mental lexicon. The child's developmental lexicon stores information about words. This includes the meaning of words (semantics), how words come together to form sentences (syntax), and their spelling and associated sounds (word morphology). These lexicon elements are organized into a grammar that involves syntactical and morphological elements to produce meaningful communication. The practical way we communicate is referred to as the pragmatics of language. *Pragmatics* refers to social language skills—that is, what we say, how we say it, how we engage nonverbally (e.g., eye contact, body language, and facial expressions when speaking), and context. *Context* refers to conversational rules that take into account turn-taking in conversation, listening to one's partner, and then responding. Autism spectrum disorder and social (pragmatic) language disorder are disorders that involve language pragmatics. The mental lexicon facilitates our capacity to move from spoken words to written ones.

Four basic organizing principles are involved with language. First, the morpheme is the smallest unit in the mental lexicon; it is the root of a word. For example, the word "freeze" is a morpheme. Adding the prefix "un" to make the word "unfreeze" or "r" to make the word "freezer" changes the meaning, resulting in three morphemes. Second, frequently used words are accessed more quickly. Third, the phoneme is the smallest unit of sound. The lexicon includes words that differ from one another by a single letter with a single phenome. Examples are "cat," "hat," and "sat." Such words are clustered in the developing mental lexicon. Fourth, the mental lexicon is organized by relationships between words. Therefore, when a word is heard, a lexical decision is made regarding whether the word is a real word or a pseudoword. Accuracy in word recognition improves when a real word is primed by a semantically related one. For example, in semantic priming studies, the prime word might be "car" and the categorically related target word is "truck" as the response rather than a word unrelated to the vehicle category, such as "night." Thus, lexical organization in the brain facilitates responsiveness to words. Word meanings are represented in semantic networks in the brain, with conceptual nodes in these networks connected to one another. Such storage of mental word meanings is essential to language comprehension and production.

The mental lexicon has been examined in people with language disorders, as discussed in Part IV. There are brain differences in these disorders. The mental lexicon is organized in the brain. Word meanings (semantics), word usage (syntax), and the forms of words (spelling and sound patterns related to words) are stored in the brain. The brain is activated by a wide variety of word inputs. One study demonstrated that storage of semantic information was not restricted to the left perisylvian cortex or to the left hemisphere of the brain (Huth et al., 2016). Semantic information was distributed throughout both brain hemispheres. However, other studies have found that categories of semantic information are predominantly represented in the left temporal lobe. Progression from posterior to anterior brain regions goes from general to more specific information.

## Language Comprehension

Understanding written and spoken language is a developmental process. Spoken words must be decoded and acoustically analyzed into the phonological code. Word grammar sentences are stored in the mental lexicon. Reading involves establishing meaning, which involves perception of words as recognizable written symbols for words and recognizing their orthography when reading. Words may be directly mapped as whole words in the mental lexicon or words broken down into phonological units in the mental lexicon.

There are approximately 40 phenomes in the English language. Infants can perceptually distinguish all of these possible phenomes in the first year of life. During that first year, perceptually infants become attuned to the phenomes of their home language (Kuhl et al., 1992). Infants aged 6–12 months articulate phonemes they hear most often. By age 2 years, infants in English-speaking countries no longer produce, and possibly no longer perceive, phenomes that are not part of the English language. Understanding speech differs from reading because speech varies among speakers and is not clearly segmented, so it may be difficult to discern where a word begins and where an earlier spoken word ends. In speech, we typically produce approximately 15 phenomes, roughly 180 words per minute (Gazzaniga et al., 2019). Thus, there may be a segmentation problem in distinguishing spoken words. We are helped in decoding other's speech by attending to the pitch and rhythm of speech, referred to as prosody. Prosody involves attending to the duration of words and attending to the pauses between them. For example, we detect prosody when the speaker asks us a question or places greater emphasis on one word and not another one, raises voice frequency at the end of a question, or speaks more loudly for emphasis. Word boundaries are also created when spoken syllables have an accent or receive greater stress (Tyler & Cutler, 2009).

Understanding speech involves particular brain systems and circuits; the superior temporal cortex is essential for sound perception. People with brain lesions involving the superior temporal lobe have problems in recognizing speech sounds; however, they can recognize other sounds normally. Their recognition to speech sounds is limited; these are phonemic deficits. The auditory association cortex is located in Heschl's gyrus, which is in the superior temporal gyrus in both brain hemispheres. Heschl's gyri are activated by both speech and non-speech sounds; however, the superior temporal sulcus is modulated bilaterally by auditory speech sounds.

As shown in Figure 5.1, acoustic sensitivity is greatest in the primary auditory cortex. It is activated by all auditory inputs. Intelligibility of speech increases and acoustic sensitivity decreases moving anteriorly, inferiorly, and posteriorly away from the primary auditory cortex. Overall, the anterior and posterior regions of the superior temporal sulcus are increasingly more speech sensitive. Accessing or integration of semantic representations involves the left posterior inferior temporal cortex. Regions of the frontal cortex contribute to the comprehension of speech (Gazzaniga et al., 2019). There is a hierarchy of word recognition (Binder et al., 2000). In this hierarchal model, auditory information moves from Heschl's gyri into the auditory cortex to the superior temporal gyrus. Speech and non-speech sounds are distinguished in the middle part of the superior temporal sulcus, but semantic information is not. The final step in distinguishing words from non-words involves the middle temporal gyrus, inferior temporal gyrus, angular gyrus, and temporal pole.

Written-word processing occurs in the occipitotemporal cortex in the left hemisphere of the brain. When this area is injured in adults, a person cannot read words

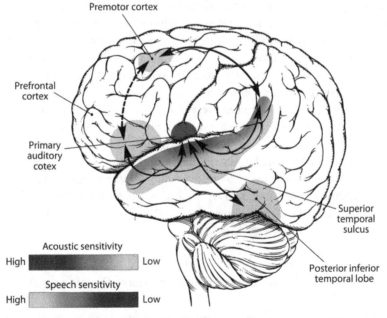

**Figure 5.1** Organization of the cortical auditory system. The figure shows hierarchal parallel processing pathways that spread out from the primary auditory cortex to motor, premotor, and prefrontal cortex. Anterior and posterior regions of the superior temporal sulcus show greater speech specificity. Regions of the frontal cortex are involved in speech comprehension.

From Gazzaniga, Ivry and Mangun (2019); redrawn by Tim Phelps (2021).

(alexia). However, other features of language are normal. Written information processing begins with visual awareness with input into the contralateral right occipital cortex. From there, visual information passes to the left hemispheric visual form recognition region via the corpus callosum. The visual form recognition center is interconnected to areas of the left perisylvian language system. This also includes regions of the inferior frontal, temporal, and parietal cortical regions (Gazzaniga et al., 2019). Once visual input is identified as a word, its semantic meaning must be accessed. Thus, integration of syntactic and semantic information is necessary to understand words in context. Following lexical access to words, lexical selection to put words into context is influenced by both sensory and higher level contextual information. The role of higher level contextual information in lexical selection is supported by an fMRI study involving word recognition which found that lexical access and selection involve a particular brain network (Zhuang et al., 2011). This network includes the medial temporal gyrus, superior temporal gyrus, and ventral inferior and bilateral dorsal inferior frontal gyri. The first two of these brain regions are involved in the translation of speech sounds into word meanings.

The next step is to process words into sentences. This involves activating grammatical and semantic information from the mental lexicon. Whole sentences are not stored in the brain. Therefore, instead of such storage, the brain works to assign syntactic structure for words that appear in sentences, the so-called syntactic parsing that builds sentences. How this occurs in the brain is studied by neuropsychologists. Ultimately, linguistic competence during development involves language use. Models of how language use facilitates linguistic development are referred to as cognitive–functional linguistics or simply usage-based linguistics. These terms emphasize how language structure emerges from language use. These models hold that in essence there is a symbolic dimension to language with grammar derived from it. In contrast to formal approaches such as generative grammar usage-based ones, grammar develops from historical usage. Collectively, this process is referred to as grammaticalization. In the usage-based approach, competence in language involves ongoing mastery of word usage. Thus, a speaker fluent in the English language effectively uses highly abstract syntactic constructions—for example, the past tense, "-ed," passive construction along with concrete expressions based on words or phrases that are used in ritualized greetings, in metaphor, and in other word usages. Therefore, children can use language functions or meanings to assist in linguistic word constructions as well as in the use of individual words. This usage-based approach is described in detail in Michael Tomasello's (2003) book, *Constructing a Language: A Usage-Based Theory of Language Acquisition*.

## Event-Related Potentials and Language Development

Electrophysiologic studies of event-related brain potentials (ERPs) are used to investigate the neural bases of semantic and syntactic analyses in sentence processing for language development in children. Changes in ERPs to familiar and unfamiliar words have been shown at different stages in early language development. An ERP is a measured brain response to a sensory, cognitive, or motor stimulus. ERPs provide a noninvasive approach to evaluate brain functioning. Importantly, ERP measures provide real-time temporal resolution in milliseconds that allows the study of speech perception, lexical processing, or sentence processing. Processes that underlie perceptual and linguistic processing are very fast, transient, and follow one another at rapid intervals. Moreover, ERP measures do not require overt task testing when measured in infants and toddlers.

Multiple cognitive spectra underlie language comprehension (speech perception, word recognition, and integration into syntactical structures) taking place within a few hundred milliseconds of stimulus presentation. A behavioral response alone is insufficient to identify these underlying operations. Moreover, different ERP components are linked to distinct cognitive processes. Different ERP responses (either the P150–250 or the N250–500) to phonetic contrasts can be predictors of later language development in which behavior measures are insufficient. The N400 response is an ERP component related to linguistic processes (Kutas & Hillyard, 1980). In one study of a sentence reading test, words occurring out of context were associated with specific ERPs. Semantically inappropriate words produced a late negative wave, referred to as N400 because it reaches its maximum amplitude at 400 ms following the onset of the word used as a stimulus. N400 amplitude was greater when the anomalous word was at the end of a sentence. Semantically congruent words such as those different in appearance (e.g., being presented as capital letters) produced a positive potential rather than an N400 negative one. The N400 effects are specific to semantic analysis.

The importance of the N200–500 component was demonstrated when 20-month-olds participated in a word learning experiment using novel word–object associations. The N200–500 component that is typically elected in response to familiar words becomes left-lateralized with continuous training. This suggests that lateralization of lexical processing becomes more specialized and is left-lateralized as word learning becomes more efficient in children. Such changes in cognitive processing are not directly observable in typical behavioral measures that include looking time and head turn preferences. Because ERP recording does not require overt behavioral responses or explicit attention to stimuli, it allows observation of cognitive processes in younger children who lack cognitive resources.

Because ERP responses are automatically elicited when exposed to linguistic stimuli, language processing can be tested and compared across age groups developmentally. This allows the study of the developmental time course of elements involved in language comprehension. This includes mechanisms involved in phonetic, lexical, and sentence processing (Friederici, 2005; Friederici & Weisenborn, 2007). It is not clear whether infants in the first 2 years of life have discrete phonological representations as they develop. The level to which sound and meaning association is established is referred to as lexical representation. For example, in regard to lexical representation, 12-month-olds show facilitation of phonological processing shown by early negativity, but they lack an N400. This suggests that infants do not retrieve appropriate meaning. However, 13- and 14-month-olds begin to show N400 responses to congruous–incongruous words, with articulated lexical representation present soon after the first year of life. Overall, how semantic memory is organized can be studied by testing to determine if the N400 can be modulated and by how much expected word and the actual word responses diverge (Kutas & Federmeier, 2000). School-age and adolescent children continue to improve in the integration and comprehension of auditory language over developmental time. Semantic processing matures earlier than syntactic processing (Schneider & Maguire, 2019).

In summary, although there are challenges in measuring ERPs in children, these methods can provide important information about the time course and distribution of neural activities that underlie language processing. This allows comparison of neural activities in children and adults at different levels of linguistic processes. ERP measures also can be used to examine social discourse. A study in adolescents examined semantically plausible sentences that they believed others would find implausible. The study demonstrated a social N400 effect. The adolescents were able to take into account the perspective of the other person (Westley et al., 2017). In addition, N400 event potential was used to compare word learning in children from lower and higher socioeconomic status homes. Children from higher socioeconomic homes, like adults, showed attention by N400 response as meaning is attached to new words. Those from the lower socioeconomic did not show such attention, suggesting a lack of language stimulation in the home setting and less support for them in language processing (Ralph et al., 2020).

ERPs have been used to study language impairments in children with developmental neuropsychiatric disorders. Approximately 25% of children with autism spectrum disorder diagnoses, despite intervention, continue to be minimally verbal. Neural mechanisms that underlie language impairment in these children might potentially enhance our ability to predict language outcomes and specify interventions. In one study, nonverbal and minimally verbal children and typically developing children participated in a semantic consequence ERP paradigm study. Pictures were displayed, followed by an expected word or an unexpected word. An N400 effect was found in all three groups but with a shorter latency in the typically developing group—that is, typically developing children responded faster. Children with autism spectrum disorder, including those with minimal language, did show evidence of semantic processing. However, such processing was characterized by delayed processing speed. Moreover, there was limited integration in children with autism spectrum disorder for mental representations (DiStefano et al., 2019).

Evidence suggests that the temporal lobe is the likely site for the generation of the N400 response. Intracranial recordings point to the temporal lobe. In one study, ERPs were recorded from cortical surface electrodes placed on the temporal lobes of people diagnosed with epilepsy. Large negative polarity responses were recorded from the ventral anterior temporal lobe to visually presented, semantically anomalous words in sentences. These measured N400-like ERPs were found to have time courses that were similar to those from scalp-recorded N400s that were generated by the same type of task (Gazzaniga et al., 2019; Nobre et al., 1994). Further support for N400 generation from left temporal lobe and surrounding areas has been found using neuromagnetic signals in magnetoencephalography (Simos et al., 1997).

## Syntactic Processing and ERP P600

Cognitive neuroscience electrophysiological methods have been used to investigate both semantic and syntactic processing. The P600 is an ERP measured, as is the N400, by electroencephalography (EEG). It is relevant to language because the P600 is elicited by hearing or reading with syntactic processing of sentences. The EEG waveform is a large peak in the positive direction that starts approximately 500 ms after a person sees or hears a language stimulus. It is referred to as the syntactic positive shift because its polarity is positive and typically elicited by syntactic stimuli (Hagoort et al., 1993; Osterhout & Holcomb, 1992). This response is elicited by ungrammatical stimuli—for example, garden path sentences that require reanalysis, complex sentences, and "fuller grasp" words that are heard at the beginning of an English language sentence but are interpreted elsewhere. Garden path sentences are sentences with no clear-cut grammatical error but must be understood in a different way than expected by the reader. The reader follows an initial interpretation but later realizes that their interpretation was wrong and must backtrack to understand the sentence (Osterhout & Halcomb, 1992). These sentences are made temporarily ambiguous by including a word group with more than one way of being understood—for example, the headline "Drunk gets 9 months in violin case" (Gazzaniga et al., 2019). The P600 effect size predicts when one is processing English syntax for future syntax learning. The N400 is related to syntax learning only in regard to vocabulary learning (Qi et al., 2017).

Overall, ERPs provide a window on how the brain is processing language. ERPs change throughout language development. ERPs are sensitive to expectation and mismatch. Such sensitivity relates to the relative timing of the N400 and P600, the semantic focus of the N400, and the syntactic focus of the P600. As previously noted, ERPs can change when comparing low socioeconomic and high socioeconomic group language development. Comprehension ERPs are related to both sentence production and language acquisition procedures and mechanisms (Fitz & Chang, 2019). Neuroimaging studies provide information on the syntactic processing of the brain. In a study by Caplan et al. (2000), positron emission tomography (PET) scans were conducted on participants who read sentences varying in syntactic complexity. There was increased activation in the left cortical cortex for more complex syntax. However, other PET studies have found activation of anterior superior temporal gyrus in syntactic processing. Thus, syntactic processing occurs in a network that involves left inferior frontal and superior temporal brain regions activated in language processing.

Changes in ERPs to familiar and unfamiliar words at different stages in early language development have been proposed (Mills et al., 1993, 1994, 1997). Mills et al. studied children who were the same chronological age but had attained different language milestones. Distinct components of ERPs that are related to familiar words were associated with independently assessed levels of comprehension ability. For example, they found that 10-month-olds who had begun to understand words differed from 10-month-olds who were still unable to comprehend speech. Furthermore, components of ERPs associated with comprehension of familiar words between 13-month-olds who could and could not produce these words were identified. At 20 months, distinct lateral and anterior–posterior brain specializations were apparent in discriminating comprehended words. Cerebral specialization for language processing is linked to the temporal and parietal regions of the left hemisphere. In addition to being related to changes in chronological age, neuronal systems that mediate language appear to change over time as a function of language learning.

## Neural Networks of Language Acquisition and Processing

Research on language learning in neural networks is a useful tool to study language acquisition and processing. Artificial neural networks are important tools in cognitive science. Neural network modes are referred to as connectionist and as parallel distribution processing models. A neural network emerges from a large number of interconnected neurons. The output of a network is determined by total activation that facilitates information processing. Each connection has a weight between two circuits that establish how strongly the first weight affects the second one. These weights can be adapted for learning or training. Network training is provided through training examples. Supervised network training involves a backpropagation algorithm that gradually builds the network toward target output. Unsupervised training makes the network adapt to input without mapping to a specific target. For example, this approach has been used to find regularities in the phonological structures of language (Frank et al., 2019). These models focus on uncovering statistical structure without knowing the underlying structure.

The best example of unsupervised neural network training is for the classical learning rule introduced by Donald Hebb (1949). Hebb's rule is a learning rule describing how neuronal activities influence the connection between neurons—that is, synaptic plasticity. The algorithm updates the weight of neuronal connection in a neural network to strengthen connections between units that are simultaneously active and to weaken connections between units if only one is active. Importantly, these cognitive network models are not claiming to simulate processing at the level of biological neurons. Rather, their value is in specifying cognitive representations while biological implementation is ignored (Frank et al., 2019).

Connectionist models have been applied to explain a variety of aspects of human language. These range from word segmentation and word meaning mapping to sentence processing and syntactic development. They are proving useful in demonstrating the extent and breadth of environmental input in language learning and contribute to the dialogue on empiricist versus nativist views of language acquisition. Moreover, artificial networks contribute to establishing knowledge needed by an information processing system to simulate human behavior. Connectionist models address the degree to which language processing is hierarchal or sequential; they address the interface between semantics and syntax and the important role of prediction in interpretation of sentence processing (Frank et al., 2019). "Deep learning" neural networks are artificial neural networks with multiple layers between input and output layers. Complex deep neural networks have multiple layers, hence the name deep networks. Deep learning networks are important in natural language processing, especially in training recurrent neural networks. For example, next word prediction methods may be applied in the future to human performance and language acquisition. Because deep learning networks might embody relevant aspects of the human language system, they have potential application for psycholinguistics (Frank et al., 2019).

## Connectionist Models: Innate Versus Domain General

Connectionist models of language acquisition and processing do differ from traditional symbolic models of human cognition. Importantly, neural networks do not make a distinction between language knowledge (language competence) and the performance of language. In networks, knowledge is incorporated in network connection weights to demonstrate language performance. The information stored is procedural in that "knowing how not" declarative knowledge refers to "knowing that." Clark and Karmiroff-Smith (1993) state, "It is knowledge in the system, but it is not knowledge to the system" (p. 495). Neural network models provide a means to study the innate nativist view that language-specific knowledge is innate compared to the language empiricist's claim that language acquisition requires only domain-general information. The connectionist approach focuses on the domain-general view that representations and involved learning mechanisms built into neural networks are not specific to language. Such networks receive no negative evidence as part of their training.

Neural networks differ from traditional linguistic approaches because they do not include language categories such as phonemics, words, or part of speech under their assigned priority units. The most relevant models allow representations to be learned in hidden layers—not assigned. Connectionists propose that symbol behavior emerges in the model from statistical regularities in language as well as from the mapping between form and meaning. Thus, the neural network approach seeks to model human language acquisition, comprehension, and production. By focusing on the discovery of structure in the long-wave environment, neural network researchers test mechanisms involved in many aspects of language. Key areas of language behavior where neural networks have been applied include language learning, comprehension, and production. Areas also include word learning, synaptic development, and sentence processing. For word learning, phonological form is included—that is, identifying words from continuous speech and mapping words to meaning. Regarding syntactic learning, network models have examined lexical category learning and how syntactic structure is learned. Empiricists propose that lexical categories are acquired as a result of experience without there being innately specified structures prior to language exposure. Neural network models examine the extent to which proposed innate knowledge is necessary for advancement in the acquisition of lexical categories. Neural network models posit that embedded syntactic structure can be learned. These models find that learning occurs without a hierarchal structure already built-in. Thus, there does not have to be an innately structured capacity. Despite the success of neural network models, it must be borne in mind that current models—for example, models of sentence production—use artificial language rather than natural stimuli. None of the sentence production models consider the phonological level of sentence production. Instead, the focus is on conceptualization in message planning and sentence formation. Finally, most models hypothesize that comprehension influences production. Although this hypothesis is supported, the exact connection is not established and requires further study.

## Language Development in Congenital Blindness

Young children acquire language rapidly without explicit training. Delays in language acquisition lead to changes in the neural bases of language processing. Early damage to left hemisphere language networks is compensated by recruitment of homologs of left hemisphere frontotemporal language regions in the right hemisphere, resulting in the affected child thereby achieving language processing in the normal range. Compensation also occurs in congenitally blind children. The language network can be augmented when individuals blind from birth are able to recruit a network of visual areas (occipital lobe) for sentence processing, lexical retrieval, reading, and the task of word production (Bedny, 2017; Watkins et al., 2012). Congenital blindness in children does modify language development. The neural basis of language differs in that typically the "visual" cortices respond to linguistic information. Frontotemporal language networks are less left-lateralized in congenitally blind children (Pant et al., 2020). Recruitment means that in blindness, "visual" cortical regions are recruited by nonvisual cognitive functions that also include spatial location and numerical processing (Bedny, 2017). In a cognitively pluripotent cortex, regions of the "visual" cortex are involved in language processing instead of other auditory or tactile tasks. Thus, some typically visual regions respond preferentially to sentences. Such language-responsive regions are sensitive to linguistic information such as semantics and grammar. In addition, there are higher responses to grammar than to simple sentences (C. Lane et al., 2015). Congenitally blind individuals may outperform people with normal site in verbal working memory tasks (Occelli et al., 2017). Plasticity in cortical response to linguistic information is consistent with there being a developmentally sensitive period that allows congenitally blind children to modify the neural basis of language differently from adult-onset blind people (Pant et al., 2020). Language and visual regions that are separate regions in those with normal sight are merged and shared in children with congenital blindness. Visual deprivation leads to a systematic large-scale reorganization of whole-brain cortical networks in regard to how occipital regions interface with other functional networks in congenitally blind people (Hasson et al., 2016).

Plasticity in brain functioning in congenital blindness indicates that the neural basis of language, although evolutionarily constrained, is established through a dynamic developmental process that includes competition for cortical territory involved in multiple cognitive functions (M. Johnson et al., 2002; Karmiloff-Smith, 2018). Further support for brain reorganization in congenitally blind people is found in studies of blind Braille readers (Kim et al., 2017). The visual word form area (VWFA), located in the left ventral occipitotemporal cortex, is specialized for the recognition of written letters and words. Unexpectedly, the anatomical location of the VWFA is active not only in sighted people but also when blind persons read Braille by touch. This indicates that vision is not required for the development of this brain region. Congenitally blind and sighted control subjects have been examined in fMRI studies that involved reading words and listening to spoken sentences varying in grammatical complexity. In blind but not sighted persons, the anatomical location of the VWFA responds to both written words and the grammatical complexity of spoken sentences. Thus, in blind individuals, the occipital region assumes high-level linguistic functions in being active in grammatical processing of spoken sentences. Experience throughout development has major effects on functional brain region specification. Intrinsic connectivity to frontotemporal language networks in blind and sighted persons seems to establish related but distinct functional brain profiles due to differences in development exposures. Whether knowledge of Braille is stored in somatosensory-sensitive areas to touch or dedicated Braille regions needs further clarification.

## Language Development in Cognitive Deafness

Language develops in a social context (Tomasello, 2003). Deaf children experience deprivation of language during the development period. Language deprivation is of particular concern when there is cognitive hearing loss early in the development period. Approximately 2 or 3 of 1,000 children have prelingual hearing loss in one or both ears. More than 90% of deaf children are born to hearing parents. When more than 98% of newborns in the United States were screened for hearing in 2016, the majority (>75%) who tested positive for hearing loss were enrolled in early intervention programs before 3 months of age. For these children, language deprivation occurred if there was a chronic lack of full access to natural language in the first 5 years of life.

Very severe language deprivation may have permanent consequences on long-term neurological development to the extent that a deaf child is unable to receive sufficient language skills for fluent language use (Leybaert & D'Hondt, 2003). Moreover, full language exposure independently influences brain development compared to auditory sound exposure from hearing loss based on timing and quality of early language access in childhood. Language processing develops and becomes more automatic for larger linguistic units (i.e., sentences) and less tied to sensory, perceptive, and phonemic units of language. Brain imaging studies reveal that the weight of neural activation shifts from posterior to more anterior brain regions in development. The timing of early language exposure affects early brain development. Thus, there is a synchrony between language development and brain growth for the classic neural network of language processing to develop properly (Mayberry et al., 2011).

In a DTI study, children with early life auditory deprivation were found to show altered white matter microstructure (Cheng et al., 2019). The authors propose that the dorsal white matter tracks that are involved in syntactic language processing show deficits in connectivity of dorsal white matter tracks, especially the left dorsal arcuate fasciculus pathway, in congenitally deaf children who are deprived of adequate language exposure. Missing a critical time window for linguistic experience seems to affect the dorsal white matter track and in turn leads to deficits in language and neural outcomes. Thus, language experience in early life may be critical for the connectivity of the brain language system.

When auditory input is absent during the developmental period, there are changes in the structure and functioning of the auditory system. The extent of change in the auditory system depends on the etiology of deafness and time hearing is lost in development. Profound hearing loss has widespread long-term consequences during a person's lifetime. Hearing loss may prevent a child from acquiring spoken language. Cochlear implants may be used during the developmental period for congenital deafness. Based on etiology, Cochlear implants may also allow expressive and receptive language skills development similar to that of typically hearing children by school age (Butler & Lomber, 2013; Svirsky et al., 2004). Successful use of Cochlear implants requires the anatomical integrity of auditory structures. Although with implants, some deaf children do develop spoken language skills approaching those of typically developing children, others do not. Moreover, auditory deprivation has effects on brain development that extend beyond the auditory system deficits in information processing (Kral et al., 2016).

Importantly, we engage the environment through sensory systems, particularly hearing and seeing. The integrity of specialized sensory reception cells to encode and transduce information is key to brain processing. Following sensory loss with deafness, the brain's connectivity is altered within the auditory system. It is altered between sensory systems and also between the auditory centers as well as those serving higher order neurocognitive functions. Basically, such congenital sensory input loss can be considered a connectome disease; it varies in individuals based on their adaptation to hearing loss. The World Health Organization estimates that globally 360 million people have disabling hearing loss, making it the fifth most important cause of years lived with disability. Fortunately, cochlea implants are effective neuroprosthetic devices for the treatment of profound sensorineural hearing loss. Their success has made the auditory system a model to investigate sensory loss. Much of what we know about changes in auditory systems involved in deafness is informed by animal models of deafness; the subcortical auditory system is highly preserved in mammals (Butler & Lomber, 2013). There is a marmoset (*Callithrix jacchus*) nonhuman primate model for cochlea implant. Marmosets are the only nonhuman animal that can hear different pitches, such as pitch heard in music and in tonal languages. Marmosets are a close proxy for human hearing studies (L. Johnson et al., 2016). The marmoset cochlea implant model is being studied to examine the failure of cochlea implants. Marmoset studies examine how information is processed in the brain. Neonatal marmosets are being studied for better cochlea implant modeling.

Most deaf children who receive bilateral cochlea implants have the best outcome when implants are placed before age 12 months. Speech will be similar to that of peers with normal hearing. However, implants do not fully restore normal hearing. The implant does not activate auditory parts of the brain in the same way that environmental speech sound does. Speech development is similar to typical speech; however, cochlea implant cases may not distinguish pitch well, may fail to pick up high-pitched sounds, and/or may fail to pick up a sound wave from background noise as well as those with typical hearing do so. Research is ongoing to better understand the cognitive effects that are not directly related to sensory input loss—for example, how hearing loss affects working memory and attention. The brain is a self-organizing system in which neural activity and environmental stimulation act reciprocally throughout brain development. Auditory input to the brain across time provides temporal patterning to the developing brain. Such input may be essential to establish sequential memory, pattern detection, and sustained attention. The role of sound in the development of cognitive sequencing is referred to as the auditory scaffolding hypothesis (Conway et al., 2009).

It is important to examine non-auditory and nonverbal cognitive abilities in deaf children with cochlea implants. This includes organizing and manipulating temporal sequences of nonverbal stimuli, thoughts, and actions. For example, a deaf person has less experience with common measures of time, such as the ticking of a clock, hearing the approaching footsteps of a friend, or a telephone ringing. The role of hearing in our capacity to automatically detect such background change is taken for granted by hearing persons. A lack of sound interferes with the development of spoken language, too. A further effect of auditory deprivation is delay in non-auditory sequencing. Children who receive sound through cochlea implants may have difficulty in the development of cognitive and perceptual sequencing skills, which may be delayed. Such delays may contribute to impairments to learning complex grammatical patterns in their spoken language. Thus, a child with a cochlea implant may accurately detect and discriminate sounds but have difficulty utilizing those sounds to learn the sequenced regularity of words, the unspoken language that is essential to base knowledge of grammar.

Electrophysiologic studies find that deaf children, unlike normally hearing children, have decreased cerebral maturation of the left frontotemporal regions and bilateral frontal regions of the brain (Conway et al., 2009). Hearing deprivation early in development prevents functional brain maturation, and it delays cortical synapse to gene relationship and later synaptic elimination that involves synaptic pruning (Kral & Shrama, 2012). This lack of auditory input also may reduce connectivity in auditory–frontal brain regions, altering prefrontal lobe neural organization and also altering sequencing skills in language development. Moreover, executive function skills, working memory, and self-regulation may be affected. In addition, a deaf child's social environment may be limited.

Deaf children are impaired in verbal short-term memory and short-term memory scanning rates for verbal material. Reduced exposure to sound and spoken language limits the ability to represent and manipulate phonological representations in working memory. Nonverbal serial memory may also be affected, as well as overall visual–motor ability and motor coordination (e.g., how quickly one catches a ball). However, deaf children with cochlea implants do reach age-typical abilities in visual–spatial and visual–motor integration. Yet, they may be impaired in fine motor sequencing skills. Moreover, such motor sequencing skills are associated with language outcomes. Individual variability in sequencing skills linked to language acquisition may also be affected (Conway et al., 2009). Fortunately, overall, cochlea implants can reverse and reorganize many of these neurocognitive effects of sensory loss in deafness (Kral & Sharma, 2012). Although most deaf children who have cochlea implants in very early life have normal cognitive ability and similar learning to hearing peers, there remains considerable variation in language function after implantation. The auditory component of the connectome incorporates the underlying substrate for nondeclarative (habit) memory (basal ganglia and cerebellum) but is also important for declarative memory, spatial orientation, fear memory, and attention (Kral et al., 2016). Variability in the establishment of these neural circuits affected by auditory deprivation may account for differences in cognitive and psychological outcomes in children who receive cochlea implantation. The complex interdependence of these brain systems is key to understanding interindividual variability in outcomes. Neuroimaging methods are important in detecting individual adaptation (Lazard et al., 2014).

Children with bilateral congenital deafness with bilateral cochlea implants (best placed before age 18 months) may reach language facility comparable to their hearing peers. However, because of variability in outcomes with cochlea implants, children with implants generally also learn American Sign Language. Signing cochlea-implanted children are reported to more consistently demonstrate better speech development, language development, and higher intelligence scores than non-signing implanted children (Amraei et al., 2017; Hall, 2017). For deaf children, it is recommended that educational priorities are best focused on language acquisition and cognitive development rather than focusing primarily on speech and spoken language outcomes (Hall et al., 2017).

## Special Issues in Language Learning

Language acquisition has been approached by studying children who were deliberately or accidentally denied language experience and congenitally blind. In some instances, the focus has been on the deaf child who is reared by deaf parents; in others, the focus has been on children who have been emotionally deprived and denied language experience and also instances in which language exposure has been minimized.

Children who are blind, children who are deaf, and children who are deprived of sensory input do develop language syntax in unique ways. Speech–language restoration interventions may be based on a sensory connectome model. This model addresses neural and neurocognitive explanations for variability in spoken language and neurocognitive outcomes following cochlea implantation. Speech–language interventions incorporate practice with executive functioning skills—for example, focusing attention on speech signals or on language components. They seek to facilitate rapid and efficient cognitive processing. Speech therapy includes computer-based auditory training and active practice using word repetition to enhance auditory and language processing skills. Targeted speech–language interventions show the greatest improvement. Interventions show a positive long-term outcome. Speech perception and language skills at ages 6 and 18 months post-implantation have been correlated with positive long-term outcomes for language, verbal working memory, and parent-reported working memory (Hunter et al., 2017).

## Language Development and Neurodevelopmental Syndromes

Another approach to language innateness involves the study of specific syndromes. In some instances, language may appear to be spared in congenital syndromes despite limitations in other cognitive abilities. Children with spina bifida, hydrocephalus, and Williams–Beuren syndrome have such disassociations. In Williams–Beuren syndrome, linguistic function is selectively preserved despite severe general cognitive deficits, suggesting that language develops independently from cognition. If so, there would be evidence of modularity of language in the brain. Subsequent investigations have reputed the view that language is disassociated from cognition in Williams–Beuren syndrome. Comprehensive studies of cognitive and language abilities in Williams–Beuren syndrome find that the overall intellectual ability in this syndrome is in the borderline to moderate intellectual developmental disorder range. Yet, with a characteristic pattern of language strengths and verbal short-term memory, the vocabulary of children with Williams–Beuren syndrome is a particular strength. Visuospatial construction is a major weakness in Williams–Beuren syndrome. Language skills are not independent of cognition; however, language skills are highly correlated with nonverbal cognitive abilities. There is a strong correlation between receptive vocabulary, receptive grammar, nonverbal reasoning, visuospatial construction, verbal short-term memory, and verbal working memory. Overall, in Williams–Beuren syndrome, there is a characteristic pattern of language strengths and weaknesses, with particular strengths in concrete vocabulary (Mervis & John, 2008). However, grammatical abilities are beyond the level of their intellectual ability. Pragmatics is a substantial weakness in Williams–Beuren syndrome. Despite early claims for their being independence in language from cognition, there is no clear evidence for dependence of language and cognition throughout development in children with Williams–Beuren syndrome (Mervis & John, 2012). Although language abilities are a relative strength in children with Williams–Beuren syndrome, language onset is delayed and the rate of vocabulary development when language begins is slower than that of typically developing children. For example, typically developing children can say approximately 100 words by age 18 months. This word level is not reached in children with Williams–Beuren syndrome until age 3 years.

A neuroconstructionist model of language development in Williams–Beuren syndrome examines the impact of early language differences (from typical language development) on later language development. The neuroconstructionist approach is distinct from earlier views that there is innate language model in the brain. The neuroconstructionist model evaluates typical development in the context of the development effect of small perturbations in the developmental trajectory of language (Karmiloff-Smith, 2006, 2009). Development, whether it is typical or atypical, is characterized by plasticity in learning. The infant brain is dynamically restructured throughout its development. Rather than designed with many static built-in modules, "the developing brain follows developmental trajectories that are the emergent property of dynamic multi-directional interactions between biological, physical and social constraints" (Farran & Karmiloff-Smith, 2012, p. 7). In Williams–Beuren syndrome, delayed early development in the verbal domain has cascading effects across verbal and nonverbal domain development. The development trajectory method is important for examining how profiles of abilities start in any neurodevelopmental disorder but especially for Williams–Beuren syndrome. Studies of delays and deviance in early developmental milestones in neurodevelopmental disorder are essential to understanding subsequent cognitive profiles.

In toddlers and preschool children with Williams–Beuren syndrome, the overall IQ score does not accurately predict their abilities. Overt performance is in the normal range for language, nonverbal reasoning, and verbal short-term memory, but it is in the moderate range of intellectual developmental disorder for visuospatial construction. Precursors to lexical development are delayed. Language-relevant abilities that are delayed in early development Williams–Beuren syndrome include the onset of babbling, early phonological development, segmentation of words from continuous speech, and comprehension of pointing gestures and full engagement in triadic joint attention with another person. Delays in each of these areas contribute to an affected child's language development. Children with Williams–Beuren syndrome show delay and immaturity in babbling, with a higher proportion producing vowel-only syllables, fewer syllables per babble, fewer consonants, and lower level of babbling. There are also delays in segmentation of words for fluent speech. In typical language development, word segmentation is correlated with both semantic and syntactic developments (Mervis & John, 2012).

Finally, in Williams–Beuren syndrome, there is a delay in comprehension and production of pointing gestures and engagement in triadic joint attention that is of importance. In triadic attention, an individual looks back to another person after looking at an object and following the other person's gaze to an object. Essentially, the individual looks to see what someone else is looking at. Pointing and triadic attention emerge before the onset acquisition of referential language—that is, communicative language in which two speakers exchange information by naming or describing something to allow the listener to identify it. Referential language allows us to learn from one another. Pointing to an object allows the child to learn the referent for a word. Typically developing pre-linguistic children, deaf children, and children with Down syndrome do point to indicate or request an object of interest, leading them to jointly attend (triadic attention). In Williams–Beuren syndrome, surprisingly, referential language precedes referential pointing by approximately 6 months. The inability to follow another person's eye gaze limits their ability to learn new words and acquire vocabulary (Becerra & Mervis, 2019).

That the onset of declarative pointing gestures precedes the onset of expressive referential language is one of the most consistent findings in the literature on language acquisition. Gestures are considered declarative when the child's goal is to direct another person's attention to something they find interesting (Colonnesi et al., 2010). By age 24 months, typically developing children produce declarative gestures before the onset of referential expressive language. These findings in Williams–Beuren syndrome suggest a divergent path to early language development. The divergence does not suggest that triadic joint attention is not a key development factor for children with Williams–Beuren syndrome to produce referential language but, rather, that other developmental means are utilized by them. The emphasis in establishing triadic joint attention apparently shifts predominantly to the child's communicative partner rather than being jointly shared in the case of Williams–Beuren syndrome. Potentially, this is be facilitated by hypersociability in Williams–Beuren syndrome, in which there is a characteristic intense drive for social contact to form affectionate bonds (Ng et al., 2014). Consistent with this proposal is the age when a child begins to produce declarative pointing gestures. The time when the child initiates triadic joint attention to their immediate interest is a stronger predictor of later lexical abilities than early expressive vocabulary (Becerra & Mervis, 2019). Thus, declarative pointing, once acquired in Williams–Beuren syndrome, as in typical language development, leads to greater engagement with communicative partners, facilitating language development. Despite earlier divergence, language development reconverges in Williams–Beuren syndrome with that of typical language development.

Although overall language is a relative strength in Williams–Beuren syndrome, it is uneven in that receptive language is more delayed than expressive or written language. Despite social interest, social pragmatic use of language is impaired, more so than lexical, phonological, and morphologic features of language. Over time, morphological errors become more apparent; the expressive–receptive gap tends to increase. Such deficits in pragmatic language in Williams–Beuren syndrome are correlated with social and behavioral problems. In these children, good expression skills can mask their true level of receptive language understanding (Rossi & Giacheti, 2017; Royston et al., 2019). Consistent with the atypical development trajectory of neurodevelopment in Williams–Beuren syndrome, the brain connectome shows altering "wiring" in the brain (Gagliardi et al., 2018).

Late adolescents and young adults with a typical Williams–Beuren syndrome profile who have overall mild cognitive impairment were studied with brain MRI. The neuroimaging included anatomical, functional (resting state), and structural (diffusion MRI) sequences. Findings were compared to those of age-matched control subjects.

Individuals with Williams–Beuren syndrome demonstrated anomalies in structural and functional connectivity consistent with their cognitive profile. On DTI, there were altered values associated with increased connectivity in anterior–posterior pathways, which link parieto-occipital pathways with frontal brain regions, and at a local level in the temporal lobe and cerebellum. These imaging findings are congruent with Williams–Beuren syndrome visual–spatial impairment. Resting-state fMRI studies showed overall lower functional connectivity in the main default mode brain network (executive control, and joint attention, sensorimotor, frontoparietal, and ventral stream). These findings are consistent with an impaired ability to integrate information from distant brain regions into coherently functional distributed networks. When functional and structural connectivity data are combined for typical control subjects, the greatest agreement is found in frontal and visual brain regions. In Williams–Beuren syndrome, the highest agreement is in posterior regions—that is, parieto-occipital and temporal areas. These preliminary findings are consistent with an altered connectome in Williams–Beuren syndrome with hyper-connectivity of posterior brain regions, not disruptions in brain connectivity in anterior brain regions. These differences in brain organization in Williams–Beuren syndrome involve sensory perception and multisensory integration, especially involving parieto-occipital networks, and impact social–emotional processing involving temporal lobe tracks and attention/control involving the frontal lobe system.

Children with Williams–Beuren syndrome require special education tailored to address their unique educational needs. Educational strategies should effectively utilize their personal interaction strengths to cope with their educational vulnerabilities in language. Thus, their educational trajectory can be modified by explicit, targeted interventions. The misleading stereotypical profile that portrays these children as having near-normal language and social skills, unfortunately, has led to some schools to discontinue language intervention for them when the children's speech is fluent. Despite an acceleration in language development following the early delay in the onset of language, their pragmatic language remains delayed during the school years (Mervis & Velleman, 2011). Atypical social development is characteristic of Williams–Beuren syndrome despite the friendliness and intense social interest they display. Affected children are indiscriminate in approaching other people, show intense gaze, are easily distracted, and chatter inappropriately and excessively. Their pragmatic language is inappropriate and superficial despite their interest in engaging in and maintaining conversation with others. Their superficial interactional skills in turn-taking and capacity to stay on topic lead to the false impression of social relevance. Language mastery and speech use depend on appropriate use of cognitive and social skills. Children with Williams–Beuren syndrome have a strong motive to interact with others but lack motivation to share meaning when speaking. They find it difficult to make their speech relevant to context. Moreover, they are impaired in monitoring and maintaining attention to the topic of conversation while inferring communicative interest in dialogue with the other speaker.

Although children with Williams–Beuren syndrome can learn to read well with phonemic instruction, they struggle to create a narrative "mental movie" when they read. In conversation, they are limited in narrative skills and have an abnormal narrative profile despite strengths in formal language and sociability. Therefore, educational interventions must target pragmatic skills for both academic performance and peer relationships. Children who are competent in narration generally do well in school. Narrative skills interventions are important components of the school curriculum for later literacy training. Narrative assessment includes assessment of vocabulary and syntax in the context of language content, organization, and language discourse. Children with Williams–Beuren syndrome and other neurodevelopmental disabilities benefit from narrative interventions (Finestack, 2012). School-age children meeting criteria for language disorder in the fifth edition of the *Diagnostic and Statistical Manual of Mental Disorders* (American Psychiatric Association, 2013) overall produce poorer narrative than typically developing children. Children with language disorders and children with Williams–Beuren syndrome show similar problems with morphology and syntax. Those with Williams–Beuren syndrome use fewer story components and less thematic integration (Reilly et al., 2004). Limited capacity in pragmatics affects building on language discourse with others to relate personal stories in everyday conversation.

Deficits in narrative competence have been addressed in a pilot intervention study for Williams–Beuren syndrome students at different levels of special education; they were studied pre- and post-intervention (Diez-Itza et al., 2018). Narrative productivity and complexity were the focus of the intervention. Children were asked to recall and sequentially order a series of scenarios, episodes, events, and characters to improve cohesion when retelling stories. Instructors used verbal scaffolding, provided context for retelling a story, and used visual supports with pictures printed from a cartoon. When reassessed for story retelling 2 weeks after the initial intervention, there was significant improvement. This study provides preliminary confirmation that children with Williams–Beuren syndrome may benefit from targeted narrative interventions. Students showed improvement in story length and narrative complexity. A follow-up study is needed to further validate the use of narrative interventions in children with Williams–Beuren syndrome.

When children with Williams–Beuren syndrome are compared to children with Down syndrome and matched for mental age, each group has a specific and complementary profile of impairments in cognition. Although these changes are in some ways analogous to differences between adult patients with damage to either the left or the right hemisphere of the brain, MRI studies in these two syndromes do not show left–right differences. However, there are group differences in brain morphology in regard to the anterior–posterior axis and cerebellar:cerebral ratios when groups are compared (Jernigan & Bellugi, 1990). There are also differences in the two syndromes in the proportionate size of the neocerebellar versus paleocerebellar structures. Studies of these specific syndromes challenge theoretic ideas about neuronal structures that mediate language and cognitive structures that relate to language.

## The Language Deprivation Syndrome

There are rare examples of children being raised without language exposure from adults during early childhood. These are usually abusive and deprivation situations. It has been difficult to separate evidence of severe neglect and abuse from either an intellectual developmental disorder or congenital language deficits when interpreting the findings.

In 1989, when the Ceausescu regime was overthrown in Romania, there were more than 170,000 children aged 6 months to 3 years (average age was 22 months) in orphanages. Many of them experienced severe physical and emotional deprivation. The babies laid in cribs all day except when fed, diapered, and bathed on a set schedule. They were not rocked or sung to. When investigators first entered the institution, they were struck by the silence; the infants seemed to have learned there would be no response to their cries. A follow-up study of 30-month-old children raised in orphanages with augmented controls was conducted. Institutionalized children showed substantial language delays, with some not yet producing intelligible words. Children placed in foster care for at least 1 year with care approximated those who were never institutionalized. However, they still showed reduced grammatical abilities and less complex language (Windsor et al., 2007).

For interventions, the best-known long-term follow-up case is that of Genie (a pseudonym). She was believed to have been functioning in the normal range of intelligence at birth. Born with hip dysplasia, she was the product of a normal gestation and delivered by caesarean section. Her pediatrician reported that at well-baby checks at ages 11–14 months, there was no indication of developmental delay or neurological disorder. At approximately age 20 months, believing that because of her hip dysplasia she was intellectually disabled, her father isolated her from the family in another room. There, she suffered severe nutritional, social, sensory, and language deprivation. She spent her days in a small closed room with curtained windows. For 11 years, Genie's days and nights were spent either strapped in a chair or placed in a covered infant crib. Her father forbade anyone to speak to her, only allowing her mother to feed her (Curtiss, 1977; Fromkin et al., 1974).

Genie came to medical attention at age 13 years, 9 months. She was taken into protective custody due to child abuse, and she was hospitalized for malnutrition and severe social and environmental deprivation. Upon admission, there was no evidence of a developmental or neurological disorder. Her EEG was normal, as was chromosomal analysis. She made no sounds, did not speak, and did not vocalize. Before admission, she "had been whipped by her father when she made noise" (Fromkin et al., 1974, p. 87). However, she could socially communicate her needs to some extent nonverbally. With support, she developed single words and recognized names but did not understand grammatical structure. After more than 2 years of speech therapy, she was able to comprehend single–plural contrasts of nouns, possessive constructions, prepositions, and conjunctions with the word "and." After 5 months of therapy, she produced single words spontaneously and eventually used sentences with a subject, object, and verb. Her grammar was similar to that of a typically developing 2½-year-old child, but her expressive speech was much poorer than that of children at that age. She could print the letters of the alphabet and decode some printed words and understand sentences using them. By 7 months of intervention, she increased cognitively from a 15-month-old to a 42-month-old level. At 14 years of chronological age, on a nonverbal test of intelligence, the Leiter International Performance Scale, she reached a peak performance at the 6- to 8-year-old level, and on the Stanford–Binet test she performed at the 6- to 8-year-old level with considerable test score scatter. Her cognitive development exceeded her linguistic development with higher performance scores. Dichotic listening studies were consistent for lateralization of language to the right hemisphere for both language and nonlanguage function. These findings seem consistent with the neuroconstructionist model that left hemisphere language stimulation is needed during a critical developmental period for left lateralization of language.

Despite intensive speech and language, Genie did not fully acquire language. Although she demonstrated the pre-2-year-old stages of language, she did not move beyond what is referred to as *protolanguage*. Her overall language consisted of two or three content words loosely linked by meaning but without grammatical items. Because language acquisition requires exposure to some form of linguistic input within a critical developmental period, Genie, who was not speaking previously, did not acquire grammatical language. If there were not a critical period for acquisition, she should have acquired better language. Some lexical input is necessary for it to develop. Still, it must be borne in mind that Genie was abused for many years and experienced both social and sensory isolation, which have been associated with brain dysfunction. After extensive language and social stimulation, her test scores on structural IQ tests were at the 8 years of age level, placing this teenage girl at the low mild to moderate level range of intellectual developmental disorder.

When Genie reached adulthood, as a ward of the state of California, she was placed in a state institution. At last report on her 27th birthday, she had regressed. Without the continued enriched language stimulation provided during her early habilitation with concerned professionals, Genie was again nonverbal and made limited eye contact (Rymer, 1993).

## Conclusion

Language exposure is essential to development throughout the life span. Language deprivation has broad implications for language development and impacts the epidemiology of mental health. Although such deprivation is most apparent in the deaf population, it may also result from environment deprivation, socioeconomic deprivation, or be a feature of neurodevelopmental disorders. Language deprivation is preventable to reduce its impact on mental health. Studies of language acquisition in children with focal brain damage show substantial plasticity of brain regions that subserve language learning. Studies of children with an intellectual developmental disorder challenge longstanding views of the relationship between language and cognition in typical development. Studies of syndromes such as Williams–Beuren syndrome raise new questions about neuronal substrates for both linguistic and cognitive development. Advances in the biological foundations of language development and language learning are based on the brain plasticity of neuronal systems in response to environmental stimulation.

## References

American Psychiatric Association. (2013). *Diagnostic and statistical manual of mental disorders* (5th ed.). American Psychiatric Publishing.

Amraei, K., Amirsalari, S., & Ajalloueyan, M. (2017). Comparison of intelligence quotients of first- and second-generation deaf children with cochlear implants. *International Journal of Pediatric Otorhinolaryngology, 92*, 167–170.

Atkinson, E. G., Audesse, A. J., Palacios, J. A., Bobo, D. M., Webb, A. E., Ramachandran, S., & Henn, B. M. (2018). No evidence for recent selection at FOXP2 among diverse human populations. *Cell*, *174*(6), 1424–1435.

Bates, E. (1992). Language development. *Current Opinion in Neurobiology*, *2*(2), 180–185.

Bates, E., & Roe, K. (2001). In C. A. Nelson & M. Luciana (Eds.), *Handbook of developmental cognitive neuroscience* (pp. 281–307). MIT Press.

Becerra, A. M., & Mervis, C. B. (2019). Age at onset of declarative gestures and 24-month expressive vocabulary predict later language and intellectual abilities in young children with Williams syndrome. *Frontiers in Psychology*, *10*, 2648.

Bedny, M. (2017). Evidence from blindness for a cognitively pluripotent cortex. *Trends in Cognitive Sciences*, *21*(9), 637–648.

Bickerton, D. (1990). *Language and species*. University of Chicago Press.

Binder, J. R., Frost, J. A., Hammeke, T. A., Bellgowan, P. S., Springer, J. A., Kaufman, J. N., & Possing, E. T. (2000). Human temporal lobe activation by speech and nonspeech sounds. *Cerebral Cortex*, *10*(5), 512–528.

Butler, B. E., & Lomber, S. G. (2013). Functional and structural changes throughout the auditory system following congenital and early-onset deafness: Implications for hearing restoration. *Frontiers in Systems Neuroscience*, *7*, Article 92.

Caplan, D., Alpert, N., Waters, G., & Olivieri, A. (2000). Activation of Broca's area by syntactic processing under conditions of concurrent articulation. *Human Brain Mapping*, *9*(2), 65–71.

Carlson, H. L., Sugden, C., Brooks, B. L., & Kirton, A. (2019). Functional connectivity of language networks after perinatal stroke. *NeuroImage: Clinical*, *23*, 101861.

Cheng, Q., Roth, A., Halgren, E., & Mayberry, R. I. (2019). Effects of early language deprivation on brain connectivity: Language pathways in deaf native and late first-language learners of American Sign Language. *Frontiers in Human Neuroscience*, *13*, Article 320.

Chomsky, N. (1957). *Syntactic structures*. Mouton.

Chomsky, N. (2006). *Language and mind*. Cambridge University Press.

Chomsky, N. (2017). The language capacity: Architecture and evolution. *Psychonomic Bulletin & Review*, *24*(1), 200–203.

Clark, A., & Karmiloff-Smith, A. (1993). The cognizer's innards: A psychological and philosophical perspective on the development of thought. *Mind & Language*, *8*(4), 487–519.

Colonnesi, C., Stams, G. J. J., Koster, I., & Noom, M. J. (2010). The relation between pointing and language development: A meta-analysis. *Developmental Review*, *30*(4), 352–366.

Conway, C. M., Pisoni, D. B., & Kronenberger, W. G. (2009). The importance of sound for cognitive sequencing abilities: The auditory scaffolding hypothesis. *Current Directions in Psychological Science*, *18*(5), 275–279.

Corballis, M. C. (2017). *The truth about language: What it is and where it came from*. University of Chicago Press.

Curtiss, S. (1977). *Genie: A linguistic study of a modern day "wild" child*. Academic Press.

Darwin, C. (1871). *The descent of man, and selections in relation to sex*. Murray.

Demontis, D., Walters, R. K., Martin, J., Mattheisen, M., Als, T. D., Agerbo, E., Baldursson, G., Belliveau, R., Bybjerg Grauholm, J., Baekvad-Hansen, M., Cerrato, F., Chambert, K., Churchhouse, C., Dumont, A., Eriksson, N., Gandal, M., Goldstein, J., Grasby, K., Glove, J., . . . Neale, B. (2019). Discovery of the first genome-wide significant risk loci for attention deficit/hyperactivity disorder. *Nature Genetics*, *51*(1), 63–75.

Diez-Itza, E., Martínez, V., Pérez, V., & Fernández-Urquiza, M. (2018). Explicit oral narrative intervention for students with Williams syndrome. *Frontiers in Psychology*, *8*, 2337.

DiStefano, C., Senturk, D., & Jeste, S. S. (2019). ERP evidence of semantic processing in children with ASD. *Developmental Cognitive Neuroscience*, *36*, 100640.

Enard, W., Przeworski, M., Fisher, S. E., Lai, C. S., Wiebe, V., Kitano, T., Monaco, A., & Pääbo, S. (2002). Molecular evolution of FOXP2, a gene involved in speech and language. *Nature*, *418*(6900), 869–872.

Farran, E. K., & Karmiloff-Smith, A. (Eds.). (2012). *Neurodevelopmental disorders across the lifespan: A neuroconstructivist approach*. Oxford University Press.

Finestack, L. H. (2012). Five principles to consider when providing narrative language intervention to children and adolescents with developmental disabilities. *Perspectives on Language Learning and Education, 19*(4), 147–154.

Fitz, H., & Chang, F. (2019). Language ERPs reflect learning through prediction error propagation. *Cognitive Psychology, 111*, 15–52.

Frank, S. L., Monaghan, P., & Tsoukala, C. (2019). Neural network models of language acquisition and processing. In P. Hagoort (Ed.), *Human language* (pp. 277–292). MIT Press.

Friederici, A. D. (2005). Neurophysiological markers of early language acquisition: From syllables to sentences. *Trends in Cognitive Sciences, 9*(10), 481–488.

Friederici, A. D., & Weissenborn, J. (2007). Mapping sentence form onto meaning: The syntax-semantic interface. *Brain Research, 1146*, 50–58.

Fromkin, V., Krashen, S., Curtiss, S., Rigler, D., & Rigler, M. (1974). The development of language in Genie: A case of language acquisition beyond the "critical period." *Brain and language, 1*(1), 81–107.

Gagliardi, C., Arrigoni, F., Nordio, A., De Luca, A., Peruzzo, D., Decio, A., Leemans, A., & Borgatti, R. (2018). A different brain: Anomalies of functional and structural connections in Williams syndrome. *Frontiers in Neurology, 9*, Article 721.

Gazzaniga, M. S., Ivry, R. B., & Mangun, G. R. (2019). *Cognitive neuroscience: The biology of the mind* (5th ed.). Norton.

Gonen, T., Gazit, T., Korn, A., Kirschner, A., Perry, D., Hendler, T., & Ram, Z. (2017). Intraoperative multi-site stimulation: Expanding methodology for cortical brain mapping of language functions. *PLoS One, 12*(7), e0180740.

Hagoort, P. (2013). MUC (memory, unification, control) and beyond. *Frontiers in Psychology, 4*, Article 416.

Hagoort, P., Brown, C., & Groothusen, J. (1993). The syntactic positive shift (SPS) as an ERP measure of syntactic processing. *Language and Cognitive Processes, 8*(4), 439–483.

Hall, W. C. (2017). What you don't know can hurt you: The risk of language deprivation by impairing sign language development in deaf children. *Maternal and Child Health Journal, 21*(5), 961–965.

Hall, W. C., Levin, L. L., & Anderson, M. L. (2017). Language deprivation syndrome: A possible neurodevelopmental disorder with sociocultural origins. *Social Psychiatry and Psychiatric Epidemiology, 52*(6), 761–776.

Hasson, U., Andric, M., Atilgan, H., & Collignon, O. (2016). Congenital blindness is associated with large-scale reorganization of anatomical networks. *NeuroImage, 128*, 362–372.

Hebb, D. O. (1949). *The organization of behavior: A neuropsychological theory*. Wiley.

Hunter, C. R., Kronenberger, W. G., Castellanos, I., & Pisoni, D. B. (2017). Early postimplant speech perception and language skills predict long-term language and neurocognitive outcomes following pediatric cochlear implantation. *Journal of Speech, Language, and Hearing Research, 60*(8), 2321–2336.

Hurst, J. A., Baraitser, M., Auger, E., Graham, F., & Norell, S. (1990). An extended family with a dominantly inherited speech disorder. *Developmental Medicine & Child Neurology, 32*(4), 352–355.

Huth, A. G., De Heer, W. A., Griffiths, T. L., Theunissen, F. E., & Gallant, J. L. (2016). Natural speech reveals the semantic maps that tile human cerebral cortex. *Nature, 532*(7600), 453–458.

Jernigan, T., & Bellugi, U. (1990). Anomalous brain morphology on magnetic resonance images in Williams syndrome and Down syndrome. *Archives of Neurology, 47*, 529–553.

Johnson, L. A., Della Santina, C. C., & Wang, X. (2016). Selective neuronal activation by cochlear implant stimulation in auditory cortex of awake primate. *Journal of Neuroscience, 36*(49), 12468–12484.

Johnson, M. H., Halit, H., Grice, S. J., & Karmiloff-Smith, A. (2002). Neuroimaging of typical and atypical development: A perspective from multiple levels of analysis. *Development and Psychopathology, 14*(3), 521–536.

Karmiloff-Smith, A. (2006). The tortuous route from genes to behavior: A neuroconstructivist approach. *Cognitive, Affective, & Behavioral Neuroscience, 6*(1), 9–17.

Karmiloff-Smith, A. (2009). Nativism versus neuroconstructivism: Rethinking the study of developmental disorders. *Developmental Psychology, 45*(1), 56–63.

Karmiloff-Smith, A. (2012). Brain: The neuroconstructivist approach. In E. K. Farran & A. Karmiloff-Smith (Eds.), Neurodevelopmental *disorders across* the *lifespan*: A *neuroconstructivist approach* (pp. 37–58). Oxford University Press.

Karmiloff-Smith, A. (2018). Development itself is the key to understanding developmental disorders. In A. Karmiloff-Smith, M. S. C. Thomas, & M. H. Johnson (Eds.), *Thinking developmentally from constructivism to neuroconstructivism* (pp. 97–117). Routledge.

Kendon, A. (2017). Reflections on the "gesture-first" hypothesis of language origins. *Psychonomic Bulletin & Review, 24*(1), 163–170.

Kim, J. S., Kanjlia, S., Merabet, L. B., & Bedny, M. (2017). Development of the visual word form area requires visual experience: Evidence from blind Braille readers. *Journal of Neuroscience, 37*(47), 11495–11504.

Kral, A., Kronenberger, W. G., Pisoni, D. B., & O'Donoghue, G. M. (2016). Neurocognitive factors in sensory restoration of early deafness: A connectome model. *Lancet Neurology, 15*(6), 610–621.

Kral, A., & Sharma, A. (2012). Developmental neuroplasticity after cochlear implantation. *Trends in Neurosciences, 35*(2), 111–122.

Kuhl, P. K., Williams, K. A., Lacerda, F., Stevens, K. N., & Lindblom, B. (1992). Linguistic experience alters phonetic perception in infants by 6 months of age. *Science, 255*(5044), 606–608.

Kutas, M., & Federmeier, K. D. (2000). Electrophysiology reveals semantic memory use in language comprehension. *Trends in Cognitive Sciences, 4*(12), 463–470.

Kutas, M., & Hillyard, S. A. (1980). Reading senseless sentences: Brain potentials reflect semantic incongruity. *Science, 207*(4427), 203–205.

Lane, C., Kanjlia, S., Omaki, A., & Bedny, M. (2015). "Visual" cortex of congenitally blind adults responds to syntactic movement. *Journal of Neuroscience, 35*(37), 12859–12868.

Lane, H. (1977). *The wild boy of Aveyron*. Harvard University Press.

Lazard, D. S., Innes-Brown, H., & Barone, P. (2014). Adaptation of the communicative brain to post-lingual deafness: Evidence from functional imaging. *Hearing Research, 307*, 136–143.

Leybaert, J., & D'Hondt, M. (2003). Neurolinguistic development in deaf children: The effect of early language experience. *International Journal of Audiology, 42*(Suppl. 1), 34–40.

Mayberry, R. I., Chen, J. K., Witcher, P., & Klein, D. (2011). Age of acquisition effects on the functional organization of language in the adult brain. *Brain and language, 119*(1), 16–29.

McCann, J., & Peppé, S. (2003). Prosody in autism spectrum disorders: A critical review. *International Journal of Language & Communication Disorders, 38*(4), 325–350.

Mervis, C. B., & John, A. E. (2008). Vocabulary abilities of children with Williams syndrome: Strengths, weaknesses, and relation to visuospatial construction ability. *Journal of Speech, Language, and Hearing Research, 51*(4), 967–982.

Mervis, C. B., & John, A. E. (2012). Precursors to language and early language. In E. K. Farran & A. Karmiloff-Smith (Eds.), *Neurodevelopmental disorders across the lifespan: A neuroconstructivist approach* (pp. 187–204). Oxford University Press.

Mervis, C. B., & Velleman, S. L. (2011). Children with Williams syndrome: Language, cognitive, and behavioral characteristics and their implications for intervention. *Perspectives on language Learning and Education, 18*(3), 98–107.

Mills, D. L., Coffey-Corina, S. A., & Neville, H. J. (1993). Language acquisition and cerebral specialization in 20-month-old infants. *Journal of Cognitive Neuroscience, 5*(3), 317–334.

Mills, D. L., Coffey-Corina, S. A., & Neville, H. J. (1994). Changes in cerebral organization in infancy during primary language acquisition. In G. Dawson & K. Fischer (Eds.), *Human behavior and the developing brain*. Guilford.

Mills, D. L., Coffey-Corina, S. A., & Neville, H. J. (1997). Language comprehension and cerebral specialization from 13 to 20 months. *Developmental Neuropsychology, 13*(3), 397–445.

Newport, E. L., Landau, B., Seydell-Greenwald, A., Turkeltaub, P. E., Chambers, C. E., Dromerick, A. W., Carpenter, J., Berl, M., & Gaillard, W. D. (2017). Revisiting Lenneberg's hypotheses about early developmental plasticity: Language organization after left-hemisphere perinatal stroke. *Biolinguistics, 11*, 407–422.

Ng, R., Järvinen, A., & Bellugi, U. (2014). Toward a deeper characterization of the social phenotype of Williams syndrome: The association between personality and social drive. *Research in Developmental Disabilities, 35*(8), 1838–1849.

Nobre, A. C., Allison, T., & McCarthy, G. (1994). Word recognition in the human inferior temporal lobe. *Nature, 372*(6503), 260–263.

Occelli, V., Lacey, S., Stephens, C., Merabet, L. B., & Sathian, K. (2017). Enhanced verbal abilities in the congenitally blind. *Experimental Brain Research, 235*(6), 1709–1718.

Ojemann, G., Ojemann, J., Lettich, E., & Berger, M. (1989). Cortical language localization in left, dominant hemisphere: An electrical stimulation mapping investigation in 117 patients. *Journal of Neurosurgery, 71*(3), 316–326.

Osterhout, L., & Holcomb, P. J. (1992). Event-related brain potentials elicited by syntactic anomaly. *Journal of Memory and Language, 31*(6), 785–806.

Pant, R., Kanjlia, S., & Bedny, M. (2020). A sensitive period in the neural phenotype of language in blind individuals. *Developmental Cognitive Neuroscience, 41*, 100744.

Petitto, L. A., & Marentette, P. F. (1991). Babbling in the manual mode: Evidence for the ontogeny of language. *Science, 251*(5000), 1493–1496.

Pinker, S., & Bloom, P. (1990). Natural language and natural selection. *Behavioral and Brain Sciences, 13*(4), 707–727.

Price, T., Wadewitz, P., Cheney, D., Seyfarth, R., Hammerschmidt, K., & Fischer, J. (2015). Vervets revisited: A quantitative analysis of alarm call structure and context specificity. *Scientific Reports, 5*, 13220.

Qi, Z., Beach, S. D., Finn, A. S., Minas, J., Goetz, C., Chan, B., & Gabrieli, J. D. (2017). Native-language N400 and P600 predict dissociable language-learning abilities in adults. *Neuropsychologia, 98*, 177–191.

Ralph, Y. K., Schneider, J. M., Abel, A. D., & Maguire, M. J. (2020). Using the N400 event-related potential to study word learning from context in children from low- and higher-socioeconomic status homes. *Journal of Experimental Child Psychology, 191*, 104758.

Reilly, J., Losh, M., Bellugi, U., & Wulfeck, B. (2004). "Frog, where are you?" Narratives in children with specific language impairment, early focal brain injury, and Williams syndrome. *Brain and Language, 88*(2), 229–247.

Reuter, M. S., Riess, A., Moog, U., Briggs, T. A., Chandler, K. E., Rauch, A., Stampfer, M., Steindl, K., Glaser, D., Joset, P., DDD Study; Krumbiegel, M., Rabe, H., Schulte-Mattler, U., Bauer, P., Beck-Wodl, S., Kohlhase, J., Reis, A., & Zweier, C. (2017). FOXP2 variants in 14 individuals with developmental speech and language disorders broaden the mutational and clinical spectrum. *Journal of Medical Genetics, 54*(1), 64–72.

Rilling, J. K., Glasser, M. F., Preuss, T. M., Ma, X., Zhao, T., Hu, X., & Behrens, T. E. (2008). The evolution of the arcuate fasciculus revealed with comparative DTI. *Nature Neuroscience, 11*(4), 426–428.

Rossi, N. F., & Giacheti, C. M. (2017). Association between speech–language, general cognitive functioning and behaviour problems in individuals with Williams syndrome. *Journal of Intellectual Disability Research, 61*(7), 707–718.

Royston, R., Waite, J., & Howlin, P. (2019). Williams syndrome: Recent advances in our understanding of cognitive, social and psychological functioning. *Current Opinion in Psychiatry, 32*(2), 60–66.

Rymer, R. (1993). *Genie: An abused child's flight from silence*. HarperCollins.

Savage-Rumbaugh, E. S., & Lewin, R. (1994). *Kanzi: The ape at the brink of the human mind*. Wiley.

Savage-Rumbaugh, E. S., Murphy, J., Sevcik, R. A., Brakke, K. E., Williams, S. L., Rumbaugh, D. M., & Bates, E. (1993). Language comprehension in ape and child. *Monographs of the Society for Research in Child Development, 58*(3–4), 1–222.

Schneider, J. M., & Maguire, M. J. (2019). Developmental differences in the neural correlates supporting semantics and syntax during sentence processing. *Developmental Science, 22*(4), e12782.

Seyfarth, R. M., & Cheney, D. L. (2003). Meaning and emotion in animal vocalizations. *Annals of the New York Academy of Sciences, 1000*, 32–55.

Seyfarth, R. M., Cheney, D. L., & Marler, P. (1980). Vervet monkey alarm calls: Semantic communication in a free-ranging primate. *Animal Behaviour, 28*(4), 1070–1094.

Simos, P. G., Basile, L. F., & Papanicolaou, A. C. (1997). Source localization of the N400 response in a sentence-reading paradigm using evoked magnetic fields and magnetic resonance imaging. *Brain Research, 762*(1–2), 29–39.

Sterelny, K. (2012). Language, gesture, skill: The co-evolutionary foundations of language. *Philosophical Transactions of the Royal Society B: Biological Sciences, 367*(1599), 2141–2151.

Svirsky, M. A., Teoh, S. W., & Neuburger, H. (2004). Development of language and speech perception in congenitally, profoundly deaf children as a function of age at cochlear implantation. *Audiology and Neurotology, 9*(4), 224–233.

Tomasello, M. (2003). *Constructing a language: A usage-based theory of language acquisition.* Harvard University Press.

Trauner, D. A., Eshagh, K., Ballantyne, A. O., & Bates, E. (2013). Early language development after peri-natal stroke. *Brain and Language, 127*(3), 399–403.

Trevarthen, C. (1979). Communication and cooperation in early infancy: A description of primary intersubjectivity. In M. Bullowa (Ed.), Before *speech*: The beginning of interpersonal communication (pp. 530–571). Cambridge University Press.

Tyler, M. D., & Cutler, A. (2009). Cross-language differences in cue use for speech segmentation. *Journal of the Acoustical Society of America, 126*(1), 367–376.

Vargha-Khadem, F., Gadian, D. G., Copp, A., & Mishkin, M. (2005). FOXP2 and the neuroanatomy of speech and language. *Nature Reviews Neuroscience, 6*(2), 131–138.

Watkins, K. E., Cowey, A., Alexander, I., Filippini, N., Kennedy, J. M., Smith, S. M., Ragge, N., & Bridge, H. (2012). Language networks in anophthalmia: Maintained hierarchy of processing in "visual" cortex. *Brain, 135*(5), 1566–1577.

Westley, A., Kohút, Z., & Rueschemeyer, S. A. (2017). "I know something you don't know": Discourse and social context effects on the N400 in adolescents. *Journal of Experimental Child Psychology, 164*, 45–54.

Windsor, J., Glaze, L. E., & Koga, S. F. (2007). Language acquisition with limited input: Romanian institution and foster care. *Journal of Speech, Language, and Hearing Research, 50*(5), 1365–1381.

Zhuang, J., Randall, B., Stamatakis, E. A., Marslen-Wilson, W. D., & Tyler, L. K. (2011). The interaction of lexical semantics and cohort competition in spoken word recognition: An fMRI study. *Journal of Cognitive Neuroscience, 23*(12), 3778–3790.

# 6

# Memory

Our modern word for memory derives from the Latin *memoria*, which means "recollection and retrieval from a store," yet in its original Greek origins, memory was bestowed by Mnemosyne, the goddess who, as the mother of the Muses, was the source of inspiration and creative invention. Barth (1992) writes that "if Zeus in this allegorizing myth, represents fertilizing power, life force, creative energy, it is Memory—fertilized, energized, and by no mean creator herself, who gestates, shapes and delivers."

The original Greek meaning then implied something more—namely that the retrieval of narrative information, the "spinning" of a tale, is a creation from universal stores of plots, rather than a rote reproduction from memorized facts. Such is the source of the inspiration that may be linked to various regions of the brain and their integrated functioning. Perhaps narrative memory links affect, image, motor skills, and consciousness, whereas the mnemonic is limited only to factual stores from semantic sources, rather than the broader ranging, multiply placed episodic events.

We have come to understand how there are multiple memory systems, how cognitive declarative memory is consolidated, where it resides in the brain, and that it may be disrupted. Moreover, there is a developmental sequence in the production of declarative memory. Memory includes both storage and retrieval of facts and events. Consolidation and retrieval of declarative memories involve specific brain regions. Facts may be reproduced as rote learning, but consolidated memories of events are re-experienced (events) when retrieved and reconstructed paralleling the two modes of thinking—the analytical and the narrative—necessary for their meaningful application and adaptation to everyday life. Cognitive processes and linked cognitive–affective processes must be considered in the study of memory (Holland & Kensinger, 2010).

Motor patterning or habit training is the basis of a form of noncognitive memory, nondeclarative, that is involved in classical and operant conditioning; it is referred to as "habit formation" by Mishkin et al. (1984) to distinguish it from memory that involves conscious cognition or knowing. Habit learning has been studied in sea slugs (*Aplysia*; Kandel, 2009), the octopus (which responds differently depending on the sensory system approached; e.g., touch or sight), and other species (Lorenz, 1981). Studies in these simple species have contributed to an understanding of the basic mechanisms of nondeclarative memory.

This chapter discusses the current classification of multiple memory systems. It reviews specific definitions in the classification of memory, reviews its neuroanatomy and synaptic basis, discusses animal models, highlights the relationship of sleep and memory, discusses emotional and autobiographical memory, and considers how disturbance of memory may be pertinent to neurodevelopmental disorders.

## Definition and Classification

A memory system can be defined as an organized relationship among brain structures involving processes that make possible memory acquisition, consolidation/retention, and utilization (Squire, 2004). Memory has been referred to in a general way to describe the ability to conserve and later remember experiences. Piaget and Inhelder (1973) wrote of memory in this wider sense, which includes its role in the acquisition of skills, vocabulary, and adaptive responses. In the stricter sense, memory describes both the cognitive functions, the ability to consciously store and subsequently reflect on past incidents, and also nonconscious habit or nondeclarative memory. An infant's performance on tasks such as habituation, object search, novelty preference, and conditioning is accounted for by the wider concept of memory that includes both declarative (cognitive) and nondeclarative (habit) memories.

Historically, William James (1890) proposed that there were two kinds of memory, primary and secondary. Primary memory referred to keeping information in mind, and secondary memory referred to stored information that remains available for retrieval. Using current terminology, primary memory is short term and includes working memory, and secondary memory is long-term, declarative memory. James discussed habits separately in his textbook of psychology and in a short book he wrote simply titled *Habit*. He describes habits broadly as follows (James, 1890):

> When we look at living creatures from an outward point of view, one of the first things that strikes us is that they are bundles of habits. In wild animals, the usual round of daily behavior seems a necessity implanted at birth; in animals domesticated, and especially in humans, it seems, to a great extent, to be the result of education. The habits to which there is an innate tendency are called instincts; some of those due to education would by most persons be called acts of reason. (p. 104)

He went on to write,

> Any sequence of mental action which has been frequently repeated tends to perpetuate itself; so that we find ourselves automatically prompted to think, feel, or do what we have been before accustomed to think, feel, or do, under like circumstances, without any consciously formed purpose, or anticipation of results.

Memory may be categorized in several ways (Maurer, 1992). General classifications have included (a) by the subprocesses used in storage (i.e., ultra-short-term, short-term, and long-term), (b) by the process used in retrieving memories (through thought, action, or perception), and (c) by the modality of cognitive memory that is lost in amnesia (i.e., global, partial, or specific). These approaches are summarized in Box 6.1.

The anatomical brain regions involved in memory are shown in Figure 6.1. Brain regions essential to attention include areas of the frontal and parietal lobes and regions of the thalamus and the superior colliculi.

The classification of memory and brain regions linked to each are specified in greater detail in Figure 6.2. Memory is classified into multiple memory systems with

## Box 6.1  Dimensions Used in Classifying Memory

By the Process Used in Retrieval of the Memory

   Retrieval through thought
      Cognitive memory
      "Conscious" or "psychological" memory
      "Unorganic" ("unorganized" and "semi-organized") memory
      Declarative memory
      Representational memory
      Explicit memory
      Anterograde and retrograde memory (taken together)

   Retrieval through action or through perception
      Habit formation (through action) and priming (through perception)
      "Unconscious" memory
      "Organic" ("organized") memory
      Procedural memory (through action)
      Nonrepresentational memory
      Implicit memory

By the Modality of Cognitive Memory Lost in Amnesia

   All modalities
      Global amnesia
      "General" amnesia

   Some modalities
      Partial amnesia
      Domain-specific memory
      Material-specific memory

   Specific "metamodalities"
      Memories localized in time
         Episodic memory
         "Unorganized" memory
      Memories not localized in time
         Semantic memory
         "Semi-organized" memory

By the Subprocess of Cognitive Memory Used in Storage of the Memory

   Ultra-short-term storage
      Ultra-short-term memory
      Sensory memory

Short-term storage
    Short-term memory
    Working memory
    Attentional memory
    Immediate memory

Long-term storage
    Long-term memory
    Secondary memory
    Recent memory (anterograde, sometimes called "short-term") and remote
        memory (retrograde, sometimes called "long-term")
    Reference memory

*From* Maurer (1992).

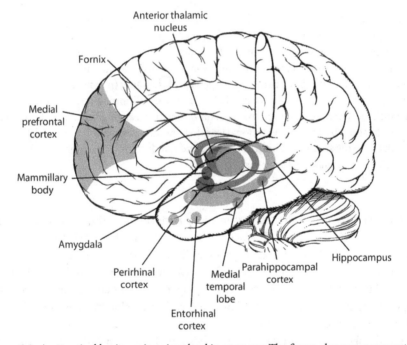

**Figure 6.1** Anatomical brain regions involved in memory. The figure shows components of the medial temporal lobe system. The prefrontal cortex and other brain regions shown are involved in the storage and retrieval of memories.

From Gazzaniga, Ivry and Mangun (2019); redrawn by Tim Phelps (2021).

underlying brain systems (Squire, 2009). The figure illustrates declarative memory and nondeclarative memory systems and related brain regions and pathways. The classification of memory in this chapter generally follows a developmental sequence as memory continues to develop from infancy to childhood to adulthood. This development allows for increasing cognitive reflection in making choices and actions and for the mastery

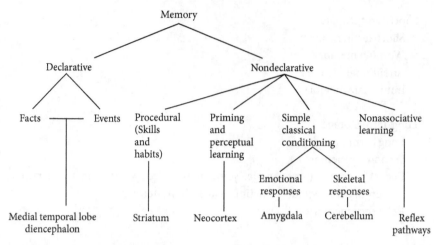

**Figure 6.2** Classification of long-term memory systems. The figure lists the brain structures thought to be especially important for each form of declarative and nondeclarative memory. Declarative (explicit) memory refers to conscious recollections of facts and events and depends on the integrity of the medial temporal lobe. In nondeclarative memory, experience alters behavior nonconsciously without providing access to any memory content. Nondeclarative (implicit) memory refers to a collection of abilities and is independent of the medial temporal lobe. Nondeclarative memory involves the striatum (procedural skills and habits), priming and perceptual learning (neocortex), simple classical learning for emotional responses (amygdala), classical conditioning (cerebellum), and nonassociative learning (reflex pathways). Nonassociative learning includes habituation and sensitization. In its role in emotional learning, the amygdala is able to modulate strength above the strength of both declarative and nondeclarative memory.
From Squire (2004); redrawn by Tim Phelps (2021).

of nondeclarative procedural (habit) memory performance. These forms of memory involve different cognitive and noncognitive systems and have different characteristics (Squire, 2004). Nondeclarative (procedural) memory systems are the first to appear, and fact and event (episodic/autobiographical) memory systems are the last to develop. Many of the higher and later developing memory functions depend on and are supported by the operations of the lower and earlier developing ones. Still, the lower systems can operate independently.

Procedural (nondeclarative) memory, the first to develop, includes skill learning and simple classical conditioning. It is followed by the establishment of a perceptual representation system (PRS), which is involved in perceptual priming and the identification of objects. Next is semantic memory, which refers to a general knowledge of the world, and episodic memory (memory for facts and events), the last to appear, which includes conscious memory consolidation and recollection of personal past experiences. Semantic and episodic memory are categorized together as declarative or propositional memory because they share common features.

Memory is distinguished as nondeclarative (implicit) or declarative (explicit), the terms used in this chapter. Nondeclarative memory refers to information acquired without personal awareness of its acquisition. In nondeclarative memory, the individual expresses what they know but does not necessarily remember how, when, or where knowledge was acquired. On the other hand, declarative cognitive memory addresses the conscious expression of both short-term memory, which includes working memory (highly accessible information of recent origin and input), and episodic memory. Declarative memory is the expression of what a person consciously remembers as a personal experience. Procedural memory, PRSs, and semantic memory are classified as nondeclarative.

From a developmental perspective, episodic memory can be described as embedded in semantic memory. Meaningful episodes are described as entering consciousness as scripts (Nelson, 1986) that later may contribute to autobiographical memory. At approximately age 4 years, children begin to demonstrate autobiographical memory in describing their daily experiences. Self-recollection is a developmental landmark for this age 4 transition.

## Description of Specific Memory Systems

The procedural system is an action system, and its operations are expressed in behavior that is independent of cognition (Kandel, 2009). Simple stimulus–response connections are examples of tasks requiring procedural memory that are expressed in behavior. Performance of perceptual–motor tasks and simple stimulus–response are characteristic behaviors. Procedural memory (nondeclarative) refers to memory for perceptional, motor skills, and other forms of nondeclarative memory involved in a number of brain systems. Whereas declarative memory involves the hippocampus and medial temporal lobe, nondeclarative memory involves several brain systems, including the cerebellum, striatum, amygdala, and simple reflex pathways. Operant behavioral approaches to the treatment of neurodevelopmentally disabled children and adolescents emphasize this form of memory. Reinforcement by conditioning relies on a basic property of the nervous system to respond to reinforcement (Lorenz, 1981). This kind of learning is preserved after hippocampectomy because procedural memory is not based on the context of the experience. Declarative memory with contextual memory retrieval requires representational storage and the integrity of the hippocampal system.

Perceptual priming refers to a special form of learning, which is expressed in enhanced identification of objects as "structured entities" (Tulving & Schachter, 1990). Priming refers to improvement in memory ability to process a stimulus following an encounter with the same or a similar stimulus (Squire, 2009). Perception at Time 1 primes the perception of the same or a similar object at Time 2. Consequently, subsequent identifications require less information and less time when priming has occurred. Priming is an unconscious memory system that is independent of the medial temporal lobe. Priming and perceptual learning involve the neocortex (Squire, 2009).

Short-term memory, also referred to as primary memory and includes working memory, provides the means to register and temporarily retain information in a highly accessible form but for only a short time. Working memory is used to support reasoning, learning, and preparation to act. Working memory is essential to select and carry out executive functioning—that is, goal-directed behavior. Semantic memory makes possible acquisition and retention of factual information and makes general knowledge of the world available to thought. It includes the classification of events, situations, objects, or symbolic descriptions of them and also knowledge of the location of objects in nonperceived space.

Finally, episodic memory makes possible the remembrance of personal past experiences. Consequently, events can be recalled as occurring in subjective time. Episodic memory depends on semantic memory but goes beyond it. The unique awareness and recollection of personal past experiences are different from those kinds of awareness that follow perceptual input and the retrieval of semantic facts. This form of memory is associated with consciousness of an enduring self-experience over time.

## General Event Representation and Autobiographical Memory

Autobiographical memory is an inclusive term describing recollections of specific personal experiences and events (Holland & Kensinger, 2010). Autobiographical memory is generally categorized as a form of episodic memory. Episodic memory is generally considered to be consolidated, stored, and retrieved using temporal and spatial cues. Declarative (or conceptual) knowledge, of which general event representation is a part, is thought to be consolidated, stored, and retrieved through other processes. In the child development literature, the term "general event representation" [GER] is used to describe the acquisition of facts and events into memory. GER represents information, including lists of people or objects that can fill slots for alternative approaches, and optional pathways. A single event that already has adequate representation in GER would not be stored separately.

On the other hand, autobiographical memory that deals with the specific representation of a particular experience may be thought of as embedded in GER because it requires the structural background of GER. Hudson (1986) has suggested that specific events are recalled not by time and space cues but, rather, in terms of a link with GER. Subsequently, routine events are not attended to but are forgotten or are absorbed into general event representational memory. However, novel experiences are better remembered. They may be linked to general representations and indexed by their distinctive features so that the context is established in a more general way.

Repeated novel experiences, as they are attended to over time, may be incorporated into GER. Attention to detail and memory for details result in the formation of new pathways. Linton (1975, 1982) describes this as a transition from episodic to semantic memory; here, the episodic memory is less intense as the more typical features are abstracted from experience. Therefore, an autobiographical memory may include both discrete details and information from general event knowledge. However, reconstruction from GER may be faulty or confused as to "what must have happened." The general representation may become confused regarding the specific details. In this way, what happened may be confused with what must or could have happened.

When speaking of remembering, we may be remembering facts or experiences. Autobiographical memory is typically used to refer to a particular memory. The emotional content of experiences may influence how an event is remembered. Moreover, emotions and emotional goals experienced when the autobiographical event is retrieved may influence how it is recalled.

In autobiographical memory, reference may be made to the self, personal goals, emotions, and personal meaning of experiences. It refers to facts about the self (semantic information) and personal episodic information (remembering events in one's life; e.g., the first day of school). Of these, personal episodic information requires recollecting and re-experiencing specific past events through integrating sensory information, language, emotion, and narrative (Rubin, 2006). These events may focus on the sense of self, social life, problem-solving, and planning. Such recall may be sufficiently vivid that one believes the event is being re-experienced—an experience that has been referred to as automatic memory (Tulving, 1985). Our autobiographical memories may be organized in a life story narrative that is referred to from childhood to adolescence to adult life. In retrieving autobiographical memories, the search begins at a general level, moving on to specific events. However, autobiographical memories are not stored as perfect records of specific events but, rather, reconstructed (Conway, 2005; Conway & Pleydell-Pearce, 2000). A constructivist approach to retrieval predicts that retelling of the same event may differ related to one's current goals and motivation.

## Neuroanatomy of Autobiographical Memory: The Case of H.M.

The medial temporal lobe, specifically the hippocampal complex, is central to the autobiographical memory system (Moscovitch et al., 2005). Larry Squire (2009) writes, "The modern era of memory research can be said to have begun in 1957 when Brenda Milner described the profound effects on memory of bilateral medial temporal lobe resection performed to relieve epilepsy in a patient known an H.M." (see also Scoville & Milner, 1957, p. 12711). Despite profound forgetfulness, H.M.'s perceptual and intellectual systems were largely intact.

H.M.'s case established that (a) memory is a distinct cerebral capacity; (b) the medial temporal lobe is not needed for short-term working memory; and (c) because H.M.'s childhood memories were intact, the hippocampus is not the final resting place for memory. Thus, memory is not unitary but, rather, involves multiple systems (Squire, 2009). Other cortical regions store past experiences. Thus, hippocampal damage results in anterograde amnesia (the capacity to form the next long-term memories). It also can result in retrograde amnesia because the link to components of past experiences needed to re-experience events is impaired.

These memories are not stored within a single brain area but, rather, are stored in a distributed network (Cabeza & St. Jacques, 2007). The network includes the medial and lateral prefrontal cortex, the medial and lateral parietal cortex, the amygdala, and sensory cortices in the occipital and temporal lobes (Svoboda et al., 2006). Our goal in remembering the past is not simply to re-experience past events. Instead, in self-reflection, we draw on past experiences to guide behavior in the present and plan for the future based on our past.

## Neuroanatomy of Other Memory Functions

A fundamental distinction is between declarative memory that is consciously recollected and procedural (nondeclarative) memory that is not consciously recollected

(Squire, 2009; Squire & Wixted, 2011). Declarative memory systems modify behavior through recollection of past facts and events, and they involve the medial temporal lobe and diencephalon, as shown on the left in Figure 6.2. However, with nondeclarative memory, experience modifies behavior without there being conscious memory control, even the knowledge that memory is being used. Nondeclarative memory in memory systems is represented in the neostriatum, neocortex, amygdala, cerebellum, and the reflux pathways, as shown in Figure 6.2. Research is ongoing to establish which neuronal circuitry is necessary for a particular type of memory, its formation, storage, and retrieval. Neuronal circuits involved in certain forms of learning have been identified. Thus, there is evidence for localization of memory.

The various forms of memory are mediated by separate brain systems. Conscious memory for facts and events (declarative or explicit memory) and nonconscious memory (acquisition of skills, habits, and other procedures; i.e., nondeclarative or implicit memory) use different brain systems, as shown in Figure 6.2. The hippocampus and its related structures are essential for declarative or explicit memory, but other structures are necessary for nondeclarative or implicit memory. The hippocampus and related medial temporal lobe structures are needed for the establishment of enduring memory. However, long-term memory storage involves the neocortex and other brain regions. Nondeclarative memory involves the striatum (procedural skills and habits) and neocortex (priming and perceptual learning). The amygdala is involved in the modulation of the strength of both declarative and nondeclarative memory (Squire, 2004). Moreover, the cerebellum is an important site for classical conditioning of both emotional and motor responses.

Computationally oriented developmental cognitive neuroscience emphasizes neural network computer models. These approaches attempt to formulate detailed models of actual neural circuits. For example, there are neural network models that address how an individual performs specific tasks; networks are constructed and trained to interpret work-like inputs. This model is then damaged, and error patterns are examined. In some respects, these model circuits mirror brain damage, so the modeling potentially accounts for difficulties in brain-damage models that allow new hypotheses to be evaluated. The use of neural networks may have more general application in understanding the process of memory storage. Moreover, there is cell biology of memory-related synaptic plasticity. Changes in gene expression and protein synthesis that relate to memory are essential in long-term sensitization and studied in animal models and human studies in invertebrates (Kandel, 2009). Long-term potentiation is an important mechanism in memory consolidation.

## Animal Models of Memory Function

Human memory has been modeled in nonhuman primates. Monkeys are prepared with bilateral lesions limited to a particular structure or combination of structures. The effects of the surgical lesions on memory are then determined by evaluating the monkeys' performance on tasks that are either identical or analogous to tasks of memory impairment in humans. To establish if the impairment in monkeys is long-lasting, as it is in humans who have had damage to the medial temporal lobe, these monkeys can be tested again several years after their surgery. Because there are multiple memory systems, specific systems can be tested in animals whose performance corresponds to that of humans with amnesia.

One model in the monkey involves large bilateral lesions of the medial temporal lobe, which approximates damage in known amnesic human patients. The damaged area includes the hippocampal formation, dentate gyrus, and the cornu ammonis (CA) regions. The CA is anatomically differentiated into four subfields along with the surrounding perirhinal and parahippocampal cortices. One region, CA3, has a specific role in memory processes. Following its lesion, monkeys are impaired on several declarative and amygdala memory tasks and, like human patients, are entirely normal on nondeclarative memory tasks involving acquiring and retaining skills. The best test to demonstrate impaired memories in monkeys is the delayed nonmatching to sample task. This is a task of recognition memory in which a single object is presented, and then after a delay, two objects are presented—the original object and a new one. The animal must choose the new object to obtain a food reward. The testing is done in multiple trials, and unique pairs of objects are used for each trial. The results in this primate model have demonstrated that structures of the medial temporal lobe—that is, the hippocampus embedded in the medial temporal lobe—rather than adjacent areas are critical for recognition memory (Squire & Zola-Morgan, 1991).

Moreover, the main components of the medial temporal lobe memory system have been identified. This memory system consists of the hippocampal formation, which includes the entorhinal cortex along with adjacent anatomically related regions. The amygdaloid complex is not a component of the medial temporal lobe memory system. It does not contribute to declarative memory per se but may modulate the strength of declarative memory. As noted in Chapter 4, the amygdala is important for conditioned fear and attachment of affect to neutral stimuli. The amygdala may also have a role in establishing links between stimuli and in making associations between various sensory modalities, as well as in the recognition of emotion in facial expressions. In the monkey model discussed previously, damage to the amygdaloid complex caused alterations in emotional behavior, in that the monkeys were less fearful than normal and willing to touch and interact with novel stimuli.

In summary, the medial temporal lobe cortex in animal models participates in memory functions through its extensive reciprocal connections with memory storage sites in the neocortex and other brain regions. Systematic research with monkeys and related research in humans has identified the connections and components of the medial temporal lobe memory system. This system is fast, has limited capacity, and performs crucial functions during the time of learning to establish long-term explicit memory. Moreover, its role continues following memory reorganization and consolidation. Memories are stored in the neocortex and eventually become independent of the medial temporal lobe memory system. Thus, long-term (permanent) memory storage is gradually assumed by the neocortex and other brain regions, to allow the medial temporal lobe memory system to be always available for the acquisition of new information. With this understanding about how memory relates to the neocortex, studies using neural networks for computational modeling are advancing.

Procedural (nondeclarative) memory has been studied in the cat using the flexion reflex; in rabbits using the eyeblink response; and in invertebrates using the gill-withdrawal

reflex in *Aplysia*, *Drosophila* (fly), and several other species. These studies seek to identify the cellular basis of neural circuits to further our understanding of learning and
memory. *Aplysia* has approximately 20,000 neurons in its central nervous system (CNS)
and *Drosophila* has approximately 300,000 neurons in the CNS identified as linked to
learning. For example, the gill-withdrawal reflex in *Aplysia* can be modified in several
kinds of learning, including nondeclarative habituation, dishabituation, sensitization,
and classical and operant conditioning (Kandel, 2009). One mechanism for learning
and short-term memory in *Aplysia* is change in synaptic strength resulting from modulation of the release of a neurotransmitter. Studies of the connections between sensory
and motor neurons led to the discovery of a biochemical mechanism for the release
of serotonin and other neurotransmitters, which activate $Ca^{2+}$/calmodulin-dependent
protein kinase.

## Long-Term Potentiation and Memory

Long-term potentiation (LTP) is a neuronal mechanism underlying learning and
memory. Most excitatory presynaptic terminals form synapses on dendritic spines on
cortical pyramidal neurons. Dendrites provide both anatomical and biochemical isolation of a synapse, allowing for synaptic specificity for LTP. LTP refers to long-lasting
strengthening of excitatory synaptic neurotransmission between nerves. Memories
are stored or encoded in neural networks in the brain. It is thought that new or novel
experiences lead to neuronal firing in these networks. Subsequently, when we attempt
to recall an experience or are reminded of one, the same firing pattern that represents
that memory may be triggered. This memory system in the brain can store and retrieve
massive amounts of information. New memory information is encoded in seconds,
stored, and remains persistently encoded.

A time period of several minutes is needed to stabilize or consolidate the memory
of a newly acquired experience or information. This encoding process is stimulated by
patterns of electrophysiologic activity in the brain that are acquired during the learning
process and are accompanied by actual morphological change. All of these aspects of
memory are consistent with the LTP model originally proposed by Hebb (1949). Hebb
hypothesized that a synaptic modification takes place with learning and memory.

LTP refers to how changes in synaptic efficiency occur in association with memory.
LTP was confirmed in 1973 when it was shown that intense neuronal firing in the hippocampus on one occasion established a pattern in which neurons fired more readily with
subsequent stimulation of the same neuron (Bliss & Lømo, 1973). Thus, when neurons
were activated, synaptic connections were strengthened by this process. In LTP, a neuron
that is repeatedly depolarized "remembers" the robust signal, laying down a "memory."
Changes also take place within the neurons and their synaptic junctions during LTP
as a result of trafficking of "occult" α-amino-3-hydroxy-5-methyl-4-isoxazolepropionic
acid (AMPA) receptors to the synapse and expression of proteins involved in excitatory
neurotransmission. With the strengthening of the affected synapses, these neurons respond to specific stimuli (Ma & Zuo, 2022).

Five characteristic features of LTP make it the major candidate for being the substrate of forms of memory. First, LTP is synaptically specific, so induction in one group

of contacts on a neuron does not affect other cellular contacts. This property allows for substantial memory capacity. Second, LTP begins to develop within 10 s of stimulation and is established by 20–30 s. Third, LTP can persist for weeks or more, allowing for long-term storage of memory. Fourth, there is a consolidation phase, also referred to as a vulnerable phase, lasting several minutes. Finally, brain activity patterns that emerge during learning are directly related to cellular events that initiate LTP (Lynch & Granger, 1992; Nicoll, 2017).

LTP has been demonstrated in many brain regions, although it has been studied most extensively in the hippocampus. The early work of Bliss and Lømo (1973) showed an increase in the size of excitatory postsynaptic potentials after a brief period of high-frequency (tetanic) electrical stimulation of the perforant path glutamatergic axons that synapse on pyramidal neurons in the hippocampus. The primary form of LTP involves activation of the $N$-methyl-D-aspartate (NMDA) subtype of glutamate. This process is shown in Figure 6.3.

The activation of the synaptic NMDA receptors results in an influx of $Ca^{2+}$ into the postsynaptic spine. The elevated $Ca^{2+}$ causes more AMPA subtype of glutamate receptors to be inserted in the postsynaptic complex; AMPA receptors are glutamate receptors that cause neuronal depolarization and then generate action potentials. The induction of LTP requires concurrent pre- and postsynaptic receptor activation and may be prevented by blocking postsynaptic NMDA receptors with dissociative anesthetics, so named because they impair memory formation in apparent clear consciousness. LTP occurs throughout the nervous system, although other glutamatergic mechanisms aside from NMDA receptors can be responsible. Persistent activation after LTP can induce the formation of new receptive postsynaptic spines, leading to additional glutamatergic synapses for a specific pathway. Thus, the NMDA receptor represents the cornerstone of neuronal plasticity in the brain.

The maintenance of LTP can involve, in part, presynaptic enhancement of glutamate release. Thus, postsynaptic neurons can release one or more retrograde messengers to presynaptic nerve terminals. The main retrograde messengers are the soluble gases nitric oxide (Bradley & Steinert, 2016) and carbon monoxide (Zhuo et al., 1998). Nitric oxide and carbon monoxide are proposed to play different roles in LTP. Nitric oxide plays a phasic signaling role, whereas carbon dioxide provides background tonic stimulation (Zhuo et al., 1998). In certain circumstances, carbon monoxide is critical for initiating LTP (Hanafy et al., 2013). Nitric oxide–induced post-translational modifications are involved in homeostatic plasticity signaling pathways; nitric oxide directly or indirectly affects receptor function by modulating the AMPA receptor translocation to the membrane (Bradley & Steinert, 2016).

These synaptic mechanisms are important for acquiring and storing memory but do not play a major role in retaining it. Fusi et al. (2005) propose that memory retention involves a cascade of states, with each state more stable than the one that precedes it. Using this model, progressive stabilization in the synapse has been documented during the transition from short-term to long-term memory. Computational neuroscience models such as these have been confirmed experimentally (Fusi, 2017; Kandel, 2009).

Memory is complex, and synaptic plasticity is an important brain mechanism to store memories. Synaptic plasticity is a dynamic system with many intermediate molecular states. Computational models are key to advancing our understanding of memory.

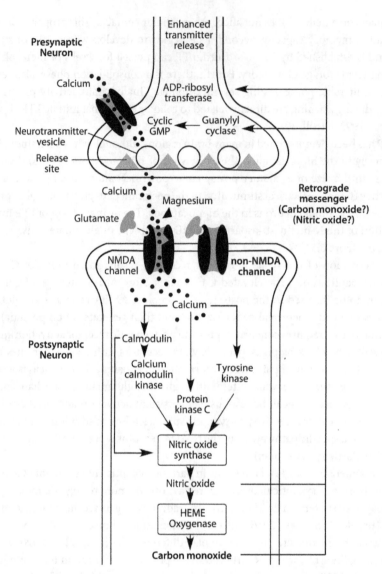

**Figure 6.3** The NMDA receptor and long-term potentiation. In long-term potentiation, the postsynaptic membrane is depolarized by the actions of the non-NMDA receptor channels. The depolarization relieves the magnesium blockade of the NMDA channel, allowing calcium to flow through the channel. The calcium triggers calcium-dependent kinases that lead to the induction of long-term potentiation. The postsynaptic cell is thought to release a retrograde messenger—nitric oxide or carbon monoxide—capable of penetrating the membrane of the presynaptic cell. This messenger is believed to act in the presynaptic terminal to enhance transmitter (glutamate) release, perhaps by activating guanylyl cyclase or ADP-ribosyl transferase.

Adapted from Harris (1998); redrawn by Tim Phelps (2021).

Importantly, the hippocampus is not the final storage state for memory. Ultimately, all the forms of declarative memory will be stored independently in areas of the neocortex. How this occurs is a subject of continuing investigation. One promising area of study is the role of non–rapid eye movement (non-REM) and REM sleep in the memory storage in neocortical regions (Ackermann & Rasch, 2014).

How memory is recalled also is a subject of ongoing study (Frankland et al., 2019). Regarding fear memory, neurons activated in the amygdala during the acquisition of learned fear are reactivated during retrieval of such memories (Kandel, 2009). Moreover, the extent of neuronal reactivation correlates with behavioral expression of learned fear (Mayford et al., 1996). Thus, associative memory has a stable neural correlate (Reijmers et al., 2007). Yet, declarative memory requires conscious attention for recalling memories. Dopamine and acetylcholine facilitate the formation of declarative memories and may be involved in recall (Kandel, 2009).

## Sleep and Memory

The earliest scientific report of the role of sleep in memory was in the 1920s when Jenkins and Dallenbach (1924) reported that sleep facilitated the memory of nonsense syllables presented before sleep. This line of research continued throughout the 20th century and advanced following the recognition of distinct sleep stages (Aserinsky & Kleitman, 1953). Advances in the developmental neuroscience of memory have facilitated the study of memory consolidation in sleep (Feld & Born, 2020; Rasch & Born, 2013).

Sleep is essential for the long-term storage of memories. Memory consolidation in sleep begins with encoding (Figure 6.4). Encoding establishes the memory trace for later retrieval. The memory trace is stabilized in sleep to actively consolidate it, maintaining the memory trace transiently in storage in the hippocampus. The trace is gradually redistributed to more permanent storage in the cerebral cortex (Feld & Born, 2020; Feld & Diekelmann, 2015). For declarative memory, slow-wave sleep is the stage most important in consolidation of memories acquired during waking. Memories newly acquired in wakefulness are reactivated during sleep periods. Sleep also promotes encoding memories following sleep. This involves renormalization of "synaptic weights" during sleep, consistent with synaptic homeostasis theory (Tononi & Cirelli, 2020).

The most widely studied model of memory consolidation in sleep is the active system consolidation theory (Feld & Born, 2020). This theory proposed the active neuronal replay of memory representations during slow-wave sleep. This replay strengthens memory traces encoded during wakefulness on the day before sleep. Sleep following learning tasks increases synaptic signaling associated with prior learning (Yang et al., 2014). Moreover, sleep may restore learning capacity by downscaling synapses that were highly potentiated during earlier periods of wakefulness (Tononi & Cirelli, 2014, 2020).

During sleep, new memory traces are reactivated in both the hippocampus and cortex. The cortical representations of the memory trace are reactivated until they are sufficiently strengthened to be stored independently from the hippocampus. Neural reactivation was first documented in rodents following a spatial learning task that

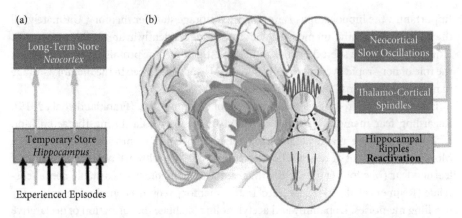

**Figure 6.4** Memory consolidation and sleep. (A) Memory consolidation during slow-wave sleep (SWS). Newly encoded declarative memories initially enter temporary storage in the hippocampal system and are subsequently reactivated and redistributed into long-term storage in the neocortex. (B) Memory system consolidation during SWS relies on an interactive dialog between neocortex and hippocampus under top-down control by the neocortical slow oscillations shown in red. The depolarizing phases of the slow oscillations drive the repeated reactivation of hippocampal memory representations together with sharp-wave ripples, shown in green, in the hippocampus and thalamocortical spindles. This synchronous drive leads to the formation of spindleppocampus under top-down control by the neocortical slow oscillations shown in reare then nested into single troughs of a spindle (shown at larger scale in the figure). Spindle–ripple events are believed to be a mechanism that supports the integration of reactivated memory information into the neocortex.
From Wilhelm et al. (2012).

activated hippocampal spatial location cells in the hippocampus during waking. The investigators found that these same spatial location cells fired together again during subsequent sleep (Wilson & McNaughton, 1994). Interestingly, the reactivation followed the same sequence as the orientation activity during wakefulness. Moreover, it was coordinated with the cortex. Also, other brain regions in the rodent model showed replays of neuronal activity during waking (striation, motor cortex, and thalamus) (K. Harris, 2014).

Sleep reactivation has been documented in humans in neuroimaging studies with functional magnetic resonance imaging (fMRI). Human subjects, similar to animals that have been studied, learned tasks that activated specific brain regions when awake. Activation of the same brain region as in waking was observed while asleep (Maquet et al., 2000; Peigneux et al., 2004). During slow-wave sleep, the slow oscillations that were measured by polysomnography were generated in the cerebral cortex and synchronized in the hippocampus. Moreover, the reactivated memory reached the cortex with sleep spindles (Feld & Diekelmann, 2015). Thus, sleep spindles enhanced plasticity in the cortex, leading to the integration of new memories into long-term storage (Ribeiro et al., 2007) for later recall of memories.

In addition to being strengthened, memories are transformed and reorganized. The reorganization of memories may allow them to be placed in context to generalize to new situations. In infants, naps may promote abstraction in language learning (Gómez et al., 2006). Thus, memory replay continues to build cognitive schema during development. Sleep is important for preserving and transforming episodic memories (Inostroza & Born, 2013). Moreover, sleep can facilitate problem-solving. In one study, participants given a serial numerical transformation task were not told a hidden rule that facilitated task mastery. Following sleep, nearly three times as many participants gained insight into the hidden rule compared to controls (Wagner et al., 2004). Insight following sleep may lead to mental restructuring. This restructuring leads to a gain in declarative knowledge when a problem is presented before sleep and then "sleeping on it." However, memories are not stored as direct copies of our life experiences, leading to loss, distortions, and inaccuracies in memory.

Because sleep plays an important role in consolidating memories, its role in the development of false memories has been examined. Payne et al. (2009) studied subjects following a night of sleep using the Deese–Roediger–McDermott (DRM) paradigm, a task that reliably produces false memories of critical words semantically associated with study words, and compared the results to an equivalent period of wakefulness. They found that verifiable memory deteriorated across both wake and sleep but that false memories were preferentially preserved by sleep. Sleep both stabilizes memories and transforms them, possibly for adaptation to new circumstances. Declarative memory that includes both episodic memory (context-specific event memory) and semantic memory (context-independent conceptual knowledge) has been studied. Both false and truthful memory rely on an association with semantic processing that uses the left ventrolateral prefrontal cortex. Truthful memory that is verified also relies on the medial temporal lobe, primarily the hippocampus. The DRM paradigm may draw on several neural systems and on different sleep stages to produce results. False memories have been examined with regard to the effects of post-encoding stress on performance in the DRM paradigm.

Pardilla-Delgado et al. (2016) measured memory consolidation following the encoding of 15 semantically related word lists (DRM false memory task) and tested memory again 24 hr later in stressed and not stressed subjects. They found that not only did stress decrease recognition of the words studied but also stress increased false recognition of semantically related words (false memory). Moreover, unlike control subjects, those who were stressed remembered more false words than true words. The authors concluded that "stress supports gist memory formation in the DRM task, perhaps by hindering detail-specific processing in the hippocampus" (p. 46).

Although it is generally believed that memory is an exact recall of experiences, we now know that memory is reconstructed when recalled and in the process can be distorted. These research findings about stress and memory are important, for example, in judging eyewitness evidence but also in how we remember meaningful life events, such as the death of a loved one, an assault, divorce, and other stressful experiences. For example, Smeets et al. (2008) found enhanced memory consolidation under stress of real-life emotional experience while impairing memory for neutral information.

The amygdala is more involved in emotional memory consolidation, whereas the hippocampus is more involved in neutral memory consolidation. These two brain regions are differentially impacted by stress. Changes in cortisol levels with stress disrupt hippocampal function but potentiate the function of the amygdala. Thus, stress hormone release may account for the differences in memory for functional versus emotional words. As such, accurate memory consolidation is affected by stress.

## Restoration of Synaptic Homeostasis in Sleep

Synaptic potentials during wakefulness impact storage of information in the brain. During sleep, there is a normalization of synaptic strength or "synaptic weight," which is called synaptic downscaling. During our waking hours, synaptic signaling increases; during sleep, it decreases (Vyazovskiy et al., 2008). These changes in restoring synaptic homeostasis largely occur during slow-wave sleep. An important consequence of synaptic downscaling during sleep is an improvement in learning after a period of sleep, even after a brief nap (Mander et al., 2011).

That suppression of slow-wave sleep in a sample of elderly subjects decreased their capacity to encode information the next morning supports the importance of slow-wave sleep in synaptic downscaling (Van Der Werf et al., 2009). The timing of sleep is important for memory function. The shorter the interval between sleep and new learning of declarative tasks, the greater the enhancement effect of sleep on memory. If there is a long interval between new learning and sleep time, reviewing material learned that day at bedtime can be beneficial. To be optimally consolidated, some types of memory require a full night sleep involving both slow-wave and REM sleep periods.

Memory consolidation during sleep may be selective for memories that one knows will be needed the following day (Wilhelm et al., 2011). Emotional engagement leads to stronger memory consolidation during sleep such that emotional memories can be vividly remembered (Groch et al., 2013, 2015). REM sleep is also reported to improve creativity by priming associative memory networks (Cai et al., 2009). Although REM sleep may also facilitate procedural memory consolidation, the biological and molecular mechanisms are not known (Rasch & Born, 2013). A two-stage memory consolidation process is involved for both declarative and nondeclarative memory. For example, the acquisition of procedural skills, such as language learning and finger sequence tapping, involves both declarative and procedural memory components (Krakauer & Shadmehr, 2006; Peigneux et al., 2001). Cerebellar circuits are substantially involved in motor learning storage (Krakauer & Shadmehr, 2006).

## Memory and the Development

During development, there are changes in memory processing. Memory functions are stabilized with structural and functional maturation of the brain, especially changes in the prefrontal cortex and medial frontal lobe (Ofen et al., 2016). Age-related differences in memory capacities, prior knowledge, and use of metacognitive abilities at different ages have been examined with neuroimaging. There are considerable differences between children and adults for memories that depend on contextual details.

## Memory in Infancy

The systems responsible for procedural memory appear to be present at birth. Procedural (nondeclarative) memory involves changes in performance based on experience and engages the striatum, cerebellum, and brain stem, which are functional at the time of birth. Thus, term infants demonstrate learning based on visual expectation and operant and classical conditioning. However, declarative memory tasks that depend on the hippocampus, such as visual paired-comparison mastery, do not develop until approximately 8–12 months of age (Richmond & Nelson, 2008). The earliest hippocampal memory function is viewed as predeclarative memory and appears as a transition toward the adult declarative memory system. Declarative (explicit) and nondeclarative (implicit) memory systems develop gradually and in parallel from birth. Hippocampal neurogenesis continues in the dentate gyrus throughout life, with high numbers of proliferating neurons in infancy but slowing of neurogenesis throughout childhood (Rovee-Collier et al., 2001). The pattern of neuronal connectivity in memory circuits is constantly being remodeled in the immature hippocampus.

The maintenance of synaptic connectivity is required for the persistence of memory. The constant production of new neurons during infancy appears to "erase" infantile memories, which accounts for infantile amnesia (Ramsaran et al., 2019). With maturation of the hippocampus, memory retention increases as neurogenesis declines. Yet, it is unclear whether memories formed in infancy can be recovered in adulthood, invalidating the concept of infantile amnesia. Guskjolen et al. (2018) performed a clever study to determine whether memories acquired by the infant mouse could be recovered in adulthood by transfecting the neurons activated in the dentate gyrus of the infant mouse with channelrhodopsin-2 (ChR2) during memory formation. Three months later, the same dentate neurons transfected with ChR2 were activated by illuminating the dentate, resulting in the restoration of the memories.

The other element in brain immaturity is timing of the development of NMDA receptors, which are important in synaptic plasticity and stabilization. Because the striatum, cerebellum, and brain stem are functionally mature in early childhood, simple conditioning is possible in newborns. Regarding declarative memory, as described previously, development of the dentate gyrus of the hippocampus, important for memory storage, lags behind that of other regions of the hippocampus. The migration of GABAergic neurons into the hippocampus during development is also prolonged. The dentate gyrus does not reach the adult configuration until the end of the first year of life. However, the differentiation of inhibitory neurons within the dentate to adult cellular morphology is not achieved until after age 2 years. These GABAergic interneurons are critical for both attention and memory.

Memory involves encoding, retention, and retrieval. Older infants encode new information faster than younger ones. Thus, 6-month-olds require twice as long as 12-month-olds on the delayed (nonmatch)-to-sample task. Developmental changes in encoding are related to the speed of information processing, which increases with age. These changes in processing speed are linked to the increasing myelination of axons, which accelerates the flow of action potentials. The most rapid phase of myelination is in the first year of life (Paus et al., 2001). Myelination occurs sequentially from the occipital cortex to the frontal and parietal lobes by approximately age 8 months and to the temporal lobe by age 12 months. Changes are most rapid in the first 6 months of life, with continuing but slowing up to 24 months and stability after that.

Compared to younger infants, older infants retain information longer in memory. For example, both 6- and 9 month-olds retain information immediately after testing, but 9-month-olds also retain information when tested after a delay (Hayne, 2004). The continuing development of the dentate gyrus throughout the first years of life may account for increased capacity to consolidate memories into long-term storage. Greater activation of the hippocampal CA2 and CA3 subfields in the dentate gyrus is important in the consolidation of associative memories. Greater activity of the subiculum is involved for retrieval (Zeineh et al., 2003). These changes are linked to the gradual maturation of the dentate gyrus, facilitating learning and memory consolidation. Memory retrieval matures later in development. It is not until the middle of the second year of life that memory retrieval becomes more consistent. For example, in a puppet memory task, 12-month-olds failed to reproduce puppet actions after a 24-hr delay if the color or form of the puppet was changed (Barr & Hayne, 2000). It is not until age 24 months that infants can generalize actions that they learned with different stimulus toys.

Although the memories of the infants can be very specific, small changes in context or the cued stimulus lead to memory failure. How do we understand memory failure in nonverbal infants? Eichenbaum's (2011) relational memory hypothesis is an explanation applicable in both human and animal research. This hypothesis posits that for nonverbal individuals and animals, relational representations with flexible expression are characteristic features.

Hippocampal networks form patterns of items that are related causally, logically, or temporally. Such hippocampal relational networks make inferences while regions outside the hippocampus (i.e., entorhinal, perirhinal, and parahippocampal cortices) support only very specific representations of individual items in memory. Memories that are hippocampal dependent are only expressed if the specific conditions present at the time of learning are re-established (Eichenbaum, 2011). Infants' failure to use memories flexibly results from an inability to form relational connections. Because the hippocampus is immature, infants bind details to test cues and context into a unity rather than establish relational representations. This prevents flexibility in memory use.

## Memory in Childhood

Declarative memory develops with the enhanced memory performance throughout early and middle childhood. Strategies focus on efficient encoding rather than on retrieving. Episodic memory, especially autobiographical memory, improves over time. The capacity to establish a complex relational context in memory begins between 4 and 7 years of age and is refined by adulthood (Yim et al., 2013). Episodic memory refers to the formation of relational structures that bind information about experiences to the context in which they are experienced. Their formation and retrieval as episodic memories were confirmed in a study of 7- to 11-year-old children. However, relational binding depended on relational type (e.g., in time, in space, and in relationships). In one study, the "space" item reached adult performance by age 9½ years, whereas the "time" and the item–item relations improved later (J. Lee et al., 2016). Behavioral evidence demonstrates that age effects are clear when more demanding aspects of memory are tested. Children may rely more on memory representations that retain less details, especially details about the context in which information was assessed.

Developmental cognitive neuroscience seeks to map the development changes and relate them to the brain. Two key brain areas of interest in the study of memory in children are the medial temporal lobe and prefrontal cortex. Development of the prefrontal cortex underlies the increase in prefrontal recruitment in children for memory coding and retrieval (Güler & Thomas, 2013). Changes in the medial temporal cortex are not as extensive (Gogtay et al., 2006). A longitudinal study did not find gender differences in hippocampal development; however, it did demonstrate that subregions of the hippocampus show different developmental trajectories. Gogtay et al. (2006) performed MRIs on 31 children aged 6–10 years every 2 years. They found that the overall volume of the hippocampus was unchanged between 4 and 25 years in adult comparison groups. Nevertheless, there were substantial differences within the subregions of the hippocampus. The posterior portion gradually increased in volume with age, but more so in the left hemisphere, whereas the anterior half decreased in volume, more so in the right hemisphere.

Maturation of medial temporal lobe and cortical brain areas, especially the prefrontal cortex, is also important in increasing the capacity for the strategic use of memory. Left prefrontal cortex activation predicts subsequent story recall in children aged 7 and 8 years. Activation of both the medial temporal lobe and the prefrontal lobe is associated with successful story recall in 10- to 18-year-olds (Chiu et al., 2006). Increased involvement of the medial temporal lobe in memory in older children may help us understand age-related improvements in memory-based rehearsal for encoding memory across middle childhood. With age, decreased involvement of the medial temporal cortex with increased interaction between the medial temporal cortex and prefrontal structures leads to improved strategy use, access to source memory, and greater self-awareness. One study involved children aged 11–19 years who had brain scans while encoding pictures of outdoor scenes. The investigation found that although the extent of encoding-related activation in the left posterior hippocampus and entorhinal cortex decreased with age, there were age-related increases on the functional connectivity of the left entorhinal cortex and left dorsal prefrontal cortex (Menon et al., 2005). The enhancement of relational memory capacities in childhood is related to improvements in both episodic memory and autobiographical memory. In another study, children aged 4–6 years and adults were presented with pictures of animals in a natural setting. Later, they were tested for recognition of the animal, the environment, and animal–environment combination. The 4- and 6-year-olds did not differ in the first two tasks; however, the 4-year-olds remembered fewer animal–environment combinations. The 6-year-olds did not differ from adults. The authors proposed that ongoing development of children for binding items relationally in memory may facilitate episodic recall (Sluzenski et al., 2006).

In summary, evidence supports the view that age-related advances in memory ability are tied to functional maturation of the prefrontal cortex with differential recruitment of the medial temporal lobe. Thus, there is increased connectivity between these two main brain regions during development. There is relative stability from middle childhood for memory recognition tasks requiring few contextual details. There are continual gains after middle childhood on tasks that require retention of detailed information. The sources of these development advances and individual differences are working memory capacity, prior knowledge, metacognitive knowledge, and the use of learned mnemonic strategies. Scientific study of memory development in children has been greatly facilitated by neuroimaging methods, which advances our mechanistic understanding of what links age and memory performance.

## Working Memory: Development in Children

Working memory is critically important for progress in learning by children, especially in mastering reading and mathematics. Working memory refers to a memory system responsible for retaining and processing information over short periods of time. It is important in the acquisition of complex academic skills. There are deficits in working memory in attention-deficit/hyperactivity disorder (ADHD), dyslexia, and language disorders (Bathelt et al., 2018). Adult working memory involves several interacting temporal memory systems. The central executive system, which is responsible for a range of regulatory systems, is the essential component of the most studied model for working memory. This model includes attention, control of action, and problem-solving (Baddeley, 1996). The working memory model has been refined by proposing "the episodic buffer." It is a multidimensional representational system that integrates temporal representations from other cognitive systems along with working memory (Baddeley, 2000).

In addition to the central executive system, there are two other components in the working memory model. These are systems that are specialized to manipulate and retain information. For example, there is a phonological code important in the phonetics of reading. This is a subvocal rehearsal process that recodes pictures or printed works that are not phonological inputs into a phonological form, allowing entry into the phonological store (Gathercole et al., 2004). This rehearsal process refreshes decaying representations in the phonological store. The third process, the visuospatial sketchpad, is used to store information consisting of visual–spatial features (Logie, 1986).

Working memory development continues throughout early and middle childhood, with the maturation of the brain systems utilized to support working memory skills in adulthood (Tamnes et al., 2013). This working memory model has been continually refined to include inhibitory processes that protect activated memory traces from being disrupted. Other enhancements include better understanding of updating, set-shifting, and relational binding of information as well as the relationship to fluid intelligence (Bathelt et al., 2018; Engle et al., 1999; Hornung et al., 2011). Overall, this three-factor structure has been widely replicated in many working memory studies and for various age groups. Working memory substantially increases throughout childhood and into adolescence. Adult levels are reached in adolescence. For example, as children grow older, there is greater brain storage capacity and enhanced attentional ability.

## Working Memory and the Brain

During development, there are substantial changes in the brain that accompany the maturation of working memory. Sowell et al. (2004) repeatedly brain-imaged 45 children between ages 5 and 11 years. Brain size was found to increase each year, especially in the frontal and occipital regions. Gray matter thinning coupled with cortical expansion occurred, which was highly significant in the right frontal and bilateral parieto-occipital regions. In the left hemisphere, gray matter thickness was correlated with changing cognitive abilities. Moreover, functional neuroimaging studies revealed that enhancement of working memory correlated with reorganization in brain networks (Houdé et al., 2010).

In adults, increased blood oxygenation during working memory tasks has been shown to include bilateral parietal, cingulate, and prefrontal brain regions. In a large meta-analysis, Wager and Smith (2003) considered spatial, verbal, and object storage and three types of executive functions. Children aged 7–12 years showed activation involving similar hemisphere specialization as adults (Thomason et al., 2009). However, their ability to bring needed neural resources to maintain verbal or spatial information in working memory was immature. Children also engaged nonspecific brain regions outside the core networks used by adults. Structural brain correlates of working memory, involving gray and white matter, showed differences during development. Neural structures and networks linked to executive working memory changed as children matured. Brain regions that contributed most to the executive aspect of working memory were the corpus callosum, bilateral posterior temporal white matter, and the left occipital temporal cortex. These brain regions contributed differently to executive working memory according to the age of the child (Bathelt et al., 2018).

The latent structure of working memory has also been examined. Factors have been identified for verbal and visuospatial storage and executive involvement pertinent to both (Kane et al., 2004, 2007). White matter organization, not cortical thickness, shows development differences with age. Differences in microstructural properties of myelin are also key elements. These differences are measured using diffusion tensor neuroimaging (DTI). Fractional anisotropy (FA), a DTI measure of brain connectivity, is linked to cognitive development and related to age (Bathelt et al., 2018). FA was found to be a more sensitive indicator of brain maturation than cortical thickness in the 6- to 16-year-old age groups (Bathelt et al., 2018).

Brain morphology and age interact in the development of executive working memory. Younger children use general brain systems, whereas in adulthood, established specialized networks are used. In children, there is higher blood oxygenation in regions other than the core working memory regions active in adults, suggesting an inefficiency in processing (Vogan et al., 2016). Working memory in children is more tightly linked with microstructural integration of white matter components. Thus, younger children are more reliant on microstructural integration of white matter and dependent on a distributed system, whereas in older children, cortical thickness of the left posterior temporal lobe also is implicated in working memory (Bathelt et al., 2018).

The research literature on development of working memory is consistent with two hypotheses (Bathelt et al., 2018). First, interhemispheric connections of the corpus callosum result in inhibition between functionally related regions in the left and right hemispheres. Reduced lateralization has been associated with lower performance in executive functioning and mastery of cognitive tasks (Nagel et al., 2013). Second, posterior temporal lobe white matter is important in establishing connections for integration between regions of the temporal lobe that are specialized for verbal and visuospatial working memory and linked to the parietal executive attention network. Posterior temporal white matter is important for working memory in adults. In younger children, there is a shift from the contributions of callosal and temporal white matter to working memory to greater reliance on working memory involving left temporal cortex in older children.

In summary, there are changes in the neural systems associated with working memory throughout childhood. Working memory and attentional impairments are frequent in neurodevelopmental disorders, especially in syndromes in which attention-deficit disorder is a feature, such as fragile X syndrome, phenylketonuria, and velocordiofacial syndrome (Holmes et al., 2014; Martinussen et al., 2005). Differences in working memory capacity are linked to different combinations of neural systems depending on the age of the child and according to differences in neural development in neurodevelopmental disorders.

## Sleep and Memory in Children

Sleep is beneficial to learning in children, as has been documented in 6- to 8 year-olds. Sleep enhances memory performance in children, impacting declarative rather than procedural tasks; memory consolidation also depends on the developmental stage (Wilhelm et al., 2008). As in adults, slow-wave sleep is essential for memory consolidation in early development. Longer and deeper sleep produces strengthening of hippocampal-dependent declarative memories. Infants aged 6–16 months consolidate new word meanings as they nap. Learning new words from storybooks read to preschool children increases when the children are allowed to nap after being read a story (Williams & Horst, 2014). The extraction of declarative memory information with sleep may be more beneficial in children than in adults. Improving sleep in children is important to enhance school performance (Ribeiro & Stickgold, 2014).

Slow-wave sleep is especially important for sleep consolidation in children. Infants and children sleep longer than adults. Sleep stages emerge during development progressing from quiet sleep to more evenly divided REM and non-REM sleep in infants to the emergence of the four sleep stages. REM sleep time is increased in the first 6 months of life in comparison to adults' duration. From the preschool years until adolescence, the proportion of slow-wave sleep is increased compared to that of adults—increasing to levels clearly longer than those of adults until the beginning of puberty. Thereafter, throughout adolescence, the amount of slow-wave sleep progressively decreases throughout the Tanner stages of puberty. Because young children have greater amounts of deep sleep (slow-wave sleep), memory consolidation is more efficient in children. Thus, children have considerable gains in declarative knowledge and increasingly better memory performance as they mature (Backhaus et al., 2008), which is shown by enhancement in declarative memory consolidation.

In one study, recall after sleep in children was better after intervals of wakefulness, and recall performance was also better. Other studies have documented sleep benefits in 7- to 14 year-olds for word memory, learning novel words, and integrating words into the knowledge base for that child (Potkin & Bunney, 2012). When sleep was restricted to 5 hr per night for four nights, adolescents increased the proportion of their slow-wave sleep during the shortened sleep period, suggesting that when sleep is restricted, there is an increase in the depth of sleep. A study in 6- to 8-year-old children documented consolidation of visuospatial memory in a task known to involve hippocampal functioning (Wilhelm et al., 2008). The size of the effect was similar to adult performance; however, the amount of slow-wave sleep found in children was twice that of adults. These studies confirm the importance of high amounts of slow-wave sleep for memory in childhood.

When children aged 10–16 years were compared to age-matched children diagnosed with ADHD, the neurotypically developing children performed better on the restoration of memory for pictures task than those with ADHD (Prehn-Kristensen, Göder, et al., 2011). Although time spent in slow-wave sleep did not differ between the two groups, the typically developing children showed a positive correlation between slow oscillation power during non-REM sleep. In comparison to children with ADHD, there were also differences in the contribution of the prefrontal cortex. The final encoding of hippocampal-dependent memories relies on the prefrontal cortex, which tags these memories during memory encoding. Tagging facilitates access to encoding during deep sleep. In children with ADHD, tagging for prefrontal selection may be compromised during slow-wave sleep. This comparison marking decreases the benefit of declarative coding in the hippocampus, making children with ADHD less efficient in selecting emotional over neutral memories in consolidation (Wilhelm et al., 2012). Nevertheless, children with ADHD benefited from sleep-associated consolidation of motor skills (nondeclarative memory) more so than did neurotypical children in the study by Wilhelm et al. Studies such as these draw attention to the competitive interaction between declarative and procedural components of memory. Neurotypical children show preferential strengthening of declarative memory rather than nondeclarative memory in sleep.

The effects of sleep on nondeclarative (procedural) memories have also been examined in children. These are memories of skills and habits acquired during daytime by repeated practice. Sensorimotor procedural skills include riding a bicycle, playing a musical instrument, and writing; earlier skills include learning to walk and to speak. Unlike in adults, studies in children do not find sleep-dependent gains in performance of skill tasks. The anatomical structures that underlie procedural memory formation mature during the first 3 years of life. Immaturity does not allow immediate and accurate integration of complex sensory and sensorimotor inputs into premotor programs, such as sleep reactivations of the behavior. Still, sleep led to performance enhancement on a motor tapping task in 4- to 6 year-olds if children had received enhanced pretraining over several days. Therefore, improvement in nondeclarative (procedural) performance depends on there being earlier representations of the task and building on earlier experience. In animal models that show a similar lack of nondeclarative (procedural) response in sleep, prior disturbance in skill performance in early life predicts a higher level of performance at a later stage in training. Most studies of sleep-dependent nondeclarative (procedural) memory formation in children show impairing instead of improving effects of sleep on skills. Essentially, low initial skill level is a factor in children; skill learning is slower and less accurate than in adults and less automated in children. Thus, for sleep to lead to gains in performance, pre-sleep practice enhancement is needed. Children may show sleep-dependent benefits if they have extensive earlier training of the task. Therefore, sleep is important for consolidation of both declarative and nondeclarative (procedural) memory.

Because declarative memory consolidation involves both the hippocampus and the prefrontal cortex, sleep was examined in children with a diagnosis of ADHD; ADHD is characterized by deficits in the prefrontal activity. The study involved 16 children with a diagnosis of ADHD and 16 neurotypical children aged 9–12 years. The modified serial reaction time test was administered in the evening, with retesting following a night's sleep. In the sleep condition, there was retesting after a night's sleep. The wake condition comparison was tested in the morning with memory retrieval in the evening before sleep. Children with ADHD demonstrated improved motor skills after the sleep condition compared to wakefulness. Gains in reaction time were correlated with the amount of Stage 4 deep sleep and with REM density. In contrast, sleep did not benefit motor performance in neurotypical children. The authors conclude that children with ADHD (prefrontal involvement) have enabled sleep-dependent gains in motor skills because there is reduced competitive interference between components of the motor task when declarative memory tagging is compromised in ADHD. In neurotypical children with normal prefrontal activity, there is no such competition (Prehn-Kristensen, Göder, et al., 2011).

## Amnesia due to Brain Damage

Modern memory research began with the recognition that damage to the medial temporal lobe results in profound forgetfulness despite intact perceptual and intellectual functioning (Squire, 2009). H.M. had bilateral resection of the medial portion of his temporal lobe, including the hippocampus, because of intractable temporal lobe epilepsy. Post-surgery, H.M. had severe anterograde amnesia so that he did not remember events that occurred following his surgery. For example, when asked to study a list of words and recall them, he showed impaired memory. However, when the words were presented along with the stem-priming fragment of a meaningful word, he demonstrated the same priming effects as normal subjects do. Moreover, nondeclarative (procedural) memory was intact; only H.M.'s declarative memory was affected. Studies of H.M. revealed that (a) memory is a specific cerebral function distinct from other cognitive abilities; (b) because H.M.'s immediate memory persisted, his temporal lobe was not needed for immediate memory functioning; and (c) the temporal lobe is not the final repository for memory storage because H.M. remembered his stored childhood experiences (Squire, 2009).

Prosopagnosic patients demonstrate a deficit in facial recognition following bilateral lesions of the medial portions of the occipital and temporal cortex. These patients are unable to recognize previously encountered faces as familiar. Yet, they show differential autonomic responses to old and new faces, as measured by skin conductance measures. Although their responses to seeing faces may not be overly emotional, the degree of physiologic arousal suggests an emotional response.

## Amnesia in Children

Infantile hypoxia results in memory impairment in children (De Haan et al., 2006). Children with bilateral hippocampal atrophy following neonatal hypoxia–ischemia typically have preserved semantic memory and factual knowledge about remembered life events. However, they do have a severe impairment in episodic memory (Elward

& Vargha-Khadem, 2018). In a well-documented case of developmental amnesia, the patient, Jon, experienced severe hypoxia–ischemic bilateral hippocampal damage in the neonatal period. Throughout childhood and his adult life, he had problems in remembering past life episodes. When originally diagnosed, a volumetric MRI study demonstrated bilateral hippocampal atrophy. Brain volume in this case and two others with neonatal hypoxia was 39–57% below normal. Neuropsychological testing revealed IQs in the normal range; however, scores on standardized memory tests were significantly lower than predicted based on intelligence. The memory pattern in these children was like that of adult amnesic patients. Although scores on tests of immediate memory were normal, these children had severe deficits in recall of information after a delay. They had difficulty finding their way when navigating familiar surroundings. They were not able to remember appointments or messages that they had received earlier in the day, forgot where they left objects, and could not describe life events that had involved them earlier the same day. All attended mainstream schools and academically were at grade and IQ level in reading, spelling, and writing. On IQ subtests, they showed normal performance on vocabulary, information, and comprehension test measures. Thus, they had an isolated, severe impairment in episodic declarative memory but relatively spared and normal semantic memory (Richmond and Nelson, 2008; Vargha-Khadem et al., 1997).

Behavioral recognition ability was less affected in these children than in amnesia in adults. A subsequent study of Jon involved using a virtual reality paradigm in which Jon had to navigate through a virtual town where he collected objects from people. When tested on the task, he performed well in individual object recognition but was impaired in memory for contextual aspects of the experimental virtual environment—that is, when asked where, when, and who gave him the objects, he was impaired. His deficit was linked to relational memory; that is, he did not learn the relations between objects and places, where they were, and when they were acquired (Richmond & Nelson, 2008; Spiers et al., 2001).

Hypoxic–ischemic injury resulted in similar effects in 6- to 14-year-olds in another study. Neuropathology was similar, as were psychological test findings, in these children with insults to the brain in middle childhood and during puberty (Vargha-Khadem et al., 2003). Both injury before age 1 year and injury between ages 6 and 14 years have been studied in typically developing children using neuroimaging. Both groups had bilateral deficits in the hippocampus, posterior thalamus, and right retrosplenial cortex and similar reductions in the volume of the hippocampus. The only differences between infants and children aged 6–14 years were on tests of immediate memory. Importantly, the profiles in long-term memories were similar in both groups.

In children with developmental amnesia, the normal developmental trajectory for acquisition of typical cognitive functions is not dependent on the hippocampus. Thus, vocabulary, conceptual language, reading, grammar, and number skills follow the typical developmental progression. The neuronal networks maintaining these cognitive functions are not hippocampal mediated. Moreover, their working memory is intact. Yet, despite IQ tests in the normal range, the memory quotient was exceptionally low (average score of 64) compared to matched control groups of typically developing children (average score of 108) (Dzieciol et al., 2017). In addition, there was severe impairment on a test of episodic memory that tests memory for everyday events (e.g., remembering a name, simple route around a room, and delivering a message). Reduction in hippocampal volume parallels the severity of impairment of episodic memory. In short, semantic memory may develop normally in both childhood and adolescence despite early, severe, selective damage to the hippocampus (Elward & Vargha-Khadem, 2018).

## Developmental Amnesia and Autobiographical Memory

Jon, the classic case of developmental amnesia, can describe "personal" experience but is unable to describe underlying facts. Further examination using fMRI was performed to study Jon's episodic and factual memory (Maguire et al., 2001). Episodic and fact memories include autobiographical facts, public events, and general knowledge. With autobiographical memory, a person remembers not only facts about an event but also that they were personally present and experienced the event. Jon had a very limited number of memories of autobiographical events. However, Jon did report a "genuine autobiographical memory" for facts. For most autobiographical life events, he knew the fact that the event took place, but he did not recall it as personally experienced.

In the fMRI study, Jon showed greater activation for autobiographical events that he remembered than for those he simply knew as facts. Maguire et al. (2001) concluded that Jon was able to retrieve semantic memories of life events that do not depend on the same hippocampal support as recollected episodes. Other studies of autobiographical memory conclude that personally relevant facts linked to specific episodic memories depend on the hippocampal system (Grilli & Verfaellie, 2016). However, personal facts not associated with a unique experience can be retrieved independent of hippocampal support (Elward & Vargha-Khadem, 2018). These findings are supported by a meta-analysis showing that episodic autobiographical factual information was indeed associated with the hippocampus, but that semantic information was not. Instead, semantic memory of autobiographical information was associated with a network of cortical areas, including the parahippocampal cortex (Martinelli et al., 2013).

How do people with developmental amnesia acquire semantic knowledge that allows them to reach levels of semantic memory like typically matched controls? Studies of Jon and others with developmental amnesia indicate that acquisition of some aspects of new semantic learning may result from the integrity of the recognition memory process. This is based on the nondeclarative (procedural) memory sense of familiarity, even when the circumstances in which the information was acquired are not available to recall. This dissociation of recognition and recall has been confirmed in developmental amnesia (Blumenthal et al., 2017). In a study involving 12 cases of developmental amnesia and 12 typical control subjects, recall, but not recognition, was correlated with the extent of hippocampal atrophy. Recognition is used as a means of compensation in developmental amnesia, thus explaining how near-normal capacities can be restored following injury.

Current evidence indicates that the hippocampus is very important for fast acquisition of new information and making it available to recall. Repeat exposure is a compensatory mechanism that allows people to use semantic representation despite hippocampal atrophy. Patients with developmental amnesia must rely on direct consolidation of the "gist" of experiences, using a slow, cortically mediated memory system.

With repeated practice, novel factual information can be incorporated into the existing generalized semantic system, allowing patients to progress to reach comparable levels of the typically developing child.

## Memory in Neurodevelopmental Disorders

The study of memory and learning is an essential component of the neurodevelopmental neuroscience in developmental disorders. The severity, developmental trajectories, and basic mechanisms of impairments in memory are not homogeneous across the neurodevelopmental syndromes and may be linked to differences in etiology and abnormality in brain development. Therefore, it is important to compare qualitative profiles of memory impairment across neurodevelopmental syndromes.

Memory in Down syndrome has the been most extensively studied among neurodevelopmental disorders across the life span. In Down syndrome, there is a gradual decline in IQ during childhood; essentially, gains in cognition do not keep pace with chronological age. Expressive language and executive functioning are more impaired than overall cognition. The presence of impaired long-germ memory is characteristic of Down syndrome. This is of interest due to increased prevalence of early onset Alzheimer's disease in Down syndrome. The gene encoding the precursor to β-amyloid, amyloid precursor protein (APP), is localized to the Down region of chromosome 21 (HSA 21) and is overexpressed in Down syndrome as a consequence of its triplication. This amyloid accumulation begins in the striation and progresses to the frontal lobe and the temporal lobe (Lott & Head, 2001). By age 45 years, almost all adults with Down syndrome show the pathology of Alzheimer disease, but only 9% of them show symptoms at this age. By age 72 years, two-thirds of people with Down syndrome will meet criteria of Alzheimer's disease compared to 5% of typically developing adults (Godfrey & Lee, 2018).

A developmental approach to Down syndrome focuses on examining memory change in adults over time. Long-term nondeclarative memory (procedural memory), long-term declarative memory, short-term memory, and working memory have been studied in Down syndrome. Nondeclarative memory is generally found to be mental age appropriate in Down syndrome. There is a functional dissociation between nondeclarative and declarative memory in people with Down syndrome (Vicari et al., 2000). Moreover, nondeclarative memory performance in Down syndrome is superior to that of peers with Williams–Beuren syndrome. A study compared 32 subjects with Williams–Beuren syndrome, 26 with Down syndrome, and 49 typically developing children with mental age comparable in the two syndrome groups on a serial reaction time task. Williams–Beuren syndrome children showed poor implicit learning, whereas those with Down syndrome were comparable to the mental age-matched typically developing controls. The results document that nondeclarative (procedural) learning in people with an intellectual developmental disorder depends on the etiology of the syndrome. These differences were not due to differences in level of cognitive development when the groups were compared on both chronological and mental age. The basal ganglia and cerebellum are involved in visual motor skills. In Williams–Beuren syndrome, unlike Down syndrome, there is atrophy of the basal ganglia with intact cerebellum. But in Down syndrome, the basal ganglia is intact, whereas there is cerebellar hypoplasia (Vicari et al., 2005).

With regard to declarative memory, 14 Down syndrome subjects and 20 mental age-matched typically developing children were examined using tests of verbal and visioperceptual declarative memory in the two groups. For declarative memory, typically developing children scored consistently higher than those with Down syndrome. Yet, results were comparable on all nondeclarative memory tests, including those requiring verbal processing. Nondeclarative learning did not correlate with intellectual level. Such automatic processes use a low expenditure of attention, whereas declarative memory uses effortful conscious learning (Vicari et al., 2000). These findings have implications for habilitation in which nondeclarative operant conditioning interventions are commonly employed.

In Down syndrome, conscious short-term memory, long-term memory, and working memory have also been studied. Those with Down syndrome have significantly impaired verbal and nonverbal working memory; however, they do not typically or consistently show impaired functioning on nonverbal short-term memory when verbal (spatial) short-term memory is impaired. Short-term memory and working memory must be evaluated separately in Down syndrome.

With regard to long-term memory, preschool children with Down syndrome may have nonverbal long-term memory comparable to that of mental age-matched typically developing children when tested after a short delay (24 hr). There is a worsening of performance compared to controls after a month-long delay in testing (Godfrey & Lee, 2018). In adolescents with Down syndrome, there are significant long-term memory impairments. However, overall, adolescents with Down syndrome perform at a comparable level or better than other intellectual developmental disorder groups. Those with Down syndrome perform worse than mental age-matched typical controls on nonverbal long-term memory tests. This is consistent with children with Down syndrome having language deficits that are worse that their global cognitive delay (Nichols et al., 2004). Adults with Down syndrome perform below mental age expectations on long-term memory tasks, especially on verbal long-term memory tasks.

With regard to short-term memory, there is consistent evidence for verbal short-term memory impairment in Down syndrome relative to mental age-matched comparison groups from school age into adulthood (Godfrey & Lee, 2018). Moreover, adults with Down syndrome perform worse than mental age-matched typically developing individuals on verbal work memory tasks but not significantly different than other intellectual developmental disorder groups. With regard to nonverbal working memory, adults with Down syndrome are similar to mental age-matched typically developing individuals (Belacchi et al., 2014). However, with aging in Down syndrome, there is declining executive functioning beginning in middle adulthood. In fact, they are the first cognitive skills to deteriorate in the early stages of Alzheimer dementia in Down syndrome (Adams & Oliver, 2010).

Individuals with different intellectual development disorder syndromes have been compared to one another. Both Down syndrome and Williams–Beuren syndrome have demonstrated deficits across verbal, spatial, and cognitive domains, including memory deficits that can be linked to the hippocampus and prefrontal cortex. Profiles of memory function were studied in adolescents and young adults diagnosed with Down syndrome

($n$ = 27) and Williams–Beuren syndrome ($n$ = 28), who were matched for chronological age and IQ with controls (Edgin et al., 2010). Profiles were compared for the two syndromes on immediate memory, working memory, and associative memory. Memory functions for the combined sample age, IQ, and adaptive behavior were assessed. The authors found significant differences in verbal memory, immediate memory in Down syndrome but less so in Williams–Beuren syndrome, spatial immediate memory (Down syndrome deficits greater than Williams–Beuren syndrome deficits), and combined spatial and verbal associative memory (Down syndrome deficits greater than Williams–Beuren syndrome deficits). For Down syndrome, verbal immediate memory corelated with IQ, and spatial associative memory corelated with adaptive behavior. For Williams–Beuren syndrome, verbal and associative memory were primarily corelated with IQ, and verbal working memory correlated with adaptive behavior. Thus, these two syndromes have very different relative strengths and differences in memory measures. Such differences in patterns of memory dysfunction, respectively, may help account for the long-term outcomes in these syndromes.

Comparisons have also been made of memory domains and executive function in Down syndrome, Williams–Beuren syndrome, and fragile X syndrome. A literature review confirmed that there is consistent evidence for impairments across groups in memory domains (short-term and long-term) and executive function (working memory, inhibition, and cognitive flexibility); subjects were all below expected mental age. For fragile X syndrome, there is the most consistent evidence for impairment across memory domains and executive function. For nonverbal long-term memory, there is insufficient evidence. In Down syndrome, there is evidence for impairments across all memory domains and executive function, as previously described; however, findings were mixed for nonverbal short-term memory and nonverbal inhibition. Poor performance in Down syndrome also may be linked to language impairment. Findings in Williams–Beuren syndrome in this review are more complicated. In Williams–Beuren syndrome, there are mixed findings for verbal long-term memory, verbal working memory, and verbal and nonverbal cognitive shifting. Verbal short-term memory is not significantly below mental age expectations in Williams–Beuren syndrome (N. Lee et al., 2016). There are differences in IQ trajectory among these three syndromes. There is relative stability in IQ from childhood to adulthood in Williams–Beuren syndrome, whereas there is lack of stability in Down syndrome and fragile X syndrome. Memory and executive deficits might be contributors in Down syndrome and fragile X syndrome.

Prospective neuroimaging studies find atypical hippocampal development in all three syndromes. In Down syndrome, hippocampal volume is reduced both in early and later development and may be linked to later development of Alzheimer's disease (Pinter et al., 2001). In Williams–Beuren syndrome and fragile X syndrome, there may be either an enlarged hippocampus (Sampaio et al., 2010) or atypical hippocampal shape (Meyer-Lindenberg et al., 2005). Overall, because of the consistency of memory deficits across all three syndromes, hippocampal dysfunction may be a key factor in all of these syndromes because the hippocampus is essential for rapid error-driven learning for associations. Basically, intellectual developmental disorder is characterized by slowness and less efficiency in learning. In these syndromes, the hippocampus and associative nuclei are central to memory for spatial navigation—that is, wayfinding. Wayfinding is important for independence in adaptive functioning in all three syndromes.

With regard to working memory, neural correlates are found in frontoparietal and frontostriatal brain regions. There are demonstrable frontal abnormalities in Down syndrome and fragile X syndrome (N. Lee et al., 2010), parietal abnormalities in Williams–Beuren syndrome (Boddaert et al., 2006), and striatal abnormalities in fragile X syndrome (Hazlett et al., 2012). Functional imaging studies link anatomical regions to brain physiology. Two functional brain imaging studies of cognitive control in Williams–Beuren syndrome and fragile X syndrome link task performance to abnormalities in frontal lobes and other brain regions (Tamm et al., 2002).

There are different age-related effects on brain aging (Koran et al., 2014). Compared to typically developing individuals, those with Down syndrome show significantly different age-related changes in gray matter development. There are substantial differences in gray matter volume in the orbitofrontal and parietal cortex in Down syndrome. Also, there was a significant difference between Down syndrome and Williams–Beuren syndrome in the left and right total lateral ventricle size. Those with Down syndrome showed a unique pattern of brain change with age apparent in gray matter and in ventricular volume. Results suggest that rather than a general pattern of atypical neurodevelopment in the two syndromes, there is a unique pattern of age-related change in gray matter and in ventricular volume. Ventricular volume changes are associated with dementia with deterioration in memory in Down syndrome.

Working memory deficits in the inherited metabolic disorder, phenylketonuria, are responsive to dietary restrictions of phenylalanine. The dietary treatment is generally effective in normalizing immediate memory impairment. However, in later childhood and in adulthood in people with phenylketonuria, in at least 25% of cases there are deficits in manipulation of working memory that persist despite following dietary recommendations (Palermo et al., 2017).

## Conclusion

Memory research in intellectual developmental disorders is providing important information regarding cognitive profiles. Still, there are limits to existing studies that may be considered in future research. There are limits in the use of neuropsychological tests to measure cognition; those with severe deficits may not be able to be examined for executive functioning. Investigations of brain–behavior relationships show limitations in establishing the underlying brain basis for neuropsychological impairments. Thus, examining developmental trajectories of cognitive domains in the early stages must be pursued in these syndromes. Additional research is needed to examine neuropsychological domains and real-world functioning as well. Finally, systemic treatment studies are needed to examine long-term memory, working memory, and other cognitive domains in neurodevelopmental disorders.

## References

Ackermann, S., & Rasch, B. (2014). Differential effects of non-REM and REM sleep on memory consolidation? *Current Neurology and Neuroscience Reports*, *14*(2), Article 430.

Adams, D., & Oliver, C. (2010). The relationship between acquired impairments of executive function and behaviour change in adults with Down syndrome. *Journal of Intellectual Disability Research*, *54*(5), 393–405.

Aserinsky, E., & Kleitman, N. (1953). Regularly occurring periods of eye motility, and concomitant phenomena, during sleep. *Science*, *118*(3062), 273–274.

Backhaus, J., Hoeckesfeld, R., Born, J., Hohagen, F., & Junghanns, K. (2008). Immediate as well as delayed post learning sleep but not wakefulness enhances declarative memory consolidation in children. *Neurobiology of Learning and Memory*, *89*(1), 76–80.

Baddeley, A. (1996). Exploring the central executive. *Quarterly Journal of Experimental Psychology Section A*, *49*(1), 5–28.

Baddeley, A. (2000). The episodic buffer: A new component of working memory? *Trends in Cognitive Sciences*, *4*(11), 417–423.

Barr, R., & Hayne, H. (2000). Age-related changes in imitation: Implications for memory development. In C. Rovee-Collier, L. P. Lipsitt, & H. Hayne (Eds.), *Progress in infancy research* (pp. 21–67). Erlbaum.

Barth, J. (1992). *Once upon a Time. Johns Hopkins Magazine*. 33–38.

Bathelt, J., Gathercole, S. E., Johnson, A., & Astle, D. E. (2018). Differences in brain morphology and working memory capacity across childhood. *Developmental Science*, *21*(3), e12579.

Belacchi, C., Passolunghi, M. C., Brentan, E., Dante, A., Persi, L., & Cornoldi, C. (2014). Approximate additions and working memory in individuals with Down syndrome. *Research in Developmental Disabilities*, *35*(5), 1027–1035.

Bliss, T. V., & Lømo, T. (1973). Long-lasting potentiation of synaptic transmission in the dentate area of the anaesthetized rabbit following stimulation of the perforant path. *Journal of Physiology*, *232*(2), 331–356.

Blumenthal, A., Duke, D., Bowles, B., Gilboa, A., Rosenbaum, R. S., Köhler, S., & McRae, K. (2017). Abnormal semantic knowledge in a case of developmental amnesia. *Neuropsychologia*, *102*, 237–247.

Boddaert, N., Mochel, F., Meresse, I., Seidenwurm, D., Cachia, A., Brunelle, F., Lyonnet, S., & Zilbovicius, M. (2006). Parieto-occipital grey matter abnormalities in children with Williams syndrome. *NeuroImage*, *30*(3), 721–725.

Bradley, S. A., & Steinert, J. R. (2016). Nitric oxide-mediated posttranslational modifications: Impacts at the synapse. *Oxidative Medicine and Cellular Longevity*, 2016, 5681036.

Cabeza, R., & St. Jacques, P. (2007). Functional neuroimaging of autobiographical memory. *Trends in Cognitive Sciences*, *11*(5), 219–227.

Cai, D. J., Mednick, S. A., Harrison, E. M., Kanady, J. C., & Mednick, S. C. (2009). REM, not incubation, improves creativity by priming associative networks. *Proceedings of the National Academy of Sciences of the USA*, *106*(25), 10130–10134.

Chiu, C. Y. P., Schmithorst, V. J., Brown, R. D., Holland, S. K., & Dunn, S. (2006). Making memories: A cross-sectional investigation of episodic memory encoding in childhood using fMRI. *Developmental Neuropsychology*, *29*(2), 321–340.

Conway, M. A. (2005). Memory and the self. *Journal of Memory and Language*, *53*(4), 594–628.

Conway, M. A., & Pleydell-Pearce, C. W. (2000). The construction of autobiographical memories in the self-memory system. *Psychological Review*, *107*(2), 261–288.

De Haan, M., Wyatt, J. S., Roth, S., Vargha-Khadem, F., Gadian, D., & Mishkin, M. (2006). Brain and cognitive–behavioural development after asphyxia at term birth. *Developmental Science*, *9*(4), 350–358.

Dzieciol, A. M., Bachevalier, J., Saleem, K. S., Gadian, D. G., Saunders, R., Chong, W. K., Banks, T., Mishkin, M., & Vargha-Khadem, F. (2017). Hippocampal and diencephalic pathology in developmental amnesia. *Cortex*, *86*, 33–44.

Edgin, J. O., Pennington, B. F., & Mervis, C. B. (2010). Neuropsychological components of intellectual disability: The contributions of immediate, working, and associative memory. *Journal of Intellectual Disability Research*, *54*(5), 406–417.

Eichenbaum, H. (2011). *The cognitive neuroscience of memory: An introduction*. Oxford University Press.

Elward, R. L., & Vargha-Khadem, F. (2018). Semantic memory in developmental amnesia. *Neuroscience Letters, 680*, 23–30.

Engle, R. W., Tuholski, S. W., Laughlin, J. E., & Conway, A. R. (1999). Working memory, short-term memory, and general fluid intelligence: A latent-variable approach. *Journal of Experimental Psychology: General, 128*(3), 309–331.

Feld, G. B., & Born, J. (2020). Neurochemical mechanisms for memory processing during sleep: Basic findings in humans and neuropsychiatric implications. *Neuropsychopharmacology, 45*(1), 31–44.

Feld, G. B., & Diekelmann, S. (2015). Sleep smart: Optimizing sleep for declarative learning and memory. *Frontiers in Psychology, 6*, Article 622.

Frankland, P. W., Josselyn, S. A., & Köhler, S. (2019). The neurobiological foundation of memory retrieval. *Nature Neuroscience, 22*(10), 1576–1585.

Fusi, S. (2017). Computational models of long term plasticity and memory. arXiv, 1706.04946.

Fusi, S., Drew, P. J., & Abbott, L. F. (2005). Cascade models of synaptically stored memories. *Neuron, 45*(4), 599–611.

Gathercole, S. E., Pickering, S. J., Ambridge, B., & Wearing, H. (2004). The structure of working memory from 4 to 15 years of age. *Developmental Psychology, 40*(2), 177–190.

Gazzaniga, M. S., Ivry, R. B., & Mangun, G. R. (2019). *Cognitive neuroscience: The biology of the mind* (5th ed.). Norton.

Godfrey, M., & Lee, N. R. (2018). Memory profiles in Down syndrome across development: A review of memory abilities through the lifespan. *Journal of Neurodevelopmental Disorders, 10*(1), Article 5.

Gogtay, N., Nugent, T. F., III, Herman, D. H., Ordonez, A., Greenstein, D., Hayashi, K. M., Clasen, L., Toga, A. W., Giedd, J. N., Rapoport, J. L., & Thompson, P. M. (2006). Dynamic mapping of normal human hippocampal development. *Hippocampus, 16*(8), 664–672.

Gómez, R. L., Bootzin, R. R., & Nadel, L. (2006). Naps promote abstraction in language-learning infants. *Psychological Science, 17*(8), 670–674.

Grilli, M. D., & Verfaellie, M. (2016). Experience-near but not experience-far autobiographical facts depend on the medial temporal lobe for retrieval: Evidence from amnesia. *Neuropsychologia, 81*, 180–185.

Groch, S., Wilhelm, I., Diekelmann, S., & Born, J. (2013). The role of REM sleep in the processing of emotional memories: Evidence from behavior and event-related potentials. *Neurobiology of Learning and Memory, 99*, 1–9.

Groch, S., Zinke, K., Wilhelm, I., & Born, J. (2015). Dissociating the contributions of slow-wave sleep and rapid eye movement sleep to emotional item and source memory. *Neurobiology of Learning and Memory, 122*, 122–130.

Güler, O. E., & Thomas, K. M. (2013). Developmental differences in the neural correlates of relational encoding and recall in children: An event-related fMRI study. *Developmental Cognitive Neuroscience, 3*, 106–116.

Guskjolen, A., Kenney, J. W., de la Parra, J., Yeung, B. R. A., Josselyn, S. A., & Frankland, P. W. (2018). Recovery of "lost" infant memories in mice. *Current Biology, 28*(14), 2283–2290.

Hanafy, K., Oh, J., & E Otterbein, L. (2013). Carbon monoxide and the brain: Time to rethink the dogma. *Current Pharmaceutical Design, 19*(15), 2771–2775.

Harris, J. C. (1998). *Developmental neuropsychiatry: Fundamentals*. Oxford University Press.

Harris, K. D. (2014). Sleep replay meets brain–machine interface. *Nature Neuroscience, 17*(8), 1019–1021.

Hayne, H. (2004). Infant memory development: Implications for childhood amnesia. *Developmental Review, 24*(1), 33–73.

Hazlett, H. C., Poe, M. D., Lightbody, A. A., Styner, M., MacFall, J. R., Reiss, A. L., & Piven, J. (2012). Trajectories of early brain volume development in fragile X syndrome and autism. *Journal of the American Academy of Child & Adolescent Psychiatry, 51*(9), 921–933.

Hebb, D. O. (1949). *The organization of behavior: A neuropsychological theory*. Wiley.

Holland, A. C., & Kensinger, E. A. (2010). Emotion and autobiographical memory. *Physics of Life Reviews, 7*(1), 88–131.

Holmes, J., Hilton, K. A., Place, M., Alloway, T. P., Elliott, J. G., & Gathercole, S. E. (2014). Children with low working memory and children with ADHD: Same or different?. *Frontiers in Human Neuroscience, 8,* Article 976.

Hornung, C., Brunner, M., Reuter, R. A., & Martin, R. (2011). Children's working memory: Its structure and relationship to fluid intelligence. *Intelligence, 39*(4), 210–221.

Houdé, O., Rossi, S., Lubin, A., & Joliot, M. (2010). Mapping numerical processing, reading, and executive functions in the developing brain: An fMRI meta-analysis of 52 studies including 842 children. *Developmental Science, 13*(6), 876–885.

Hudson, J. A. (1986). Memories are made of this: General event knowledge and development of autobiographic memory. In K. Nelson (Ed.), *Event knowledge: Structure and function in development* (pp. 97–118). Erlbaum.

Inostroza, M., & Born, J. (2013). Sleep for preserving and transforming episodic memory. *Annual Review of Neuroscience, 36,* 79–102.

James, W. (1890). *The principles of psychology.* (Vol. 1, No. 2). Macmillan.

Jenkins, J. G., & Dallenbach, K. M. (1924). Obliviscence during sleep and waking. *American Journal of Psychology, 35*(4), 605–612.

Kandel, E. R. (2009). The biology of memory: A forty-year perspective. *Journal of Neuroscience, 29*(41), 12748–12756.

Kane, M. J., Conway, A. R., Hambrick, D. Z., & Engle, R. W. (2007). Variation in working memory capacity as variation in executive attention and control. *Variation in Working Memory, 1,* 21–48.

Kane, M. J., Hambrick, D. Z., Tuholski, S. W., Wilhelm, O., Payne, T. W., & Engle, R. W. (2004). The generality of working memory capacity: A latent-variable approach to verbal and visuospatial memory span and reasoning. *Journal of Experimental Psychology: General, 133*(2), 189–217.

Koran, M. E., Hohman, T. J., Edwards, C. M., Vega, J. N., Pryweller, J. R., Slosky, L. E., Crockett, G., Villa de Rey, L., Meda, S. A., Dankner, N., Avery, S. N., Blackford, J. U., Dykens, E. M., & Thornton Wells, T. A. (2014). Differences in age-related effects on brain volume in Down syndrome as compared to Williams syndrome and typical development. *Journal of Neurodevelopmental Disorders, 6*(1), Article 8.

Krakauer, J. W., & Shadmehr, R. (2006). Consolidation of motor memory. *Trends in Neurosciences, 29*(1), 58–64.

Lee, J. K., Wendelken, C., Bunge, S. A., & Ghetti, S. (2016). A time and place for everything: Developmental differences in the building blocks of episodic memory. *Child Development, 87*(1), 194–210.

Lee, N. R., Maiman, M., & Godfrey, M. (2016). What can neuropsychology teach us about intellectual disability? Searching for commonalities in the memory and executive function profiles associated with Down, Williams, and fragile X syndromes. In *International Review of Research in Developmental Disabilities, 51,* 1–40.

Lee, N. R., Pennington, B. F., & Keenan, J. M. (2010). Verbal short-term memory deficits in Down syndrome: Phonological, semantic, or both? *Journal of Neurodevelopmental Disorders, 2*(1), 9–25.

Linton, M. (1975). Memory for real world events In D. A. Norman & D. E. Rumelhart (Eds.), *Explorations in cognition* (pp. 376–404). Freeman.

Linton, M. (1982). Transformations of memory in everyday life. In. U. Neisser (Ed.), *Memory observed: Remembering in natural contexts* (pp. 77–91). Freeman.

Logie, R. H. (1986). Visuo-spatial processing in working memory. *Quarterly Journal of Experimental Psychology Section A, 38*(2), 229–247.

Lorenz, K. (1981). *The foundations of ethology.* Springer-Verlag.

Lott, I. T., & Head, E. (2001). Down syndrome and Alzheimer's disease: A link between development and aging. *Mental Retardation and Developmental Disabilities Research Reviews, 7*(3), 172–178.

Lynch, G., & Granger, R. (1992). Variations in synaptic plasticity and types of memory in corticohippocampal networks. *Journal of Cognitive Neuroscience, 4*(3), 189–199.

Ma, S., & Zuo, Y. (2022). Synaptic modifications in learning and memory: A dendritic spine story. *Seminars in Cell & Developmental Biology, 125,* 84–90.

Maguire, E. A., Vargha-Khadem, F., & Mishkin, M. (2001). The effects of bilateral hippocampal damage on fMRI regional activations and interactions during memory retrieval. *Brain, 124*(6), 1156–1170.

Mander, B. A., Santhanam, S., Saletin, J. M., & Walker, M. P. (2011). Wake deterioration and sleep restoration of human learning. *Current Biology, 21*(5), R183–R184.

Maquet, P., Laureys, S., Peigneux, P., Fuchs, S., Petiau, C., Phillips, C., Aerrts, J., Del Fiore, G., Degueldre, C., Meulemans, T., Luxen, A., Franck, G., Van Der Linden, M., Smith, C., & Cleeremans, A. (2000). Experience-dependent changes in cerebral activation during human REM sleep. *Nature Neuroscience, 3*(8), 831–836.

Martinelli, P., Sperduti, M., & Piolino, P. (2013). Neural substrates of the self-memory system: New insights from a meta-analysis. *Human Brain Mapping, 34*(7), 1515–1529.

Martinussen, R., Hayden, J., Hogg-Johnson, S., & Tannock, R. (2005). A meta-analysis of working memory impairments in children with attention-deficit/hyperactivity disorder. *Journal of the American Academy of Child & Adolescent Psychiatry, 44*(4), 377–384.

Maurer, R. G. (1992). Disorders of memory and learning. In S. J. Segalowitz & I. Rapin (Eds.), *Handbook of neuropsychology: Child neuropsychology* (Vol. 6, pp. 241–260). Elsevier.

Mayford, M., Bach, M. E., Huang, Y. Y., Wang, L., Hawkins, R. D., & Kandel, E. R. (1996). Control of memory formation through regulated expression of a CaMKII transgene. *Science, 274*(5293), 1678–1683.

Menon, V., Boyett-Anderson, J. M., & Reiss, A. L. (2005). Maturation of medial temporal lobe response and connectivity during memory encoding. *Cognitive Brain Research, 25*(1), 379–385.

Meyer-Lindenberg, A., Mervis, C. B., Sarpal, D., Koch, P., Steele, S., Kohn, P., Marenco, S., Morris, C., Das, S., Kippenhan, S., Mattay, V., Weinberger, D., & Berman, K. (2005). Functional, structural, and metabolic abnormalities of the hippocampal formation in Williams syndrome. *Journal of Clinical Investigation, 115*(7), 1888–1895.

Mishkin, M., Malamut, B., & Bachevalier, J. (1984). Memories and habits: Two neural systems. In G. Lynch, J. L. McGaugh, & N. M. Weinberger (Eds.), Neurobiology of *human learning* and *memory* (pp. 65–77). Guilford.

Moscovitch, M., Rosenbaum, R. S., Gilboa, A., Addis, D. R., Westmacott, R., Grady, C., McAndrews, M., Levine, B., Black, S., Winocur, G., & Nadel, L. (2005). Functional neuroanatomy of remote episodic, semantic and spatial memory: A unified account based on multiple trace theory. *Journal of anatomy, 207*(1), 35–66.

Nagel, B. J., Herting, M. M., Maxwell, E. C., Bruno, R., & Fair, D. (2013). Hemispheric lateralization of verbal and spatial working memory during adolescence. *Brain and Cognition, 82*(1), 58–68.

Nelson, K. (1986). *Event knowledge: Structure and function in development.* Erlbaum.

Nichols, S., Jones, W., Roman, M. J., Wulfeck, B., Delis, D. C., Reilly, J., & Bellugi, U. (2004). Mechanisms of verbal memory impairment in four neurodevelopmental disorders. *Brain and Language, 88*(2), 180–189.

Nicoll, R. A. (2017). A brief history of long-term potentiation. *Neuron, 93*(2), 281–290.

Ofen, N., Yu, Q., & Chen, Z. (2016). Memory and the developing brain: Are insights from cognitive neuroscience applicable to education? *Current Opinion in Behavioral Sciences, 10*, 81–88.

Palermo, L., Geberhiwot, T., MacDonald, A., Limback, E., Hall, S. K., & Romani, C. (2017). Cognitive outcomes in early-treated adults with phenylketonuria (PKU): A comprehensive picture across domains. *Neuropsychology, 31*(3), 255–267.

Pardilla-Delgado, E., Alger, S. E., Cunningham, T. J., Kinealy, B., & Payne, J. D. (2016). Effects of post-encoding stress on performance in the DRM false memory paradigm. *Learning & Memory, 23*(1), 46–50.

Paus, T., Collins, D. L., Evans, A. C., Leonard, G., Pike, B., & Zijdenbos, A. (2001). Maturation of white matter in the human brain: A review of magnetic resonance studies. *Brain Research Bulletin, 54*(3), 255–266.

Payne, J. D., Schacter, D. L., Propper, R. E., Huang, L. W., Wamsley, E. J., Tucker, M. A., Walker, M. P., & Stickgold, R. (2009). The role of sleep in false memory formation. *Neurobiology of Learning and Memory, 92*(3), 327–334.

Peigneux, P., Laureys, S., Delbeuck, X., & Maquet, P. (2001). Sleeping brain, learning brain. The role of sleep for memory systems. *Neuroreport, 12*(18), A111–A124.

Peigneux, P., Laureys, S., Fuchs, S., Collette, F., Perrin, F., Reggers, J., Phillips, C., Degueldre, C., Del Fiore, G., Aerts, J., Luxen, A., & Maquet, P. (2004). Are spatial memories strengthened in the human hippocampus during slow wave sleep? *Neuron, 44*(3), 535–545.

Piaget, J., & Inhelder, B. (1973). *Memory and intelligence.* Basic Books.

Pinter, J. D., Brown, W. E., Eliez, S., Schmitt, J. E., Capone, G. T., & Reiss, A. L. (2001). Amygdala and hippocampal volumes in children with Down syndrome: A high-resolution MRI study. *Neurology, 56*(7), 972–974.

Potkin, K. T., & Bunney, W. E., Jr. (2012). Sleep improves memory: The effect of sleep on long term memory in early adolescence. *PLoS One, 7*(8), e42191.

Prehn-Kristensen, A., Göder, R., Fischer, J., Wilhelm, I., Seeck-Hirschner, M., Aldenhoff, J., & Baving, L. (2011). Reduced sleep-associated consolidation of declarative memory in attention-deficit/hyperactivity disorder. *Sleep Medicine, 12*(7), 672–679.

Prehn-Kristensen, A., Molzow, I., Munz, M., Wilhelm, I., Müller, K., Freytag, D., Wiesner, C., & Baving, L. (2011). Sleep restores daytime deficits in procedural memory in children with attention-deficit/hyperactivity disorder. *Research in Developmental Disabilities, 32*(6), 2480–2488.

Ramsaran, A. I., Schlichting, M. L., & Frankland, P. W. (2019). The ontogeny of memory persistence and specificity. *Developmental Cognitive Neuroscience, 36,* 100591.

Rasch, B., & Born, J. (2013). About sleep's role in memory. *Physiological Reviews, 93*(2), 681–766.

Reijmers, L. G., Perkins, B. L., Matsuo, N., & Mayford, M. (2007). Localization of a stable neural correlate of associative memory. *Science, 317*(5842), 1230–1233.

Ribeiro, S., Shi, X., Engelhard, M., Zhou, Y., Zhang, H., Gervasoni, D., Lin, S. C., Wada, K., Lemos, N. A., & Nicolelis, M. A. (2007). Novel experience induces persistent sleep-dependent plasticity in the cortex but not in the hippocampus. *Frontiers in Neuroscience, 1,* 43–55.

Ribeiro, S., & Stickgold, R. (2014). Sleep and school education. *Trends in Neuroscience and Education, 3*(1), 18–23.

Richmond, J., & Nelson, C. A. (2008). Mechanisms of change: A cognitive neuroscience approach to declarative memory development. In C. A. Nelson & M. Luciana (Eds.), *Handbook of developmental cognitive neuroscience* (pp. 541–552). MIT Press.

Rovee-Collier, C. K., Hayne, H., & Colombo, M. (2001). *The development of implicit and explicit memory* (Vol. 24). Benjamins.

Rubin, D. C. (2006). The basic-systems model of episodic memory. *Perspectives on Psychological Science, 1*(4), 277–311.

Sampaio, A., Sousa, N., Férnandez, M., Vasconcelos, C., Shenton, M. E., & Gonçalves, O. F. (2010). Williams syndrome and memory: A neuroanatomic and cognitive approach. *Journal of Autism and Developmental Disorders, 40*(7), 870–877.

Scoville, W. B., & Milner, B. (1957). Loss of recent memory after bilateral hippocampal lesions. *Journal of Neurology, Neurosurgery, and Psychiatry, 20*(1), 11–21.

Sluzenski, J., Newcombe, N. S., & Kovacs, S. L. (2006). Binding, relational memory, and recall of naturalistic events: A developmental perspective. *Journal of Experimental Psychology: Learning, Memory, and Cognition, 32*(1), 89–100.

Smeets, T., Otgaar, H., Candel, I., & Wolf, O. T. (2008). True or false? Memory is differentially affected by stress-induced cortisol elevations and sympathetic activity at consolidation and retrieval. *Psychoneuroendocrinology, 33*(10), 1378–1386.

Sowell, E. R., Thompson, P. M., Leonard, C. M., Welcome, S. E., Kan, E., & Toga, A. W. (2004). Longitudinal mapping of cortical thickness and brain growth in normal children. *Journal of Neuroscience, 24*(38), 8223–8231.

Spiers, H. J., Burgess, N., Hartley, T., Vargha-Khadem, F., & O'Keefe, J. (2001). Bilateral hippocampal pathology impairs topographical and episodic memory but not visual pattern matching. *Hippocampus, 11*(6), 715–725.

Squire, L. R. (2004). Memory systems of the brain: A brief history and current perspective. *Neurobiology of Learning and Memory, 82*(3), 171–177.

Squire, L. R. (2009). Memory and brain systems: 1969–2009. *Journal of Neuroscience, 29*(41), 12711–12716.

Squire, L. R., & Wixted, J. T. (2011). The cognitive neuroscience of human memory since H.M. *Annual Review of Neuroscience, 34,* 259–288.

Squire, L. R., & Zola-Morgan, S. (1991). The medial temporal lobe memory system. *Science, 253*(5026), 1380–1386.

Svoboda, E., McKinnon, M. C., & Levine, B. (2006). The functional neuroanatomy of autobiographical memory: A meta-analysis. *Neuropsychologia, 44*(12), 2189–2208.

Tamm, L., Menon, V., Johnston, C. K., Hessl, D. R., & Reiss, A. L. (2002). fMRI study of cognitive interference processing in females with fragile X syndrome. *Journal of Cognitive Neuroscience, 14*(2), 160–171.

Tamnes, C. K., Walhovd, K. B., Grydeland, H., Holland, D., Østby, Y., Dale, A. M., & Fjell, A. M. (2013). Longitudinal working memory development is related to structural maturation of frontal and parietal cortices. *Journal of Cognitive Neuroscience, 25*(10), 1611–1623.

Thomason, M. E., Race, E., Burrows, B., Whitfield-Gabrieli, S., Glover, G. H., & Gabrieli, J. D. (2009). Development of spatial and verbal working memory capacity in the human brain. *Journal of Cognitive Neuroscience, 21*(2), 316–332.

Tononi, G., & Cirelli, C. (2014). Sleep and the price of plasticity: From synaptic and cellular homeostasis to memory consolidation and integration. *Neuron, 81*(1), 12–34.

Tononi, G., & Cirelli, C. (2020). Sleep and synaptic down-selection. *European Journal of Neuroscience, 51*(1), 413–421.

Tulving, E. (1985). How many memory systems are there? *American Psychologist, 40*(4), 385–398.

Tulving, E., & Schacter, D. L. (1990). Priming and human memory systems. *Science, 247*(4940), 301–306.

Van Der Werf, Y. D., Altena, E., Schoonheim, M. M., Sanz-Arigita, E. J., Vis, J. C., De Rijke, W., & Van Someren, E. J. (2009). Sleep benefits subsequent hippocampal functioning. *Nature Neuroscience, 12*(2), 122–123.

Vargha-Khadem, F., Gadian, D. G., Watkins, K. E., Connelly, A., Van Paesschen, W., & Mishkin, M. (1997). Differential effects of early hippocampal pathology on episodic and semantic memory. *Science, 277*(5324), 376–380.

Vargha-Khadem, F., Salmond, C. H., Watkins, K. E., Friston, K. J., Gadian, D. G., & Mishkin, M. (2003). Developmental amnesia: Effect of age at injury. *Proceedings of the National Academy of Sciences of the USA, 100*(17), 10055–10060.

Vicari, S., Bellucci, S., & Carlesimo, G. A. (2000). Implicit and explicit memory: A functional dissociation in persons with Down syndrome. *Neuropsychologia, 38*(3), 240–251.

Vicari, S., Bellucci, S., & Carlesimo, G. A. (2005). Visual and spatial long-term memory: Differential pattern of impairments in Williams and Down syndromes. *Developmental Medicine and Child Neurology, 47*(5), 305–311.

Vogan, V. M., Morgan, B. R., Powell, T. L., Smith, M. L., & Taylor, M. J. (2016). The neurodevelopmental differences of increasing verbal working memory demand in children and adults. *Developmental Cognitive Neuroscience, 17,* 19–27.

Vyazovskiy, V. V., Cirelli, C., Pfister-Genskow, M., Faraguna, U., & Tononi, G. (2008). Molecular and electrophysiological evidence for net synaptic potentiation in wake and depression in sleep. *Nature Neuroscience, 11*(2), 200–208.

Wager, T. D., & Smith, E. E. (2003). Neuroimaging studies of working memory. *Cognitive, Affective, & Behavioral Neuroscience, 3*(4), 255–274.

Wagner, U., Gais, S., Haider, H., Verleger, R., & Born, J. (2004). Sleep inspires insight. *Nature, 427*(6972), 352–355.

Wilhelm, I., Diekelmann, S., & Born, J. (2008). Sleep in children improves memory performance on declarative but not procedural tasks. *Learning & Memory, 15*(5), 373–377.

Wilhelm, I., Diekelmann, S., Molzow, I., Ayoub, A., Mölle, M., & Born, J. (2011). Sleep selectively enhances memory expected to be of future relevance. *Journal of Neuroscience, 31*(5), 1563–1569.

Wilhelm, I., Prehn-Kristensen, A., & Born, J. (2012). Sleep-dependent memory consolidation: What can be learnt from children? *Neuroscience & Biobehavioral Reviews, 36*(7), 1718–1728.

Williams, S. E., & Horst, J. S. (2014). Goodnight book: Sleep consolidation improves word learning via storybooks. *Frontiers in Psychology, 5*, Article 184.

Wilson, M. A., & McNaughton, B. L. (1994). Reactivation of hippocampal ensemble memories during sleep. *Science, 265*(5172), 676–679.

Yang, G., Lai, C. S. W., Cichon, J., Ma, L., Li, W., & Gan, W. B. (2014). Sleep promotes branch-specific formation of dendritic spines after learning. *Science, 344*(6188), 1173–1178.

Yim, H., Dennis, S. J., & Sloutsky, V. M. (2013). The development of episodic memory: Items, contexts, and relations. *Psychological Science, 24*(11), 2163–2172.

Zeineh, M. M., Engel, S. A., Thompson, P. M., & Bookheimer, S. Y. (2003). Dynamics of the hippocampus during encoding and retrieval of face–name pairs. *Science, 299*(5606), 577–580.

Zhuo, M., Laitinen, J. T., Li, X. C., & Hawkins, R. D. (1998). On the respective roles of nitric oxide and carbon monoxide in long-term potentiation in the hippocampus. *Learning & Memory, 5*(6), 467–480.

# 7

# The Human Connectome

## Introduction

The human brain connectome refers to connectivity maps that capture patterns of activity between different brain regions. The connectome map provides a comprehensive description of the connections within the human brain, from local circuits to networks that constitute the entire nervous system. The connectome has added a new dimension to the study of neuroanatomy because it involves a systemic study of all relevant brain connectivity matrices along with a complex network analysis (Swanson & Lichtman, 2016).

The Brain Connectome Project has established a new branch of research called connectomics. *Connectomics* refers to the application of techniques of computer-assisted image acquisition and analyses to the structural mapping of sets of neural circuits. Disruptions of the normal human connectome are referred to as *connectopathies*; these are associated with a wide range of developmental neuropsychiatric and neurodevelopmental disorders. Structural neural connections at every level of analysis are defined as the structural link between two modes in a wiring diagram of the nervous system. The mode can be an individual neuron, a neuron type, or a gray matter region. These neural connections may be studied at four levels of analysis: (a) gray matter regions (macro level), (b) between neuron types (meso level), (c) between individual neurons (micro level), and (d) nanoconnections at synapses.

The National Institutes of Health's Human Connectome Project, which was initiated in 2010, provided funding to develop improved neuroimaging methods and to acquire the necessary data to begin mapping the human connectome, the connections between all areas of the brain. The initial project sought to analyze multimodal neuroimaging, behavioral, and genotype data from 1,200 healthy young adult twins and non-twin siblings and to freely share the data among investigations in user-friendly databases (Glasser et al., 2016). Within the field of connectomes, there are two main models of connectomics—structural and functional. *Structural connectomics* refers to the anatomical white matter fibers connecting brain regions. *Functional connectomics* refers to any measure of co-variation between brain signals at different locations. Tractography algorithms are used to reconstruct white matter fiber tracts—for example, using diffusion-weighted magnetic resonance imaging (dMRI) between two brain areas. These regions remain relatively constant over short timescales. The functional connectivity brain matrix is computed as the correlation between brain activity (functional MRI [fMRI] blood oxygen level-dependent [BOLD] imaging signals) estimated in two areas over the whole recording time (Cabral et al., 2017). dMRI and fMRI are noninvasive imaging technologies that allow analysis of the brain connectome. These approaches enable better diagnostics and deeper understanding of the brain.

Machine learning models are then applied to connectome data to analyze subnetworks in the brain and predict clinical outcomes. Once the connectome is created, machine learning tasks are incorporated to analyze the connectome data. There are on-going investigations for future applications (Brown & Hamarneh, 2016). For example, machine learning has been applied to the structural connectome to predict symptom reduction in depressed adolescents treated with cognitive–behavioral therapy (CBT). The classification used by the authors enabled machine learning to predict with 83% accuracy reductions of depressive symptoms with CBT, including highlighting the role of the right thalamus in predicting reduction of depressive symptoms with CBT. There was a negative correlation between changes in depressive symptoms and nodal strength of the right thalamus in this study (Tymofiyeva et al., 2019).

This chapter reviews the understanding of nervous system connectivity in classical antiquity, when the first global structural account of the organization of the nervous system was proposed, the emergence of Cajal's revolutionary neuron doctrine, a paradigm shift in neuroscience. Cajal used Golgi's anatomical methods to illustrate the basic framework of neural circuit organization that is refined in the model used today. The chapter reviews the four levels of analyses used in structural connectomes and functional connectomes, the synaptome, applications of artificial intelligence based on machine learning, brain neuronal network connectivity maps, and the development of the functional connectome.

## Historical Background: Ancient and Modern

In 500 BC, Hippocrates proposed that our brain gives rise to sensory impressions, emotional thoughts, and memories (Hippocrates, 1962). Hippocrates had knowledge of the structure of the brain, including the ventricles and subarachnoid space. Plato (429–374 BC) proposed the brain with the consistency of marrow harbored a rational soul (Schiller, 1997). Herophilos (approximately 290 BC) and Erasistratus (280 BC) conducted human dissections in Alexandria, Egypt, and were the first to describe the four cerebral ventricles and their communications (Clarke & O'Malley, 1996). Building on this knowledge of anatomy, Galen of Pergamon (130–200 AD) proposed the ventricular–pneumatic doctrine. The brain was described as the place where vital spirits (pneuma) arrived with blood from the heart and were converted to psychic pneuma or animal (derived from *anima*, the soul) spirits. The psychic pneuma was believed to be a special thought substance, with the power to account for sensory activity, feelings, and emotions ascribed to the brain (Clarke & O'Malley, 1996, pp. 10–20). Alternatively, for the church fathers, the proposed soul was located in the cerebral ventricles. Instead, Nemesius of Emesa (approximately 390 AD in Syria) placed the faculty of the imagination and its links to the senses, and intellect in the cerebral ventricles. The faculty of the intellect with "its subdivisions of judging, approving, refuting, and making choices was there" too, along with the faculty that defines the future through dreams. That faculty was located "in the middle part of the brain and the vital spirit therein contained" (Clarke & O'Malley, 1996, p. 464). All this activity was passed on to the memory in the cerebellum.

This theory conceived in the classical age was called the ventricular–pneumatic doctrine and evolved into the three-cell theory. Each ventricle was designated a seat of a special function and contained a unique spirit to carry out its function. The three-cell theory was the earliest attempt to localized mental functions in separate brain sites; for more than 1,000 years, it was accepted by Byzantine, Arabian, and Western Latin schools well into the Renaissance. In this doctrine, the two lateral ventricles represented the first cell, the third ventricle represented the second cell, and the fourth ventricle represented the third cell. Sensory information flowed into the first, as did bodily sensation.

The pneuma was believed to mediate vital functions. The ventricular–pneumatic doctrine developed into the theory of nerve physiology based on the assumption that the pneuma flowed in hollow nerves, thereby transporting sensations from the sense organs to the anterior ventricles and motor commands from the posterior ventricles to the muscles. Imagination was located in the anterior ventricle, cognition in the middle one, and memory in the posterior one (Manzoni, 1998).

It was not until the 16th century that the three-cell theory was seriously challenged and drastically revised by Renaissance and post-Renaissance experimentalists, anatomists, and scholars. Still, elements of Galenic pneumatic neurophysiology endured into the 18th century. It was only when Renaissance scholars realized the importance of direct observation of dissected cadavers that changes were made. It was Leonardo da Vinci, artist and scientist, not a physician, who provided the first accurate description of the cerebral ventricles. Da Vinci's ventriculography (study of the cerebral ventricles) was based on his ability to insert molten wax into the cerebral ventricles of cattle. This allowed him to develop an accurate model of the ventricles. Da Vinci located the soul in the brain, too. In 1489, his drawings showed the optic nerves as converging on the anterior ventricle linking vision with intellect, with the olfactory and auditory nerves coursing toward the middle ventricle; the last ventricle was labeled memoria. Da Vinci viewed sensation and action as influenced by intellect from the anterior ventricle and by memory from the third. Still, da Vinci continued to adhere to the classical theory of the three cells, labeling them imagination, cognition, and memory. He moved sensation from the first to the third ventricle.

In 1508, da Vinci injected wax into the third ventricle of the ox brain and proposed that the horns of the lateral ventricles allow air and fluid to exit. At the time of da Vinci's death in 1519, the ventricular localization of brain function was still the dogma. Andreas Vesalius (1514–1564), the founder of modern human anatomy, denounced the ventricular localization of brain function, but he had no proposal to replace this model. Finally, Rene Descartes (1596–1650), in his book *Treatise of Man* (*De Homine*), made a complete break with the medieval tradition of the three-cell module based on Plato's concept of the three-part soul. Descartes considered the human body like a machine that was directed by a rational soul. Descartes located the soul in the pineal gland based on his view that the body was a machine. He proposed that a single soul was needed to run the mechanical body. Descartes refocused anatomy by asking how physical laws applied to the cerebrum and reflex functions (Del Maestro, 1998).

Renowned English anatomist, Thomas Willis (1621–1675), disagreed with Descartes' view that the soul resided in the pineal gland. He believed that chemical, not mechanistic, concepts were basic to human brain function. In *Anima Brutorum*, Willis proposed that the corpus striatum received all sensory information and that it was the seat of the soul. Moreover, he linked the corpus callosum to the imagination, and he proposed that the cerebral cortex stored memories. Willis realigned the three-part soul with a better understanding of brain function. Willis (1965; see also Arráez-Aybar et al., 2015) wrote,

> The ventricles are only a vacuity. . . . The ancients have so magnified the importance of this cavern, that they have affirmed it the shop of animal spiritus. . . . But on the other side the moderns . . . to which opinion has been some trust given, for that these ventricles are often seen as dead to be filled with water; for excretion. (pp. 96–97)

Finally, Jean Magendie (1783–1855) stated that the spinal fluid is a natural fluid (not a vital one). The function of the brain and spinal cord and fluid was to provide mechanical protection; they functioned to carry away the products of metabolism (Sourkes, 2002). Thus, the ventricular pneumatic doctrine that arose in the 5th century and had given rise to the three-cell theory was scientifically discredited in the 19th century. What was revolutionary and replaced the doctrine in the late 19th century was the finding that deep in the brain there were connections between different kinds of neurons. Santiago Ramón y Cajal (1852–1934), Camillo Golgi, and others' studies of the brain set the stage for new knowledge and understanding of nervous system structure–function architecture (Swanson & Lichtman, 2016). Cajal initiated a paradigm shift in neuroscience by providing a framework for neural circuit organization that, with refinements during the past century, is used today in determining the brain connectome.

Cajal's proposal regarding the organization of neural circuits became the central dogma in neuroscience. He emphasized that (a) individual neurons interact with other neurons and effector cells (i.e., muscles and glands) through individual contact rather than through reticular networks and (b) the neural impulse flows with directionality through circuits and not within individual neurons. Input is through dendrites of the cell body, and output is through the axon. The neuron doctrine was confirmed in the 1950s using electron microscopy. The neural impulse flow proposal became known as the law of functional (dynamic) polarity. It was confirmed in studies documenting the physical basis of graded action potentials (Swanson & Lichtman, 2016).

Nervous system circuitry involves three major classes of neurons that contribute to the nervous system functioning: the sensory neurons, interneurons, and motor neurons. Moreover, specific brain regions are made up of different neuron types, and local connections are important. Cajal identified axon terminals and proposed that neurons communicate at a specialized region of connection, later referred to as the synapse by Sherrington (Sherrington, 1897, 1906). This connection was "the mode of nexus between neurone and neurone." Cajal had adapted and refined the Golgi histological method, sliver chromate staining—the Golgi stain identified their whole neurons, the cell body, the axon, and dendrites—in proposing the neuron doctrine.

Golgi's studies of neural communication had led him to reject Cajal's neuron doctrine and lent support to the older reticular network theory of neural connection by anastomosis. For Golgi, how quickly neurons respond to environmental sensory challenges gave him pause. He believed the neuron doctrine was inconsistent with the recovery process in some patients with neurological brain injury (J. C. Harris, 2010). Despite their differences, Golgi and Cajal shared the Nobel Prize in Physiology or Medicine in

1906. Both were recognized for their work on the structure of the nervous system. Cajal conclusively demonstrated the neuron doctrine. Unlike Golgi, Cajal studied immature and newborn animals, whose nervous systems were less complex than those of the adult animals studied by Golgi. This reduced complexity allowed Cajal to identify distinct connections to the spines along dendrites. Cajal is celebrated for pioneering the centrality of the neuron doctrine. However, Golgi, despite the evidence provided by Cajal, did not abandon the idea of a unitary action of the nervous system.

On the 100th anniversary of the Nobel Prize being awarded to Golgi and Cajal, the merits of their respective arguments were re-evaluated in light of contemporary knowledge (Kruger & Otis, 2007). Golgi's reluctance to accept Cajal's second principle of the polarity of the neuron doctrine and his views about cerebral recovery of function after injury have been re-examined. Golgi, unlike Cajal, was a clinician directing a research ward as well as a skilled neuroanatomist, whereas Cajal was primarily an outstanding neuroanatomist. Golgi's reluctance came from clinical experience with neurology patients. In an era limited to light microscopy, Cajal's views triumphed, were widely accepted, and confirmed nearly 50 years later by election microscope. Yet, in the past 100 years, Golgi's views on the functioning nervous system have gained support with advances in modern neurobiology.

In the 1960s, direct circuits were identified between the cytoplasm of one cell and the next connecting them across intercellular space. Referred to as gap junctions, these consist of hemi-channels known as connexions. The connexions are formed in the Golgi body within the cell and transported to the intercellular junction. The gap junctions are unlike the chemical synapses identified by Cajal. These are electrical synapses that provide instantaneous rapid signal transmission, usually bidirectional. These electrical conductions are ion channels. Mutations in a connectome gene, CX32, underlie X-linked Charcot–Marie–Tooth disease.

A modern re-examination considers the contributions of both Golgi and Cajal regarding the functional coupling between individual neurons and their grouping. In modern neuroscience, the findings of both Nobel laureates have been updated and define our understanding of neural interaction. Golgi and Cajal were not incorrect in their proposals. However, when separated, neither's view suffices to understand the extent of neural connections and networking patterns, especially at gap junctions. Golgi's concept of nervous activity did not derive from the activity of isolated nerve cells but instead focused on the simultaneous activity of large groups of cells. Cajal's neuronal doctrine focused on isolated nerve cell activity. Current observations of axo-axonic and dendro-dendritic synapses reveal gap junction involvement in the direction of impulse connection, that there are multiple channels along with gating, and that neural plasticity is complex. Modern science has moved beyond Cajal's polarized neuron doctrine explanations of fixed and immutable connections. We now know there are two main modalities of synaptic transmission—chemical and electrical. Without violating cell theory, these two modalities of synaptic transmission interact during development and within the brain. Receptor interactions at the level of electrical and mixed synapses play a role in the synchronization of the whole brain pertinent to the "binding phenomena" implicated in the emergence of conscious experience (J. C. Harris, 2010).

Rather than considering synaptic transmission as either/or, synaptic transmission essentially is both/and with regard to interaction. It involves many instances of interactions between these two forms of interneuronal communication (Pereda, 2014). Electrical synapses are more widespread in the brain than originally thought. Interactions of electrical and chemical synapses are diverse and take place at all stages of brain development. During development, electrical synapses are essential to the formation of neural circuits, whereas in adults, their role is more focused on the recognition of hardwired networks. Their interaction may be important functionally after brain injury. Networks of electrically coupled neurons first identified during early development may reappear after brain injury. Glutamate transmission has been shown to increase expression of connexion Cx36 and gap junctions. Communication in vivo and in vitro models of ischemic stroke and traumatic brain injury take these models into account (Belousov & Fontes, 2013).

## Neural Connections and Structural Connectomes

A strategy to study neuronal connections is hierarchal, beginning with examination of macroconnections between gray matter regions focusing on two nodes—for example, examining the connections between the retina and the suprachiasmatic nucleus. The next level of connectivity is mesoconnections. At this level, the neuron types forming each gray matter region are examined. For mesoconnectivity, the nodes are individual neurons—for example, connections between a granule cell and a Purkinje cell in the cerebellar cortical gray matter. The third level is microconnections. These are connectomes between individual neurons identified by examining connections for each neuron type. The two nodes used are between individual neurons—for example, a specific granule cell to a specific Purkinje cell. The finest grain connectivity analysis is for nanoconnections, for which the two nodes are pre- and postsynaptic elements of a synapse (Swanson & Lichtman, 2016). The macro- and mesoconnectomes are genetically determined and thus hardwired. The micro- and nanoconnectomes can be modified by various environmental events, such as life experiences, education, hormonal influences, and use of drugs. These levels of connectivity are illustrated in Figure 7.1.

## Macroconnectome

The macroconnectome is the first level of the connectome to be examined. The brain in mammals has approximately 500–1,000 gray matter regions with 25,000–100,000 macroconnections between them (Bota et al., 2003). In rat brains, a meta-analysis revealed approximately 2,400 macroconnections between 73 cerebral brain regions (Bota et al., 2015). The authors proposed this number may be sufficient to create a qualitatively accurate rat nervous system macroconnectome. A review of this literature suggests that the macro architecture of the mammalian brain is more broadly interconnected with motor, sensory, and cognitive state subsystems.

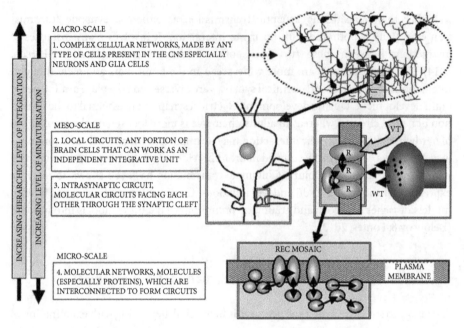

**Figure 7.1** Neural connections and structural connectomes. A three-level hierarchical model is shown based on gray matter regions, the neurons forming each gray matter region, and individual neurons forming each neuron type. Macroconnections (macroscale)—the highest, most coarsely grained complex cellular networks—connect gray matter regions. Mesoconnections (mesoscale) are the next level, showing local circuits between neuron types. Mircoconnections (microscale) are molecular connections between individual neurons. Nanoconnections are the most fine-grained intrasynaptic circuits of pre- and postsynaptic elements of a synapse.

From Agnati et al. (2007).

## Mesoconnectome

The mesoconnectome specified nodes are sets of axonal connections between specific neuron types within gray matter regions. These have been examined with regard to age, gender, or disease state. Molecular biologic methods have been used to study neural circuits and to classify neurons. Neurons are recognized in brain regions by distinct location (e.g., cerebellum and retina) and their shapes, connections, gene expression patterns, and functions (Swanson & Lichtman, 2016). At the mesoconnection level, increasing complexity in the mammalian brain is being documented. There are approximately 2,500–5,000 types of neurons, with an average of 5 neuron types in each category (Bota et al., 2003).

## Microconnectome

A synaptic connectivity matrix interconnects different types of neurons. Historically, Cajal demonstrated functional connections by indicating the classes of axions of one cell type that impinged on dendrites and soma of other classes. Currently, high-resolution anatomical or electrophysiological methods are used to study the microconnectome. The older Golgi method allowed for unambiguous identification of pre- and postsynaptic partners; both were shown in black. Golgi's pivotal discovery that the full neuron could be visualized using the "black reaction" has been revolutionized by addressing the drawbacks of a monochromatic approach. Golgi adjusted the technique so that a very small percentage of neurons were impregnated with silver so the connections of individual neurons could be discerned. But, the Golgi method required looking at a large number of cells of a specific type and pooling results. Because this approach could lead to false inferences of imputed connectivity, a multicolor Golgi-like approach has been developed using genetic techniques to identify inputs.

The Brainbow transgenic method allows genetic labeling of hundreds of connections with different hues generated with expression of a few spectrally distinct fluorescent proteins. With this technique, color profiles can be used as cellular identification tags for tracing axons through the nervous system and following individual cells during development (Weissman & Pan, 2015). This approach has also been used successfully in visualizing glia in mammalian brains. However, the number and density of neuronal inputs to cortical neurons require different approaches. Another approach is to focus on presynaptic input to a neuron with retrograde tracing techniques. Even more fine-grained approaches are required to generate a complete microconnectome that incorporates the connections of all neurons which innervate each brain neuron.

Another innovative approach to study neuronal connectivity involves the examination of adhesion molecules found on the cell surface that physically connect neurons to one another. Schroeder et al. (2018) studied three different adhesion molecules. They found that one molecule controlled the number of connections with two others that affected signal transmission, one positively and one negatively. When combined, the three adhesion molecules were precise in describing exactly how the synapse looked and functioned. Essentially, this method defines the identity of a connection like a zip code or a barcode. With refinement, this method is being used to fine-tune the characterization of different connections. Basically, adhesion molecules define not only the number but also the architecture and function of a synapse (Schroeder et al., 2018). This approach moves away from anatomical connectivity methods and replaces them with a connectivity matrix.

## Nanoconnectome

Nanoconnections are connections at the level of the synapse pre- and postsynaptically. Synapses are specialized junctions that permit a neuron to send signals to another neuron. The human brain is estimated to have 100 billion neurons and 1,000 trillion synaptic connections (Kim et al., 2016). The first clear morphological evidence for synaptic structure was established in the 1950s using the transmission electron microscope to study the ultrastructural characteristics of neurons (Blackstad, 1965). Subsequently, technical advances have made it possible to examine small-scale three-dimensional

(3D) nervous system composition using serial brain sections. Thousands of serial sections are manually traced using aligned images placed in stacks. This allows reconstruction of the geometry of neurons and identification of cellular participants at each synapse.

A major advance is brain mapping utilizing integrated neurotechnologies (Brain/MINDS). Such brain mapping is being carried out in humans and in nonhuman primates. The nonhuman primate chosen is the marmoset because the marmoset brain shares aspects of the anatomical features of the human brain and engages in a variety of complex social behaviors (Okano et al., 2015). The tiny roundworm, *Caenorhabditis elegans*, roughly the size of a comma, was the first model used to study nanoconnectivity. It is one of the simplest organisms with a nervous system. Its body is made up of only 1,000 cells; one-third are neurons that direct its movements as it searches for food. It was chosen because of its simple nervous system structure, transparent body, and genetic accessibility (Brenner, 1974).

Study of the *C. elegans* nervous system began before computers were used for mapping. The complete structure of the roundworm nervous system had to be examined using the electron microscope using manual image acquisition. The goal of mapping *C. elegans* neuronal connectivity has been to determine how its behavior results from the structure of its nervous system. *Caenorhabditis elegans* genetics is known; there are known behavioral mutants, and its life cycle is short. There are 302 neurons in the *C. elegans* nervous system. Images of its nervous system were printed from glass plates in a dark room and connections drawn by manual tracing to complete its connectome. Manual reconstruction of electron microscope images led to the full visualization of the *C. elegans* nervous system wiring diagram. This structural connectivity map subsequently was completed by genetic screening and with reconstruction of serial electron microscope images in 1986.

The millimeter-long worm's brain sections were photographed by a camera mounted on an electron microscope (White et al., 1986). The graph of the male connectome has 579 nodes (385 neurons, 155 muscles, and 39 nonmuscle end organs). There are 5,315 chemical and 1,755 gap junction edges in the male. The other sex, the hermaphrodite connectome, has 460 nodes (302 neurons, 132 muscles, and 26 nonmuscle end organs). There are 4,887 chemical (or directed) edges and 1,447 gap junctions (Cook et al., 2019). The posture of the worm results from muscle tension that arises from summed inputs of three groups of motor neurons. Quantitative connected networks are the starting point to make sense of the neural control of the behavior of *C. elegans*. The behavioral state and motor output are emergent properties of the networks. Among these, the chemical synapses and gap junctions between neurons were found to be stereotypical and reproducible. Figure 7.2 illustrates how serial sections generated the map of synaptic connectivity of the roundworm.

Although *C. elegans* is an invertebrate whose nervous system differs from those of terrestrial vertebrates, the structure of the roundworm's few hundred neurons is identical between individuals. The differences between the nervous system of *C. elegans* and those of terrestrial vertebrates have implications for nanoconnectomics. Vertebrates have many neurons of the same type; no two neurons are doing exactly the same thing. For example, in a pool of vertebrate motor neurons, each one has a unique wiring pattern. Therefore, what seems to be a stereotypical pattern at a lower level of brain resolution hides the diversity evident at higher resolution.

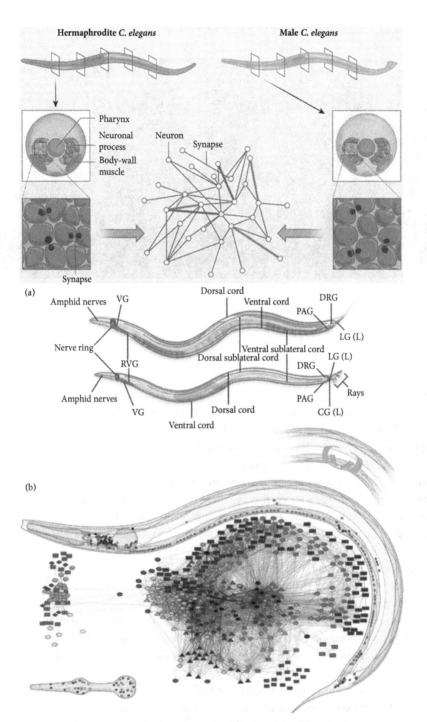

**Figure 7.2** (Top) Thousands of serial sections were taken along the body of an adult roundworm. High-resolution electron microscopic images were created to construct the roundworm nanoconnectome . CG; DRG; LG; PAG; RVG; VG. (Bottom) *Caenorhabditis elegans* adult nervous system neuroanatomy and connectivity. (a) The major nerve tracts and ganglia of the adult hermaphrodite and adult male are illustrated. The major sex difference is that the male has a larger number of neurons and muscles in the tail utilized in copulation. (b) Individual cells in the adult hermaphrodite connected to nodes in the network. Black arrows indicate chemical synapses, and red lines indicate gap junction connections. Sensory neurons (triangles), interneurons (hexagons), motor neurons (circles), and muscles (rectangles) are demarcated.

(Top) From Portman (2019); (bottom) from Cook et al. (2019).

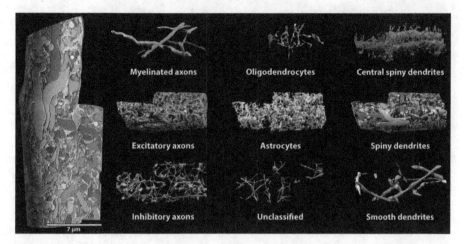

**Figure 7.3** Volumetric reconstruction of cortical connectivity in the mouse brain (segments of layer 5 pyramidal neurons in somatosensory cortex). Spiny dendrites, smooth dendrites, excitatory and inhibitory neurons, myelinated axon, astrocytes, oligodendrocytes, and unclassified cells with the reconstructed volume are shown.
From Swanson and Lichtman (2016).

Compared to studies in the roundworm, *C. elegans*, 3D electron microscopy reconstructions of neuron circuits in the brains of mammals are performed on a smaller scale due to technical challenges, as shown in Figure 7.3.

Figure 7.3 includes 1,700 synaptic connections and locations in the volume shown and location of each with their pre- and postsynaptic partners. More than 90% of the connections examined were excitatory. There were no electrical connections identified in this three-cylinder volume. Gap junction proteins (electronic synapses) have been identified in inhibitory neurons in layers 4 and 6. Studies such as these reveal the complexity of brain connectivity and the magnitude of the difficulty facing neuroscientists who seek to understand the brain (Swanson & Lichtman, 2016). That difficulty is further demonstrated in a study based on 100 trillion voxels drawn from an electron microscopy data set involving cohorts of retinal ganglia cells innervating a diverse group of postsynaptic thalamocortical neurons (Swanson & Lichtman, 2016). From this study, the authors concluded that neural circuits in the mouse thalamus are formed by experience-linked inputs onto postsynaptic cells rather than connections between intrinsically different neuronal types.

The previously mentioned studies are part of the mouse-brain cubic-millimeter project focused on a nanoscale connectome. In another mouse nanoconnectome study at the Allen Institute in Seattle, Washington, conducted over 5 months, more than 100 million sections of mouse visual cortex, each 40 nm thick, were collected. It took 3 more months to assemble the images into a 3D volume study for 1 mm³ of a mouse brain. The number and size of large-scale reconstructions of neural circuitry in the mammalian brain are expanding.

The mouse-brain cubic-millimeter project (approximately 100,000 neurons) is one attempt to map a nanoscale connectome; this is a wiring diagram of a nervous system at the synaptic level. A nanoscale connectome of the whole brain is aspirational and seems almost inconceivable. The human brain has $10^{15}$ connections of approximately 100 billion neurons. This is roughly similar to the number of stars estimated to be in the Milky Way (Deweerdt, 2019). With current imaging technology, data collection would take thousands of years. Yet, daunting as the task of the mouse-brain cubic-millimeter project is, approximately 500 mm$^3$ connectivity might be possible in another decade. Other animal models eventually will be considered with advances in imaging methods using artificial intelligence (AI).

The mouse-brain project focuses on examining complete neural circuits instead of single neurons (J. A. Harris et al., 2019). Now that 1 mm$^3$ of a mouse has been imaged, the next step is to align the images, annotate the resulting images, and trace an estimated 4 km of nerve fibers in this cubic-millimeter volume. Tracing the path of a single neuron through stacked electron micrographs took nearly a decade in *C. elegans* with tracing or segmenting done by hand. Now AI is utilized for tracing. This involves using a machine-learning algorithm designed to examine images pixel by pixel to establish the location of neurons. Each step must be examined to ensure accurate reconstruction.

Because computers may make errors, human and artificial intelligence are being combined. Crowdsourcing is employed utilizing an online game called *Eyewire*. Crowdsourcing includes "citizen scientists" who join the crowd along with computer scientists to add to the number of people working. *Eyewire* puzzles are used to increase person power to map the mammalian connectome. The reason for crowdsourcing, using citizen scientists, is that it takes neuroscientists tens of hours to reconstruct a single cellular connection. The online game *Eyewire* is used to crowdsource the data analyses of the neurons. This approach acknowledges that people are better than computers at pattern recognition. *Eyewire* is essentially a game introduced to use person power to map the brain. A background in science is not needed to participate; curiosity and finding joy in solving puzzles are key. The goal is to map neurons, help investigations, and identify new cell types and synapses. Players are asked to map branches of a neuron from one side of the cube to another. Thus, players scroll through the mouse-brain cubic-millimeter imaging cube and reconstruct neurons in segments, tracing them using an artificial algorithm. In the game, multiple players map each cube. Subsequently, comparisons of work among them in their mapping are used to achieve consensus. *Eyewire* has nearly 300,000 registered users. By mid-2017, users had put in the equivalent work of 32 people working for 7 years and contributed to the discovery of six types of neurons in the mouse retina. As the work progresses from one brain region to another, new versions of *Eyewire* are created. There is continuing refinement in imaging technology as investigations move from serial-section electron microscopy to focused ion beam microscopy. These methods are being continuously refined to find the greatest accuracy.

With these advances in technology, new problems arise. Maps are being created at the different scales described: macro, meso, micro, and nano scales. An ongoing challenge is how to put them all together. The connectome maps are continuously providing new information on the location of synapses but not their composition. Synaptic molecular composition is important to link to the genome. It is essential to develop optimal specimen preparation methods for volume electron microscopy. Optimal imaging parameters are needed for enhanced detector sensitivity. It is important to combine ultrastructural data with structural information. The activity patterns of neuronal populations in freely behaving animals can be recorded with genetically engineered calcium indicators. This is combined with multiphoton and in vivo confocal imaging correlated with light and electron microscopy to identify neural circuits that are associated with behavior. The goal is to decode the brain perceiver internally along with externally generated stimuli. Once perceived, the multiple sensory inputs are integrated, stored, and examined for their role in emotion regulation and in the execution of motor movements (Kim et al., 2016).

## Synaptome

The term *synaptome* refers to the set of all synapses in the brain. Synapses connect axons and dendrites into a global anatomical network, the structural connectome. The linking of the connectome with the synaptome is an aspirational goal in neuroscience. Genetic labeling and imaging methods map synaptic molecular composition and diversity across the whole mouse brain (Zhu et al., 2018). Each subtype of synapse is being found to have a unique anatomical distribution in the mouse brain. Each mouse brain region is characterized by a distinct signature of synapse subtypes. The mapping of circuits demonstrates correspondence between synapse diversity and the structural and functional connectomes. Researchers studying the mouse brain have found that behaviorally relevant patterns of neuronal activity initiate spatiotemporal postsynaptic responses, pertinent to the structure of synaptome maps (Zhu et al., 2018). The greatest synaptic diversity found is in areas controlling higher cognitive function. Of importance, mutations that lead to cognitive disorders may show reorganized synaptome maps.

Homozygous knockin mice expressing enhanced green fluorescent protein labeled postsynaptic proteins have been studied. A semiautomatic standard image capture and analysis approach is used. Specific synaptic subtypes were identified in discrete circuits and connected regions on the mesoscale for the mouse structural connectome (Oh et al., 2014). The wiring diagram of the brain connects specialized local synaptome maps into a global brain network. To map the mesoconnectomes, axonal projections from brain regions were traced using green fluorescent protein markers. The results are registered to a common 3D space identifying a matrix of connection strengths between 213 brain regions. The nucleus accumbens was found to be connected to the entire brain by loops. There are thousands of such loops through the isocortex, striatum, and thalamus; the medulla contains more than 100 loops (Grange, 2018).

In summary, in the mouse synaptome, specific synaptic subtypes have been identified in discrete circuits and connected regions of the mesoscale structural connectome of the mouse (Zhu et al., 2018). The mouse synaptome studies circuits across the brain that can be defined by their synaptic composition. The mouse brain wiring diagram demonstrates connections between specialized local synaptome maps onto a global brain network.

## Development of the Functional Connectome

The structural and functional connectomes are constructed as the brain develops from the prenatal period to the postnatal period, throughout childhood into adult

life. Developmental trajectories of brain network formation, although genetically programmed, are modified epigenetically with environmental influences (Keunen et al.,
2017). Initially, developmental processes begin in the prenatal embryonic period and
continue throughout early infancy with ongoing contextualized brain network formation. The blueprint of the adult human brain is present in the neonatal brain. In the
postnatal period, brain connections are continually sculpted and organized to become
more like a replica of the adult human brain. Thus, the neonatal cerebral cortex reveals
a complex gyrification pattern similar to that of the adult brain. The basic white matter
large-scale connections are in place in the neonatal brain. Utilizing high-quality neuroimaging methodology, especially diffusion-weighted imaging, fMRI), and electrophysiology (EEG), early human brain development can be examined in detail in vivo
noninvasively (Gao et al., 2017).

Resting-state connectivity studies are particularly important. Resting-state fMRI
(rs-fMRI) utilizes spontaneous fluctuations in BOLD imaging signals across the entire
brain at a resolution of 1 mm. Brain regions are viewed to be functionally connected
when synchronous activity is demonstrated (i.e., temporal fluctuations in BOLD signals are highly correlated connected supporting synapses). Moreover, these approaches
are being applied to typically developing children and for early identification of altered
neurodevelopment in neurodevelopmental disorders (Gao et al., 2017). Disruptions in
early brain development may be genetically programmed in neurogenetic syndromes,
mediated epigenetically, and subject to environmental influences.

Brain development begins in the embryonic and early fetal period. The human brain
is made up of 86 billion neurons and an astonishing number of connected supporting
synapses, dendrites, and axons. The brain emerges from the neural tube. Neural tube
closure begins at embryonic day 21 and ends at embryonic day 27. The neural tube, the
precursor of the developing human brain, expands through neuronal proliferation, ongoing neurogenesis, and underlying genetic programming. By the second trimester or
middle of human gestation (20–30 weeks of gestation), neurogenesis is essentially complete. When neurons arrive at their destination in the cortical plate, axons and dendrites
extend to form the internal capsule, corpus callosum, and other brain structures.
Synaptogenesis, dendrite sprouting, and axonal pathfinding in the second trimester
lead to neuronal circuit formation and eventual functional communication within
the brain. For example, thalamocortical and corticothalamic fibers establish transient
circuits with subplate neurons and then grow into the developing cortex and thalamus
(Keunen et al., 2017).

In the third trimester, these corticothalamic connections are consolidated and long-
range association fibers extend into the cortical plate. An rs-fMRI study documents that
thalamocortical connections are established by the time of birth (Kostović & Jovanov-
Milošević, 2006). During the late fetal period in the third trimester, the overlying cortices' relatively smooth surface is transformed into a highly convoluted structure with
sulci that looks like the adult human brain. Neuroimaging studies of preterm infants
show the brain continuing to develop postnatally. There is a fivefold increase in cortical
surface area and changes in cortical curvature in a comparable time frame matching
the third trimester of pregnancy (Moeskops et al., 2015). Concurrently, myelination,
synaptogenesis, formation of dendrites, and development of dendrite spines continue
throughout the third trimester. Myelination proceeds from the back of the brain to

the front, moving centrally to peripherally. Brain areas involved in primary functions myelinate before association areas. Such myelination increases conduction speed.

Just as in the adult connectome, the developing human brain connectome may be studied at different levels. At the macro level, the focus is on the whole brain network development. At the micro level, advances are made in delineating the establishment of neural circuits in the cortex, subplate, thalamus, and cerebellum in the perinatal and postnatal brain (Kostović et al., 2014). Like the adult brain, the neonatal brain displays short path lengths. Newborn infants' brains show clustering of neurons to form connections that lead to triangles of interconnected nodes. The term *modularity* is used to describe subnetworks on modules that make up the connectome. The highest degree nodes, referred to as hub nodes, are more tightly connected to each other. The overall layout of the spatial structural hub nodes in the neonatal connectome shows considerable overlap with the adult human brain. In the neonate, functional hubs are immature (Keunen et al., 2017). The neonatal connectomes are basically confined to primary brain regions, including the sensorimotor and primary visual cortex. Refinements in structure are linked to communication efficiency with enhanced connection strength. This results in shorter characteristic path length and increasing functional anisotropy. Subsequently, during postnatal development, the functional brain's architecture reorganizes its spatial arrangement as brain hubs advance from primary brain order regions to higher order association areas (Keunen et al., 2017).

## Postnatal Brain Development

By the end of normal gestation, all major white matter tracts are in place. Networks for specialized information processing are in place, with brain regions with the most dense connections forming a central core. In premature birth, the overall layout is in place, but the quality of connections differs, an issue of importance for ongoing development. Short-range cortico-cortical connections continue to develop with increasing reinforcement of connections of existing connections. During the postnatal period, there is ongoing dendritic arborization and a massive increase in synaptogenesis. This results in abundant overproduction of synapses and connections that will be pruned in the ensuing years to form a more concentrated mature connectivity. *Pruning* refers to the selective elimination of synapses, a process that continues throughout childhood and adolescence. Pruning occurs as a result of competition for neurotrophic factors that are transferred to the innervating neuron with a completed synapse on the receptive neuron.

The competition for synaptic connections involves brain-derived neurotrophic factor (BDNF), with synapses receiving insufficient BDNF being pruned (Keunen et al., 2017). Neurotrophins signal through membrane-associated tyrosine kinases (Trk) that become active when the neurotrophin causes their dimerization to engage intracellular signaling pathways, including nuclear factor-κB, extracellular signal-regulated kinase, and phosphoinositide 3-kinase. The neurotrophin family comprises nerve growth factor acting at TrkA, BDNF and neurotrophin-4 binding to TrkB, and neurotrophin-3 binding to TrKC. By activating TrkB, BDNF induces the expression of additional AMPA receptors that are then inserted in the postsynaptic density, further enhancing their excitatory response to synaptic glutamate. In this case, BDNF is behaving as an autocrine substance—that is, acting on the neuron that released it. Synaptic BDNF also binds to TrkB receptors on the presynaptic terminals for retrograde transport in endosomes to the afferent cell body, where it ensures its survival. Afferents that do not make appropriate synaptic connections, thus lacking trophic support, undergo apoptotic (i.e., programmed) cell death (Yamashita, 2021).

Synaptic plasticity is not merely functional. If the excitatory input remains persistently quite active, the postsynaptic dendrite can sprout addition synaptic spines that form new synapses (Ma & Zuo, 2022). The proliferation of synapses is driven in part by increased BDNF synthesis and release. This sprouting of new synapses with robust presynaptic glutamatergic input has been observed in real time in vivo in the hippocampus of mice that have been transfected with green fluorescent protein which it is expressed only in pyramidal neurons, revealing their 3D structure replete with dendritic spines like a Golgi stain.

Recent research indicates that complement C4, a protein involved in innate immunity, labels vulnerable, poorly connected synapses, which are phagocytized by microglia (Whitelaw, 2018). Notably, the gene encoding complement C4 is the most robust risk gene for schizophrenia, which is characterized by a significant reduction in glutamatergic synapses on cortical neurons (Germann et al., 2021). There is an ongoing and increasing integration of the neonatal connectome. Modules, too, are increasingly shaped and interconnected in the early postnatal years. Myelination increases with the increased diameter of axons to promote efficient axonal transmission. Connectivity is stabilized within modules.

## Functional Network Development

The study of early functional connectome development has progressed largely through the use of rs-fMRI, which reveals the "default network." The default mode is made up of discrete bilaterally symmetrical areas of the brain and measures ongoing intrinsic activity in quiet response with eyes closed or in simple visual fixation. rs-fMRI is being used to determine functional brain architecture in the neonatal brain with the goal of understanding the functional development of the brain in utero. Intrauterine imaging might identify infants at risk for neurodevelopmental disorders. Interhemispheric connectivity has been studied in the fetal brain as early as 24 weeks post-conception. Connectivity increases in the ensuing weeks of gestation following a medial to lateral trajectory (Thomason et al., 2015).

Initial formation and reorganization of the functional connection has been studied in detail in the second trimester. It is an important time window and a vulnerable time in connectome development. In one study, 105 pregnant women (fetal gestational age between 20 and 40 weeks) were enrolled (Turk et al., 2019). The basic principles of the functional connectome were found to be established in the late second trimester. Maternal viral infection, extensive stress during pregnancy, gestational use of alcohol, and other events may have long-lasting effects on later-life functional connectivity. Mapping the healthy fetal connectome and understanding its development will permit early detection of functional alterations in the early developing brain in autism spectrum disorder

(Girault et al., 2022). The results of this large fetal functioning resting-state study (Turk et al., 2019) confirmed the presence of a blueprint of the functional brain connectome in utero in the second and third trimesters of pregnancy. This study provided the first evidence of higher order networks and identified primary motor and sensory networks. These connections are later pruned with the emergence of cognition postpartum. High overlap between adult and fetal functional organization was confirmed in this study. Major white matter pathways were shown to be established in the third trimester. The most densely functionally connected areas identified by the authors are hubs that are confined to the temporal cortex along with midline cortical regions of the insula, frontal lobes, and primary sensorimotor cortex. The functional hub organization involves medial temporal, fusiform, and primary somatosensory regions, along with inferior frontal and orbitofrontal regions and insular cortexes. These hubs coordinate activity linked to primary functions.

Overall, four functional modules were identified: (a) occipital and parietal visuo-somatosensory module, (b) midline prefrontal–temporal insular module, (c) temporal module, and (d) an extensive lateral and midline frontal module (Turk et al., 2019). In utero studies such as these have certain technical imaging limitations, including the need for spatial normalization and realignment of fMRI volumes to a standard average 32-week gestation template brain. These adjustments account for variation within the fetal group to age-specific brain templates.

When imaging the fetal brain in vivo, maternal respiration, movement, and changing positions of the fetus must be considered and addressed to reduce motion artifact. Despite these challenges, technical limitations such as these have been successfully addressed. Imaging in normal pregnancies of fetal brain functional architecture provides the baseline for further examination of prenatal risk factors, including maternal stress, gestational abuse of alcohol and other drugs, and premature birth, and it may potentially lead to early identification of neurodevelopmental and neurological disorders with the prospect of in utero interventions. The most comprehensive studies of the functional fetal connectome have utilized rs-fMRI, EEG, magnetoencephalography, and near-infrared spectroscopy (Vasung et al., 2019).

In typically developed, healthy adults, distinct resting-state networks have been demonstrated. Networks are widely distributed across the cortex and involve multiple regions of the brain. These networks are for primary functions including sensorimotor, auditory, and visual processing. Primary networks are linked to cognitive functions such as self-awareness, attention, future planning, memory, theory of mind, understanding the perspective of others, and executive functioning (Damoiseaux et al., 2006). The default mode network extends to the posterior cingulate cortex, ventral and dorsal medial prefrontal cortex, inferior parietal lobule, lateral temporal cortex, and hippocampal regions (Buckner et al., 2008).

In the neonatal brain, primary networks are evident, whereas higher order networks are fragmentary (Damoiseaux et al., 2006). The medial frontal cortex, frontal association cortices, and posterior cingulate cortex have been studied at 35 weeks of gestation (Thomson et al., 2015). Immature forms of sensorimotor visual and auditory networks were detected. In early life, the most dramatic development of the functional brain network occurs in the first postnatal years. In one study, 65 normally developing infants were examined with multiple longitudinal rs-fMRI scans every 3 months in the first year of life. The authors sought to establish maturation of nine key brain functional networks in the first year and examine socioeconomic status (SES) correlations. They identified a maturational sequence from primary sensorimotor/auditory to visual to attention/default mode, to executive control networks. Network-specific periods for cortical growth were found at age 6 months. Marginally significant positive brain correlations were identified for both the sensorimotor and default mode networks taking into account the impact of family SES and potentially the role of early life social engagement on functional network development. These approaches are an important focus for ongoing and future network research (Gao et al., 2015). In another study, the sensorimotor network, visual processing network, and auditory language network showed adult-like topology at birth with minimal changes in the first years. The dorsal attention network and the default mode network developed later, showing increasing synchronization with spatially remote brain regions. These are in networks attaining mature topology after 1 year of age. The last networks to mature are higher cognitive networks, including the salience network and bilateral frontoparietal networks. The latter are involved in executive functions, decision-making, and working memory. These higher cognitive networks are not mature at 1 year; their configuration is incomplete. Overall, the sequence of maturation of functional resting-state networks follows the developmental maturation of myelination and synaptogenesis. It parallels developmental–behavioral milestones in visual and sensorimotor function typical in the first year of life.

The last to develop are major cognitive functions involved in executive control and mature social cognition. These functions continue to develop well into adolescence and the early adult years (Casey et al., 2000). Associated brain networks for these higher cognitive and social–cognitive networks are the last to become fully operational.

## Functional Connectivity and Behavior

Functional operative network architecture has been identified in neonates at the whole-brain level. This architecture is genetically based and sculpted by environmental input and personal learning. There is a complex interplay in development of these networks modified by environmental experience with epigenetic changes. Activity in language areas including Broca's area emerges long before speech production. Genetic unfolding of the blueprint for brain development is incorporated into the brain structure in two ways: experience-expectant development changes and experience-dependent development changes (Greenough et al., 1987). Experience influences the developing brain, and these two mechanisms are involved in integrating them. The experience-expectant stage refers to the incorporation of environmental information that is ubiquitous and experienced in everyday life. For example, common to all species is pattern perception. Pattern and light information exposure facilitates low-level visual ability, which is important for depth perception, and supports high-level visual abilities important for face reception. Auditory information is essential for the development of speech and language brain regions. Availability of caregivers facilitates brain regions involved in personal social attachment. These experience-expectant processes have evolved as a neuronal preparation for the incorporation of specific information needed to drive circuit development. In many sensory systems, the synaptic connections between nerve cells are overproduced. The experience-expectant process allows ongoing sensory experiences to stabilize the circuitry for the connectivity remaining after synapse pruning.

Experience-dependent information processing refers to the incorporation of environmental information that is unique to a particular individual rather than universal—for example, learning about one's home or adding new words to one's vocabulary. Experiences such as these lead to the active formation of new synaptic connections, unlike the experience-expectant systems that are defined by eliminating overabundant ones by pruning to refine the synaptic architecture. Experience-dependent synaptogenesis continues throughout the life span when we remember and reconstruct events, acquire vocabulary, and refine the quality of attachment relationships.

Neonatal functional hubs, as noted above, are primarily confined to brain regions supporting primary functions, such as sensorimotor and visual cortex. There are a few neonatal hubs linked to the association cortex and regions such as the insula and posterior cingulate cortex (Keunen et al., 2017). In a prenatal study involving 33 pregnant women, a modular composition was identified in the fetal brain network architecture. It was less evident in the youngest fetuses at 24–31 weeks post-conception compared to somewhat older fetuses at 31–39 weeks post-conception, demonstrating functional brain integration increases during development (Keunen et al., 2017).

Electrophysiological connectivity, too, advances in the prenatal period. Functional activity patterns in early development have been extracted from recorded EEGs. Early on, a bimodal connectivity pattern is recognized. There is strong electrophysiological functional coupling of spatially remote brain regions during times of heightened brain activity but minimal function synchronizing during times of relative quiescence. The bimodality decreases with increasing postnatal age with the emergence of sensory-driven oscillations, reflective of ongoing cortical activity (Omidvarnia et al., 2014).

## Functional Brain Networks in Childhood and Adolescence

Coordinated neuronal activity between regions of the brain continues to mature after the first year of life into childhood and adolescence. During those years, it is clear that default networks predict patterns of interregional brain activity across several tasks (Grayson & Fair, 2017). Interregional functional connectivity results from the strength of anatomical connections, synaptic receptor densities, and correlated expression of genes. Such connectivity is sculpted by experience-dependent and activity-dependent modulation throughout the life span. The relationship between structural and functional connectivity is linked to ongoing neurodevelopmental events—neurogenesis, cell death, myelination, synaptic pruning, and glial development. Many of the network changes noted in infancy reflect long-term trajectories that continue to mature in childhood and adolescence. Connectivity continues to strengthen from early childhood throughout development, especially regarding long-range anterior–posterior links.

An ongoing technological problem for fMRI studies in children is in the interpretation of head motion artifact. Head motion increases nonspecific local coupling and decreases long-range coupling. Taking motion artifact into account, functional network maturation follows precise spatiotemporal trajectories. This is consistent with the fact that systems with different functional roles follow different trajectories. Thus, sensorimotor systems known to be well developed in childhood show little change into adulthood. However, default mode networks involved in cognitive tasks, including the salience network, frontoparietal executive network, and attentional network, become increasingly segregated, and the default mode network is increasingly synchronized. Figure 7.1 illustrates sensorimotor, cingulo-opercular, and frontoparietal default networks and occipital and cerebellum regions.

Within-network and between-network connections are activated to accomplish more complex task demands. Integration between cingulo-opercular/salience and the somatomotor modules extends as the age range increases from 10 to 26 years. The cingulo-opercular network is made up of the anterior insula/operculum, dorsal anterior cingulate cortex, and thalamus. Its central role is to sustain alertness with cognitive control (Coste & Kleinschmidt, 2016). Network structure continues to evolve after late childhood coincidental with later cognitive development.

Regarding structure–function relationships in later teenage years, these relationships are increasingly integrated compared to those in younger children. These enhanced relationships are consistent with white matter bundles increasing capacity to transfer information with increasing myelination and the increasing diameter of the axons. Although the most substantial changes in network connectivity take place in the first 2 years of life, networks continue to be refined throughout childhood and adolescence. In particular, there is strengthening of connections around functional hubs. Refinements in imaging technology and linking different imaging studies will lead to a better understanding of heterogeneity in connectivity in typically and atypically developing populations.

## Applications of Machine Learning Models to Predict Clinical Outcome

Applications of AI, especially machine learning, to connectome data may facilitate the diagnosis and treatment of mental and neurodevelopmental disorders. Machine learning is being applied to predict clinical outcomes and analyze subnetworks in the brain (Brown & Hamarneh, 2016). Standard medical imaging provides static topography of the brain. Biomarkers for disorders based on the connectome focus on brain regions as interconnected nodes that are either structurally or functionally connected. For the connectome, consideration must be given to changes in brain structure with development over a lifetime. Importantly, brain connectivity is altered by learning and life experiences. Brain injury and neurodevelopmental genetic disorders impact connectivity. Structural connectomes, derived from diffusion MRI, identify connections between pairs of nodes to designate the extent of white matter connectivity between associate pairs of regions of interest. Tractography is used to define structural connectivity. For the functional connectome, fMRI is used to measure the BOLD signal. This signal measures neural activity of each voxel over time. Signals are averaged within each region of interest. Subsequently, functional connectivity is computed between pairs of regions of interest.

An important application of machine learning is to predict outcomes. For example, connectome features with applied machine learning methods have been used to identify patients with attention-deficit/hyperactivity disorder (Cheng et al., 2012), major depression, and schizophrenia. Moreover, machine learning using connectome data has been used for early diagnosis of autism spectrum disorder (Wee et al., 2016). In conducting these studies, machine learning tools are adapted to make use of the unique properties of connectome data. Machine learning also has been applied to predict which individuals with a mental disorder will respond to a particular intervention. In one study, machine learning was applied to a depressed adolescent's brain imaging data to predict symptom reduction with CBT (Tymofiyeva et al., 2019). Supervised machine learning was applied to diffusion MRI-based structural connectome data to predict symptom reduction in 30 adolescents with depression following 3 months of CBT. Inputs included baseline depression score, age, gender, two global network properties, along with node strengths of brain regions previously implicated in depression. The classifiers led to 83% accuracy in the prediction of depression symptom reduction. The role of node strength within the right thalamus was identified in predicting symptom reduction with CBT (Tymofiyeva et al., 2019). Ongoing research is exploring structural and functional connectome data in machine learning to model different disorders and conditions.

# References

Agnati, L. F., Genedani, S., Leo, G., Rivera, A., Guidolin, D., & Fuxe, K. (2007). One century of progress in neuroscience founded on Golgi and Cajal's outstanding experimental and theoretical contributions. *Brain Research Reviews, 55*(1), 167–189.

Arráez-Aybar, L. A., Navia-Álvarez, P., Fuentes-Redondo, T., & Bueno-López, J. L. (2015). Thomas Willis, a pioneer in translational research in anatomy (on the 350th anniversary of Cerebri anatome). *Journal of Anatomy, 226*(3), 289–300.

Belousov, A. B., & Fontes, J. D. (2013). Neuronal gap junctions: Making and breaking connections during development and injury. *Trends in Neurosciences, 36*(4), 227–236.

Blackstad, T. W. (1965). Electron microscopy and biological structure research. Tidsskrift for den Norske *Laegeforening: Tidsskrift* for *Praktisk Medicin, ny Raekke, 85*, 97–103.

Bota, M., Dong, H. W., & Swanson, L. W. (2003). From gene networks to brain networks. *Nature Neuroscience, 6*(8), 795–799.

Bota, M., Sporns, O., & Swanson, L. W. (2015). Architecture of the cerebral cortical association connectome underlying cognition. *Proceedings of the National Academy of Sciences of the USA, 112*(16), E2093–E2101.

Brenner, S. (1974). The genetics of *Caenorhabditis elegans. Genetics, 77*(1), 71–94.

Brown, C. J., & Hamarneh, G. (2016). Machine learning on human connectome data from MRI. arXiv, 1611.08699.

Buckner, R. L., Andrews-Hanna, J. R., & Schacter, D. L. (2008). The brain's default network: Anatomy, function, and relevance to disease. *Annals of the New York Academy of Sciences, 1124*, 1–38.

Cabral, J., Kringelbach, M. L., & Deco, G. (2017). Functional connectivity dynamically evolves on multiple time-scales over a static structural connectome: Models and mechanisms. *NeuroImage, 160*, 84–96.

Casey, B. J., Giedd, J. N., & Thomas, K. M. (2000). Structural and functional brain development and its relation to cognitive development. *Biological Psychology, 54*(1–3), 241–257.

Cheng, W., Ji, X., Zhang, J., & Feng, J. (2012). Individual classification of ADHD patients by integrating multiscale neuroimaging markers and advanced pattern recognition techniques. *Frontiers in Systems Neuroscience, 6*, Article 58.

Clarke, E., & O'Malley, C. D. (1996). *The human brain and spinal cord: A historical study illustrated by writings from antiquity to the twentieth century* (2nd ed.). Norman Publishing.

Cook, S. J., Jarrell, T. A., Brittin, C. A., Wang, Y., Bloniarz, A. E., Yakovlev, M. A., Nguyen, K., Tang, L., Bayer, E., Duerr, J., Bülow, H. E., Hobert, O., Hall, D., & Emmons, S. (2019). Whole-animal connectomes of both *Caenorhabditis elegans* sexes. *Nature, 571*(7763), 63–71.

Coste, C. P., & Kleinschmidt, A. (2016). Cingulo-opercular network activity maintains alertness. *NeuroImage, 128*, 264–272.

Damoiseaux, J. S., Rombouts, S. A., Barkhof, F., Scheltens, P., Stam, C. J., Smith, S. M., & Beckmann, C. F. (2006). Consistent resting-state networks across healthy subjects. *Proceedings of the National Academy of Sciences of the USA, 103*(37), 13848–13853.

Del Maestro, R. F. (1998). Leonardo da Vinci: The search for the soul. *Journal of Neurosurgery, 89*(5), 874–887.

Deweerdt, S. (2019). Deep connections. *Nature, 571*, 56–58.

Gao, W., Alcauter, S., Elton, A., Hernandez-Castillo, C. R., Smith, J. K., Ramirez, J., & Lin, W. (2015). Functional network development during the first year: Relative sequence and socioeconomic correlations. *Cerebral Cortex, 25*(9), 2919–2928.

Gao, W., Lin, W., Grewen, K., & Gilmore, J. H. (2017). Functional connectivity of the infant human brain: Plastic and modifiable. *The Neuroscientist, 23*(2), 169–184.

Germann, M., Brederoo, S. G., & Sommer, I. E. C. (2021). Abnormal synaptic pruning during adolescence underlying the development of psychotic disorders. *Current Opinion in Psychiatry, 34*(3), 222–227.

Girault, J. B., Donovan, K., Hawks, Z., Talovic, M., Forsen, E., Elison, J. T., Shen, M. D., Swanson, M. R., Wolff, J. J., Kim, S. H., Nishino, T., Davis, S., Snyder, A. Z., Botteron, K. N., Estes, A. M., Dager, S. R., Hazlett, H. C., Gerig, G., McKinstry, R., . . . Piven, J.; IBIS Network. (2022). Infant visual brain development and inherited genetic liability in autism. *American Journal of Psychiatry, 179*(8), 573–585.

Glasser, M. F., Smith, S. M., Marcus, D. S., Andersson, J. L., Auerbach, E. J., Behrens, T. E., Coalson, T., Harms, M., Jenkinson, M., Moeller, S., Robinson, E. C., Sotiropoulos, S., Xu, J., Yacoub, E., Ugurbil, K., & Van Essen, D. (2016). The Human Connectome Project's neuroimaging approach. *Nature Neuroscience, 19*(9), 1175–1187.

Grange, P. (2018). Topology of the mesoscale connectome of the mouse brain. arXiv, 1811.04698.

Grayson, D. S., & Fair, D. A. (2017). Development of large-scale functional networks from birth to adulthood: A guide to the neuroimaging literature. *NeuroImage, 160*, 15–31.

Greenough, W. T., Black, J. E., & Wallace, C. S. (1987). Experience and brain development. *Child Development, 58*(3), 539–559.

Harris, J. A., Mihalas, S., Hirokawa, K. E., Whitesell, J. D., Choi, H., Bernard, A., & Feiner, A. (2019). Hierarchical organization of cortical and thalamic connectivity. *Nature, 575*(7781), 195–202.

Harris, J. C. (2010). Camillo Golgi, Nobel laureate: The olfactory bulb. *Archives of General Psychiatry, 67*(10), 983–984.

Hippocrates. (1962). *Heraclitus, of Ephesus* (W. H. S. Jones & E. T. Withington, Trans.). Harvard University Press.

Keunen, K., Counsell, S. J., & Benders, M. J. (2017). The emergence of functional architecture during early brain development. *NeuroImage, 160*, 2–14.

Kim, G. H., Gim, J. W., & Lee, K. J. (2016). Nano-resolution connectomics using large-volume electron microscopy. *Applied Microscopy, 46*(4), 171–175.

Kostović, I., & Jovanov-Milošević, N. (2006). The development of cerebral connections during the first 20–45 weeks' gestation. Seminars in Fetal and Neonatal Medicine, *11*(6), 415–422.

Kostović, I., Jovanov-Milošević, N., Radoš, M., Sedmak, G., Benjak, V., Kostović-Srzentić, M., Vasung, L., Culjat, M., Radoš, M., Huppi, P., & Judaš, M. (2014). Perinatal and early postnatal reorganization of the subplate and related cellular compartments in the human cerebral wall as revealed by histological and MRI approaches. *Brain Structure and Function, 219*(1), 231–253.

Kruger, L., & Otis, T. S. (2007). Whither withered Golgi? A retrospective evaluation of reticularist and synaptic constructs. *Brain Research Bulletin, 72*(4–6), 201–207.

Ma, S., & Zuo, Y. (2022). Synaptic modifications in learning and memory—A dendritic spine story. *Seminars in Cell & Developmental Biology, 125*, 84–90.

Manzoni, T. (1998). The cerebral ventricles, the animal spirits and the dawn of brain localization of function. *Archives Italiennes de Biologie, 136*(2), 103–152.

Moeskops, P., Benders, M. J., Kersbergen, K. J., Groenendaal, F., de Vries, L. S., Viergever, M. A., & Išgum, I. (2015). Development of cortical morphology evaluated with longitudinal MR brain images of preterm infants. *PLoS One, 10*(7), e0131552.

Oh, S. W., Harris, J. A., Ng, L., Winslow, B., Cain, N., Mihalas, S., Wang, Q., Lau, C., Kuan, L., Henry, A., Mortrud, M. T., Ouellette, B., Nguyen, T., Sorensen, S., Slaughterbeck, C., Waeman, W., Li, Y., Feng, D., Ho, A., . . . Ng, L. (2014). A mesoscale connectome of the mouse brain. *Nature, 508*(7495), 207–214.

Okano, H., Miyawaki, A., & Kasai, K. (2015). Brain/MINDS: Brain-mapping project in Japan. *Philosophical Transactions of the Royal Society B: Biological Sciences, 370*(1668), 20140310.

Omidvarnia, A., Fransson, P., Metsäranta, M., & Vanhatalo, S. (2014). Functional bimodality in the brain networks of preterm and term human newborns. *Cerebral Cortex, 24*(10), 2657–2668.

Pereda, A. E. (2014). Electrical synapses and their functional interactions with chemical synapses. *Nature Reviews Neuroscience, 15*(4), 250–263.

Portman, D. S. (2019). Neural networks mapped in both sexes of the worm. *Nature, 571*(7763), 40–42.

Schiller, F. (1997). The cerebral ventricles: From soul to sink. *Archives of Neurology, 54*(9), 1158–1162.

Schroeder, A., Vanderlinden, J., Vints, K., Ribeiro, L. F., Vennekens, K. M., Gounko, N. V., Wierda, K., & de Wit, J. (2018). A modular organization of LRR protein-mediated synaptic adhesion defines synapse identity. *Neuron, 99*(2), 329–344.

Sherrington, C. S. (1897). The central nervous system. In *A text book of physiology*. Macmillan.

Sherrington, C. S. (1906). *The integrative action of the nervous system*. Charles Scribner's Sons.

Sourkes, T. L. (2002). Magendie and the chemists: The earliest chemical analyses of the cerebrospinal fluid. *Journal of the History of the Neurosciences, 11*(1), 2–10.

Swanson, L. W., & Lichtman, J. W. (2016). From Cajal to connectome and beyond. *Annual Review of Neuroscience, 39*, 197–216.

Thomason, M. E., Grove, L. E., Lozon, T. A., Jr., Vila, A. M., Ye, Y., Nye, M. J., Manning, J., Pappas, A., Hernadez-Andrade, E., Yeo, L., Mody, S., Berman, S., Hassan, S., & Romero, R. (2015). Age-related increases in long-range connectivity in fetal functional neural connectivity networks in utero. *Developmental Cognitive Neuroscience, 11*, 96–104.

Turk, E., van den Heuvel, M. I., Benders, M. J., de Heus, R., Franx, A., Manning, J. H., Hect, J., Hernandez-Andrade, E., Hassan, S., Romero, R., Kahn, R. S., Thomason, M., & van den Heuvel, M. (2019). Functional connectome of the fetal brain. *Journal of Neuroscience, 39*(49), 9716–9724.

Tymofiyeva, O., Yuan, J. P., Huang, C. Y., Connolly, C. G., Blom, E. H., Xu, D., & Yang, T. T. (2019). Application of machine learning to structural connectome to predict symptom reduction in depressed adolescents with cognitive behavioral therapy (CBT). *NeuroImage: Clinical, 23*, 101914.

Vasung, L., Turk, E. A., Ferradal, S. L., Sutin, J., Stout, J. N., Ahtam, B., Lin, P., & Grant, P. E. (2019). Exploring early human brain development with structural and physiological neuroimaging. *NeuroImage, 187*, 226–254.

Wee, C. Y., Yap, P. T., & Shen, D. (2016). Diagnosis of autism spectrum disorders using temporally distinct resting-state functional connectivity networks. *CNS Neuroscience & Therapeutics, 22*(3), 212–219.

Weissman, T. A., & Pan, Y. A. (2015). Brainbow: New resources and emerging biological applications for multicolor genetic labeling and analysis. *Genetics, 199*(2), 293–306.

White, J. G., Southgate, E., Thomson, J. N., & Brenner, S. (1986). The structure of the nervous system of the nematode *Caenorhabditis elegans*. *Philosophical Transactions of the Royal Society of London Series B: Biological Sciences, 314*(1165), 1–340.

Whitelaw B. S. (2018). Microglia-mediated synaptic elimination in neuronal development and disease. *Journal of Neurophysiology, 119*(1), 1–4.

Willis, T. (1965). *The anatomy of the brain and nerves: Tercentenary Ed., 1664–1964*. McGill University Press.

Yamashita, N. (2021). NGF signaling in endosomes. *Advances in Experimental Medicine and Biology, 1331*, 19–29.

Zhu, F., Cizeron, M., Qiu, Z., Benavides-Piccione, R., Kopanitsa, M. V., Skene, N. G., Koniaris, B., DeFelipe, J., Fransen, E., Komiyama, N., & Grant, S. G. (2018). Architecture of the mouse brain synaptome. *Neuron, 99*(4), 781–799.

# 8

# Consciousness

Consciousness is at the center of the study of both objective and subjective experience; to experience existence is to be conscious (Flanagan, 1992). Fundamentally, consciousness is subjectively experienced from the first-person perspective. Looking outward, we perceive the visible world; looking inward, we feel emotions, think, and reflect on our thoughts before acting (Revonsuo, 2018). Consciousness is an internal sense organ for perception of psychological content focused on the surface of the conscious mind (Revonsuo, 2018). *Consciousness* refers to a general state of a person—it is a particular capability found in living systems—whereas *awareness* refers to the experience of exercising consciousness in a particular situation—for example, being aware of a sensory stimulus. Attention is linked to consciousness and refers to focusing the direction of consciousness to the selection of the contents of awareness (Tulving, 1985). Consciousness traditionally was discussed in psychological or functional terms (Dennett, 1991). Currently, consciousness studies focus on evolutionary neurobiology and affective cognitive neuroscience (Damasco, 1998; Gazzaniga et al., 2019; MacLean, 1990; Merker, 2007; Panksepp & Biven, 2012; Revonsuo, 2018). Consciousness has long been considered to arise from the brain's responses to sensory stimuli from the outside world. However, empirical evidence indicates that consciousness is actively generated within the brain. Moreover, sensory signals from the outside environment may constrain the internal generation of consciousness (Hong et al., 2018; Solms, 2019). Important aspects of consciousness studied are phenomenal consciousness (awareness of existence, of being alive), reflective (or access) consciousness, and self-awareness.

This chapter introduces the study of consciousness. It reviews the history of the study of consciousness, current concepts of consciousness, consciousness from an evolutionary standpoint, various concepts of consciousness and the brain, consciousness and memory, and the relationship between sleep and consciousness. It also reviews clinical situations in which consciousness is affected, and it summarizes recent views on the neurobiology of consciousness.

## History of the Study of Consciousness

The scientific study of consciousness has three major stages. The first of these (1860s–1920s) defined consciousness as the study of the conscious mind and focused on sensation, perception, and attention. Physicist Gustav Fechner (1801–1887) focused on psychophysics, the relationship between physical stimuli and consciousness, demonstrating that consciousness could be empirically studied. The father of the experimental science of psychology is Wilhelm Wundt, who founded a laboratory of experimental psychology in Leipzig, Germany, in 1879. He focused on introspection, the verbal descriptions of experienced physical sensations. He measured the time it took to detect a stimulus and identify it. Edward Titchener (1867–1927) was Wundt's most prominent student. Titchener proposed that the mind is a subjectively experienced stream of mental processes, whereas consciousness is the sum of mental processes in the present. Titchener's approach to psychology, structuralism, proposed that consciousness is made up of simple elements. The goal of structuralism was to break down overall experience into its simplest qualities. However, structuralism ultimately was found to be misguided and failed as a model of consciousness when the number of elements comprising it could not be agreed upon. Moreover, consciousness is not made up of simple elements; it is experienced holistically (Revonsuo, 2018).

William James (1842–1910) challenged the basis of the structuralist position, proposing that psychology should not begin with sensations as the simplest mental elements when examining consciousness. James proposed that consciousness is holistic. It is a dynamic ever-changing stream of consciousness. James (1890) wrote that consciousness "is nothing jointed; it flows . . . let us call it stream of thought, of consciousness, or of subjective life" (p. 239). James used introspective observation as his method to discover states of consciousness, both everyday and altered states of consciousness. Similarly, in the early 20th century, Gestalt psychologists argued for a holistic conception of consciousness, noting that consciousness is not built up from simple sensations that come together like the elements of a mosaic. Localized sensations instead are experienced in the context that surrounds them; the smaller parts depend on the whole rather than the whole being built from independent sensory units. For example, in visual illusions, a part of a figure looks different—bigger, smaller, or distorted—than it really is because of what else surrounds it in the visual field. Although they did not have the tools to prove it, Gestalt psychologists proposed that perceptual consciousness is tightly connected to large-scale patterns of neuronal activity in the brain (Revonsuo, 2018).

Although the early introspectionists were interested in experiment psychology in the study of consciousness, it was abandoned as central to psychology with the rise of behaviorism and psychoanalysis. The behaviorists' critique of consciousness in psychology stated that psychology should be an objective natural science and not a subjective one (Watson, 1913). Leading behaviorist John Watson's background was in animal psychology; animal models (rats, pigeons, and dogs) could not report on subjective experiences. So, introspection was not an appropriate methodology to study them. Psychology was redefined by these behaviors as the science of behavior whose focus should be to predict and control behavior. Watson proposed unobservable subjective approaches should be replaced with objective study of behavior in both animals and humans. However, the cognitive approach to the mind challenged behaviorism in the 1960s and 1970s by emphasizing information processing in the mind. Cognitive psychology advanced with the development of brain imaging and advancements in neuropsychologic testing, ending the dominance of behaviorism and shifting the focus to cognitive approaches. Brain imaging provided an objective means to study the conscious brain.

Freudian psychoanalysis also shifted the focus away from the study of consciousness, seeking to study instead the unconscious. For Sigmund Freud, the role of consciousness was less significant. Freud proposed the unconscious mind influences the contents of consciousness. Freud's theory of mind emphasized altered states of mental activity such as dreams. He proposed that dreams could not be explained unless unconscious mental life was considered. The goal of psychoanalysis is to examine how the unconscious mind helps understand human behavior. Although Freudian psychoanalysis became the dominant approach in psychiatry in the mid-20th century, analytic psychologist Carl Jung's approach to the unconscious, with its emphases on archetypes of the collective unconscious, re-established the primacy of consciousness (Edinger, 1984). Jung's approach to dreaming and the role of active imagination in psychotherapy emphasized the creation of consciousness as a goal of psychotherapy (Edinger, 1984).

## Concepts of Consciousness

Consciousness "is a state of awareness of the self and the environment" (Fish, 1967). Sims (1988) suggested that consciousness is best used as an adjective because a conscious person does not possess consciousness but is a conscious being. This consciousness is not separable from what one is conscious of; that is, consciousness implies sentience, the capacity to feel, perceive, or know subjectively. Clinically, consciousness refers to an inner awareness of bodily experience, a potential intentional response, and the experiencing of a conscious self. Consciousness principally operates at three levels: (a) the level of phenomenal consciousness, consciousness as felt, as subjective experience in the here and now; (b) the level of reflective consciousness with regard to thinking about experiences, evaluating their importance and acting upon them; and (c) the level of self-awareness, which refers to awareness of experiences and their continuity from past to present to future.

Unconsciousness refers to a lack of inner existence or experience. The term "unconscious" (Sims, 1988) refers to three situations in which there may be no subjective experience: (a) in brain disease, in which a person may be classified on a continuum from normal consciousness to coma;(b) in sleep, in which there is a continuum from wakefulness to deep sleep (there is, however, conscious awareness in in lucid dreaming); and (c) in processes that cannot be observed through introspection, such as nondeclarative (implicit) memory functions. Each of these processes is out of awareness.

Vigilance, lucidity, and self-awareness are all aspects of consciousness. Vigilance is on a continuum with drowsiness. It may be linked to threat, anxiety, or basic affects. It may be heightened with interest, pleasure, anger, or fear and reduced during boredom and depression. These changes may be most evident in the cognitively impaired or brain-damaged person. The sensorium (consciousness or full awareness of internal and external events) may be clear or clouded. "Clouded" refers to a slight impairment of consciousness on the alertness–coma continuum. With clouding, intellectual functions (e.g., attention, concentration, recognition, judgment, speech, and planned action) may be impaired.

Consciousness of the self is an emerging capacity that accompanies alertness and awareness. In psychiatric disorders, there may be an impairment in self-awareness regarding the ability to distinguish the "I" from the "Not I" (Jaspers, 1963). Jaspers outlines four characteristics of self-awareness: (a) the feeling of awareness of activity (carrying out an activity provides an awareness of carrying it out), (b) an awareness of unity (I am one person, not many), (c) an awareness of identity (continuity of being one person all the time), and (d) an awareness of the boundaries of the self (distinguish myself from the outside world, which is not self).

Self-awareness may be expressed as self-concept and self-image. Self-concept refers to conscious abstract awareness of one's self, whereas the body image may refer to physical aspects and those that are not in awareness. Developmental phases of self-awareness begin in early life with differentiation of the self from one's surroundings (ages 1–3 years), followed by the emergence of an externally derived self-image and establishment of a social role (ages 4–10 years), the re-establishment of the body image at puberty (ages 11–14 years), and the establishment of mature roles of the social self in adolescence.

## Consciousness and Brain Evolution

Consideration of consciousness begins with the evolution of the subjective brain (MacLean, 1990). The neocortex receives sensory input through the five senses. It is oriented toward the external world. Consciousness was long viewed as being the brain's passive response to sensory stimuli from the external world. However, we now understand that consciousness is generated within the brain. The overall level of consciousness is mediated through the reticular activating system, a diffuse network of nerve pathways that connect the spinal cord, cerebrum, and cerebellum.

Central to our individuality is the subjective self. MacLean (1990) contrasted epistemology, which is objective knowledge that is acquired through analytic methodology, with epistemics, a term he proposes for the study of subjectivity. Epistemics is the study of the evolution of the subjective self and its relation to the internal and external world. Moreover, MacLean furthered our understanding of the evolution of consciousness by tracing brain evolution from reptiles to mammals. The oldest part of the brain includes the matrix of the brain and makes up the majority of the reticular formation, midbrain, and basal ganglia. MacLean is best known for identifying and naming the limbic system, the emotional brain, and his views on tracing the evolution of the brain and behavior (MacLean, 1952, 1990).

Importantly, MacLean considered the role of the cerebral cortex in brain evolution by examining the developmental consequence of radical decortication in infancy in animals. Decortication has been studied in neonatal rats, cats, and hamsters. These studies demonstrate that species-typical behavior (social, maternal, aggressive, and sexual behavior) is preserved after removal of the cortex in early life. For example, developing hamsters without a cortex resemble littermates regarding weight gain; physical development; and the onset of species-typical behaviors such as nest building, digging, hoarding, and scent marking. The males show species-typical territorial defense and aggression when confronted by another male. Despite decortication, male hamsters show a strong sexual preference for their own species, display sexual arousal, and impregnate females. Females were normally receptive to males, conceived, gave birth, and nursed (Murphy et al., 1981).

In humans, an extreme form of cortical decortication, hydranencephaly, has been examined. This is a rare, inherited neurodevelopmental disorder in which infants are born without cerebral hemispheres. With proper care and stabilization, affected children can live for years and remain responsive to their surroundings (McAbee et al., 2000). An infant born with hydranencephaly may show no obvious symptoms at birth and may even not be recognized with a brain disorder until normal developmental milestones are missed. However, in the first year of life, these children typically develop seizures and gastrointestinal reflux. Although there is a high mortality rate, those successfully treated survive and may live for years. When stabilized, these children are responsive to the environment, orienting to it and emotionally responsive to it (Figure 8.1). They

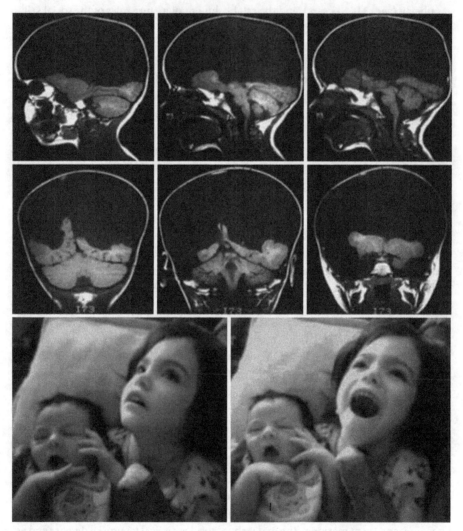

**Figure 8.1** Sagittal and frontal magnetic resonance images of the head of a child with hydranencephaly (top) and the child's responsiveness when her baby brother is placed in her arms (bottom). In the top panel, most of the brain is missing. The cranium is largely filled with cerebrospinal fluid. Spared regions of the ventromedial occipital and midline cortical matter overlie an intact cerebellum and brain stem. The bottom panel shows the emotional responsiveness of an awake and alert 3-year-old girl with hydranencephaly when her younger brother is placed in her arms.
From Merker (2007).

can express pleasure through smiling and laughing and aversion by "fussing" and emotional facial expressions. They may show preferences for familiar toys, music, or videos. Hearing is typically preserved, whereas vision is compromised (Merker, 2007).

Examination of these children allows study of the functions of a human brain stem regarding phenomenal consciousness despite the loss of both cerebral hemispheres. Children with the loss of both cerebral hemispheres demonstrate that the "human brain stem is specifically human"—that is, "the children laugh and smile in a specifically human manner" (Merker, 2007, p. 80).

Essentially, these children possess primary phenomenal consciousness. Sensory information related to bodily action (e.g., orienting) and motivation/learning takes place through the brain stem. The brain stem evolved long before the evolutionary expansion of the neocortex in the human brain. In the normal brain, the human brain stem performs the functions needed to integrate information necessary for decision-making. The brain stem is involved in the integration of environmental experiences, emotions, and behaviors. Merker (2007) proposes that anatomically, the brain stem function that supports phenomenal consciousness involves a structural complex with three domains that interact to allow the organism to determine what to do next. Conscious functioning produces a neural simulation of real-world external reality. Bodily activities are influenced by feelings that reflect current needs. The three domains of the *selection complex* are composed of the periaqueductal gray matter, superior colliculus, substantia nigra, and surrounding midbrain reticular complex. Thus, subjective phenomenal consciousness in both animals and humans is determined by the neural simulation of reality based on momentary needs. Brain stem–level functions involve vigilance, orienting, and phenomenal consciousness. Phenomenally, conscious persons are sentient beings who are able to feel and perceive. A phenomenally conscious mind is a feeling mind (Revonsuo, 2018).

MacLean (1985) proposed the term *evolutionary psychiatry*, whose focus is the subjective self; it emphasizes the importance of integrated functioning of the evolving brain. MacLean emphasized that empathy is an outcome of integrated brain functioning in brain evolution. He spoke of how brain evolution links the cold sense of vision with the warmth of emotion that allows us to consciously look toward others with genuine feeling (Harris, 2003). MacLean (1990) examined the evolution of the emotional brain in the transition from reptiles to human primates. He emphasized that in the transition, the paleo-mammalian brain limbic system plays an important role in the emergence of affective consciousness. Virtually all conscious experience has an affective tone. Affective tone influences information processing and facilitates attention, memory, and decision-making; all of these are associated with consciousness (Damasio, 1999). Brain evolution illustrates how secondary cognitive forms of consciousness emerged from phenomenal (primary) emotional consciousness. Panksepp proposed that raw emotional experiences arising subcortically make up the neural ground from which conscious processes emerge (Panksepp and Biven, 2012; Panksepp & Panksepp, 2000). For example, patients with psychomotor epilepsy report feelings of enhanced reality and increased awareness linked to affective emotional feeling (MacLean, 1990). Paleo-mammalian subcortical networks linked to emotions provide the sense of sentience—that is, phenomenological awareness that provides meaning to experiences. The paleo-mammalian brain consists of the septum, amygdala, hypothalamus, and cingulate cortex. The neocortex is superimposed on the paleo-mammalian brain. The cortex is essentially the "thinking cap" of the brain; it allows both reflective consciousness and self-consciousness. Neocortical reflective consciousness and subsequent self-consciousness comprise the most advanced stage of brain evolution.

Concurrently, in the evolution of the autonomic nervous system, phylogenetically there are areas of convergence where core brain regions impact affective consciousness. At the instinctual brain stem level of phenomenal consciousness, the nonmyelinated vagus nerve is the first to respond to overwhelming threats that lead to, at this most basic level, immobilization in animals (death feigning) and psychological dissociation in humans (Porges, 2001). This parasympathetically determined immobilization is mediated through an instinctual response to threat. The paleo-mammalian or emotional brain copes with threat at a higher level of functioning that is modulated by the sympathetic nervous system through fight-or-flight behaviors that are mediated by neuroendocrine mechanisms (Van Honk & Schutter, 2005). This response is largely mediated through the extended amygdala via its connections with subcortical and cortical systems involved in emotion, motivation, and emotional regulation. Through the activation of emotions, the amygdala responds to threat by initiating fight-or-flight behaviors. Finally, at the neocortical level, the myelinated vagus facilitates social cognition and social engagement in consort with the release of the social bonding hormones oxytocin and vasopressin (Porges, 2001).

Affective consciousness is modulated from the cortex top-down. Emotional affective consciousness is nonverbal. Damacio (1999) refers to affective consciousness as a "feeling of what happens" and conscious introspection as providing a cognitive account of cognitive experience. Such introspection involves the orbitofrontal cortex, which is interconnected with other cortical and subcortical brain areas (Damasio, 1999).

Both MacLean's (1990) proposal of an evolutionary evolving brain system and Porges' (2001) polyvagal theory offer insight into consciousness. Both examine brain systems that are evolutionarily separate physiologically and behaviorally. Merker's (2007) examination of consciousness without a cortex contributes to understanding phenomenal (basic) consciousness (Van Honk et al., 2007). MacLean's evolutionary model links the paleo-mammalian brain to affective consciousness. Ledoux (2012) provides a further refinement of our understanding of the amygdala in affective consciousness and a critique of Maclean's approach. However, MacLean's triune brain continues to be a useful metaphor to stimulate further evolutionary brain research into consideration of how mature brains have evolved and function as an integrated whole. The brain model proposed is a cortico-centric model in which consciousness is viewed as transient synchronized thalamo-cortico-cortical neural activity (Baars et al., 2003).

Cognitive content is available in the global workspace that includes attention, evaluation, memory, and verbal expression. Global availability allows for the continuous nature of consciousness. In humans, information stored in the cortex is essential to our sense of self. The self places an individual in historical time as self-consciousness autobiographical self that draws on memories of past lifetime experiences and anticipates the future (Gazzaniga et al., 2019).

## Consciousness and Memory

Remembering is a conscious experience; to remember is to be consciously aware of past events. Primary memory is identified with cognitive self-consciousness; the rehearsal of an idea is a conscious process; activated memory is conscious (James, 1890).

In considering cognitive reflective consciousness, working short-term memory (a few seconds) and very short-term memory (a fraction of a second) may be the most pertinent. Working short-term memory is limited by the number of items that it may hold at one time—approximately seven—yet the storage potential of memory is far greater than this. An ambiguous event may have only one interpretation at a time in consciousness; generally, tasks are carried out one at a time. Because consciousness is linked to the executive function of attention, it can inhibit automatic responses generated through perceptions and affects that are linked to nondeclarative (procedural) memory. Furthermore, information processing may occur out of awareness, resulting in solutions subsequently becoming available to consciousness.

Long-term episodic memory apparently is not necessary for consciousness because those with brain injury, who may not be able to lay down new episodic memory, are conscious. The complexity of our capacity to consciously and unconsciously process information linking life experiences requires a brain layered analysis such as that proposed by Tulving (1985, 2002). Tulving links the three basic memory systems—procedural, semantic, and episodic—to three kinds of consciousness: anoetic (non-knowing, unthinking), noetic (knowing and thinking consciousness linked to perception and cognition), and autonoetic (self-knowing consciousness) with conscious awareness and reflection. Anoetic consciousness, which is characteristic of procedural nondeclarative (implicit) memory, is temporally and spatially bound to the current situation. This form of consciousness registers perceptions, internally represents them, and allows behavioral response to internal and external aspects in the present. Noetic consciousness is the characteristic of semantic memory. It allows one to be aware of and cognitively process objects, events, and the relations among objects and events when these objects and events are absent. This allows flexible action upon symbolic knowledge of the world. Noetic consciousness accompanies information being entered into and retrieved from semantic memory. It may be associated with "involuntary memory" when experience comes into awareness without our conscious choice.

Autonoetic consciousness is correlated with episodic memory and is necessary to remember personally experienced events. To remember an event, one is aware of it as part of one's past existence. This form of consciousness gives the phenomenological quality to remembrance and distinguishes it from other forms of awareness (e.g., perceiving, thinking, imagining, or dreaming).

Tulving (1985) studied case N.N., who had profound amnesia for personal events before and after a closed head injury. N.N. could not recall a single personal event or incident from his past. His knowledge of the past had an impersonal quality, as did his knowledge of other aspects of the world, yet his language skills and general knowledge skills remained intact. His awareness of chronological time was intact, but his awareness of subjective time was severely impaired. This patient lacked autonoetic consciousness and had severely impaired episodic memory. His difficulty was in the ability to "apprehend and to contemplate extended subjective time." His case suggests that amnesia may be characterized by an abnormality in consciousness as well as in the memory of past events. Tulving emphasizes the distinction between knowing and remembering so that the prior occurrence of specific events is meaningful. People do make judgments about the accuracy of their performance when asked about their memories. People can know something happened by remembering the event as their own experience. Tulving suggests that episodic memory has subjective certainty that leads to more effective action in the present and better planning for the future. Understanding consciousness and its emergence from the brain as consciousness of self is an ongoing challenge in the study of consciousness.

Regarding brain function, anoetic conscious involves the upper brain stem to the septum. Noetic (knowing) consciousness and learning involve the lower subcortical and upper limbic brain regions—for example, cortical midline structures. Autonomic consciousness (self-knowing) involves higher neocortical functions which include all association cortices that facilitate everyday awareness.

At a cortical level, mental events are the product of underlying neural capacity. This neural circuitry has both physical and symbolic structure. The mental event controls what is being constructed. We are born with a physical brain that is modified by experience in a continually evolving brain. Gazzaniga (2018) proposes that although we may describe its progression from the phenomenal brain stem to paleo-mammalian reflective (affective) consciousness to cortical self-awareness, "consciousness is inherent throughout the brain" (p. 231). Removing part of the cerebral cortex changes its contents but does not block consciousness. Consciousness is not localized as speech or vision; it is essential to all cognitive processing.

## Consciousness and the Split Brain

In split-brain subjects, when the corpus callosum is severed, typically as a last resort for treatment for refractory epilepsy, each hemisphere has separate perception, concepts, and behavior impulses (Gazzaniga, 2000; Figure 8.2).

Each hemisphere has its own conscious experiences. Consciousness has two independent sources. What are the implications of such split-brain studies? They suggest that there is no single brain circuit for consciousness. Because both cortical hemispheres are connected to the requisite hemispheric subcortical brain systems, there is consciousness. Subcortical processing alone is sufficient to produce conscious experience, albeit with more limited conscious content (Merker, 2007; Panksepp, 2004, 2005). Subcortical brain regions emerged early in evolution; they are autonomically, neurochemically, and functionally similar (MacLean, 1990; Panksepp, 2005). Thus, we can feel without a cognitive reporting of the feeling (Gazzaniga, 2018). Language enhances our conscious experiences, yet we may be conscious without it. Consciousness is sustained with language deprivation in the profoundly deaf and in children, who lack language exposure during development. Classic examples are Victor of Aveyron, the French feral (wild) child (Lane, 1976) who spent his childhood in the forest without exposure to language. He was studied by Itard at the behest of the French Academy of Sciences to test Étienne Bonnot, Abbé de Condillac's theory that all knowledge is acquired through the senses. Victor made limited gains over 5 years but did not develop normal language. Yet, he was

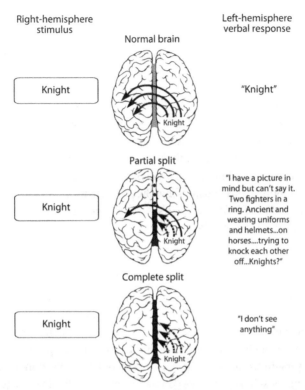

Right-hemisphere stimulus

Left-hemisphere verbal response

Normal brain

Knight

"Knight"

Knight

Partial split

Knight

"I have a picture in mind but can't say it. Two fighters in a ring. Ancient and wearing uniforms and helmets...on horses....trying to knock each other off...Knights?"

Knight

Complete split

Knight

"I don't see anything"

Knight

**Figure 8.2** Schematic representation of callosal resection in a spilt-brain patient. The location of callosal resection establishes what information is transferred between the cerebral hemispheres. (Top) In the normal brain, when the word "knight" is shown as a stimulus word to the right hemisphere, his left hemispheric verbal response is the word l hemis." (Middle) With partial callosal resection, when the word "knight" is presented to the right hemisphere, his left hemispheric verbal response is shown to be "I have a picture in my mind, but I can't say what it is." (Bottom) When the callosal resection is complete, when the "knight" stimulus word is presented to the right hemisphere, his left hemispheric verbal response is "I didn't see anything."

From Gazzaniga et al. (2019).

cooperative and fully conscious. Similarly, Genie, the child who was abused and systematically language deprived from at least age 20 months to age 13 years, never developed grammatical language despite at least 5 years of language instruction (Rymer, 1993). Another classical case is that of Phineas Gage, a railroad worker. A construction explosion forced a metal rod through his skull into the median and through the left frontal lobe. Yet, he did not lose consciousness in the moments after the accident. Despite the loss of a large part of the cognitive cortex, Gage could carry out his daily activities. However, he did develop social behavior deficits. He was not socially appropriate in his relationships but was no less conscious. Gage had poor emotional control. He was more easily agitated and aggressive, indicating less regulation of subconscious emotions.

Gazzaniga (2000) accounts for conscious preservation in these examples by proposing the adult brain, in which brain functions have already been localized in the brain systems because the specified layered cortical networks in the language area of the left cerebral cortex are already established. Losing these regionally specific brain regions results in the loss of brain functions. Yet, the mind persists and maintains continuous consciousness. These relatively independent specified brain regions essentially provide a localized link to consciousness for that function, which are supported by subcortical processing. Therefore, local specified brain circuits provide the contents of consciousness. How, then, do these specialized brain regions that are organized in layers, each of which is linked to consciousness, result in the mental experiences that follow from one moment to the next over time? How is the gap between objective neuronal events and subjective mental events so consistently bridged? It is important to keep in mind that consciousness, as we are defining it in animals and humans, must have been present throughout evolution. Consciousness has been present in human evolution, from *Australopithecus* to *Homo habilis* (stone tool use) to *Homo erectus* to modern *Homo sapiens*, and has become increasingly refined.

Over evolutionary time, the brain has become larger and more complex with the establishment of new adaptive capacities. This has led to different layers of brain organization. Consciousness develops in these different layers of brain organization that operate on their own timescale. Unlike neural events, mental states emerge from bottom-up neuronal changes. Emergent mental states (thoughts, desires, and beliefs) subsequently regulate neuronal events top-down. There is ongoing reciprocity between bottom-up activity and top-down choices. The whole brain constrains its parts; overall, there is a hierarchy of layers linked to cell biology and physiology involved in the emergence of conscious and unconscious processes (Gazzaniga et al., 2019). The integration of these hierarchically organized layers is a subject of ongoing study.

In theoretical biology, Howard Pattee (2012) proposed that genotype–phenotype modeling of gene replication provides an example of upward and downward causation. In his example, genes determine sequences that produce enzymes, and in turn, the enzyme is involved in the next step in development. He writes, "The parts represented by codons are in part, controlling the construction of the whole (enzymes) but the whole is in part controlling the identification of the parts (genetic translation) and the construction of itself (protein synthesis)."

Gazzaniga (2018) suggests viewing mind–brain layers helps in understanding how mental states and beliefs act. In psychiatry, Adolf Meyer's psychobiology approach and George Engel's biopsychosocial model focus on hierarchal systems at the social level of interaction and emphasize the context of interpersonal relationships (G. Engel, 1980; Muncie, 1948). For example, a functional magnetic resonance imaging (fMRI) study concurrently measured activity in the brains of two people speaking to one another. In this study, the activity of the listener's brain mirrored that of the person speaking to them. Brain regions anticipated the responses of the other brain. One person's behavior affected the other's behavior (Hasson et al., 2012).

At the social level of analyses, the layers of brain organization are beyond basic neuronal functions. Social engagement and socially responsive behavior are social concepts. When whole brain integration is between two people, the study found that a person's behavior is not simply determined by the brain bottom-up; it can be regulated by social constraints.

Consciousness is the product of thousands of specialized brain systems with specialized neuronal circuits. These circuits enable mental representation of the features of conscious experience. From moment to moment, these specialized systems vie with others for conscious attention. This dynamic movement fluctuates as consciousness moves freely from one thought to the next to create a unified narrative.

## Autobiographical Consciousness

The unified narrative we create is mediated through language into an extended narrative framework that culminates in autobiographical consciousness (Nelson & Fivush, 2020). The narrative framework draws on autobiographical memory that develops in the context of social relationships. It encompasses memories of a child, who interacts with a changing interpersonal and physical environment. This interaction leads to increased organization and integration at the interface of the developing mind with the external world. *Autobiographical memory* is defined as "an explicit memory of an event that occurred in a specific time and place in one's personal past" (Nelson & Fivush, 2004, p. 486).

Autobiographical memory gradually develops across the preschool years. Its emergence takes place in the context of language use, memory, and the developing self. There are individual and gender differences and cultural factors that characterize autobiographical memory. The components that come together in autobiographical memory include basic memory systems, acquisition of complex language, narrative comprehension, narrative production, talking about memories with parents and other people, an understanding of past and present time, personal selfhood, and psychological understanding of intentionality (theory of mind). Autobiographical memory emerges developmentally from these components. Emergence refers to the arising of a new structural layer of complexity from the interaction of existing structural layers located in the brain at levels of layered organization (MacWhinney, 1999).

Emergence can be witnessed during human development. A newborn infant emerges from a single cell (the zygote) because of interactions that involve the molecular level (DNA), the cellular level, and organ growth within the uterus. Similarly, emergence applies to psychological development as new autobiographical memories are formed. Emergence and human structural context are important in neuroconstructionist models of development. Autobiographical memory is the developmental outcome of a culturally embedded cognitive system. In this system, the components are experienced over time and, in particular contexts, for each individual. Autobiographical memory is significant because of its personal meaning, making it functionally distinct from other forms of memory (see Memory chapter). Typically, children by age 4 or soon after have mastered the elements for establishing of autobiographical memory. Important among them are self-representation, the ability to understand the perspective of others (theory of mind), narrative structure and context, episodic memory, and conversations with others about past and future.

When we consider autobiographical consciousness, both autobiographical memory and language are key components. Language is important in the development of autobiographical consciousness because it is used to engage others outwardly through explicit verbal communication and inwardly with interior thought. Language provides the means for personal engagement with others and self-reflection. The linguistically mediated understanding of mind allows a narratively structural perceptive for autobiographical consciousness. Autobiographical consciousness has its beginnings in mother–child narratives. These narratives facilitate the child's emergent sense of the self–other dialogue. The narrative might begin with reminiscences of past experiences in the pre-school years. Throughout childhood and adolescence, such dialogue culminates in reflective awareness of one's consciousness of lived experiences. Autobiographical consciousness moves beyond memories of specific past events to the establishment of a self, extended through time with an enhanced capacity to find meaning in one's life (Nelson & Fivush, 2020).

## Generation of Consciousness Within the Brain

Consciousness is actively generated within the brain. Neurons of the brain stem reticular formation play a central role in maintaining consciousness. An alert individual visually scans the environment, shifts attention to objects of interest, and integrates sensory information to generate a simulation of the sensory world that results in phenomenal sensory consciousness (Merker, 2007). The model generated within the brain is a virtual reality–based model based on our perceptions.

The neural correlates of consciousness have been examined in identified brain areas involved in producing consciousness in the normal healthy brain using functional brain imaging methodologies (fMRI, resting-state fMRI, positron emission tomography [PET], electroencephalography [evoked EEG], and magnetoencephalography [MEG]). Studies with fMRI and PET show where the neural correlates of consciousness are located in the brain, and EEG and MEG measures indicate when a perceived stimulus reaches consciousness (Revonsuo, 2018). EEG and MEG measures reveal that it takes 200–300 ms to process a stimulus entering consciousness. Transcranial magnetic stimulation releases brief magnetic pulses to the cortex that interfere with ongoing brain activity in that brain region, thus briefly inhibiting regional brain activity, and show whether that region is needed for conscious perception.

Brain regions necessary for consciousness have been examined by administering anesthetic drugs. fMRI and PET reveal that consciousness is abolished by anesthetics and then resumes on waking. These studies find that when consciousness is extinguished by anesthetics, there are changes in the thalamus (Alkire et al., 2008; Alkire & Miller, 2005). The thalamus is the primary brain center through which sensory information enters the cortex. Information regularly converges between the thalamus and cortex; anesthesia prevents neural activity in these thalamocortical loops. Anesthesia affects diffusely distributed nonspecific global connections from the thalamus to cortex (Liu et al., 2013). This global network of connectivity integrates information throughout the brain and establishes the background state of waking consciousness. Fast brainwave activity in thalamocortical connections integrates the different contents of consciousness into a unified consciousness (Alkire et al., 2008).

Visual consciousness is the main mode of continuous perception in awake humans. There are two distinct visual systems (Milner & Goodale, 2008). The ventral "perceptual" stream establishes a detailed map of the world from visual input that is used for cognitive engagement with the everyday world. The dorsal "action" stream transforms visual information into a coordinating system for skilled visual action planning and co-ordination. The ventral visual system is the "what" system—that is, the use of vision to recognize and identify. The dorsal system is the "where" system—that is, vision for ac-tion that involves visual guidance of actions and recognition of where they are in space. The ventral visual system involves a complex set of cortical areas. It is proposed that the temporal lobe creates a coarse sketch of what we see that is refined with details added from V1 and adjacent visual areas (Revonsuo, 2018).

Other brain areas activated in visual consciousness are regions of the frontal and parietal cortex (Dehaene & Changeux, 2011). The frontoparietal region involved in attention and working memory is also involved in reflective consciousness. Thus, im-mediately after information enters phenomenal consciousness, it is moved into reflec-tive consciousness, where information is needed to make a decision or to accomplish a task to meet a goal.

Conscious experience begins in infancy and develops throughout childhood into adult life as the individual becomes increasingly conscious of the external world and reflects on their life experiences. Self-reflection strengthens the capacity for self-control and personal decision-making. Everyday visual consciousness is a single, unified visual spatial world in three-dimensional consciousness. Objects having color and shape are perceived in motion. How does the brain bind color and shape together? Wolf Singer ( C. Engel & Singer, 2008) proposes that a unique feature of waking consciousness is its coherence. There is a continuous change in the contents of consciousness of the present that varies from one moment to the next. There is growing coherence in phe-nomenal awareness as contents of consciousness are related to one another. There is a close relationship between consciousness and the binding of brain systems together. Only contents bound together will simultaneously enter consciousness (Metzinger, 2009). This binding is referred to as the "binding problem" because we do not know how binding occurs; it links consciousness to attention and short-term memory. Stimuli must be attended to be perceived and to access short-term memory. The reason that binding must be considered relates to consciousness being organized as a highly dis-tributed system; large numbers of mental operations are carried out in parallel. There is no single center for convergence when parallel compilations can be bound coherently. Multiple brain modules are interconnected in densely reciprocal connections. There are at least 30–40 brain areas that process aspects of visual information. These connections generate order through self-organizing mechanisms. Moreover, representations of such complex cognitive contents are distributed within the brain. Conscious contents in-clude perceived objects, thoughts, plans for action, and memories that are reactivated into consciousness.

Neuronal systems recognize the present moment as made up of parts of such dis-tributed systems. This recognition is signaled by changes in neuronal discharge frequency. However, it remains to be clarified how neurons signal and how they co-operate. This cooperation involves the synchronization of discharges from individual neurons. Such synchronization involves neuronal engagement in rhythmic oscillatory discharges. These were first described in the visual cortex in the 1990s. Current evi-dence indicates that the synchronization of oscillatory activity is the mechanism for the binding of distributed brain processes. Oscillatory frequencies are different for dif-ferent brain modules. For example, in the cerebral cortex, the typical range of beta and gamma oscillation is 20–80 Hz. Synchronization takes place in association with various functions that are pertinent for conscious experience (Metzinger, 2009). Oscillations occur when perceptual objects are encoded as coherent representations of them. Oscillations are recorded when a person directs their attention toward an object and returns information about the object in working memory. Such oscillations are consistent and distinctive correlations of conscious perception. The evidence for this is that during conscious perception, very widely distributed regions of the cerebral cortex are observed to transiently engage one another through precisely synchronized high-frequency oscillations.

When a stimulus is not consciously perceived, although the regions still engage some high-frequency oscillation, this localized processing does not enter into globally synchronized patterns. Focused conscious attention is required for global synchronization and consciousness. Therefore, access to consciousness requires the engagement of a sufficiently large number of processing areas semantically bound by synchronization so that coherent states of mind can be maintained over time. This synchronization accounts for the unity of consciousness (Metzinger, 2009).

Further research is expected to lead to even more detailed descriptions of these states. The eventual goal is to reveal the semantic content—that is, the actual meaning. It is hoped that it will eventually become possible to understand how altering the contents of consciousness is linked to neuronal activity and the contents of phenomenal awareness. These patterns of neuronal activation that give rise to subjective feelings, emotions, etc. "will probably remain a conundrum for quite some time, even if we arrive at precise descriptions for neuronal states of consciousness" (Metzinger, 2009, p. 69). The challenge is to understand how information is encoded in distributed networks. A related challenge is to determine how subjective feelings emerge from such distributed neuronal activity. Coordinated research is needed because phenomena that are traditionally the subject matter of the humanities (e.g., empathy, altruism, and shared attention) are being studied using neuroscientific methods.

When we examine consciousness and the brain, direct evidence is drawn from two sources: measures of brain activity during waking and sleeping in healthy persons and studies of neuropsychological patients who have experienced a brain lesion that affects an aspect of consciousness. Features of consciousness involve specific areas of the brain associated with particular aspects of consciousness. Brain injury may result in a distortion or loss of subjective experience (Revonsuo, 2018). When a healthy person performs a task involving this type of consciousness, brain experience is revealed; injury eliminates that particular aspect of consciousness. For example, visual consciousness loss is found in visual agnosia, loss of vision for coherent visual objects, with damage to the visual cortex. In unilateral spatial neglect, elements of perceptual space disappear from consciousness due to damage to the right posterior parietal lobe. Brain-damaged patients may also dissociate and lose subjective experience of an environmental stimulus. They report that they do not perceive objective measurements of revealed stimulus. Therefore, information is still being processed by the brain but outside their conscious awareness. Thus, there can be differences between conscious and unconscious information processing in the brain.

Other examples are blindsight dissociation involving neural damage to the primary visual cortex ($V_1$). These include blindsight (loss of conscious vision coupled with the ability to accurately guess visual features); prosopagnosia (defect in face recognition), in which familiar faces look like complete strangers; and neglect, in which the individual loses awareness of the left side of perceptual space (damage to the right posterior parietal lobe). In these instances, the brain processes information of the a situation at both the conscious level and the nonconscious level. Finally, self-awareness may be distorted after brain damage. In this instance, there is loss of self-awareness that the brain is injured. When self-aware, we have momentary consciousness of ourselves as persons.

The self is a lasting self with a past and a future. This loss of awareness occurs with amnesia. Amnesia is a disorder of self-awareness as much as it is of memory. In the other deficits described, something is gone from phenomenal consciousness. With loss of self-awareness, we lose our capacity to perceive ourselves as embodied persons with a sense of continuity in time. Loss of self-awareness in amnesia is retrograde when there is loss of old memories before a head injury. If one cannot form new memories after an accident, it is referred to as anterograde amnesia. People with both retrograde and anterograde amnesia have global amnesia. In summary, once the brain is injured, the conscious mind is affected as well. The change in consciousness depends on the size and location of the brain damage.

## Dreaming and Consciousness

Dream consciousness involves mental activity that is remarkably like waking consciousness. That dreaming generates consciousness without external sensory stimuli is consistent with consciousness being an internally generated and constructive process.

David Foulkes (1985) proposed that dreaming is a mental phenomenon that is important in processing and consolidating cognitive information. Viewed cognitively, dreams are a form of consciousness that is coherently organized to simulate waking reality. Viewed across time, a series of dreams develops a continuous narrative. A cognitive-psychological approach to dreaming is largely based on examining dreams recorded in dream diaries, and content is systematically analyzed. With the rise of the cognitive approach, dream consciousness is examined as a form of consciousness that studies subjective mental experiences as psychological phenomena and views dreaming as a virtual reality simulator. Dream consciousness is linked to neural events that involve brain activity in space and time (Nir & Tononi, 2010). The medial prefrontal cortex, as part of the default brain network, is very active in dreaming activity (and is correlated with rapid eye movement [REM] sleep), just as it is in wakefulness when at rest.

Dreaming is more closely related to imagination. In imagination, brain activity moves in a top-down manner. If dream images are viewed as imagination, this may account for dream features including sudden transitions, poor subsequent recall, and disconnectedness. Since the discovery of REM sleep in humans (Aserinsky & Kleitman, 1953) and its correlation with dream activity (Dement & Kleitman, 1957), researchers have sought to identify the neuronal mechanisms of dreaming. Hobson (2009) has proposed a theory of consciousness based on the study that dreaming constitutes a proto-consciousness state important to adaptive waking consciousness. Consciousness varies throughout the sleep–wake cycle.

## The Functions of Dreams

There are four leading theories regarding the functions of dreams: (a) Dreams are random and have no function, (b) dreams are essential to problem-solving, (c) dreams are important to mental health through emotion regulation and imaginative imagery, and (d) dreaming is the brain's reality generator that provides a variety of narrative scenarios to prepare us to adapt to the everyday world. Among these, mood regulation and problem-solving are encompassed in the important role that REM sleep and dreaming play in virtual reality and adaptation.

Dreaming has been viewed as serving no meaningful function, essentially a side effect of brain activations, but more recently it has been viewed as playing a meaningful role in adaptive functioning. Random activation theory views dreams as random and not meaningful. Conversely, dreaming has been viewed as not random but, rather, as having a creative purpose whose goal is to find solutions to problems; this is the problem-solving theory of dreaming. Dreaming also has been proposed as important to mental health and for psychotherapy, its purpose being to regulate our emotions and enhance our sense of well-being. Importantly, dreaming has been proposed as a virtual reality simulation of the waking world. Virtual simulation allows us to rehearse social scenarios in dreams to prepare for life challenges.

Hobson (2009) has proposed a virtual simulation theory of consciousness based on the study of dreaming. Hobson's model constitutes a state of proto-consciousness in preparation for the next day's waking consciousness. Hobson proposes that abundant REM sleep in infants produces a simulation of reality preparing the infant to engage the real world on waking and that virtual reality simulation continues throughout life.

We are consciously aware when we are awake and also aware of being aware. When asleep, we are consciously aware when dreaming and have perceptions and emotions in dreaming that may be more vivid in lucid dreams. During waking, various states of consciousness arise as we adapt to psychosocial and environmental challenges and reflect on them. Unlike waking, in dreams, we are isolated and single-minded and nonreflective. There is generally a thematic coherence in the dream narrative. When dreaming, a single train of related thoughts and images persists in dreams and may continue over an extended period to be recorded in dream diaries (Rechtschaffen, 1978).

Dreaming is most reliably reported during REM sleep. In the sleep laboratory, 80–90% of awakenings in REM sleep result in dream narrative reports. Imagery is reported in 25–50% of awakenings. Referred as sleep mentation (not dreaming), these typically are static images of a visual object or scene. As shown in Figure 8.3, there is a continuum of consciousness during a night's sleep. Consciousness may be totally absent (dreamless sleep), or there may be simple and repetitive thoughts or images (sleep mentation) and the appearance of static scenes intermediate with sleep mentation and dreaming. Finally, during genuine dreams, the person is conscious and involves themself in a dream narrative.

REM sleep is present in development long before dreams are reported. Ultrasound imaging allows visualization of fetal eye movements consistent with REM being identified in utero as early as 23 weeks of gestation and makes up the majority of sleep throughout pregnancy, peaking in the last trimester. REM sleep predominates sleep in the third trimester of pregnancy and in the first year of life, but it progressively decreases

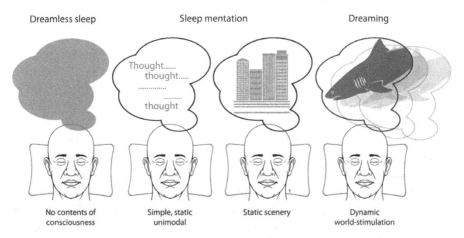

| Dreamless sleep | Sleep mentation | | Dreaming |

| No contents of consciousness | Simple, static unimodal | Static scenery | Dynamic world-stimulation |

**Figure 8.3** The continuum of consciousness during sleep: dreamless sleep, sleep mentation, and dreaming sleep. Consciousness is totally absent in dreamless sleep. Images and thoughts are present in sleep mentation. In dreaming, animated virtual reality narratives are experienced by the dreamer.

From Revonsuo (2018); redrawn by Tim Phelps (2021).

as waking time during the day increases. Concurrently, non-REM sleep, much like waking time, increases following birth. Despite its decline, REM sleep occupies approximately 1.5 hr per day throughout life (Hong et al., 2018). In animal studies, REM sleep is reported to be involved in synaptic pruning and synaptic maintenance (Li et al., 2017). Thus, REM sleep is essential for brain–mind development and equally important throughout life in the maintenance of the mind–brain.

After birth, the amount of REM sleep steeply declines until age 9 or 10 years, more gradually during the adolescent years, and more or less stabilizes in late adult life but persists throughout the lifetime. However, dream consciousness is not associated with REM sleep until the brain has developed to the point where the narrative organization of subjective experience is possible. When do children report dreams? In preschool children, dreams are simple and tend to be static images, such as thinking about eating or seeing an animal. There is little feeling or fear, no social interactions, and the child is not a character in the dream. Children aged 2–5 years do not report dreams about people or events. Autobiographical memory is not established until age 4 or 5 years. This is the beginning appearance of episodic memories and the early creation of an autobiographic narrative. Between ages 5 and 7 years, dreams may contain sequences of events with characters, who move around and interact but are infrequent with limited narration. At approximately age 7 years, children identify themselves as a character participating in a dream whose thoughts and feelings may be expressed. Notably, night terrors, which occur in young children, are not dreams; they are arousal disorders from deep sleep (Nir & Tononi, 2010).

Based on dream reports recorded in children by Foulkes (2009), dreams were reported only 20% of the time when children were awakened from REM sleep compared to 80–90% for adults. Based on extensive studies of children's dreams during development, Foulkes (2009) regarded dreams as creating analogs in experiences in the everyday world. Dreams are an organized form of consciousness that simulates daily life experiences. Children with the most highly developed visual–spatial skills, not those with the best verbal or memory abilities, have the most developed mental imagery. Visuospatial ability may be tested using the block design test on the Wechsler Intelligence Scales. Visuospatial skills correlate with children's dream reports. Visuospatial skills are linked to the development of the parietal lobe, which is not fully myelinated before age 7 years.

REM sleep is important in the development of behaviors that become automatic and self-organizing. In a classic experiment, Michael Jouvet (1973) lesioned the pontine to inhibit movement during REM sleep in the cat. To his surprise, the sleeping cat moved during REM sleep when typically it should be immobile. The cat movements were those of stalking prey, grooming, and acting aggressively. Jouvet proposed that in REM sleep, the cat was practicing behavior preparatory for action. Similarly, threat stimulation theory states that dreaming about threatening events is anticipatory (Revonsuo, 2000; Valli & Revonsuo, 2009). Threat simulation theory proposes that dreaming simulates the virtual reality of threatening situations by activating emotional memories to prepare us for future danger (Metzinger, 2009). Effective threat simulation in dreams could increase survival by dream practice—for example, through dreams of chases, escapes, attacks, or floods. Moreover, nonthreatening situations may also be rehearsed in dreams, such as social interactions with others. These studies are consistent with the notion that sleep is preparatory for daily activity.

Hobson proposes that both waking consciousness and consciousness in dreams are constructive (Hobson, 2009; Hobson et al., 2014). In this model, dreaming prepares and informs everyday consciousness. Dreaming and waking consciousness states are complementary mental states both necessary for adaptation (Hobson et al., 2014). Waking consciousness responds and adapts to external sensory input to the brain. In dreaming, the brain generates consciousness without external sensory stimuli. Basically, consciousness is an internally constructive process that takes place in waking and sleeping. The brain perceives and infers the causes of sensory input, making conscious experience exclusively internal. Whether awake or dreaming, the brain is motivated by sensory input. The world that we perceive is a world generated by the hierarchal and parallel processing systems in the brain that infers our world; the perceived world we see is a "virtual reality." What we perceive as the bodily self in wakefulness is a construct of the brain that emerges from multisensory integration of the bodily self. A bodily self, generated in neural networks, is supported by reports that at least 20% of people born without limbs (phocomelia) experience phantom limbs without sensory input from the limbs (Melzack et al., 1997). Thus, our waking perception is based on a reconstruction of a model of the world by the brain. That capacity to model or infer this world underlies perception both in waking and in dreaming (Hobson et al., 2014).

Helmholtz proposed in 1860 that perception anticipates knowledge-driven probabilities for making choices in facing challenges (Clark, 2013). His insights have been updated in modern computational neuroscience, resulting in predictive coding theory—that is, built-in neuronal implementation of active inference models. Predictive coding is a theory that the brain is constantly generating and updating a mental model of the environment that is compared to actual sensory input. Predictive coding proposes how the sentient brain makes inferences about the world and examines false inferences in psychopathology (Fletcher & Frith, 2009; Quattrocki & Friston, 2014). The brain infers causes of sensations, constructing explanations that minimize surprise (i.e., reduce prediction error). Overall, the brain generates a hypothesis about what causes sensory input (i.e., predictive coding) and essentially tests the hypothesis by comparing it with already sampled data to clarify if there is a discrepancy. In doing so, it updates its ongoing internal model of the world, passing messages between the higher and lower level of cortical circuits.

The human brain has a hierarchal structure so that output at one level is the input of the next higher one. This results in progressively higher but also deeper levels of explanation; the higher, the more integrated. The hierarchal approach to human cognition (understanding the mind in action) may be integrated into narrative psychology. This entails placing the personal narrative at the top of a mental personal knowledge hierarchy. Narratives direct our attention to and structure our expectations about life events as they unfold; this may occur at the highest levels of the predictive hierarchy. New sensory information is interpreted to anticipate the unfolding of events over time, sequence and plan goal-directed action, determine the emotional significance of an event in present time, and maintain personal identity. Also, active inference and predictive coding models can integrate interoceptions, our sense of the internal physiology of the body. For example, one mechanism of interoceptive predictive coding addresses emotional responses (Seth et al., 2011) and multisensory integration of the self (Seth, 2013). Here, the brain infers its bodily self from visual, tactile proprioceptive, and vestibular input. Conversely, predictive interoceptive coding helps to understand the failure of predictive integration—for example, understanding the disturbed perception of the bodily self in anorexia nervosa and body dysmorphic disorder (Gaudio et al., 2014).

The awake brain is modulated by sensory stimuli, in keeping with predictive coding theory, by engaging the external world and recognizing internal bodily states. Thus, our working perception reconstructs the external and interior world in waking life. However, the capacity to predict the world is guided not only by waking perception but also by dreaming. There is evidence that a dream is a prelude to our waking perception. In waking, we link conscious and unconscious perceptions with the production of sensory input generated by internal stimuli emanating from the brain. There is evidence that this mechanism is optimized in sleep to generalize to new situations that arise during waking life. This optimization facilitates greater efficiency in interpretation of sensory data (Hobson et al., 2014). Importantly, optimization in sleep is based on the same neuronal mechanisms that are utilized with our waking perception: synaptic activity and synaptic plasticity. Thus, dreaming is a mechanism for optimizing in which dream imagery and narrative utilize the perceptional inference construct. Because dreaming is very highly correlated with REM sleep, its functions underlie the neurobiology of conscious and unconscious processing. The isolation and encapsulation of dreaming consciousness during sleep allow the freedom to rehearse imaginative scenarios that could be encountered in waking life (Revonsuo, 1995, 2006). Thus, the embodied self—that is, first-person consciousness—is dynamically constructed during dreaming and carried forth renewed and prepared to adapt to daily life challenges. REM sleep in this hypothesis is an opportunity to clarify and potentially optimize a generative model of the self that integrates experience from the previous day to prepare for the next.

## Differences in Waking and Dreaming

Support for the previously discussed explanations of dreaming is based on formal analyses of the phenomenology and not on the traditional psychological views of dream content and interpretation. The focus is on the formal structure of dreaming and, importantly, on the neuroanatomy involved in subjective processing. Thus, emphasis is placed on formal analysis of the form of the dream, not dream content. Such formal analysis allows for the study of how virtual reality is generated in the brain. For example, formal analysis of dreams includes sensory perception (visually, whether the dream is in color or black and white, etc.), visual scanning, language, motor control, multisensory binding, and organization of intrinsic brain networks (Hobson et al., 2014; Hong et al., 2009; Koike et al., 2011). Formal analyses recognize the vividness of a dream, lack of cognitive reflection during a dream, intensity or absence of feeling in a dream, and the lack of ability to predict what might come next in a dream. Dreams, as first-person accounts, notify our waking self what to expect; waking experiences either confirm or refute such expectations. In summary, dreams are not simply the replay of remembered experiences from daily life. Instead, dreams synthesize daily life experiences. Dreaming tends to be associated with a greater depth of emotion than waking.

Hobson's (2009) virtual reality dream theory calls for exploration of the vast repertoire of predictive dream scripts. Hobson proposes that these dream scripts and scenarios are continuously rehearsed during dreaming. Such rehearsal provides preparatory adaptive resources to be taken up by the awake sensorium to pursue. Hobson's hypothesis emphasizes that dreaming and REM sleep are conscious. Inference is important in optimizing virtual reality scenarios in the brain. Hobson proposes that the system is optimized to minimize complexity and redundancy by reducing the complexity of synaptic connections in the brain. These scenarios are rehearsed during dreaming. Therefore, dreaming prepares the brain for the unpredictable range and variety of real-world situations that one may encounter while awake. While awake, daydreaming may also provide creative solutions by temporarily suspending cognitive judgment. Basically, the brain in daydreaming is doing something similar to dreaming in sleep. The difference is that there is no sensory input during sleep to distract the dreamer.

Experiences while awake are revised during dreaming to allow different hierarchal representations to become more consistent with fewer errors. This process ends with a revised hierarchal inference scenario that may generalize to the wide variety of sensory experiences encountered while awake. The physiology of sleep that underlies these functions must also be considered. The transition from wakefulness to sleep is based on selective gating of sensory inputs inherent in the neurochemistry of the sleep–wake cycle (Hobson, 2009).

Studying eye movements during sleep is important in understanding how REM sleep is associated with higher levels of consciousness. They are key for identifying multisensory recruitment into dream consciousness that occurs during REM sleep (Hong et al., 2009). Hong et al. found changes in brain regional activation that were correlated during REM sleep. It was found to be widespread using fMRI to study REM-locked brain activation. Peak brain activity was found in both primary visual cortex and nonvisual sensory cortex—that is, in the regions that are implicated in perceptual binding of attributes of visual perception of shape, movement, and color. This perceptual binding creates both a visual and a nonvisual perception. Neural correlates of binding during wakefulness and during REM sleep involve synchronous gamma oscillations (Crick & Koch, 2003; Gross & Gotman, 1999; Hong et al., 2009). It is proposed by Crick and Koch, Gross and Gotman, and Hong et al. that the thalamic reticular nucleus and claustrum are crucial for the binding of information. In the fMRI study of REM sleep by Hong et al., there was peak activation in both the thalamic nucleus and the claustrum. The claustrum is densely connected to other brain regions, making it important in salience detection (Smythies et al., 2014). The claustrum is important in sensorimotor integration and in generating consciousness in both awake and dreaming states. Dreaming ceases after a prefrontal lobotomy, which disrupts thalamocortical projections. In individuals with posterior left hemisphere damage, the capacity to generate visual imagery from their long-term memory while awake is lost. In individuals whose corpus callosum is surgically severed in the treatment for refractory epilepsy, left posterior localization is affected (Farah et al., 1985).

The same neuronal systems are shared in awake visual perception and dreaming. Scanning eye movements play a generative role in the awake visual life and in dreaming. In dreaming, rapid eye movements may re-enact the scan path of the eyes in awake visual perception of the same scene and thus retrieve the visual information encoded by the scan path (Hong et al., 2009). Image generation from scanning eye movements is consistent with active inference and predictive coding theory. Rapid eye movement–locked activation in supplemental eye fields in the left hemisphere provides evidence that rapid eye movements scan visual imagery. The left supplemental eye fields are involved in sequencing saccadic eye movements (rapid eye movement between eye fixation points) in awake vision. It has been demonstrated that single-unit neuronal activity and intracranial EEG time-locked to the rapid eye movements in neurosurgical epilepsy patients can be measured (Andrillon et al., 2015). Regions scanned included structures in the ventral visual pathway, the so-called "why" pathway associated with visual memory processing, which revealed that the most robust REM-locked activation is localized to the primary visual cortex, the thalamic reticular nucleus, and the visual claustrum.

Hong et al. (2018) proposed that rapid eye movements provide a unique probe into dreaming consciousness. Essentially, active vision is internalized during sleep. As evidence, there is a homology in ponto-geniculo-occipital (PGO) waves in REM sleep and a neurophysiological response that follows oculomotor reflexes during saccadic searches of a visual scene. PGO waves during REM sleep are internally generated phasic activation signals for the dreaming brain–mind. They also convey to the thalamus and cortex feedforward information about the direction of upcoming eye movements. Thus, they are efferent copies of stimuli from oculomotor circuits to the visual forebrain. Continuity of awake consciousness is in part regarded to be a function of wave dampening, whereas the discontinuity of dream consciousness is regarded as a function of PGO wave disinhibition. Efferent copies play a key role in saccadic suppression of sensory attenuation. In predictive coding theory, the efferent copy is equivalent to a discharge that mediates top-down predictions and sensory attenuation. This suggests that REM sleep reflects rehearsal of active visual engagement and provides a perceptual synthesis engaging the outside world from a first-person perspective. During sleep onset, the same neuronal systems are engaged to experience the same images in dreaming (Horikawa et al., 2013).

EEG and fMRI studies provide promising evidence for a common neural architecture for virtual experience across REM sleep, non-REM sleep, and wakefulness. Recognition of virtual reality and conscious inference in dreaming and their neural underpinning supports a theory of consciousness derived from the study of dreaming. This hypothesis provides compelling support for Hobson's (2009) proposal that REM sleep may constitute a protoconscious state that offers a virtual reality model of the world—one that is used to facilitate the development and maintenance of waking and consciousness for social adaptation. This primary consciousness provides a building block on which secondary consciousness is constructed utilizing self-awareness, abstract thinking, and metacognition. Dream consciousness (a subjective, psychological state) integrates perception and emotion to create a rich and reliable representation of the world by integrating disparate images and themes into a dream scenario.

Awake and REM sleep states both involve activation of the corticothalamic and limbic systems that are responsible for conscious experience (Hobson, 2009). Dreaming is hyperassociative in that it moves quickly from one image to another, and it is also synthetic because only 20% of a dream is remembered by the dreamer as related to specific life history (Fosse et al., 2003). Hobson (2009) proposes that dreaming introduces the "set of foreordained scripts or scenarios" (p. 807) to organize our waking experience. Consistent with Carl Jung's (1968) views of the objective or archetypal unconscious, dreams provide narrative charts that draw on mythological motifs. These motifs allow us to navigate the world by drawing on a library of alternative adaptive plots with sufficient verisimilitude to make meaningful choices. The activation of the forebrain without external environment input during sleep may provide an automatic built-in sense of self-organization that offers a solution to the binding problem of consciousness.

## Consciousness and the Binding Problem

The binding problem is central to modern theories of consciousness. It asks how brain mechanisms construct moment-to-moment continuity in the experience of consciousness (Singer, 2001). Dreaming is proposed to link primary to secondary adaptive consciousness. For binding, neurons must be corrected and activated in temporal unison. With intrinsic activation of the brain, a proto-self is established in REM sleep. Dreams are experienced as a first-person narrative, leading us to believe that we are the central figure in the dream. On waking, we are aware that we were dreaming.

In lucid dreaming, aspects of waking consciousness are restored (Voss et al., 2009). Lucid dreaming is rare but involves both primary and secondary consciousness circuits. In the shift from nonlucid to lucid dreaming, changes in frontal EEG activity may indicate synchronization of such cortical activity as to result in temporal binding characteristics of awake consciousness (Voss et al., 2009). The cortex is more synchronized in the lucid dream. Lucid dreamers are aware they are dreaming and do as they choose in a dream world. Lucidity occurs during continuous REM sleep with no disruption in sleep continuity. Lucidity is a skill that can be learned. When a dreamer is lucid, parts of the brain typically suppressed become activated (Dresler et al., 2012). The dreamer enters a dream stage that allows them to exercise control or reflect on the dream experience. Voss et al. (2014) used external electrical stimulation during REM sleep on sleeping subjects at frequencies varying from 2 to 100 Hz while monitoring participants using EEG. Stimulation between 25 and 100 Hz induced reflective consciousness while dreaming. This study documented that lucid dreaming can be induced, allowing a framework to study changes in self-awareness as they take place (Voss et al., 2014; see also Revonsuo, 2018).

## Conclusion

The study of dream consciousness is important in modern cognitive neuroscience. It involves subjective dream reports along with objective studies of brain activity. While sleeping without sensory input, the brain generates dream experiences that involve multisensory brain activation. Reflective consciousness, other than in lucid dreaming, is diminished. Hobson's (2009) protoconscious proposal provides evidence that the ongoing development of awake consciousness and higher brain functioning is dependent on brain activation during REM sleep. This proposal emphasizes that the cooperative interaction between dreaming and awake states facilitates optimal adaptation. Hobson's findings substantially advance our understanding of the relation between the mind and brain functioning.

As we learn more from progress in developmental cognitive neuroscience about the emergence of mental functions from complex neuronal interactions, new insights will be gained toward our understanding of the mind–body problem, as well as a greater understanding of the brain's place in the valuation of experiences and how it distinguishes between appropriate and inappropriate behavior (Metzinger, 2009). The study of consciousness and how it emerges from the subjective brain is expected to continue to offer rich rewards to those who pursue the neurobiology of consciousness.

## References

Alkire, M. T., Hudetz, A. G., & Tononi, G. (2008). Consciousness and anesthesia. *Science*, *322*(5903), 876–880.

Alkire, M. T., & Miller, J. (2005). General anesthesia and the neural correlates of consciousness. *Progress in Brain Research*, *150*, 229–597.

Andrillon, T., Nir, Y., Cirelli, C., Tononi, G., & Fried, I. (2015). Single-neuron activity and eye movements during human REM sleep and awake vision. *Nature Communications*, *6*(1), 1–10.

Aserinsky, E., & Kleitman, N. (1953). Regularly occurring periods of eye motility, and concomitant phenomena, during sleep. *Science*, *118*(3062), 273–274.

Baars, B. J., Ramsøy, T. Z., & Laureys, S. (2003). Brain, conscious experience and the observing self. *Trends in Neurosciences*, *26*(12), 671–675.

Clark, A. (2013). Whatever next? Predictive brains, situated agents, and the future of cognitive science. *Behavioral and Brain Sciences*, *36*(3), 181–204.

Crick, F., & Koch, C. (2003). A framework for consciousness. *Nature Neuroscience*, *6*(2), 119–126.

Damasio, A. R. (1998). Investigating the biology of consciousness. *Philosophical Transactions of the Royal Society of London Series B: Biological Sciences*, *353*(1377), 1879–1882.

Damasio, A. R. (1999). *The feeling of what happens: Body and emotion in the making of consciousness*. Houghton Mifflin Harcourt.

Dehaene, S., & Changeux, J. P. (2011). Experimental and theoretical approaches to conscious processing. *Neuron, 70*(2), 200–227.

Dement, W., & Kleitman, N. (1957). The relation of eye movements during sleep to dream activity: An objective method for the study of dreaming. *Journal of Experimental Psychology, 53*(5), 339–346.

Dennett, D. C. (1991). *Consciousness explained*. Little, Brown.

Dresler, M., Wehrle, R., Spoormaker, V. I., Koch, S. P., Holsboer, F., Steiger, A., Obrig, H., Samann, P., & Czisch, M. (2012). Neural correlates of dream lucidity obtained from contrasting lucid versus non-lucid REM sleep: A combined EEG/fMRI case study. *Sleep, 35*(7), 1017–1020.

Edinger, E. F. (1984). *The creation of consciousness: Jung's myth for modern man*. Inner City Books.

Engel, C., & Singer, W. (2008). Better than conscious. In C. Engel & W. Singer (Eds.), Better *than conscious?* Decision *making,* the *human mind,* and *implications* for *institutions*. MIT Press.

Engel, G. L. (1980). The clinical application of the biopsychosocial model. *American Journal of Psychiatry, 137*(5), 535–544.

Farah, M. J., Gazzaniga, M. S., Holtzman, J. D., & Kosslyn, S. M. (1985). A left hemisphere basis for visual mental imagery? *Neuropsychologia, 23*(1), 115–118.

Fish, F. (1967). *Clinical psychopathology*. Wright.

Flanagan, O. (1992). *Consciousness reconsidered*, p. 220. MIT Press, Cambridge, MA.

Fletcher, P. C., & Frith, C. D. (2009). Perceiving is believing: A Bayesian approach to explaining the positive symptoms of schizophrenia. *Nature Reviews Neuroscience, 10*(1), 48–58.

Fosse, M. J., Fosse, R., Hobson, J. A., & Stickgold, R. J. (2003). Dreaming and episodic memory: A functional dissociation? *Journal of Cognitive Neuroscience, 15*(1), 1–9.

Foulkes, D. (1985). *Dreaming: A cognitive–psychological analysis*. Erlbaum.

Foulkes, D. (2009). *Children's dreaming and the development of consciousness*. Harvard University Press.

Gaudio, S., Brooks, S. J., & Riva, G. (2014). Nonvisual multisensory impairment of body perception in anorexia nervosa: A systematic review of neuropsychological studies. *PLoS One, 9*(10), e110087.

Gazzaniga, M. S. (2018). *The consciousness instinct: Unraveling the mystery of how the brain makes the mind*. Farrar, Straus & Giroux.

Gazzaniga, M. S. (2000). Cerebral specialization and interhemispheric communication: Does the corpus callosum enable the human condition? *Brain, 123*(7), 1293–1326.

Gazzaniga, M. S., Ivry, R. B., & Mangun, G. R. (2019). *Cognitive neuroscience: The biology of the mind* (5th ed.). Norton.

Gross, D. W., & Gotman, J. (1999). Correlation of high-frequency oscillations with the sleep–wake cycle and cognitive activity in humans. *Neuroscience, 94*(4), 1005–1018.

Harris, J. C. (2003). Social neuroscience, empathy, brain integration, and neurodevelopmental disorders. *Physiology & Behavior, 79*(3), 525–531.

Hasson, U., Ghazanfar, A. A., Galantucci, B., Garrod, S., & Keysers, C. (2012). Brain-to-brain coupling: A mechanism for creating and sharing a social world. *Trends in Cognitive Sciences, 16*(2), 114–121.

Hobson, J. A. (2009). REM sleep and dreaming: Towards a theory of protoconsciousness. *Nature Reviews Neuroscience, 10*(11), 803–813.

Hobson, J. A., Hong, C. C.-H., & Friston, K. J. (2014). Virtual reality and consciousness inference in dreaming. *Frontiers in Psychology, 5*, 1133.

Hong, C. C.-H., Fallon, J. H., Friston, K. J., & Harris, J. C. (2018). Rapid eye movements in sleep furnish a unique probe into consciousness. *Frontiers in Psychology, 9*, 2087.

Hong, C. C.-H., Harris, J. C., Pearlson, G. D., Kim, J. S., Calhoun, V. D., Fallon, J. H., Golay, X., Gillen, J. S., Simmonds, D. J., van Zijl, P. C., Zee, D. S., & Pekar, J. J. (2009). fMRI evidence for multisensory recruitment associated with rapid eye movements during sleep. *Human Brain Mapping, 30*(5), 1705–1722.

Horikawa, T., Tamaki, M., Miyawaki, Y., & Kamitani, Y. (2013). Neural decoding of visual imagery during sleep. *Science, 340*(6132), 639–642.

James, W. (1890). *The principles of psychology*. Harvard University Press.

Jaspers, K. (1963). *General psychopathology* (J. Hoenig & M. W. Hamilton, Trans.). Manchester University Press.

Jouvet, M. (1973). Essai sur le rêve. *Archives Italiennes de Biologie, 111*(3–4), 564–576.

Jung, C. G. (1968). *The archetypes and the collective unconsciousness*. Princeton University Press.

Koike, T., Kan, S., Misaki, M., & Miyauchi, S. (2011). Connectivity pattern changes in default-mode network with deep non-REM and REM sleep. *Neuroscience Research, 69*(4), 322–330.

Lane, H. (1976). *The wild boy of Aveyron* (Vol. 149). Harvard University Press.

LeDoux, J. (2012). Rethinking the emotional brain. *Neuron, 73*(4), 653–676.

Li, W., Ma, L., Yang, G., & Gan, W. B. (2017). REM sleep selectively prunes and maintains new synapses in development and learning. *Nature Neuroscience, 20*(3), 427–437.

Liu, X., Lauer, K. K., Ward, B. D., Li, S. J., & Hudetz, A. G. (2013). Differential effects of deep sedation with propofol on the specific and nonspecific thalamocortical systems: A functional magnetic resonance imaging study. *Anesthesiology, 118*(1), 59–69.

MacLean, P. D. (1952). Some psychiatric implications of physiological studies on frontotemporal portion of limbic system (visceral brain). *Electroencephalography & Clinical Neurophysiology, 4*(4), 407–418.

MacLean, P. D. (1985). Evolutionary psychiatry and the triune brain. *Psychological Medicine, 15*(2), 219–221.

MacLean, P. D. (1988). Evolution of audiovocal communication as reflected by the therapsid-mammalian transition and the limbic thalamocingulate division. In J. D. Newman (Ed.), *The physiological control of mammalian vocalization* (pp. 185–201). Springer.

MacLean, P. D. (1990). *The triune brain in evolution: Role in paleocerebral functions*. Springer.

MacWhinney, B. (1999). The emergence of language from embodiment. In B. MacWhinney (Ed.), *The emergence of language* (pp. 213–256). Erlbaum.

McAbee, G. N., Chan, A., & Erde, E. L. (2000). Prolonged survival with hydranencephaly: Report of two patients and literature review. *Pediatric Neurology, 23*(1), 80–84.

Melzack, R., Israel, R., Lacroix, R., & Schultz, G. (1997). Phantom limbs in people with congenital limb deficiency or amputation in early childhood. *Brain, 120*(9), 1603–1620.

Merker, B. (2007). Consciousness without a cerebral cortex: A challenge for neuroscience and medicine. *Behavioral and Brain Sciences, 30*(1), 63–81.

Metzinger, T. (2009). *The ego tunnel: The science of the mind and the myth of the self*. Basic Books.

Milner, A. D., & Goodale, M. A. (2008). Two visual systems re-viewed. *Neuropsychologia, 46*(3), 774–785.

Muncie, W. (1948). *Psychobiology and psychiatry: A textbook of normal and abnormal human behavior* (2nd ed.). Mosby.

Murphy, M. R., MacLean, P. D., & Hamilton, S. C. (1981). Species-typical behavior of hamsters deprived from birth of the neocortex. *Science, 213*(4506), 459–461.

Nelson, K., & Fivush, R. (2004). The emergence of autobiographical memory: A social cultural developmental theory. *Psychological Review, 111*(2), 486–511.

Nelson, K., & Fivush, R. (2020). The development of autobiographical memory, autobiographical narratives, and autobiographical consciousness. *Psychological Reports, 123*(1), 71–96.

Nir, Y., & Tononi, G. (2010). Dreaming and the brain: From phenomenology to neurophysiology. *Trends in Cognitive Sciences, 14*(2), 88–100.

Panksepp, J. (2004). *Affective neuroscience: The foundations of human and animal emotions*. Oxford University Press.

Panksepp, J. (2005). Affective consciousness: Core emotional feelings in animals and humans. *Consciousness and Cognition, 14*(1), 30–80.

Panksepp, J., & Biven, L. (2012). *The archaeology of mind: Neuroevolutionary origins of human emotions* (Norton Series on Interpersonal Neurobiology). Norton.

Panksepp, J., & Panksepp, J. B. (2000). The seven sins of evolutionary psychology. *Evolution and Cognition, 6*(2), 108–131.

Pattee, H. H. (2012). Causation, control, and the evolution of complexity. In *Laws, language and life* (pp. 261–274). Springer.

Porges, S. W. (2001). The polyvagal theory: Phylogenetic substrates of a social nervous system. *International Journal of Psychophysiology, 42*(2), 123–146.

Quattrocki, E., & Friston, K. (2014). Autism, oxytocin and interoception. *Neuroscience & Biobehavioral Reviews, 47,* 410–430.

Rechtschaffen, A. (1978). The single-mindedness and isolation of dreams. *Sleep, 1,* 904–921.

Revonsuo, A. (1995). Consciousness, dreams and virtual realities. *Philosophical Psychology, 8*(1), 35–58.

Revonsuo, A. (2000). The reinterpretation of dreams: An evolutionary hypothesis of the function of dreaming. *Behavioral and Brain Sciences, 23*(6), 877–901.

Revonsuo, A. (2006). *Inner presence: Consciousness as a biological phenomenon.* MIT Press.

Revonsuo, A. (2018). Afterword. In *Foundations of consciousness* (pp. 154–156). Routledge.

Rymer, R. (1993). *Genie: A scientific tragedy.* HarperCollins.

Seth, A. K. (2013). Interoceptive inference, emotion, and the embodied self. *Trends in Cognitive Sciences, 17*(11), 565–573.

Seth, A. K., Suzuki, K., & Critchley, H. D. (2012). An interoceptive predictive coding model of conscious presence. *Frontiers in Psychology, 2,* Article 395.

Sims, A. (1988). *Symptoms in the mind: An introduction to descriptive psychopathology.* Bailliere Tindall.

Singer, W. (2001). Consciousness and the binding problem. *Annals of the New York Academy of Sciences, 929*(1), 123–146.

Smythies, J. R., Edelstein, L. R., & Ramachandran, V. S. (2014). Hypotheses relating to the function of the claustrum. In J. R. Smythies, L. R. Edelstein, & V. S. Ramachandran (Eds.), *The claustrum* (pp. 299–352). Academic Press.

Solms, M. (2019). The hard problem of consciousness and the free energy principle. *Frontiers in Psychology, 9,* 2714.

Tulving, E. (1985). Memory and consciousness. *Canadian Psychology, 26*(1), 1–12.

Tulving, E. (2002). Episodic memory: From mind to brain. *Annual Review of Psychology, 53*(1), 1–25.

Valli, K., & Revonsuo, A. (2009). The threat simulation theory in light of recent empirical evidence: A review. *American Journal of Psychology, 122*(1), 17–38.

Van Honk, J., Morgan, B. E., & Schutter, D. J. (2007). Raw feeling: A model for affective consciousness. *Behavioral and Brain Sciences, 30*(1), 107–108.

Van Honk, J., & Schutter, J. L. G. (2005). Dynamic brain systems in quest for emotional homeostasis. *Behavioral and Brain Sciences, 28*(2), 220–221.

Voss, U., Holzmann, R., Hobson, A., Paulus, W., Koppehele-Gossel, J., Klimke, A., & Nitsche, M. A. (2014). Induction of self-awareness in dreams through frontal low current stimulation of gamma activity. *Nature Neuroscience, 17*(6), 810–812.

Voss, U., Holzmann, R., Tuin, I., & Hobson, A. J. (2009). Lucid dreaming: A state of consciousness with features of both waking and non-lucid dreaming. *Sleep, 32*(9), 1191–1200.

Watson, J. B. (1913). Psychology as the behaviorist views it. *Psychological Review, 20*(2), 158–177.

# PART III
# SOCIAL NEUROSCIENCE

# 9

# Attachment

Social attachment is the decisive evolutionary event that establishes human social bonds. It is the intensity of secure early infant bonding that ensures sociability and predicts optimal social adaptation. Parental care and mutual engagement between mother and infant are the origin of sociability. Attachments are characterized by linking coordinated nonverbal behavior with coordinated physiological responses among partners. This biobehavioral synchrony is a key feature in the establishment of infant–mother attachments. Social bonds are established from the beginning of life. These bonds are not derived from the need for food, sex, or dependency. Social bonding is protective; it is essential to care-seeking or in caregiving. The formation of these bonds requires the infant's accessibility to the adult; a secure, socially engaged base is essential to attachment and, once the infant's safety is established, it leads the infant to explore their environment. Exploration involves leaving close proximity of the secure base, which can be returned to at times of threat. A secure base facilitates play and peer contact. The secure base in humans is maintained throughout childhood and adolescence. As the child matures, the time away from close contact with the parent that can be tolerated becomes greater—from half days at age 3 years to weeks or months in adolescence.

John Bowlby (1988) proposed that analogous to physiological models of homeostasis, attachment behavior is a form of environmental homeostasis regulating distance and personal accessibility. Homeostasis is essential for survival throughout evolution from unicellular organisms to human life. It ensures that life is regulated not only to allow survival but also to flourish (Damasio, 2018). Attachment behavior is activated by fear of harm and by the need for care when tired or hungry; it is relieved by reunion with the caregiver, which provides reassurance and comfort. Such behavioral control systems themselves are sources of motivated behavior, rendering general theories of drive or psychic energy obsolete. A failure to respond to an infant's care-eliciting behavior by the parent causes stress reactions in the infant, separation anxiety in the younger child, and sometimes the experience of betrayal in the adolescent. An attachment relationship in children and adolescents inhibits aggressive behavior—a change that may be neurochemically modulated.

The attachment system is most efficient when interacting with the person whom the child believes is the most likely to respond. A failure in response by the family caregiver causes stress and may be traumatic. Attachment is based on the reciprocity of care-eliciting behavior by the child with responsive caregiving by the parent. Thus, caregiving is complementary to attachment behavior. Altruistic care of the young promotes survival of offspring and one's own genes. Thus, social engagement at a cultural level emphasizes altruism and sociability throughout life.

As a consequence of early experiences, a child increasingly develops internal working models of relationships with parents as attention and memory emerge with cognitive and emotional maturation. These working models foster planning for future events in the real world. By age 5 years, children's working models may have evolved to include awareness that caregivers have their own interests, moods, and intentions. The parents develop complementary working models of the child. Some working models are in constant use; others may be incorporated in memory and operate largely out of awareness over long periods of time. Attachment may be discordant between the child and the mother or father.

## Patterns of Attachment

The theoretical work of Bowlby (1969) and the methodological contributions of Mary Ainsworth and colleagues (Ainsworth, 1985a, 1985b; Ainsworth et al., 1978) have provided a means to test the quality of mother–infant attachment and to extend these observations to better understand the antecedents, stability, construction, and long-term sequelae of patterns of attachment. Ethology, evolutionary biology, control systems theory, and insights from contemporary developmental cognitive psychology and social psychology have provided a framework to investigate the long-term implications of the parent–infant bond. The initial work on attachment theory emphasized the quality of the caregiver's response to the infant's cues and the important role of attachment in personality development. Ainsworth extended Bowlby's research by emphasizing the importance of both security and insecurity in the attachment relationship and devised a methodology for testing secure and insecure attachment—that is, the Strange Situation Procedure (Ainsworth et al., 1978). This paradigm has become the primary means for assessing the security of infantile attachments. The research on attachment has been extended to evaluate the representational aspects of attachment relationships in children and adults, cross-cultural influences on the functioning of the attachment system, and the role of temperament in the establishment of attachment.

Early lifetime experiences leave a lasting legacy. Constructs of attachment and personality are critical in the study of child development. Early experience, parent and infant bonding, and peer relationships are important. Progress has been made in establishing an integrated view of the importance of neurophysiology and experience in attachment research. Early experience retains the potential to influence later developmental changes. Attachment representations carry on and preserve early experiences. Attachment experiences are foundational in regard to individual difference in personality (Sroufe, 2016).

Four basic patterns of attachment have been reliably described (Ainsworth, 1985a, 1985b; Ainsworth et al., 1978; Main et al., 1985; Main & Stadtman, 1981; Main & Weston, 1981). Which pattern develops depends on treatment by the parental figure and the child's responsiveness. These patterns of attachment were identified in infants using the Strange Situation procedure developed by Ainsworth et al. (1978). The Strange Situation procedure is a semi-standardized, easy-to-use, and easily scorable means to identify infants/toddlers (ages 12–20 months) who are securely or insecurely attached to their caregivers. In the Strange Situation procedure, attachment security is evaluated by creating conditions with gradually escalating stress that activate the infant's attachment behavior system. The Strange Situation procedure consists of eight episodes, lasting 21 min, in which various social changes are observed to occur in an experimental playroom setting while the infant is playing with toys. These changes include a stranger's presence or absence and the caregiver's departure and return, in addition to other social events, while the infant's response to the caregiver is directly observed. The episodes are as follows:

1. The mother and infant are introduced to the playroom together for 1 min.
2. The infant explores the room for 3 min.
3. A stranger, unknown to the infant, enters the room and sits for 1 min, talks to the mother, and gets down on the floor to play with the infant for 1 min.
4. The mother leaves the room, leaving the child alone with the stranger, who plays with the infant for 3 min and then withdraws from interaction with the child (first separation).
5. The mother returns to the room, and the stranger leaves quietly and unobtrusively. The mother settles the child and sits down for 3 min (first reunion).
6. The mother leaves the infant alone in the room for 3 min (second separation).
7. The stranger comes into the room, attempts to settle the child for 3 min, and then disengages.
8. The mother returns, and the stranger again leaves quietly and unobtrusively. The mother settles the infant and sits down (second reunion), and the session ends after approximately 20 min.

If there is a strong attachment relationship, the infant will use the mother as a secure base to explore the room in episodes 2, 3, and the end of episode 5. However, the infant will be stressed by the mother's absence in episodes 4, 6, and 7. These episodes are terminated if the infant becomes very upset or if the mother wishes to return sooner. Focused attention is given to the infant's behavior in reunion episodes 5 and 8 to clarify if the infant is effectively comforted by the mother's presence (Cowie et al., 2015; George & Solomon, 2016).

Classification is based on the infant's behavior toward the caregiver during the two reunion episodes. The infant's behavior during reunion is also rated on scales focused on infant–caregiver interactive behavior. This is used in assessing classification. These are proximity and contact seeking, contact maintaining, avoidance and resistance to contact, and interaction.

As shown in Table 9.1, attachment is classified as securely attached; insecure-avoidant, -resistant, or -ambivalent attachment; insecure-resistant or -ambivalent attachment (Ainsworth et al., 1978); and "attachment-disorganized/disoriented" attachment (Main et al., 1985; Main & Solomon, 1986, 1990):

Secure: The infant uses the mother as a secure base for exploration. When separated, the infant shows signs of missing the parent, especially during the second separation from her. In reunion activity, the infant greets the parent with a smile, vocalization, or gestures; however, if the infant has become upset on separation, the infant seeks contact with the parent. When comforted, the infant begins to explore again. Any distress shown in separation is related to the absence of the mother.

**Table 9.1** Infant and Adult Attachment Classification[a]

| Infant | Adult |
| --- | --- |
| Secure | Secure |
| Avoidant | Dismissive |
| Ambivalent | Preoccupied |
| Disorganized | Fearful |

| Secure Attachment | |
| --- | --- |
| Children | Adults |
| Able to separate from parent | Have trusting relationships |
| Seek comfort from parents if frightened | Tend to have good self-esteem |
| Return of parents is met with positive emotions | Comfortable sharing feelings with others |
| Prefer parents to strangers | Seek out social support |

| Ambivalent Attachment | |
| --- | --- |
| Children | Adults |
| May be wary of strangers | Reluctant to become close to others |
| Become greatly distressed when the parent leaves | Worry that their partner does not love them |
| Do not appear to be comforted by the return of the parent | Become very distraught when a relationship ends |

| Avoidant Attachment | |
| --- | --- |
| Children | Adults |
| May avoid parent on reunion | May have problems with intimacy |
| Do not seek much comfort or contact from parents on reunion | Invest little emotion in social and romantic relationships |
| Show little or no preference between parent and stranger | Unable or unwilling to share thoughts and feelings with others |

| Disorganized Attachment | |
| --- | --- |
| Age 1 year | Age 8 years |
| Show a mixture of avoidant and resistant behaviors | May take on a parental role |
| May seem dazed of confused or apprehensive | Some children act as caregiver toward parent |

[a]The infant categories are based on the Strange Situation test. Adult categories are based on the Adult Attachment Inventory. The top portion of the table lists the infant and adult categories. The lower panels describe secure, ambivalent, avoidant, and disorganized feature in infants and adults.

*Avoidant*: The infant readily explores the room showing little displayed affect or emotion and does not focus on the mother as a secure base. The infant shows minimal visual distress when left alone. On reunion, the infant actively avoids the parent by looking away, generally focusing on toys. The infant may stiffen if picked up and leans away from the mother. The infant is apparently not distressed with the separation nor distressed when seemingly to be left alone during the mother's personal absence.

*Ambivalent or resistant*: The infant is visibly distressed on initially entering the room. The infant may be fretful or passive, failing to engage in exploration. On separation, the infant appears distressed and unsettled. On reunion with the mother, the infant may alternately seek contact with the mother or have an apparently angry reaction, tantrum, or appear to be upset to make contact. The child does not find comfort in the mother's approach.

*Disorganized/disoriented*: The infant's behavior seems to lack any observable goal or intention. It is difficult to explain. There may be contradictory sequencing in behavior, interruptions, movements, freezing, or indications of fear or apprehension while being with the mother. The infant appears confused and disoriented. Overall, there is no clear pattern of attachment, with inconsistent or odd responses to both separation and reunion.

Box 9.1 shows the definitions for adult attachment from the Adult Attachment Interview. If the pattern of attachment is secure, it is likely to be associated with healthy future development and lead to subsequent socially competent behavior. With secure attachment, the parent is available, is sensitive to the child's signals, and is appropriately and lovingly responsive when the child needs protection. An insecure or anxious pattern may emerge if there is uncertainty as to the parent's availability or responsiveness. Because of this uncertainty, attachment is potentially insecure and the child is prone to experience separation anxiety, a form of anxiety that is associated with anxious attachment, (i.e.,

---

**Box 9.1  Adult Attachment**

*Secure*: It is relatively easy for me to become emotionally close to others. I am comfortable depending on others and having others depend on me. I don't worry about being alone or having others not accept me.

*Dismissive*: I am comfortable without close emotional relationships. It is very important to me to feel independent and self-sufficient, and I prefer not to depend on others or have others depend on me.

*Preoccupied*: I want to be completely emotionally intimate with others, but I often find that others are reluctant to get as close as I would like. I am uncomfortable being without close relationships, but I sometimes worry that others don't value me as much as I value them.

*Fearful*: I am somewhat uncomfortable getting close to others. I want emotionally close relationships, but I find it difficult to trust others completely or to depend on them. I sometimes worry that I will be hurt if I allow myself to become too close to others.

anxious-resistant or anxious-ambivalent attachment). With insecure attachment, there is anxiety about exploration and about moving away from the secure parental base.

Box 9.2 illustrates attachment throughout development from infancy to the transition to adulthood with major attachment issues and subsidiary issues. A development task to be mastered is shown for each age period: infancy (establishing an attachment relationship), toddler (parent-guided self-regulation), preschool (personal self-regulation), school years (competence in social and cognitive tasks), and adolescence (individuation with establishment of a personal identity and intimacy in relationships). In the transition to adulthood, the task to be mastered is emancipation in launching a personal life course. Subsidiary tasks are involved for overall task mastery at any age.

Separation anxiety is unlike other forms of anxiety in that it may be terminated by contact with the parent, especially when securely attached. However, with an anxious attachment, in which the parent is randomly available or unavailable, the child experiences uncertainty, and separation anxiety is enhanced on separation. Experiences of uncertainty and potentially of abandonment or threats by the parent of abandonment may lead to chronic anxious attachment. Moreover, a punitive parent who uses threat of abandonment as a means of control increases the insecurity of attachment. Insecure or anxious-avoidant attachment occurs when the child, through experience, learns to expect to be continuously rejected and has no confidence in being helped. This pattern of constant rejection may lead to compulsively self-reliant behavior in children and may be a precursor for delinquency as the individual attempts to survive without the consistent support of a caregiver. Finally, children with the disorganized/disoriented form of attachment are fearful of their caregiver. They may be unable to use their caregiver as a secure base and may be socially inhibited. Winnicott (1958) described disturbances in interpersonal attachment as characteristic of children with an antisocial tendency. Children who exhibit the antisocial tendency have a history of early positive attachment followed by perceived parental rejection. They continually seek attention, hoping to gain support, but do so in an inappropriate or antisocial way, such as through stealing or socially disruptive.

---

### Box 9.2  Attachment in Development

*Infancy*
    Major issue: Formation of an effective attachment relationship
    Subsidiary issues
        Beginning reciprocity
        Dyadic affect regulation
        Attachment–exploration balance

*Toddler*
    Major issue: Guided self-regulation
    Subsidiary issues
        Increased autonomy
    Increased awareness of self and others
        Awareness of standards for behavior
            Self-conscious emotions

*Preschool*
> Major issue: Self-regulation
> Subsidiary issues
>> Self-reliance with support (agency)
>> Self-management
>> Expanding social world
>> Internalization of rules and values

*School years*
> Major issue: Competence
> Subsidiary issues
>> Personal effectance
>> Self-integration
>> Competence with peers
>> Place in group
>> Functioning in group
>> Loyal friendships
>> Competence in school

*Adolescence*
> Major issue: Individuation
> Subsidiary issues
>> Autonomy with connectedness
>> Identity
>> Peer network competence
>> Place in network
>> Functioning in network
> Intimate relationships
> Coordinating school, work, and social life

*Transition to adulthood*
> Major issue: Emancipation
> Subsidiary issues
>> Launching a life course
>> Financial responsibility
>> Adult social competence
> Coordinating partnerships and friendships
> Coordinating colleagues, partners, and friends
> Stable relationships
> Coordinating work, training, career, and life

Patterns of attachment persist through time and may be predictive of later behavior. Early attachment relationship assessments predict later relationship functioning or individual behavior better than any other measure of child characteristics used in the first 2 years of life (Sroufe et al., 2005). Main et al. (1985) reported that the pattern of attachment to the parent established at age 12 months persisted with few exceptions at 6 years. Sroufe et al. (1983) found that the pattern of attachment in infancy at age 12 months was predictive of behavior in a nursery school group at age 3½ years. In this study, the children with a secure pattern at age 12 months were described by teachers as cooperative, resourceful, and able to socialize well with other children. Infants were followed longitudinally from ages 9 to 33 months, and observations were made in a laboratory study designed to elicit fear, anger, and joy. Their responses differed by attachment style. Avoidant infants became more fearful, resistant infants became less joyful, and the disorganized type became angrier. The secure infants showed less fear, anger, or distress to challenges in this study (Kochanska, 2001). The relationship of attachment status and later measures of internalizing and externalizing behaviors also have been studied. A subset of children enrolled in the National Institute of Child Health and Development (NICHD) Study of Early Child Care and Youth Development ($N = 1,364$) participated in the Strange Situation procedure at age 15 months. For older children, the Q-sort behavior rating was issued for attachment construct measurement. Q-sort follow-up ratings of attachment were conducted by mothers at 24 months. Q-sort is a measure of individual differences in attachment as assessed by the child's use of the parent as a secure base to explore, affective responsiveness, and social cognition, especially social referencing to the parent. Social referencing correlations of security dependency and sociality scores are derived in this test (Waters & Deane, 1985). The Q-sort ratings of child–mother attachment security at 24 months predicted internalizing and externalizing behavior problems at age 3 years, demonstrating that attachment is associated with behavior problems. Attachment security predicted rating of internalizing problems for boys and girls and externalizing problems for boys. Maternal defensive symptoms predicted mother's ratings of internalizing and externalizing problems. Finally, there were meaningful associations of attachment insecurity and behavior problems when assessed by both mothers and caregivers.

Those with an early anxious attachment were described as attention-seeking, hostile, and lacking in spontaneous emotionality. Those in the anxious-resistant group were described as tense, easily frustrated, impulsive, and often passive. Secure attachment at 12 months predicted curiosity and problem-solving ability at age 2 years, social confidence in nursery school at age 3 years, empathy and independence at age 5 years, and fewer behavioral problems at age 6 years (Oppenheim et al., 1988).

Overall, once patterns of attachment are established, they tend to persist and to be self-perpetuating. The securely attached child is easier to care for and less demanding. The anxious-ambivalent or anxious-resistant child tends to whine and cling, and the anxious-avoidant child tends to be bad-tempered and often bullies others. Negative behavioral cycles may emerge from these interactions.

Although patterns are most likely to persist, they do not necessarily do so. During the early years of life, the stability of the attachment depends on the consistency of the parental relationship. Attachment security is a dyadic measure and a characteristic of a relationship. Not only may the mother–child and father–child pattern differ but also, if a parent treats a child differently, the pattern may change as the child grows older. Moreover, stability of attachment cannot be simply attributed to temperament (Sroufe,

1985). Ainsworth et al. (1973) found that placid newborns may become anxious and de-manding if their mothers subsequently become rejecting and insensitive. Still, as a child grows older, the pattern of attachment and personality features becomes more resistant to change.

There is a tendency to impose earlier patterns of attachment experience and the working models self-derived from them onto new relationships and to persist in these patterns despite an "absence of fit" (Bowlby, 1988). This "transference" of attachment patterns of relating to new situations supports an object relations or interpersonal view of psychoanalytic theory rather than the classical form of psychoanalysis. This attach-ment model considers internal models of the self and of psychological bonding as in-teractional models between individuals. Studies of attachment lead to questions about continuity and discontinuity in development.

## Attachment and Internal Working Models

Attachment is a developmental construct that may be measured at different stages of de-velopment throughout the life span. The Strange Situation procedure measures the se-curity of attachment by behavioral analysis—that is, how the infant behaves at reunion following a separation. Typically, the Strange Situation is carried performed with chil-dren aged 12–24 months. For preschool-age children, attachment relationships are less dependent on physical proximity to the parent. In those years, attachment is internalized cognitively as working mental models of their earlier caregiving experiences. These models focus on more abstract qualities of relationship, such as interpersonal affection, trust, and approval by the parent. Although younger children may spend considerable time in day care, parents remain as the main figures in their lives. In middle childhood, the world of the child has expanded, with the parent having less influence over their social environments and social contacts. Peers become important, rather than parents, as playmates. Children become more self-reliant, with greater self-awareness, meta-cognition, and memory, and they have greater cognitive flexibility and capacity to regu-late emotions (Kerns & Brumariu, 2016).

Kerns and Brumariu (2016) suggest four defining features of attachment in middle childhood. First, the goal of the attachment system changes from proximity to the at-tachment figure, allowing longer separations and greater distance. Second, parents re-main the principal attachment figures in middle childhood despite play preferences with peers. When an 11- or 12-year-old is afraid or sad, parents are preferred over peers (Seibert & Kerns, 2009). Third, in middle childhood, there is a shift toward more co-regulation of secure base contact between child and parent. Bowlby (1988) noted that a fourth phase of attachment, termed the goal-corrected partnership, emerges after age 3 years and is further refined in middle childhood when the child has greater cognitive understanding of the parent's desires. The child uses this information in planning goals. Securely attached children are more likely to "check in" with parents regarding their activities, an aspect of co-regulation. Increasingly, parents and chil-dren work together in problem-solving, resulting in a collaborative alliance between children and parents by the end of middle childhood. By that time, the child uses the parent as a resource rather than fully relying on the parent to solve their problems. Last, in middle childhood, parents, as attachments figures, act as safe havens when the child is upset or distressed and as a secure base for support of the self-confident child's explorations. When challenged, the mother may provide a more emotionally confiding safe haven and the father a more secure base protection (showing confidence in the child's ability to master challenges) as each parent provides complementary support (Kerns et al., 2015).

The role of these mental representational features, internal working models, has been emphasized by Bretherton and Munholland (2008) and Main et al. (1985), who portray attachment as not only a behavioral system but also a conceptual system that governs social relations throughout life. These authors suggest that through the history of interactions with the caregiver, an infant generates a rudimentary conceptual representation of the attachment figure. These "working models" have provided the basis for secure and insecure attachment by the end of the first year of life and are maintained to guide subsequent behavior at later ages. Representations of significant relationships may be stored and operate outside conscious awareness, becoming more stable over time. Such consistent, long-term models not only may affect the parent–child relationship but also are carried on as caregiving tendencies to the next generation. The child has internalized the role of caregiver and for the one to be cared for.

If attachment may be described as an internalized conceptual model, then individual differences in attachment security may lead to social expectations that differ from those of the caregiver. A working model suggests expectations by children of a caregiver's responsiveness and accessibility to them. By the end of the first year of life, early primitive representation regarding a caregiver's behavior may have become consolidated as it is relevant to the infant's security and the support provided.

Another aspect of the working model of representational theory considers whether a mother's quality of care for her infant is related to her own representations of her life experience as a child. This hypothesis is supported by studies by Main et al. (1985), Main and Goldwyn (1984), and Ricks (1985). These authors suggest that attachment, as an internalized representation, provides working models for both the caregiver's own earlier life and the infant receiving care. Thus, these models may be maintained and reproduced in caregiving roles in later life. In reviewing parents' memories of early experiences of care, particularly recollections of security and comfort along with fears of abandonment and separation, the authors found that, overall, an infant's attachment status bore a relation to the parents' own conceptualization of attachment-related issues, especially including their own acceptance or rejection as children and their current level of self-esteem. The parents' reports are a recollection of memories of their childhood that serve as the source of the parents' contemporary working model of attachment as it relates to their own children.

Adult attachment status is measured using the Adult Attachment Interview administered over an hour (Hesse, 2016). It examines how a secure or insecure parent–infant attachment reflects the adult's representations of their own attachment-related experiences. Just as sensitive parenting facilitates security in a child, a child who is securely attached may also affect a parent's perceptions of their own parenting ability, their self-esteem, and perhaps their reflections on their own earlier experience. Thus, the behavior of the infant or child may reciprocally affect the parent's own beliefs. In this sense, attachment demonstrates mutually reinforcing influences between parents and offspring that persist over time, provided that there are not major changes in family relationships.

The relationship between attachment in infancy, preschool, school age, adolescence, and adulthood is receiving continued emphasis. Studies of various ages emphasize the continuity of functioning based on the working model hypothesis of internalized representations. If infants do construct working models of their caregivers that result in secure or insecure attachment, such working models might exert an ongoing influence on how children cope with attachment concerns at later ages. Internal working models are cognitions based on memories of day-to-day interactions with the attachment figure. These become "event scripts" or cognitive "narratives" that guide action based on prior interactions, expectations, or emotional experiences (Cowie et al., 2015). Those whose attachment is secure may have internal working models of affection and trust. If so, the securely attached child may communicate early and openly regarding attachment-related issues, such as being lost or left alone by a parent who has gone shopping. Conversely, a child with avoidant attachment style may not expect to be comforted if distressed when found after being lost and expresses rejection to the parent. Those with an ambivalent style may not know what to expect when found after being lost and may find it difficult to communicate feelings.

One measure used to evaluate attachment security in school-age children is the Separation Anxiety Test. Children or adolescents are shown photographs of separation experiences. The child is asked how the child in the picture would feel or act in the scene shown. They are asked how they would feel in this situation (Main et al., 1985). A revised version of the Separation Anxiety Test that is shown to be reliable for use with 8- to 12-year-olds is available (Wright et al., 1995). Large differences were identified between children in treatment for behavior disorders and a control group. Overall, securely attached children acknowledged the anxiety resulting from separation and provided coherent narratives describing how they might cope. Children who were insecurely attached typically either identified anxiety or suggested inappropriate coping strategies.

Secure attachment in middle childhood is associated with sensitive, responsive, and accepting parenting behavior along with realistic support for autonomy. Secure attachment is highly correlated with the child's attitude toward school and classroom behavior. These findings are confirmed in cross-sectional and longitudinal studies using a variety of attachment measurements (Kerns & Brumariu, 2016). Children aged 8–12 years who are securely attached report higher self-esteem and social self-efficacy (Coleman, 2003). They positively view other's actions and tend to propose more prosocial solutions when asked to solve peer problems. They report more positive and less negative mood throughout the day and greater awareness of their emotional state. When faced with challenges, securely attached children use more appropriate coping strategies, such as seeking support from others. However, the behavior of those with avoidant attachment has been linked to emotional suppression and ambivalent attachment associated with emotion dysregulation (Brenning et al., 2012). In regard to coping in middle school children, children with disorders of attachment typically do not use active coping strategies. They are more likely to catastrophize if things go wrong (Brumariu et al., 2012).

In one study, children who were more securely attached showed lower electrodermal reactivity to a social stress test. Two groups of children ages 4 and 7 years were shown the same fear-inducing film clips. Concurrently, skin conductance and heart rate variability were measured. Both age groups responded with increased skin conductance and a decrease in heart rate variability. A secure attachment relationship was linked to fearful temperament in more fearful children but not in less fearful children, regardless of the children's age. The study is supportive of the role of attachment in the differential susceptibility to social context model, because children with high negative emotion are more susceptible to positive as well as negative rearing influences (Gilissen et al., 2008).

## Attachment in Middle Childhood and Peer Relationships

Attachment status predicts the quality of peer relationships in middle childhood. Secure attachment enhances the exploration of peer relationships, and securely attached children show greater interest in and motivation to engage peers. Emotional regulation facilitates emotional control with peers. Attachment is more related to the quality of children's friendships rather than number of friends, responsiveness to one another, and conflict resolution (Abraham & Kerns, 2013). Overall, secure attachment is associated with higher popularity with peers (Kerns & Brumariu, 2016). Moreover, securely attached children demonstrate greater social participation and social engagement with peers. Regarding patterns of unsecure attachment, ambivalent children were found to have poor efficacy in peer relations. Avoidant children were more isolated from peers (Shulman et al., 1994). Moreover, both avoidant and disorganized children showed the greatest problems, especially regarding exclusion and aggression with peers. Ambivalent children had fewer peer problems (Seibert & Kerns, 2015).

Attachment security is correlated with lower levels of externalizing and internalizing problems in middle childhood. Self-report measures of internalizing problems show positive correlation of internalizing problems with both avoidant and ambivalent preoccupied attachment (Brenning et al., 2012). Children with secure attachment to their mothers have reduced likelihood of developing internalized symptoms and conduct and attention problems. A meta-analysis of 46 studies involving 8,907 children with insecure attachment and anxiety from early childhood to adolescence found that attachment was moderately correlated with anxiety ($r = 0.30$). The strongest correlation was with ambivalent attachment (Colonnesi et al., 2011).

Most studies focus on the child's attachment profile. Multiple components of parenting style outcomes were examined in a meta-analysis that focused on parents of children aged 5–18 years. Parents whose children had secure attachment were more supportive of their child's autonomy, and they used more behavioral control strategies and less harsh parent control strategies. Parents whose children were more avoidant were found to be less responsive and used less behavior control strategies; ambivalent attachment was not significantly related to any of the parent behavior strategies. There were insufficient numbers of children with disorganized attachment to evaluate correlation (Koehn & Kerns, 2018).

## Genetics and Attachment

Are infants genetically predisposed to an attachment style just as they may be to a particular temperament? Does environment experience matter most? Behavioral genetic studies of attachment have been conducted to address these questions. Twin studies are an important source of information in behavioral genetics to address these issues. In twin studies, monozygotic (MZ) twins whose DNA genes are identical are compared with dizygotic (DZ) twins or fraternal twins who share an average of half of their DNA. If MZ twin pairs are more similar to one another in attachment states (or other traits) than DZ twin pairs, then genetic factors influence attachment (Bakermans-Kranenburg & van IJzendoorn, 2016). With strong similarity between MZ twins and much smaller similarity between DZ twins, attachment would be shown to be highly heritable as long as both MZ and DZ twins were not treated differently during their rearing. Several twin studies have been carried out with infants and preschool children. The majority of these did not find differences in attachment similarity when MZ and DZ twins were compared. Overall, 50% of attachment variance was attributed to shared environments—that is, parental care factors that make children in the same family similar. For example, one twin study that evaluated attachment status in twin pairs using the Strange Situation procedure found 70% of MZ twins and 64% of DZ twins were not significantly different in this paradigm. Only 14% of the variance was due to genetic factors; 32% was due to shared environments and 53% to nonshared environments (O'Connor & Croft, 2001). In the NICHD Study of Early Child Care and Youth Development, which involved enrollment of approximately 14,000 children with follow-up long-term in the United States, 485 same-sex twin pairs were assessed. Both shared and nonshared environments contributed to attachment security measured by the Q-sort technique, whereas the genetic contribution was small to negligible (Cowie et al., 2015; Roisman & Fraley, 2008). Shared environment variance in attachment security has been found to substantially overlap with variance in observed maternal sensitivity, suggesting that parental sensitivity is important in shaping attachment sensitivity (Fearon et al., 2006).

A study conducted with foster mothers found concordance between the foster mother's state of mind and infant attachment measured by the Strange Situation procedure (Meins et al., 2001), just as was found with biological mother–infant pairings; environmental rather than genetic influence is key (Dozier et al., 2001). Others propose that how the mother views the infant matters most. Mind-mindfulness is another important construct in the mother–infant relationship. Mind-mindfulness refers to the mother treating the infant as a person with a mind of their own. The emphasis is on the mother responding to an infant's inferred state of mind, not simply behavior. In a study of 71 mother–infant pairs, maternal sensitivity (i.e., responsiveness to their infant's cues) along with a focus on mind-mindfulness was examined (Meins et al., 2001). Mind-related comments by the mother have been measured at 6 months of age. The infant's mind focuses independently-predicted security of attachment at 12 months.

Viewing the infant as a person is very important in sensitive caregiving for infants with developmental disabilities who exhibit fewer cues to social engagement.

There is an extensive literature on maternal sensitivity and attachment outcomes. Deans (2020) reviewed 687 articles along with a meta-analysis. Secure attachment between mother and child is an essential condition for the child's well-being (Ainsworth et al., 1971). The operationalization of secure attachment focuses on the concept of maternal sensitivity. Maternal sensitivity is measured by viewing live or videotaped interactions and coding accuracy of reading the infant's or child's signals and also acceptance and warmth toward the infant's or child's lead. There is a robust correlation between maternal sensitivity and attachment. Statistically, the correlates are modest in predicting attachment states based on the meta-analysis (Deans, 2020). There are multiple longitudinal studies linking attachment to maternal sensitivity (Whipple et al., 2011). However, the link was not found for infants in low-quality non-maternal care (Aviezer et al., 2003). There is ongoing research about whether maternal sensitivity has a direct or less direct mediating effect on behavioral and cognitive outcomes (Deans, 2020). On a measure of maternal sensitivity, the maternal responsiveness scale, the strongest convergent and productive ability was on the nonresponsiveness subscale (Leerkes & Qu, 2017). Disorganized attachment also has been examined using a twin design. Disorganized attachment is typically found in children who are mistreated, abused, or frightened by parental behavior (Lyons-Ruth & Jacobvitz, 2016). Disorganized infants and children show frightened facial expressions, freezing behavior, or social withdrawal and avoidance on reunion in the Strange Situation. In a study of 157 MZ and DZ twins, environmental influences on attachment were examined using the Strange Situation procedure (Bokhorst et al., 2003). There was negligible correlation with heritability or shared environments for disorganized attachment. For secure and insecure attachment styles, 52% of the variance on attachment security was explained by shared environment and 48% of the variance was explained by nonshared environment and measurement error. Attachment theory consistently considers environmental influences, especially the effects of parenting on individual differences in an attachment relationship and internal working models. These models are a dyadic construct shaped by parents and subsequently psychologically internalized by the child. For the most part, behavioral genetics, twin and adoption studies, document and highlight the dominant role of environment in attachment security.

It is also important to be cautious in drawing conclusions from behavioral genetics for several reasons. First, twin studies break down variation in attachment within a specific environment and specific population. Thus, the result is situation- and sample-specific, relatively independent of environmental variation. Second, behavioral genetic results are at the group level and not necessarily indicative of individuals. Third, the effects of genetics increase with age. Alternatives to twin studies are genome-wide association studies and genome-wide complex trait analysis (GCTA) (C. Lee, 2022). GCTA extends behavior genetics, not being dependent on twin studies. However, like twin studies, GCTA results in estimates of heritability but does not point to specific genes or gene pathways involved in the phenotype. Despite the application of molecular genetic approaches for identifying "attachment genes," none have been found in the sample sizes studied to date.

The study of genes is associated with neurotransmitter pathways involved in endophenotypes of attachment, such as the dopamine system involved in social reward; the serotonin system involved in mood regulation; and the neuropeptides, oxytocin and vasopressin, involved in social sensitivity and social engagement. These association studies, which sample small numbers of subjects, attempt to link statistically specific behaviors or phenotypes to allelic variants of genes encoding proteins involved in the disposition of the neurotransmitter of interest, such as synthetic enzymes, catabolic enzymes, transporters, and receptors. Several limitations of this approach have been raised, including biased selection of genes; underpowered data sets given the multiple comparisons involved in these studies; and publication bias, which tends to favor positive studies (Edwards et al., 2016).

Dopamine has been shown to play a critical role in motivation and reward and in regulating positive and negative emotions (Schultz, 2006). Because having an infant is rewarding to parents, parents are motivated to socially engage. Variations in the dopamine system may impact parenting behavior. A study on parenting behavior and the dopamine system examined 200 mother–child dyads (S. Lee et al., 2010). The association between the dopamine transporter gene was examined in three observed patterns of maternal behavior: positive parenting, negative parenting, and total maternal commands to control behavior. Children diagnosed with attention-deficit/hyperactivity disorder (ADHD) were matched to children without ADHD. Children were observed in free play and in challenging tasks, including cleanup, settling and counting geometric shapes, and play while ignored by the mother. The dopamine transporter was chosen because it plays a key role in modulating dopamine-mediated behavior.

In this study, the maternal dopamine transporter gene was negatively associated with negative parenting and commands for control for disruptive behavior and other factors in the child's behavior. Mothers with the 9/9 and 10/10 genotype showed less negative parenting than mothers with the 9/10 genotype. Mothers with the 9/10 genotype used more fear commands than the other two groups. The dopamine transporter genotype was unrelated to positive parenting (S. Lee et al., 2010). These findings are consistent with the relationship of dopamine transporter genotype influencing negative emotionality. The role of dopamine transporter genotype in the child evoking negative parenting behavior was examined in another study (Hayden et al., 2013). In this study, 365 children (197 male) were genotyped for variants of dopamine transporter. They participated with their primary caregiver in standardized interactions. The study found that children with the dopamine transporter 9-repeat variant demonstrated negative affect toward the parent when interacting. Moreover, parents with the dopamine transporter 9-repeat allele exhibited more hostility and less guidance/encouragement than parents without this allele. The results are consistent with the dopamine transporter 9-repeat allele's potential importance in eliciting negative parenting. The dopamine transporter 9-repeat allele is associated with greater dopamine transporter striatal expression in humans. The 9-repeat allele has been linked to personality traits with a fivefold greater likelihood of exhibition of angry impulsive traits. Not only is dopamine related to impulsivity and anger but also it influences the extent to which the child processes affective and social cues. In addition, children with the 9-repeat allele had mothers who responded with less warmth and negative parenting style. There was a trend of mothers demonstrating more negative parenting style, suggesting a pattern of mother–child transaction that becomes more apparent over time and strengthens in middle childhood. Genetic information on the dopamine transporter allele was not available for parents in this study, only for children. Finally, children with the 9-repeat allele may also be at risk for poor peer relationships.

The 9-repeat allele in a child is not the only factor driving the negative relationships. Its role must be put into context of the child's larger environment exposure that may modulate its effects (Hayden et al., 2013). Mothers with better working memory and better attention are more engaged with their infant. Investigators examined dopamine receptor gene alleles in the Maternal Adversity, Vulnerability and Neurodevelopment (MAVAN) study. In this study, there was an association with allelic variants of the dopamine DRD1 and DRD2 receptor genes and the mother's orientation away from the infant and infant-directed vocalizing toward her during 20 min of free play at age 6 months. These finding suggest that dopamine mediated distractibility in the infant. However, looking more broadly, the association with dopamine DRD1 and DRD2 genetic polymorphisms was not linked to global maternal sensitivity ratings. The association was only in these discrete maternal engagement behaviors, accounting for 2% of the 7% of total variance in outcomes (Mileva-Seitz et al., 2012). Other studies of human parenting have reported similar variance. The findings of orienting away by the mother and infant-directed vocalization are endophenotypes that are separate but overlapping parts of a complex maternal phenotype and must be considered in the broader context of the parent–infant relationship. Maternal sensitivity, mother–infant synchrony, and overall maternal infant stimulation must all be considered in attachment studies. Allelic variants of the DRD4 gene, which is implicated in attention, have also been studied and found to be correlated with differential sensitivity to early life experiences (Belsky & Pluess, 2009). Overall, all these studies support a role for the dopamine system in the regulation of maternal behavior (Mileva-Seitz et al., 2012). Although firm conclusions from these studies about specific behavioral phenotypes must be tempered, the dopamine transporter and dopamine D2 receptor genes are significantly associated with behavioral pathology (Trubetskoy et al., 2022).

The serotonin system has also been implicated in mother–infant behavior. In the MAVAN study, mothers who carried the short allele of the serotonin transporter gene were found to be more sensitive with their infants at age 6 months; they were less likely to orient away from their infants (Mileva-Seitz et al., 2011). The serotonin transporter gene 5-HTTLPR has been studied extensively in regard to mood disorders-based attention involving amygdala activation when responding to emotional stimuli. Short alleles of transporter gene are associated with reduced transcriptional efficiency of the serotonin transporter. Carriers of this short allele may be more attentive to children's emotional signals, responding more quickly to them than carriers of long alleles. This study is consistent with the short allele's association with greater maternal sensitivity to infant signals. However, sensitive mothers might also be overwhelmed by negative child signals that could compromise parenting and withdrawal.

Attachment relationships in rhesus monkeys parallel those in humans. Researchers have identified factors in rhesus monkey mother–infant attachment that influence the development trajectory of different attachment relationships. Relationships have been studied in infant rhesus monkey outcomes with supportive, rejecting, and abusive mothers along with peer rearing in the absence of opportunity for attachment with an adult. The serotonin transporter gene in rhesus monkeys is homologous structurally and functionally to the human one. The short (LS; 9-repeat) allele of the serotonin transporter gene confers low transcriptional efficiency to the serotonin transporter. Studies of the 9-repeat allele show striking differences for peer-reared and mother-reared monkeys (Champoux et al., 2002). The relationship of early rearing history and serotonin transporter gene on neonatal behavior was studied during the first month of life. Benefits of maternal behavior toward the infant in these studies are referred to as maternal buffering. Infants with the LS allele, who were raised in the laboratory neonatal nursery, were found to have deficits in measures of activity, attention, and motor maturity compared to those with the long (LL) allele. Yet, both LS allele and LL allele infants reared with competent mothers showed normal developmental findings on activity, attention, and motor maturation. Thus, competent mother-rearing apparently buffered the LS allele deficits. Moreover, the serotonin metabolite 5-hydroxyindoleactic acid (5-HIAA) measured in cerebrospinal fluid did not differ in the securely attached. Significantly lower cerebral spinal fluid 5-HIAA was found in those with the LL allele. Similarly, in regard to aggressive behavior, peer-reared infants with the LS allele showed high levels of aggression, whereas LS allele infants reared by mothers did not (Barr et al., 2003).

Overall, peer-reared monkeys demonstrated deficits in behavioral development during the early weeks of life and reduced serotonin metabolism. Mother-reared monkeys with the LS allele showed normal early neurodevelopmental development and normal serotonin metabolism. Although these findings suggest there is a risk of LS allele for later psychopathy, mother-rearing of LS allele monkeys leading to secure early attachment may compensate. In later life, these monkeys may survive longer because they are risk averse.

## Oxytocin–Vasopressin and Attachment

The oxytocin–vasopressin pathways facilitate social sensitivity and attachment in mother–infant attachment (Carter, 2014). There are associations between maternal behavior and oxytocin-regulated genes linked to polymorphisms in the oxytocin receptor gene (OXTR). A meta-analysis examined the association between the oxytocin receptor polymorphism, rs3576, and sensitive parenting. The study involved mothers who were socially engaged with their 2-year-old toddlers, examining externalizing behavior problems. When maternal discord, education, and depression history were taken into account, parents with the A allele had lower levels of sensitivity to their toddlers. The association between OXTR/rs3576 was replicated in a twin study of behavioral and emotional development (Bakermans-Kranenburg & van IJzendoorn, 2008). This study included 500 families with twins. The twins, aged 6–10 years, were examined for warmth, negativity, and parental control. Both parents and children were genotyped for OXTR/rs3576. In this study, the mother's genotype was found to correlate with maternal warmth. The mothers with the AA genotype showed less warmth when interacting with their children compared to mothers with the CG or AG genotype. Moreover, the maternal OXTR genotype associated with warmth was unaffected, controlling for the child-driven evocative effects and the child's OXTR genotype, age, and gender. The child OXTR genotype did not predict the type of parenting given, nor was the father's genotype associated with parenting behavior (Klahr et al., 2015).

Overall, the role of oxytocin in parenting is clear and undisputed. Studies of the relationship of oxytocin polymorphisms are ongoing, although replication is needed with larger sample sizes. Dopamine and oxytocin work together to regulate behavior responses to social stimuli. Dopamine affords motivation and oxytocin facilitates sensitivity to social cues and regulates the hypothalamic–pituitary–adrenal stress axis. Oxytocin may mediate social salience, promoting a wide range of social behaviors. Thus, oxytocin may increase attention and orientation toward social stimuli and improve social recognition. By modulating activity in the mesocorticolimbic dopaminergic network, oxytocin may facilitate alterations in social salience and valiance with increase in positive behavior (Love, 2014).

Continuing research on the interaction of genes and environment must take into account that some children may be more affected by parenting experiences than others, based in part on their genetic makeup. Differential susceptibility to child-rearing and other environmental experiences provide a model to examine such effects. Differential susceptibility posits that individuals vulnerable to adversity may also make them disproportionally more likely to benefit from social support, depending on social context. In positive environments, they may thrive, whereas in stressful environments, they decompensate. Thus, these genes are considered to be susceptibility genes reflecting synaptic plasticity rather than Mendelian genes. A meta-analysis that included 15 studies involving dopamine-related genotypes found that genotypes in adverse contexts increased risk for behavior problems, whereas in supportive contexts, they provided substantial benefit (Bakermans-Kranenburg & van IJzendoorn, 2011).

Life experiences lead to epigenetic changes in gene expression. For example, epigenetic methylation blocks gene expression. The caring giving environment may alter methylation. Gene expression-altered methylation induces long-term changes in the stress response in animal models that can be transmitted to the next generation (Zhang & Meaney, 2010). Genetic differential susceptibility to context, taking into account epigenetics, may provide an opportunity to refine the interplay of genes and environment in attachment studies.

## Attachment in Adolescence

Adolescence brings substantial changes in expression of attachment-related cognition, behavior, and affect. Attachment measures of the quality of adolescent relationships with parents change over time during the adolescent years. Moreover, during adolescence, there is a refinement of romantic relationships. Adolescents seek to establish emotional self-sufficiency and independence from parental attachment figures. They seek to find a new balance between attachment behaviors and exploration. The coordinated goal-corrected partnership of infancy is replaced in adolescence by an often challenging negotiated partnership with parents as adolescents seek behavioral autonomy. In healthy adolescents, the attachment hierarchy shifts to become more flexible as they move away from parents to engage first peers and then romantic partners. The shift involves directing attention away from childhood memories of dependency on parents toward emotional independence and intimate peer relationships. The Attachment Interview for Childhood and Adolescence (AICA) has been used to examine how the transition from late childhood to early adolescence influences attachment organization. The interview is based on the Adult Attachment Interview, with minor adaptations suited for the early adolescent age group. In the adult interview, the secure category is maintained, but the adult avoidant attachment category becomes dismissive, the ambivalent category becomes preoccupied, and the disorganized category becomes fearful. In the study by Ammaniti et al. (2000), participants (14 girls and 17 boys) completed the AICA at ages 10 and 14 years. The stability of secure attachment between these ages was 78%. Secure and dismissive attachment were more stable than preoccupied and unresolved categories. More dismissive strategies appeared over the 4 years; there also was a greater tendency to report rejection by parents. This rejection may be a defense to keep parents at a distance when seeking personal identity. There were no gender differences (Ammaniti et al., 2000). In a systematic review of more than 200 studies that included adolescents, differences were found from adult reports. In normative nonclinical groups of adolescents, 35% reported dismissive attachment and 13% preoccupied attachment. These findings may reflect adolescent struggles with independence. The findings were similar for adolescents who had moved out of their family home and those who remained at home (Bakermans-Kranenburg & van IJzendoorn, 2009). Overall, adolescent attachment overidentifies dismissive states of mind. Despite this, emphasis on attachment to parents is not the same as dismissive attachment because peers are a greater focus for adolescents. It is this age period when adolescents are moving away from reliance on parents; they de-idealize them and view parents in both positive and negative ways.

Adolescents integrate attachment-relevant experiences from the past to the present with past caregivers along with new relationships. They re-evaluate cognitions, memories, and affective relationships related to attachment (Allen & Tan, 2016). Outcomes in the context of new relationships are examined as adolescents evaluate their relationship to their parents more objectively. During adolescence, peer relationships more clearly become attachment relationships. By late adolescence, peers, either as close friends or romantic partners, serve as attachment figures. Peers and partners serve as attachment figures regarding proximity seeking and safe haven, but not so much with regard to separation distress and commitment. Parents remain at the top of the attachment hierarchy in situations concerning danger for adolescents (Rosenthal & Kobak, 2010). The quality of parent–adolescent communication is strongly correlated with the overall quality of the attachment relationship. Miscommunication and dyadic asynchrony are factors promoting insecure adolescent attachment. For adolescents with insecure, dismissive attachment, concordance between parent and adolescent internalizing symptoms is poor because when in a dismissive state of mind there is resistance to discuss emotionally distressing events with parents. Thus, avoidance restricts communication. Adolescents with insecure preoccupied attachment consistently report higher levels of symptoms. For the preoccupied, symptoms are cries for distress. This suggests overactivation of the attachment system when their cries go unheard. Adolescents who are securely attached are better able to deal with conflicts with parents and engage productively in problem-solving discussions. Such engagement acknowledges the secure function of attachment.

Secure adolescents with LS short allele of the serotonin transporter (the LS allele has been associated with greater emotionality and sensitivity to emotional stimuli) show more agreeability in coping with autonomy with parents. Insecure adolescents with the LS short allele may show greater hostility toward their parents (Zimmermann et al., 2009). This is consistent with parental buffering of emotional distress in the rhesus monkey model. The effect is situation specific, and there is no main effect of the LS allele in attachment security overall. Adolescents with insecure dismissive attachment show the least autonomy and relatedness among attachment groups (Becker-Stoll et al., 2008). Insecure preoccupied attachment in adolescence is associated with heightened and generally unproductive over-engagement with parents in arguments. This attachment type tends to undermine adolescent autonomy and is associated with difficulty in coping with situations such as leaving home for college.

In peer relationships, securely attached adolescents engage in more confiding relationships with close peers. Anxious-ambivalent adolescents show greater interpersonal hostility in peer relationships. Preoccupied attachment leads to greater stress in peer relationships. Dismissive attachment leads to poorer communication skills with peers (Shomaker & Furman, 2009). Individual differences in attachment style influence romantic and sexual relationships in adolescence. Those with secure-attachment, romantic relationships showed less anxiety and avoidance. However, insecurity in attachment is linked to great anxiety in romantic relationships and less enjoyment in sexual relationships. Adolescents who are overly preoccupied and insecure in relationships engaged in earlier sexual activity. Those with preoccupied attachment were at greater risk for internalizing disorders and those with insecure dismissive attachment for externalizing disorders.

Adolescents with secure attachment have lower rates of both internalizing and externalizing disorders and substance abuse. The modified Adult Attachment Interview appears to identify relatively stable classification across adolescence (Allen et al., 2004). However, adolescent attachment shows only modest continuity with measurement of attachment in early life. This may result from differences in the constructs of the Strange Situation procedure and the use of self-reports in the Adult Attachment Interview. Essentially, the Adult Attachment Interview is capturing the caregiving system more so than the attachment system as studied in infancy. However, the two are closely related (Allen & Manning, 2007). The Adult Attachment Interview predicts the parents' success as caregivers in promoting secure attachment in child-rearing. This focus on caregiving helps explain why the assessment interview is more pertinent to peer relationships than parental relationships. Infant attachment security with mothers has greater correlation and is predictive of autonomy and relatedness in adolescent–mother interactions that are linked to adolescent states of mind (Becker-Stoll et al., 2008). The adolescent world, with its social, emotional, and cognitive developmental tasks, illustrates the complexity of adolescent attachment and the importance of continuing research.

This complexity is revealed in substantial developmental change in the reorganization of the brain during the adolescent years. Changes differ in white matter and gray matter in adolescent brain development. The density of white matter steadily increases during the first two decades of life, eventually stabilizing during late adolescence. White matter myelination in the brain increases the speed of information transmission in the brain. In adolescence, one of the last regions of the brain to fully myelinate is the pre-frontal cortex, which is critical for mature cognition and self-regulation. Brain changes in gray matter follow an inverted L shape, with a development peak followed by a de-cline. The volume of gray matter peaks before the onset of puberty in boys at age 12 years and in girls at age 10 years; it is refined through synaptic pruning during adolescence to attain brain maturation during the early adult years (Giedd et al., 1999).

In addition, during adolescence, there is increased dopaminergic innervation involving the orbitofrontal ventromedial prefrontal cortex and the striatal "reward" neuronal system (Casey et al., 2008). There is a developmental increase in dopamine neuronal input to frontal brain regions during adolescence, with changing patterns of receptor subtype expression followed by greater dopaminergic activity within the ventral striatum later in adolescence. In addition. the dorsal lateral prefrontal cortex does not reach its full volume until the early 20s (Sowell et al., 1999).

White matter organization, measured by diffusion tensor imaging (DTI), has been examined in male and female adolescents with regard to impulsive behavior. DTI values correlated with self-report measures of impulse control in males but most strongly in cognitive inhibitory control in females with the Stroop Color Word Test. This suggests male/female differences in white matter microstructure are related to cognitive and be-havioral domains (Silveri et al., 2006). Sex-specific links to impulsive behavior involve the right anterior callosum in males and the right anterior splenium in females.

Functional magnetic resonance imaging (fMRI) studies have compared how adolescents process information differently than adults. Adolescents generally enlist different brain regions than adults. This difference is pertinent to executive functions involved in attention, self-monitoring, planning, judgment, and motor control. A study that compared children, adolescents, and adults found that adolescents had a greater volume of activation in dorsolateral prefrontal cortex. These maturational changes have been associated with increased risky behavior, but they also may lead to independent ac-tion against the norms prescribed by parents. Such behavior may be associated with re-warding social behaviors with friends and romantic partners (Ward, 2016). Adolescent risk-taking refers to a preference for greater sensation-seeking in adolescence than in younger children. Risk-taking is a motivated goal-directed behavior, but it is not the same as impulsivity, which is more autonomic and nonreflective.

The prefrontal cortex is involved in attentional shifting, response inhibition, pro-cessing speed, abstract thought, self-organization, decision-making, and planning. Neuroimaging studies in adolescence measure changes in brain structure and func-tion that parallel improvements in both cognitive abilities and emotional processing. Although the brain shows little change in size after age 5 years, it undergoes remodeling during late childhood and particularly during adolescence. Maturational changes in 12- to 16-year-olds and 23- to 30-year-olds are greater in the dorsal, medial, and lateral re-gions of the frontal lobes than in the parietal occipital lobes in the response inhibition task (Sowell et al., 1999). There is greater reliance on the frontal executive network in adults than children (Luna et al., 2001). Studies of executive functions in the adoles-cent years find that an increase in frontal activation results in improved performance (Yurgelun-Todd, 2007).

Adolescent social relationships improve with more accurate reading of social cues and better self-regulation of affective responses. With brain maturation, self-control also improves with progressive frontalization of inhibitory processing. Neuroendocrine changes are associated with these changes in brain organization, cognitive functioning, and cerebral metabolism (Ernst et al., 1997). Gains in frontal inhibitory activity allow better modulation of the amygdala and related subcortical and limbic emotional processing brain regions. For example, investigators find greater modulation of the amygdala on fMRI studies examining affective responses to angry and fearful faces with maturation. Functional imaging studies find that adults have greater orbitofrontal activity than adolescents when attention is focused on emotional stimuli (Monk et al., 2003). In one study, age was significantly correlated with bilateral frontal activity in adolescent females; males correlated only to right prefrontal activity. These findings provide additional support for the progressive acquisition in the prefrontal cortex of greater functional activity during the adolescent years (Yurgelun-Todd, 2007). Overall, maturation of the prefrontal brain network is critically important in the development of cognitive and emotional behaviors in adolescence. Still, differences in brain activation in adolescence need cautious interpretation. The increase found in frontal activation in adolescence may indicate these brain regions work less efficiently, requiring more effort and brain activity.

Cortical thickness in the frontal mentalizing network (theory of mind) shows a developmental reduction in adolescence (Mills et al., 2014). Mentalizing is measured beginning in the preschool years starting at approximately age 4 years. At that age, theory of mind, the ability to attribute mental states (beliefs, intents, desires, and emotions) to oneself and others, is being established. Theory of mind is important in psychological development to understand that others have mental states and perspectives different from one's own. Theory of mind deficits have been extensively evaluated in children with autism spectrum disorder (Happé & Frith, 2014). Some aspects of theory of mind competence reach adult levels in late adolescence.

Adolescent mentalization is studied using the ultimatum game. In the ultimatum game, one player, the proposer, is given money and asked to decide what proportion to give to a second player, the responder. The responder can accept or reject the offer. If accepted, the money is split between the two players at an agreed upon amount. But if the responder rejects the offer, neither player gets anything. The responder decides whether the split is fair (e.g., 50–50) or unfair (e.g., 80–20). Responders typically reject money offers below 20% because this seems unfair; the responder may decide to punish the proposer for making such an unfair offer. It is a trade-off between financial value (monetary gain) and social judgment (fairness). In brain imaging studies involving the ultimatum game, increased activity was found in the insula. The insula is a brain region linked to the emotion of disgust. Thus, when an unfair offer is made, disgust is activated. In one study, the ultimatum game responses in 9-year-old children and 18-year-old adolescents were compared (Güroğlu et al., 2009). When the responder was given the opportunity to reject the offer, there was an age-related increase in adolescence in the amount the participant proposer offered. This suggests that with development into adolescence, taking the perspective of the other person is more advanced than in childhood. With regard to social emotions, reaching sexual maturity in females influences appraisal of social emotions. In adolescents, confiding relationships have greater influence on health and in reducing stress.

## The Adult Attachment Interview

The Adult Attachment Interview is a semistructured interview that examines memoires for one's own childhood experience. Transcripts of the Adult Attachment Interview are coded based on how the adult reflects on and evaluates these early memories. The Adult Attachment Interview predicts parenting behavior and later infant–parent attachment (Bakermans-Kranenburg & van IJzendoorn, 2009). The interview alternatively asks for general descriptions of attachment relationships, specific supportive memories, and descriptions of current relationships with one's parents and other identified attachment persons. Autobiographical memories from early childhood are then evaluated in the current perspective of one's life. There are four main attachment styles (Main et al., 1985). These are coded as secure-autonomous, insecure-dismissive, insecure-preoccupied/enmeshed, and unresolved. The secure-autonomous category includes people who can recall early attachment-related experience objectively, coherently, and openly, whether they are favorable memories or not. Adults in the dismissive category minimize the importance of early attachment in their own lives or idealize them without being able to give concrete illustrations. They grade early memories as of little concern, value, or influence in their lives. Adults with preoccupied/enmeshed classification maximize the importance of attachment impact. They are preoccupied with dependency on their own parents and actively continue to struggle to please them. They are not able to describe their early relationships objectively or coherently and reflectively, in some instances with anger. The classification unresolved attached is used when there is evidence in the interview of unresolved experiences of trauma in childhood, often involving the loss or early death of attachment figures. Frequently with death of a parent in childhood, the mourning process has not been fully worked through. The unresolved classification has received empirical support as a predictor of post-traumatic stress disorder (Harari et al., 2009). In some instances in which discourse is contradictory in the Adult Attachment Interview—for example, when the parent is remembered as idealized and simultaneously described in a preoccupied angry manner—the term "cannot classify" is proposed. Examples of these four classifications are shown in Box 9.1.

In a North American study summarizing 10,000 interviews, the adult attachment classified prevalence in nonclinical adults, who completed the Adult Attachment Interview, was 58% secure, 23% dismissive, and 19% preoccupied, with 18% coded for unresolved loss or other trauma (Bakermans-Kranenburg & van IJzendoorn, 2009). There were no gender differences in the use of dismissive and preoccupied categories in this interview, but in another large-scale review, women scored higher on preoccupied states of mind and men scored higher in the dismissive category (Haydon et al., 2014).

In clinical cases with mental disorders, the insecure and unresolved classifications were more common. In a normative sample, there was evidence that secure patterns were especially stable; change in attachment patterns was only associated with significant life events (Crowell & Hauser, 2008). Overall, the secure classification is most stable, whereas the unresolved classification is least stable. In addition, there is a weak association with intelligence but no significant association with memory, social desirability, or discourse style (Crowell et al., 2016). However, despite overall stability in attachment status, change does occur based on life events. Change in attachment status varies in response to life challenges at different ages. During infancy and childhood, attachment status is related to family stress and to changes in available social support, or the waxing or waning of maternal depression. Attachment status may change across generations. Such intergenerational transmission may be linked to parent responsiveness and sensitivity. Autonomous secure adults have a greater likelihood of having secure infants, dismissive adults have a greater likelihood of having socially avoidant infants, preoccupied/enmeshed adults have a greater likelihood of having ambivalent infants, and unresolved adults have a greater likelihood of having disorganized infants.

Adult attachment status may be affected by marriage, divorce, supportive counseling, or serious reflection of one's life. One longitudinal study involved 100 mothers and fathers, who completed the Adult Attachment Inventory before their child was born. Subsequently, the Strange Situation assessment was carried out with the mother when the infant was age 12 months and with the father when the infant was age 18 months. Research staff determined the extent of deprivation and disruption the parents had experienced in their early lives. Those life experiences influenced infant attachment status and were based on how parents had coped with adversity in their own experiences of being parented. Based on background information, the research staff established a reflective self-functioning scale to ascertain potential capacity in coping. Among 17 mothers who experienced deprivation and scored low on self-reflection, 16 had insecurely attached infants. Ten mothers with deprived parenting, who were highly self-reflective, had securely attached infants. The authors concluded that the capacity for self-reflection allows changes in internal working models sufficient to enhance resilience to adversity and avoid the intergenerational transmission for insecurity in their infants (Fonagy et al., 1994). Self-reflective mothers also may have benefited from using self-reflection when receiving counseling or other supportive care. Among all attachment types, however, disruptive attachment in one generation did predict disorganized attachment in the next (Raby et al., 2015). Disorganized attachment predicts lack of resolution of trauma or loss on the Adult Attachment Interview. The lack of attachment resolution predicts the long-term risk of frightening parental behavior toward the child and the importance of recognizing attachment styles.

## Maternal Sensitivity Mental Health and Psychopathology

Maternal mental illness is a modifiable risk factor in child development. Maternal symptoms of anxiety and depression (both postnatal depression and general depression), ADHD, schizophrenia, and substance abuse (alcohol, cocaine, and opiates) have been shown to impact their sensitivity to infant social cues and overall care. The impact of maternal depression or anxiety in children has been examined in studies of temperament, behavior, brain structure, and brain connectivity (Buss et al., 2012; Lupien et al., 2009; Qiu et al., 2015). Subclinical depression in mothers is associated with irritability, interpersonal conflict, and insecure attachment.

The influence has been studied in typically developing children (Phua et al., 2020). The influence of positive maternal health impacts parenting and child outcomes, whereas depression and anxiety have negative effects. Positive mental health refers to secure autonomy, self-acceptance, meaningful relationships, and life satisfaction. Positive mental health enhances maternal sensitivity to infants, leading to greater weight gain, language acquisition, and cognitive development in infants. These findings draw attention to the importance of facilitating positive mental health. Maternal sensitivity is essential to infant mental health.

One meta-analysis included 70 published studies examining 88 maternal sensitivity measures of attachment status (Bakermans-Kranenburg et al., 2003). Attachment interventions included measures of maternal sensitivity, social support for the parent, maternal mental health supports, and enhancing reflective positive maternal representations of the infant. Most studies included in the review were randomized controlled trials measuring the effect size of the interventions on maternal sensitivity outcomes. The most effective interventions were those using video feedback to mothers; these started when infants were 6 months old. Trials that measured attachment security showed small but significant effect size on infant attachment security (Deans, 2020). The mother's age, socioeconomic status, prematurity of the infant, and risk factors were evaluated. A follow-up to this meta-analysis study searched for children younger than age 36 months over a subsequent 3-year period. These four new randomized control trials showed that the attachment-based interventions improved attachment security (Mountain et al., 2017). Meta-analyses of successful interventions in improving maternal sensitivity in mothers with psychiatric diagnoses, especially depression, have shown benefit. There is a consensus from these meta-analyses that intervention does increase maternal sensitivity. Emotional and behavioral responses learned by the mother that facilitated either interactional synchrony or better understanding of their child's emotions and behavior were shown to be effective. Longer term studies are needed to establish longitudinal benefit (Deans, 2020).

Parenting mediates the association between maternal mental health and child outcomes. In addition to research on attachment security, other studies have focused on outcomes based on parental style of child-rearing. Some parents emphasize strict discipline, whereas others are more permissive. Research studies identify global styles of child-rearing used in the United States. These styles are authoritarian, authoritative, and permissive. Authoritarian parents are dogmatic and focus on discipline and behavior; they believe in strict discipline. Authoritative parents also focus on discipline and behavior, but they are more warm and supportive. They use explanation and discuss behavior with children and adapt discipline accordingly. Permissive parents are indulgent and relaxed regarding ideas about behavior and discipline. The Parenting Styles and Dimensions Questionnaire was used to examine parental style (Robinson et al., 2001). In a longitudinal study involving 6,400 adolescents aged 14–18 years, participants were asked to report on parents' involvement in their schooling. Authoritative parenting was best correlated with school performance (Steinberg et al., 1992). In contrast, authoritarian parents and permissive parents had little involvement with schools. Four components were identified as important in authoritative parenting: parental acceptance and expressed warmth, behavioral supervision, strictness, and encouragement of psychological autonomy. A 2019 analysis of data from 270 mother–child pairs from a longitudinal birth cohort examined child outcomes at age 48 months using the Parenting Styles and Dimensions Questionnaire. Positive maternal health was strongly correlated with authoritative parenting. Authoritative parenting predicted child performance and mastery of cognitive and executive function tasks. Poorer outcomes were mediated by authoritarian and permissive parenting styles. However, there are cultural differences in parenting styles. A study in Spain found permissive/indulgent parenting common, and another in China found that more authoritarian style was common.

## Neurobiology of Maternal Mental Health and Parenting

Social neuroscience focuses on the neurobiology of social perception, social cognition, and social behavior (Stanley & Adolphs, 2013). Social neuroscience increasingly involves refined fMRI studies to measure aspects of sociability. Our understanding of individual differences in social behavior is being advanced through examination of genotype differences and the role of neuropeptides, oxytocin, and vasopressin in social affiliation. Studies of maternal behavior and parenting benefit from new knowledge from the neuroendocrinology of social engagement. These include examination of the neural circuits linked to oxytocin and vasopressin in receptors. Both peptides influence a range of social behaviors. Oxytocin underlies social engagement, and vasopressin is involved with long-term pair bonding and protective aggression in males. Intranasal oxytocin administration can increase trust and is linked to empathy and in-group altruism. Effects of both peptides are context-dependent. Oxytocin and vasopressin are important in parenting and child outcomes from parenting. The interface of dopamine and oxytocin facilitates motivation for social contact and cognitive emotional states of mind that are crucial for effective parental care. Oxytocin reduces anxiety and facilitates positive states of mind, prosocial behavior, and social well-being. Oxytocin is associated with a sense of calm linked to increased parasympathetic tone (Uvnäs-Moberg et al., 2005). Polymorphisms of the oxytocin receptor gene are correlated with the degree of expressed positive affect (Lucht et al., 2009). Single nucleotide polymorphisms in oxytocin and oxytocin receptor genes and their variants are associated with both emotional well-being and positive behaviors (Mileva-Seitz et al., 2013).

In people diagnosed with social anxiety disorders, administration of oxytocin intranasally modulates amygdala to frontal lobe functional connectivity, the amygdala–frontal resting state studied with resting-state fMRI. Oxytocin-enhanced resting-state functional connectivity was studied in a randomized double-blind crossover study that involved 18 patients with generalized social anxiety disorder and 18 control subjects (Dodhia et al., 2014). The study reported oxytocin-enhanced resting state connectivity involving the left and right amygdala. This connectivity links to the rostral anterior cingulate/medial prefrontal cortex. Oxytocin concurrently normalized (reversed) amygdala frontal connectivity. These findings demonstrate that oxytocin can modulate a neural circuit involved in threat processing and emotional regulation. Oxytocin plays an essential role in activating maternal behavior, social sensitivity, and reciprocal attachment in human child-rearing. It moderated autonomic nervous activity to facilitate social behavioral adaptation (Carter, 2014).

In a study in which plasma oxytocin levels were measured across pregnancy and the postpartum period in 62 women, oxytocin levels in early pregnancy and in the postpartum period were correlated with mother–infant positive affect, gaze, vocalizations, affectionate touch, and mother's frequent checking on the infant. Oxytocin proved important in the emergence of these nurturant behaviors and mental representations important to mother–infant bonding. The association of oxytocin levels in the first trimester of pregnancy with postpartum behaviors is consistent with oxytocin administration priming mental processes important for social bonds. These findings are consistent with oxytocin's priming function in other mammals. The oxytocin level increase from early pregnancy to late pregnancy was associated with a higher level of maternal–infant attachment in this study (Feldman, 2007).

Neuroimaging studies have also examined mothers' responses to their own infants compared to an unfamiliar infant using pictures of their child and correlated the responses with attachment style (secure or dismissive) during the second trimester of pregnancy. Postpartum brain activation patterns measured with fMRI and oxytocin levels measured in mother–infant play were correlated with attachment status. When mothers were shown a picture of their own child versus that of an unknown child, there was activation of brain regions that mediate emotional responsiveness (amygdala and insula) and those linked to theory of mind (anterior paracingulate cortex and posterior superior temporal sulcus) (Leibenluft et al., 2004). Viewing unfamiliar children versus unfamiliar adults was associated with activation of fusiform gyrus, intraparietal sulcus, precuneus, and posterior superior temporal sulcus. These patterns of differential brain activation in the orbital frontal cortex and ventral striatum are consistent with normal maternal attachment. A double-blind study using cortical event-related potentials examined the effects of intranasal oxytocin on early neural responses to emotional faces in mothers of 1-year-old infants. Thirty-eight of the mothers were presented with happy and sad infant faces, and face-sensitive and attentional brain activation were examined. The findings support the role of oxytocin to enhance perceptual salience of social and emotional stimulation (Peltola et al., 2018). Variations in gene encoding the oxytocin receptor are proposed to be related to variations in maternal parenting (Michalska et al., 2014).

Oxytocin has been shown to have a significant role in parenting by enhancing the reward value of social engagement with the infant. A genetic neuroimaging study examined activation of brain regions that mediate affect, reward, and social behavior. In response to child stimulus, these regions were significantly correlated with positive parenting. Moreover, single nucleotide polymorphisms of the oxytocin receptor (rs53576 and rs1042778) were significantly correlated with both positive parenting and hemodynamic responsiveness to presentation of child stimuli, with activation in the orbitofrontal cortex, anterior cingulate cortex, and right hippocampus. In this study, the oxytocin receptor rs53576 allele was associated with greater activation in regions of interest linked to parenting. These included (a) orienting toward, monitoring, and evaluation of cues in the child's behavior; and (b) evaluating the salience of emotional information and its regulation of emotional responses. Mother–child interactions were videotaped and coded using the dyadic parent–child interaction coding system for positive parenting (praise and positive affect) and negative parenting (critical statements and negative commands). For the neuroimaging component, photographs of the child at ages 4–6 years and photographs of unrelated matched children were used in fMRI stimuli. Orbitofrontal activation was correlated with positive parenting. The findings linking polymorphisms of the oxytocin receptor to neural functioning in maternal parenting support the feasibility of tracing biological pathways from genes to brain regions to positive maternal parenting behavior incorporating genetic imaging methodology.

Neuroimaging studies also reveal activation of brain regions high in dopamine receptors when parents view images of their children. Moreover, polymorphisms of dopamine signaling genes are linked to maternal sensitivity and infant-directed vocalizations (Mileva-Seitz et al., 2012). Genetic variation in both DRD1 and DRD2 genes was examined in 187 Caucasian mothers, and it was found to predict variation in mother–infant interaction at the age of 6 months. Consistent with the animal literature, Mileva-Seitz et al. (2012) found genetic variation in DRD1 and DRD2 and maternal orienting away and infant vocalizing, respectively. DRD1 compared to DRD2 in humans has a preferential role in visuospatial working memory correlated with executive functioning. The DRD1 polymorphism is consistent with maternal distractibility and inattention to the infant. The DRD2 polymorphism was correlated with attending to infant vocalizations during free play with the infant. The DRD2 genetic variation was linked to reward and working memory. Overall, this study is an example of translational research showing the role of the dopamine system in the regulation of mothering.

Taken together, both oxytocin and dopamine systems have been linked to maternal positive affect and to executive functions essential for effective parenting. Oxytocin facilitates social salience and social engagement between mother and infant. Dopamine systems associate positive affect to executive functions. Dopamine polymorphisms predict maternal attention to their infant during free play. Oxytocin receptor polymorphisms are linked to maternal emotional sensitivity and positive parenting; thus, dopamine and oxytocin genes act synergistically. Maternal executive functioning mediates the relationship between oxytocin and dopamine gene variants and maternal responsiveness. This interaction was examined in a study of 157 mothers recruited in the MAVAN study carried out in Canada (O'Donnell et al., 2014). In this study, single nucleotide polymorphisms related to both oxytocin receptors (rs237885 and rs2254298) and dopamine receptors (DRD1 rs686 and DRD2 rs265976) were correlated with a mother's decision-making at 48 months using the Cambridge Neuropsychological Test Automated Battery. The authors evaluated maternal responsiveness from videotaped interactions. Their analysis found that oxytocin receptor rs2254298 carriers had an indirect effect on positive parenting mediated by a mother's performance on decision-making tasks, and oxytocin receptor rs2254298 had effects on physically controlling behavior. Dopamine receptor polymorphisms were not associated with any measure of executive functioning or parenting. Earlier oxytocin studies showed the importance of oxytocin with the onset of maternal behavior and bonding, close contact, and nursing. A study of 4-year-olds extends finding to executive functioning with improved and positive parenting and decreased physical control with one polymorphism (O'Donnell et al., 2014). The polymorphism of the dopamine receptor chosen was linked to parenting. Other investigators have focused more broadly on the role of the oxytocin peptide and dopamine neuromodulation. Dopamine striatal neurons mediate general reward and reward anticipation, including social reward. Feldman et al. (2016) emphasized the roles that oxytocin and dopamine play in biobehavioral synchrony, highlighting the rewards of social engagement as related to dopamine rather than specific maternal behaviors. Feldman et al. also suggested that salience of social stimuli is increased by oxytocin (Bartz et al., 2010). The integration of oxytocin and vasopressin measures may enhance the experience of social synchrony with cycles of rewarding social bonding along with repetitive reinforcing motivation involving the dopamine system and warm social engagement from oxytocin.

Neuroimaging studies confirm that the activation of brain systems is linked to social bonding and the importance of oxytocin in facilitating social engagement. The extent to which these systems explain the quality of human attachment (secure vs. insecure) between mother and infant has also been examined. One study measured the differences in maternal reward brain activation using fMRI and peripheral oxytocin release in response to infant cues based on the mother's attachment classification. The authors hypothesized that mothers with a secure pattern of adult attachment would, when challenged, demonstrate an increased response to their own infant's face in mesocorticolimbic regions on fMRI. These include the midbrain ventral tegmental area, the ventral striatum, and medial prefrontal cortex. Moreover, this would be found to be true when viewing both happy and sad infant faces. They also hypothesized that mothers who rated securely attached on the Adult Attachment Interview would be found to have enhanced plasma oxytocin response when interacting with their infants and that these would correlate with maternal brain responses.

The study found group differences in maternal brain activation of fMRI and oxytocin response by the mother to infant cues. These differences were correlated with secure or insecure attachment self-report ratings on the Adult Attachment Interview. Mothers with secure versus insecure (dismissing) attachment could be distinguished. Mothers with secure attachment showed activation of mesocorticolimbic fMRI-based reward regions when viewing their own infant's smiling face. Their peripheral oxytocin increased when they played with their infants. Moreover, substantial differences in brain activation were found in response to their own infant's sad face. Securely attached mothers showed greater activation on brain reward processing regions, whereas insecure/dismissive mothers showed greater activation of the anterior insula. The anterior insula region is associated with feelings of disgust, unfairness, and pain (Montague & Lohrenz, 2007; Vicario et al., 2017). These findings are consistent with those of an another report that found individual differences in activation of striatum and amygdala circuits based on personal significance of facial expressions (Vrticka et al., 2008). The findings are also consistent with the finding that people with an insecure/dismissive attachment style have difficulty in inhibiting negative social emotions. Negative social emotions may lead to avoidance or rejection of negative (sad) infant cues; conversely, the motivation of securely attached mothers is to approach and console. Dismissive mothers showed greater activation of the hypothalamic–pituitary stress hormone axis. Securely attached mothers exhibited approach behavior with activation of the lateral prefrontal cortex bilaterally; the left medial prefrontal cortex (orbitofrontal cortex); and the hypothalamic–pituitary area, where oxytocin is produced and released. Securely attached mothers showed a greater response to their own infant's face than insecure mothers. Securely attached mothers showed a greater peripheral oxytocin response when interacting with their infant during free play time ($p = .01$).

In this study (Vrticka et al., 2008), the correlation of peripheral oxytocin release with activation of reward regions of the brain indicates that oxytocin release may be a mechanism whereby socially relevant social cues can activate reward-based dopaminergic pathways and reinforce positive mother–infant interaction. Although promising as a mechanism, there is no reported independent measure of oxytocin in specified brain regions nor evidence that central oxytocin is released during the time of behavior measurement; the oxytocin measured was peripheral and measured 4 months before the fMRI scanning. Importantly, the correlation between oxytocin and hemodynamic brain activation may reflect enduring trait differences and be critical with attachment security (Strathearn et al., 2009). These findings are consistent with earlier findings that insecure attachment is associated with difficulty in affect regulation.

Although intragenerational transmission of attachment has been proposed, the mechanism is not well understood (van IJzendoorn, 1995). The intragenerational transmission gap cannot be explained by genes alone or by separate accounts of genetic and environmental input. However, gene–environment interactions provide compelling evidence of their importance. The differential sensitivity model proposes that children may differ in their openness to parenting influences, and it hypothesizes that vulnerability to insecure attachment may make some children more vulnerable to stressful environments and others prone to becoming very securely attached to positive environments (Bakermans-Kranenburg & van IJzendoorn, 2016). Importantly, some focus of attachment status may endure across generations. The intragenerational transmission model proposes the study of repeated insecurity across generations, including both grandparents and great grandparents. The study by Strathearn (2009) contributes to our understanding of intragenerational transmission by its demonstration that secure attachment is associated with more intense maternal brain region reward activation to infant faces, whereas insecure mothers show greater insula responses to negative infant cues.

Oxytocin has the potential to not only modulate functional connectivity in specific circuits but also facilitate functional connectivity between these brain regions (Bethlehem et al., 2013). Additional research is needed in larger samples that include mothers with insecure/preoccupied attachment. Epigenetic studies may advance our understanding of intragenerational attachment. Studies in animals demonstrate that the maternal grooming of the newborn female rat pups also impacts the second-generation offspring of the original mother. Maternal grooming of her pups moderates the stress response of her offspring as adults (Cameron et al., 2005). This animal model may explain, in part, the human mother attachment intergenerational cycle. Rearing experiences affect gene expression; this stimulation could precipitate a cascade of developmental processes, leading to differences in parenting strategies in adulthood. These strategies then might be transmitted intergenerationally by nongenetic or epigenetic means (Simpson & Belsky, 2008).

Attachment theory is essentially an evolutionary theory of human social behavior. In *The Descent of Man*, Charles Darwin (1871) wrote,

> For with those animals which benefit by living in close association, the individuals which took the greatest pleasure in society would best escape various dangers; whilst those that care least for their comrades and lived solitary would perish in greater numbers. (p. 800)

For John Bowlby, almost 100 years later, attachment theory is an evolutionary theory of social behavior "from cradle to grave" (Bowlby, 1969, p. 129). In regard to attachment, there may be an intergenerational gap (van IJzendoorn, 1995). Despite strong meta-analysis, there is evidence that adult and child attachment are associated; mediation of parental security is partial (Bakermans-Kranenburg et al., 2003). A meta-analytic path model found the association was not fully explained by parental sensitivity—referred to as the transmission gap. A meta-analysis involving 4,819 dyads in 95 studies found the gap was nearly 50% (Verhage et al., 2016). This intergenerational transmission may depend on multiple pathways and not only caregiver sensitivity. Both caregiver sensitivity and support for maternal secure autonomy are important. Mothers with more insecure/dismissive attachment are less sensitive to their children, whereas those with insecure/preoccupied attachment provide less support for the child's autonomy.

The context of the parent–child relationship must be taken into account (family functioning, relationship between parents, and mutual support) as well as recognition of the differential sensitivity to the child–caregiver interaction. Differential sensitivity refers to differences in genetic makeup or temperamental features related to the impact of rearing environments on children. Based on this study (Verhage et al., 2016), there are multiple conditions that determine whether intergenerational transmission occurs. For example, intergenerational transmission was not found for teenage mothers; however, the involvement of active grandparents may be predictive. Cumulative adversity also may affect maternal sensitivity. Epidemiology studies of human populations in which there is generational adversity indicate higher rates of psychiatric disorders despite an absence of actual exposure (Yehuda et al., 2001).

The recapitulation of disorders or risk factors in new generations has not been adequately assessed in humans but has been demonstrated in mice mediated by epigenetic marks transmitted to offspring (Saavedra-Rodríguez & Feig, 2013). The generation of transmissible epigenetic marks has been explained through behavioral and social transmission. A compelling example is a rat model of social transmission (McGowan et al., 2011) in which enriched maternal care measured by high levels of maternal licking and grooming changes DNA methylation throughout the genome and at transcription factor binding sites in the hippocampal glucocorticoid receptor (Weaver et al., 2004). Maternal care associated with hypomethylation of the glucocorticoid receptor promotor leads to increased expression of the receptor protein and downregulation of hypothalamic–pituitary–adrenal axis reactivity, enhancing stress resilience in the offspring. This epigenetic mechanism predisposes the next generation of mothers to high levels of licking in their own pups.

Human studies have also revealed behavioral (social) transmission of acquired epigenetic marks. Differences were found in offspring of mothers affected by the Dutch Hunger Winter during the Nazi occupation of the Netherlands in World War II. Moreover, there were alterations in the expression of cortisol in children who were in utero during the September 11, 2001, terrorist attacks (Matthews & Phillips, 2012). Reprograming in the germline related to environment exposure has been demonstrated in plants, fruit flies, and mammals; however, the strongest findings are in animal models (Boyce & Kobor, 2015; Franklin et al., 2010). Finally, maternal and paternal post-traumatic stress disorder has been found to impact epigenetic regulation of the glucocorticoid receptor in the offspring of Holocaust survivors through differential methylation of the receptor's promotor. All these studies demonstrate that life experiences, especially in early life, can result in alterations of the epigenetic marks. Through this mechanism, neurodevelopment can be regulated, with impact on learning, behavior, and risk for mental disorders (Boyce & Kobor, 2015).

Importantly, the rearing environment can compensate for children at risk; compensatory parental mentalization may play a role in the establishment of secure attachment. *Parental mentalization* is defined as the degree to which parents show appropriate appreciation of their infant's mental states (van IJzendoorn & Bakermans-Kranenburg, 2019). Mentalization involves three components: parental mind-mindedness, insight, and parental reflective functioning (Zeegers et al., 2017). Mentalization is typically assessed in an interview with the parent about the child's thoughts and feelings, although it is not a dimension of parenting behavior per se. Rather, it refers to mental or cognitive capacity expressed through parental behavior toward the child. A meta-analysis found that both mentalizing and maternal sensitivity are important in child attachment security (Zeegers et al., 2017). Further studies are needed to incorporate adult attachment measures in the research design.

In summary, attachment-relevant parenting must take into account parental sensitivity, continued support to maintain secure attachment in mothers, limit setting, behavioral synchrony, and parent–child communication. In addition, the recognition of situations that are stressful for the child and the parents and providing support to cope are important for positive attachment parenting. A variety of interventions target mental health in mothers during pregnancy and in the postpartum period (Phua et al., 2020). These interventions should be tailored to specific cognitive emotional demands of pregnancy and child-rearing on maternal mental health. A common intervention is mindfulness-based intervention in the perinatal period to target emotional and cognitive demands in pregnancy (Hall et al, 2016; Taylor et al., 2016).

In the postnatal period, interventions have been developed that focus specifically on parenting skills to enhance maternal and child outcomes. One example is the Triple P-Positive Parenting Program (Sanders, 1999) to facilitate parenting skills. Overall, maternal health must also be taken into account at both perinatal and postnatal follow-up. There is a strong association of maternal mental health with birth outcomes; positive mental health during pregnancy is associated with reduced maternal cortisol levels (Pluess et al., 2012). There is an ongoing need for reliable measures of the dimensions of positive mental health and underlying biology across pregnancy, the perinatal period, and infancy. Both positive mental health measures and measures of anxiety, depression, and maternal stress should be routinely assessed in studies of child growth and development. These will serve as the foundation for evidence-based interventions targeting maternal mental health (Phua et al., 2020).

# References

Abraham, M. M., & Kerns, K. A. (2013). Positive and negative emotions and coping as mediators of mother–child attachment and peer relationships. *Merrill–Palmer Quarterly*, 59(4), 399–425.

Ainsworth, M. D. (1973). The development of mother–infant attachment. *Review of Child Development Research*, 3, 1–94.

Ainsworth, M. D. (1985a). Patterns of infant–mother attachments: Antecedents and effects on development. *Bulletin of the New York Academy of Medicine*, 61(9), 771–791.

Ainsworth, M. D. (1985b). Attachments across the life span. *Bulletin of the New York Academy of Medicine*, *61*(9), 792–812.

Ainsworth, M. D., Bell, S. M., & Stayton, D. J. (1971). Individual differences in strange-situation behaviour of one-year-olds. In H. R. Schaffer (Ed.), *The origins of human social relations* (pp. 17–58). Academic Press.

Ainsworth, M. D., Blehar, M., Waters, E., & Wall, S. (1978). *Patterns of attachment*: A psychological study of the strange situation. Erlbaum.

Allen, J. P., & Manning, N. (2007, Fall). From safety to affect regulation: Attachment from the vantage point of adolescence. *New Directions for Child and Adolescent Development*, (117), 23–39.

Allen, J. P., McElhaney, K. B., Kuperminc, G. P., & Jodl, K. M. (2004). Stability and change in attachment security across adolescence. *Child Development*, *75*(6), 1792–1805.

Allen, J. P., & Tan, J. (2016). The multiple faces of attachment in adolescence. In J. Cassidy & P. R. Shaver (Eds.), *Handbook of attachment: Theory, research, and clinical applications* (3rd ed., pp. 399–434). Guilford.

Ammaniti, M., van IJzendoorn, M. H., Speranza, A. M., & Tambelli, R. (2000). Internal working models of attachment during late childhood and early adolescence: An exploration of stability and change. *Attachment & Human Development*, *2*(3), 328–346.

Aviezer, O., Sagi-Schwartz, A., & Koren-Karie, N. (2003). Ecological constraints on the formation of infant–mother attachment relations: When maternal sensitivity becomes ineffective. *Infant Behavior and Development*, *26*(3), 285–299.

Bakermans-Kranenburg, M. J., & van IJzendoorn, M. H. (2008). Oxytocin receptor (OXTR) and serotonin transporter (5-HTT) genes associated with observed parenting. *Social Cognitive and Affective Neuroscience*, *3*(2), 128–134.

Bakermans-Kranenburg, M. J., & van IJzendoorn, M. H. (2009). The first 10,000 Adult Attachment Interviews: Distributions of adult attachment representations in clinical and non-clinical groups. *Attachment & Human Development*, *11*(3), 223–263.

Bakermans-Kranenburg, M. J., & van IJzendoorn, M. H. (2011). Differential susceptibility to rearing environment depending on dopamine-related genes: New evidence and a meta-analysis. *Development and Psychopathology*, *23*(1), 39–52.

Bakermans-Kranenburg, M. J., & van IJzendoorn, M. H. (2016). Attachment, parenting, and genetics. *Handbook of Attachment: Theory, Research, and Clinical Applications*, *3*, 155–180.

Bakermans-Kranenburg, M. J., van IJzendoorn, M. H., & Juffer, F. (2003). Less is more: Meta-analyses of sensitivity and attachment interventions in early childhood. *Psychological Bulletin*, *129*(2), 195–215.

Barr, C. S., Newman, T. K., Becker, M. L., Parker, C. C., Champoux, M., Lesch, K. P., Goldman, D., Suomi, S., & Higley, J. D. (2003). The utility of the non-human primate model for studying gene by environment interactions in behavioral research. *Genes, Brain and Behavior*, *2*(6), 336–340.

Bartz, J. A., Zaki, J., Bolger, N., Hollander, E., Ludwig, N. N., Kolevzon, A., & Ochsner, K. N. (2010). Oxytocin selectively improves empathic accuracy. *Psychological Science*, *21*(10), 1426–1428.

Becker-Stoll, F., Fremmer-Bombik, E., Wartner, U., Zimmermann, P., & Grossmann, K. E. (2008). Is attachment at ages 1, 6 and 16 related to autonomy and relatedness behavior of adolescents in interaction towards their mothers? *International Journal of Behavioral Development*, *32*(5), 372–380.

Belsky, J., & Pluess, M. (2009). Beyond diathesis stress: Differential susceptibility to environmental influences. *Psychological Bulletin*, *135*(6), 885–908.

Bethlehem, R. A., van Honk, J., Auyeung, B., & Baron-Cohen, S. (2013). Oxytocin, brain physiology, and functional connectivity: A review of intranasal oxytocin fMRI studies. *Psychoneuroendocrinology*, *38*(7), 962–974.

Bokhorst, C. L., Bakermans-Kranenburg, M. J., Pasco Fearon, R. M., van IJzendoorn, M. H., Fonagy, P., & Schuengel, C. (2003). The importance of shared environment in mother–infant attachment security: A behavioral genetic study. *Child Development*, *74*(6), 1769–1782.

Bowlby, J. (1969). *Attachment*. Basic Books.

Bowlby, J. (1988). Developmental psychiatry comes of age. *American Journal of Psychiatry*, *145*(1), 1–10.

Boyce, W. T., & Kobor, M. S. (2015). Development and the epigenome: The "synapse" of gene–environment interplay. *Developmental Science, 18*(1), 1–23.

Brenning, K. M., Soenens, B., Braet, C., & Bosmans, G. (2012). Attachment and depressive symptoms in middle childhood and early adolescence: Testing the validity of the emotion regulation model of attachment. *Personal Relationships, 19*(3), 445–464.

Bretherton, I., & Munholland, K. A. (2008). Internal working models in attachment relationships: Elaborating a central construct in attachment theory. In J. Cassidy & P. R. Shaver (Eds.), *Handbook of attachment: Theory, research, and clinical applications* (pp. 102–127). Guilford.

Brumariu, L. E., Kerns, K. A., & Seibert, A. (2012). Mother–child attachment, emotion regulation, and anxiety symptoms in middle childhood. *Personal Relationships, 19*(3), 569–585.

Buss, C., Davis, E. P., Shahbaba, B., Pruessner, J. C., Head, K., & Sandman, C. A. (2012). Maternal cortisol over the course of pregnancy and subsequent child amygdala and hippocampus volumes and affective problems. *Proceedings of the National Academy of Sciences of the USA, 109*(20), E1312–E1319.

Cameron, N. M., Champagne, F. A., Parent, C., Fish, E. W., Ozaki-Kuroda, K., & Meaney, M. J. (2005). The programming of individual differences in defensive responses and reproductive strategies in the rat through variations in maternal care. *Neuroscience & Biobehavioral Reviews, 29*(4–5), 843–865.

Carter, C. S. (2014). Oxytocin pathways and the evolution of human behavior. *Annual Review of Psychology, 65*, 17–39.

Casey, B. J., Getz, S., & Galvan, A. (2008). The adolescent brain. *Developmental Review, 28*(1), 62–77.

Champoux, M., Bennett, A., Shannon, C., Higley, J. D., Lesch, K. P., & Suomi, S. J. (2002). Serotonin transporter gene polymorphism, differential early rearing, and behavior in rhesus monkey neonates. *Molecular Psychiatry, 7*(10), 1058–1063.

Coleman, P. K. (2003). Perceptions of parent–child attachment, social self-efficacy, and peer relationships in middle childhood. *Infant and Child Development, 12*(4), 351–368.

Colonnesi, C., Draijer, E. M., Stams, G. J. J. M., Van der Bruggen, C. O., Bögels, S. M., & Noom, M. J. (2011). The relation between insecure attachment and child anxiety: A meta-analytic review. *Journal of Clinical Child & Adolescent Psychology, 40*(4), 630–645.

Cowie, H. A., Smith, P. K., & Blades, M. (2015). *Understanding children's development* (6th ed.). Wiley.

Crowell, J. A., Fraley, R. C., & Roisman, G. I. (2016). Measurement of individual differences in adult attachment. In J. Cassidy & P. R. Shaver (Eds.), *Handbook of attachment: Theory, research, and clinical applications* (3rd ed., pp. 598–635). Guilford.

Crowell, J. A., & Hauser, S. T. (2008). AAIs in a high-risk sample: Stability and relation to functioning from adolescence to 39 years. In H. Steele & M. Steele (Eds.), *Clinical applications of the Adult Attachment Interview* (pp. 341–370). Guilford.

Damasio, J. (2018). *The strange order of things: Life, feeling, and the making of cultures.* Pantheon.

Darwin, C. (1871). *The decent of man and selection in relation to sex* [Electronic version]. Appleton.

Deans, C. L. (2020). Maternal sensitivity, its relationship with child outcomes, and interventions that address it: A systematic literature review. *Early Child Development and Care, 190*(2), 252–275.

Dodhia, S., Hosanagar, A., Fitzgerald, D. A., Labuschagne, I., Wood, A. G., Nathan, P. J., & Phan, K. L. (2014). Modulation of resting-state amygdala–frontal functional connectivity by oxytocin in generalized social anxiety disorder. *Neuropsychopharmacology, 39*(9), 2061–2069.

Dozier, M., Stoval, K. C., Albus, K. E., & Bates, B. (2001). Attachment for infants in foster care: The role of caregiver state of mind. *Child Development, 72*(5), 1467–1477.

Edwards, A. C., Bacanu, S. A., Bigdeli, T. B., Moscati, A., & Kendler, K. S. (2016). Evaluating the dopamine hypothesis of schizophrenia in a large-scale genome-wide association study. *Schizophrenia Research, 176*(2–3), 136–140.

Ernst, M., Cohen, R. M., Liebenauer, L. L., Jons, P. H., & Zametkin, A. J. (1997). Cerebral glucose metabolism in adolescent girls with attention-deficit/hyperactivity disorder. *Journal of the American Academy of Child & Adolescent Psychiatry, 36*(10), 1399–1406.

Fearon, R. M., van IJzendoorn, M. H., Fonagy, P., Bakermans-Kranenburg, M. J., Schuengel, C., & Bokhorst, C. L. (2006). In search of shared and nonshare environmental factors in security of attachment: A behavior–genetic study of the association between sensitivity and attachment security. *Developmental Psychology, 42*(6), 1026–1040.

Feldman, R. (2007). Parent–infant synchrony and the construction of shared timing; Physiological precursors, developmental outcomes, and risk conditions. *Journal of Child Psychology and Psychiatry, 48*(3–4), 329–354.

Feldman, R., Monakhov, M., Pratt, M., & Ebstein, R. P. (2016). Oxytocin pathway genes: Evolutionary ancient system impacting on human affiliation, sociality, and psychopathology. *Biological Psychiatry, 79*(3), 174–184.

Fonagy, P., Steele, M., Steele, H., Higgitt, A., & Target, M. (1994). The Emanuel Miller Memorial Lecture 1992: The theory and practice of resilience. *Journal of Child Psychology and Psychiatry, 35*(2), 231–257.

Franklin, T. B., Russig, H., Weiss, I. C., Gräff, J., Linder, N., Michalon, A., Vizi, S., & Mansuy, I. M. (2010). Epigenetic transmission of the impact of early stress across generations. *Biological Psychiatry, 68*(5), 408–415.

George, C., & Solomon, J. (2016). The Attachment Doll Play Assessment: Predictive validity with concurrent mother–child interaction and maternal caregiving representations. *Frontiers in Psychology, 7*, 1594. https://doi.org/10.3389/fpsyg.2016.01594

Giedd, J. N., Blumenthal, J., Jeffries, N. O., Castellanos, F. X., Liu, H., Zijdenbos, A., Paus, T., Evans, A., & Rapoport, J. L. (1999). Brain development during childhood and adolescence: A longitudinal MRI study. *Nature Neuroscience, 2*(10), 861–863.

Gilissen, R., Bakermans-Kranenburg, M. J., van IJzendoorn, M. H., & van der Veer, R. (2008). Parent–child relationship, temperament, and physiological reactions to fear-inducing film clips: Further evidence for differential susceptibility. *Journal of Experimental Child Psychology, 99*(3), 182–195.

Güroğlu, B., van den Bos, W., & Crone, E. A. (2009). Fairness considerations: Increasing understanding of intentionality during adolescence. *Journal of Experimental Child Psychology, 104*(4), 398–409.

Hall, H. G., Beattie, J., Lau, R., East, C., & Biro, M. A. (2016). Mindfulness and perinatal mental health: A systematic review. *Women and Birth, 29*(1), 62–71.

Happé, F., & Frith, U. (2014). Annual research review: Towards a developmental neuroscience of atypical social cognition. *Journal of Child Psychology and Psychiatry, 55*(6), 553–577.

Harari, D., Bakermans-Kranenburg, M. J., De Kloet, C. S., Geuze, E., Vermetten, E., Westenberg, H. G. M., & van IJzendoorn, M. H. (2009). Attachment representations in Dutch veterans with and without deployment-related PTSD. *Attachment & Human Development, 11*(6), 515–536.

Hayden, E. P., Hanna, B., Sheikh, H. I., Laptook, R. S., Kim, J., Singh, S. M., & Klein, D. N. (2013). Child dopamine active transporter 1 genotype and parenting: Evidence for evocative gene–environment correlations. *Development and Psychopathology, 25*(1), 163–173.

Haydon, K. C., Roisman, G. I., Owen, M. T., Booth-LaForce, C., & Cox, M. J. (2014). Shared and distinctive antecedents of adult attachment interview state-of-mind and inferred-experience dimensions. *Monographs of the Society for Research in Child Development, 79*(3), 108–125.

Hesse, E. (2016). Adult Attachment Interview: Protocol, method of analysis, and selected empirical studies. In J. A. Cassidy & P. R. Shaver (Eds.), *Handbook of attachment: Theory, research, and clinical applications* (3rd ed., pp. 553–597). Guilford.

Kerns, K. A., & Brumariu, L. E. (2016). Attachment in the middle childhood. In J. A. Cassidy & P. R. Shaver (Eds.), *Handbook of attachment: Theory, research, and clinical applications* (3rd ed., pp. 349–365). Guilford.

Kerns, K. A., Mathews, B. L., Koehn, A. J., Williams, C. T., & Siener-Ciesla, S. (2015). Assessing both safe haven and secure base support in parent–child relationships. *Attachment & Human Development, 17*(4), 337–353.

Klahr, A. M., Klump, K., & Burt, S. A. (2015). A constructive replication of the association between the oxytocin receptor genotype and parenting. *Journal of Family Psychology, 29*(1), 91–99.

Kochanska, G. (2001). Emotional development in children with different attachment histories: The first three years. *Child Development, 72*(2), 474–490.

Koehn, A. J., & Kerns, K. A. (2018). Parent–child attachment: Meta-analysis of associations with parenting behaviors in middle childhood and adolescence. *Attachment & Human Development, 20*(4), 378–405.

Lee, C. (2022). Towards the genetic architecture of complex gene expression traits: Challenges and prospects for eQTL mapping in humans. *Genes, 13*(2), Article 235.

Lee, S. S., Chronis-Tuscano, A., Keenan, K., Pelham, W. E., Loney, J., Van Hulle, C. A., Cook, E., & Lahey, B. B. (2010). Association of maternal dopamine transporter genotype with negative parenting: Evidence for gene × environment interaction with child disruptive behavior. *Molecular Psychiatry, 15*(5), 548–558.

Leerkes, E., & Qu, J. (2017). The Maternal (non) Responsiveness Questionnaire: Initial factor structure and validation. *Infant and Child Development, 26*(3), e1992.

Leibenluft, E., Gobbini, M. I., Harrison, T., & Haxby, J. V. (2004). Mothers' neural activation in response to pictures of their children and other children. *Biological Psychiatry, 56*(4), 225–232.

Love, T. M. (2014). Oxytocin, motivation and the role of dopamine. *Pharmacology Biochemistry and Behavior, 119*, 49–60.

Lucht, M. J., Barnow, S., Sonnenfeld, C., Rosenberger, A., Grabe, H. J., Schroeder, W., Volzke, H., Freyberger, H., Herrmann, F., Kroemer, H., & Rosskopf, D. (2009). Associations between the oxytocin receptor gene (OXTR) and affect, loneliness and intelligence in normal subjects. *Progress in Neuro-Psychopharmacology and Biological Psychiatry, 33*(5), 860–866.

Luna, B., Thulborn, K. R., Munoz, D. P., Merriam, E. P., Garver, K. E., Minshew, N. J., Keshavan, M., Genovese, C., Eddy, W., & Sweeney, J. A. (2001). Maturation of widely distributed brain function subserves cognitive development. *NeuroImage, 13*(5), 786–793.

Lupien, S. J., McEwen, B. S., Gunnar, M. R., & Heim, C. (2009). Effects of stress throughout the lifespan on the brain, behaviour and cognition. *Nature Reviews Neuroscience, 10*(6), 434–445.

Lyons-Ruth, K., & Jacobvitz, D. (2016). Attachment disorganization from infancy to adulthood: Neurobiological correlates, parenting contexts, and pathways to disorder. In J. A. Cassidy & P. R. Shaver (Eds.), *Handbook of attachment: Theory, research, and clinical applications* (3rd ed., pp. 667–695). Guilford.

Main, M., & Goldwyn, R. (1984). Predicting rejection of her infant from mother's representation of her own experience: Implications for the abused–abusing intergenerational cycle. *Child Abuse & Neglect, 8*(2), 203–217.

Main, M., Kaplan, N., & Cassidy, J. (1985). Security in infancy, childhood, and adulthood: A move to the level of representation. *Monographs of the Society for Research in Child Development, 50*(1–2), 66–104.

Main, M., & Solomon, J. (1986). Discovery of an insecure–disorganized/disoriented attachment pattern. In T. B. Brazelton & M. W. Yogman (Eds.), *Affective development in infancy* (pp. 95–124). Ablex.

Main, M., & Solomon, J. (1990). Procedures for identifying infants as disorganized/disoriented during the Ainsworth Strange Situation. In M. T. Greenbert, D. Cicchetti, & E. M. Cummings (Eds.), *Attachment in the preschool years: Theory, research, and intervention* (pp. 121–160). University of Chicago Press.

Main, M., & Stadtman, J. (1981). Infant response to rejection of physical contact by the mother. *Journal of the American Academy of Child Psychiatry, 20*(2), 292–307.

Main, M., & Weston, D. R. (1981). The quality of the toddler's relationship to mother and to father: Related to conflict behavior and the readiness to establish new relationships. *Child Development, 52*, 932–940.

Matthews, S. G., & Phillips, D. I. (2012). Transgenerational inheritance of stress pathology. *Experimental Neurology, 233*(1), 95–101.

McGowan, P. O., Suderman, M., Sasaki, A., Huang, T. C., Hallett, M., Meaney, M. J., & Szyf, M. (2011). Broad epigenetic signature of maternal care in the brain of adult rats. *PLoS One, 6*(2), e14739.

Meins, E., Fernyhough, C., Fradley, E., & Tuckey, M. (2001). Rethinking maternal sensitivity: Mothers' comments on infants' mental processes predict security of attachment at 12 months. *Journal of Child Psychology and Psychiatry and Allied Disciplines, 42*(5), 637–648.

Michalska, K. J., Decety, J., Liu, C., Chen, Q., Martz, M. E., Jacob, S., Hipwell, A., Lee, S., Chronis-Tuscano, A., Waldman, I., & Lahey, B. B. (2014). Genetic imaging of the association of oxytocin receptor gene (OXTR) polymorphisms with positive maternal parenting. *Frontiers in Behavioral Neuroscience, 8*, Article 21.

Mileva-Seitz, V., Fleming, A. S., Meaney, M. J., Mastroianni, A., Sinnwell, J. P., Steiner, M., Atkinson, L., Levitan, R., Matthews, S., Kennedy, L., & Sokolowski, M. B. (2012). Dopamine receptors D1 and D2 are related to observed maternal behavior. *Genes, Brain and Behavior, 11*(6), 684–694.

Mileva-Seitz, V., Kennedy, J., Atkinson, L., Steiner, M., Levitan, R., Matthews, S. G., Meaney, M., Sokolowski, M., & Fleming, A. S. (2011). Serotonin transporter allelic variation in mothers predicts maternal sensitivity, behavior and attitudes toward 6-month-old infants. *Genes, Brain and Behavior, 10*(3), 325–333.

Mills, K. L., Lalonde, F., Clasen, L. S., Giedd, J. N., & Blakemore, S. J. (2014). Developmental changes in the structure of the social brain in late childhood and adolescence. *Social Cognitive and Affective Neuroscience, 9*(1), 123–131.

Monk, C. S., McClure, E. B., Nelson, E. E., Zarahn, E., Bilder, R. M., Leibenluft, E., Charney, D., Ernst, M., & Pine, D. S. (2003). Adolescent immaturity in attention-related brain engagement to emotional facial expressions. *NeuroImage, 20*(1), 420–428.

Montague, P. R., & Lohrenz, T. (2007). To detect and correct: Norm violations and their enforcement. *Neuron, 56*(1), 14–18.

Mountain, G., Cahill, J., & Thorpe, H. (2017). Sensitivity and attachment interventions in early childhood: A systematic review and meta-analysis. *Infant Behavior and Development, 46*, 14–32.

O'Connor, T. G., & Croft, C. M. (2001). A twin study of attachment in preschool children. *Child Development, 72*(5), 1501–1511.

O'Donnell, K. A., Gaudreau, H., Colalillo, S., Steiner, M., Atkinson, L., Moss, E., Goldberg, S., Karama, S., Matthews, S. G., Lydon, J. E., & Silveira, P. P. (2014). The maternal adversity, vulnerability and neurodevelopment project: Theory and methodology. *The Canadian Journal of Psychiatry, 59*(9), 497–508.

Oppenheim, D., Sagi, A., & Lamb, M. E. (1988). Infant–adult attachments on the kibbutz and their relation to socioemotional development 4 years later. *Developmental Psychology, 24*(3), 427–433.

Peltola, M. J., Strathearn, L., & Puura, K. (2018). Oxytocin promotes face-sensitive neural responses to infant and adult faces in mothers. *Psychoneuroendocrinology, 91*, 261–270.

Phua, D. Y., Kee, M. Z., & Meaney, M. J. (2020). Positive maternal mental health, parenting, and child development. *Biological Psychiatry, 87*(4), 328–337.

Pluess, M., Wurmser, H., Buske-Kirschbaum, A., Papousek, M., Pirke, K. M., Hellhammer, D., & Bolten, M. (2012). Positive life events predict salivary cortisol in pregnant women. *Psychoneuroendocrinology, 37*(8), 1336–1340.

Qiu, A., Anh, T. T., Li, Y., Chen, H., Rifkin-Graboi, A., Broekman, B. F., Kwek, K., Saw, S., Chong, Y., Gluckman, P., Fortier, M. V., & Meaney, M. (2015). Prenatal maternal depression alters amygdala functional connectivity in 6-month-old infants. *Translational Psychiatry, 5*(2), e508.

Raby, K. L., Steele, R. D., Carlson, E. A., & Sroufe, L. A. (2015). Continuities and changes in infant attachment patterns across two generations. *Attachment & Human Development, 17*(4), 414–428.

Ricks, M. H. (1985). The social transmission of parental behavior: Attachment across generations. *Monographs of the Society for Research in Child development, 50*(1–2), 211–227.

Robinson, C. C., Mandleco, B., Olsen, S. F., & Hart, C. H. (2001). The Parenting Styles and Dimensions Questionnaire (PSDQ). In B. F. Perlmutter, J. Touliatos, & G. W. Holden (Eds.), *Handbook of family measurement techniques: Vol. 3. Instruments & index.* (pp. 319–321). SAGE.

Roisman, G. I., & Fraley, R. C. (2008). A behavior–genetic study of parenting quality, infant attachment security, and their covariation in a nationally representative sample. *Developmental Psychology, 44*(3), 831–839.

Rosenthal, N. L., & Kobak, R. (2010). Assessing adolescents' attachment hierarchies: Differences across developmental periods and associations with individual adaptation. *Journal of Research on Adolescence, 20*(3), 678–706.

Saavedra-Rodríguez, L., & Feig, L. A. (2013). Chronic social instability induces anxiety and defective social interactions across generations. *Biological Psychiatry, 73*(1), 44–53.

Sanders, M. R. (1999). Triple P-Positive Parenting Program: Towards an empirically validated multilevel parenting and family support strategy for the prevention of behavior and emotional problems in children. *Clinical Child and Family Psychology Review, 2*(2), 71–90.

Schultz, W. (2006). Behavioral theories and the neurophysiology of reward. *Annual Review of Psychology, 57*, 87–115.

Seibert, A. C., & Kerns, K. A. (2009). Attachment figures in middle childhood. *International Journal of Behavioral Development, 33*(4), 347–355.

Seibert, A. C., & Kerns, K. A. (2015). Early mother–child attachment: Longitudinal prediction to the quality of peer relationships in middle childhood. *International Journal of Behavioral Development, 39*(2), 130–138.

Shomaker, L. B., & Furman, W. (2009). Parent–adolescent relationship qualities, internal working models, and attachment styles as predictors of adolescents' interactions with friends. *Journal of Social and Personal Relationships, 26*(5), 579–603.

Shulman, S., Elicker, J., & Sroufe, L. A. (1994). Stages of friendship growth in preadolescence as related to attachment history. *Journal of Social and Personal Relationships, 11*(3), 341–361.

Silveri, M. M., Rohan, M. L., Pimentel, P. J., Gruber, S. A., Rosso, I. M., & Yurgelun-Todd, D. A. (2006). Sex differences in the relationship between white matter microstructure and impulsivity in adolescents. *Magnetic Resonance Imaging, 24*(7), 833–841.

Simpson, J. A., & Belsky, J. (2008). Attachment theory within a modern evolutionary framework. In J. Cassidy & P. R. Shaver (Eds.), *Handbook of attachment: Theory, research, and clinical applications* (pp. 131–157). Guilford.

Sowell, E. R., Thompson, P. M., Holmes, C. J., Jernigan, T. L., & Toga, A. W. (1999). In vivo evidence for post-adolescent brain maturation in frontal and striatal regions. *Nature Neuroscience, 2*(10), 859–861.

Sroufe, L. A. (1985). Attachment classification from the perspective of infant–caregiver relationships and infant temperament. *Child Development, 56*(1), 1–14.

Sroufe, L. A. (2016). The place of attachment in development. In J. A. Cassidy & P. R. Shaver (Eds.), *Handbook of attachment: Theory, research, and clinical applications* (3rd ed., pp. 997–1011). Guilford.

Sroufe, L. A., Egeland, B., Carlson, E., & Collins, W. A. (2005). Placing early attachment experiences in developmental context: The Minnesota Longitudinal Study. In K. E. Grossman, K. Grossman, & E. Waters (Eds.), *Attachment from infancy to adulthood: The major longitudinal studies* (pp. 48–70). Guilford.

Sroufe, L. A., Fox, N. E., & Pancake, V. R. (1983). Attachment and dependency in developmental perspective. *Child development, 54*(6), 1615–1627.

Stanley, D. A., & Adolphs, R. (2013). Toward a neural basis for social behavior. *Neuron, 80*(3), 816–826.

Steinberg, L., Lamborn, S. D., Dornbusch, S. M., & Darling, N. (1992). Impact of parenting practices on adolescent achievement: Authoritative parenting, school involvement, and encouragement to succeed. *Child Development, 63*(5), 1266–1281.

Stratern, L., Fonagy, P., Amico, J., & Montague, P. R. (2009). Adult attachment predicts maternal brain and oxytocin response to infant cues. *Neuropsychopharmacology, 34*(13), 2655–2666.

Taylor, B. L., Cavanagh, K., & Strauss, C. (2016). The effectiveness of mindfulness-based interventions in the perinatal period: A systematic review and meta-analysis. *PLoS One, 11*(5), e0155720.

Trubetskoy, V., Pardiñas, A. F., Qi, T., Panagiotaropoulou, G., Awasthi, S., Bigdeli, T. B., Bryois, J., Chen, C. Y., Dennison, C. A., Hall, L. S., Lam, M., Watanabe, K., Frei, O., Ge, T., Harwood, J. C., Koopmans, F., Magnusson, S., Richards, A. L., Sidorenko, J., . . . O'Donovan, M.; Schizophrenia Working Group of the Psychiatric Genomics Consortium. (2022). Mapping genomic loci implicates genes and synaptic biology in schizophrenia. *Nature, 604*(7906), 502–508.

Uvnäs-Moberg, K., Arn, I., & Magnusson, D. (2005). The psychobiology of emotion: The role of the oxytocinergic system. *International Journal of Behavioral Medicine, 12*(2), 59–65.

van IJzendoorn, M. H. (1995). Adult attachment representations, parental responsiveness, and infant attachment: A meta-analysis on the predictive validity of the Adult Attachment Interview. *Psychological Bulletin, 117*(3), 387–403.

van IJzendoorn, M. H., & Bakermans-Kranenburg, M. J. (2019). Bridges across the intergenerational transmission of attachment gap. *Current Opinion in Psychology, 25,* 31–36.

Verhage, M. L., Schuengel, C., Madigan, S., Fearon, R. M., Oosterman, M., Cassibba, R., Bakermans-Kranenburg, M. J., & van IJzendoorn, M. H. (2016). Narrowing the transmission gap: A synthesis of three decades of research on intergenerational transmission of attachment. *Psychological Bulletin, 142*(4), 337–366.

Vicario, C. M., Rafal, R. D., Martino, D., & Avenanti, A. (2017). Core, social and moral disgust are bounded: A review on behavioral and neural bases of repugnance in clinical disorders. *Neuroscience & Biobehavioral Reviews, 80,* 185–200.

Vrticka, P., Andersson, F., Grandjean, D., Sander, D., & Vuilleumier, P. (2008). Individual attachment style modulates human amygdala and striatum activation during social appraisal. *PLoS One, 3*(8), e2868.

Ward, J. (2016). *The student's guide to social neuroscience.* Psychology Press.

Waters, E., & Deane, K. E. (1985). Defining and assessing individual differences in attachment relationships: Q-methodology and the organization of behavior in infancy and early childhood. *Monographs of the Society for Research in Child Development, 50*(1–2), 41–65.

Weaver, I. C., Diorio, J., Seckl, J. R., Szyf, M., & Meaney, M. J. (2004). Early environmental regulation of hippocampal glucocorticoid receptor gene expression: Characterization of intracellular mediators and potential genomic target sites. *Annals of the New York Academy of Sciences, 1024*(1), 182–212.

Whipple, N., Bernier, A., & Mageau, G. A. (2011). A dimensional approach to maternal attachment state of mind: Relations to maternal sensitivity and maternal autonomy support. *Developmental Psychology, 47*(2), 396–403.

Winnicott, D. W. (1958). The antisocial tendency. In *Collected papers. Through pediatrics to psychoanalysis.* Hogarth.

Wright, J. C., Binney, V., & Smith, P. K. (1995). Security of attachment in 8–12-year-olds: A revised version of the Separation Anxiety Test, its psychometric properties and clinical interpretation. *Journal of Child Psychology and Psychiatry, 36*(5), 757–774.

Yehuda, R., Halligan, S. L., & Bierer, L. M. (2001). Relationship of parental trauma exposure and PTSD to PTSD, depressive and anxiety disorders in offspring. *Journal of Psychiatric Research, 35*(5), 261–270.

Yurgelun-Todd, D. (2007). Emotional and cognitive changes during adolescence. *Current Opinion in Neurobiology, 17*(2), 251–257.

Zeegers, M. A., Colonnesi, C., Stams, G. J. J., & Meins, E. (2017). Mind matters: A meta-analysis on parental mentalization and sensitivity as predictors of infant–parent attachment. *Psychological Bulletin, 143*(12), 1245–1272.

Zhang, T. Y., & Meaney, M. J. (2010). Epigenetics and the environmental regulation of the genome and its function. *Annual Review of Psychology, 61,* 439–466.

Zimmermann, P., Mohr, C., & Spangler, G. (2009). Genetic and attachment influences on adolescents' regulation of autonomy and aggressiveness. *Journal of Child Psychology and Psychiatry, 50*(11), 1339–1347.

# 10

# Developmental Social Neuroscience

Psychiatry is, and should be forever, a science dunked in milk of human kindness.

—Leo Kanner (1942), p. 21

Developmental social neuroscience studies the development and neural underpinnings of social behavior (De Hann & Gunnar, 2009). It seeks to specify the evolutionary, neural, hormonal, cellular, and genetic mechanisms underlying social behavior. The neurobiological approaches and methodologies of social neurosciences are described in this chapter. It examines neurobiological development and how it is related to social understanding and social behaviors. An important consideration is whether general cognitive processes involved in perception, language, attention, and memory are sufficient to explain social competence or whether more specific neurobiological processes, rather than general ones, are necessary for social interaction. Development studies are essential for answering this question.

A developmental perspective emphasizes the importance of studying the social brain and its environmental interactions. To what extent does being raised in a socially enriched environment shape the structural and functional development of the social brain? Importantly, cells and neuronal pathways grow or wither contingent on the quality and extent of social interactions during development (Ward, 2016).

Gene-based influences, *our nature*, and environmentally based experiences, *our nurture*, interact in social development. We must consider the evolution (phylogeny) of our species as we evolved from reptiles to nonhuman primates to human social behavior. We examine the emergence of sociability within three main stages of human development: infancy (birth to 18 months), childhood (18 months to puberty), and adolescence (puberty to adulthood). The underlying neural structures involved in social behavior develop throughout these three developmental stages. Some brain structures, such as the amygdala, central to the emotional regulation, are engaged early in social development in infancy, whereas others, such as the cortical system, become increasing specialized for processing social stimuli in adolescence and adulthood. Developmental studies allow the study of social behavior from the earliest time of life when infants first become socially engaged and also the examination of the emergence of social behaviors in subsequent developmental periods. Although brain structures mature at different rates, they become increasingly integrated from infancy to adolescence and beyond. There is a progressive emergence of increasingly complex social skills with maturation. Advances in noninvasive imaging (functional magnetic resonance imaging [fMRI]), electrophysiologic methods (electroencephalography [EEG] and event-related potentials [ERPs]) and other methodologies are being used to refine our understanding of developmental social neuroscience at many levels of research (genetic, neurophysiological, neurohormonal, and neuroanatomical) (De Hann & Gunnar, 2009).

This chapter reviews the findings of evolutionary biology and social behavior with an emphasis on *mutual aid* as the driving force in evolution (Kropotkin, 1989). Development takes place in the context of the family. Experience expectant systems include preference for human faces such as mimicking facial expressions of adults by infants in the first weeks of life. Social skills, including empathy, goal-based imitation, and face-specific processing, are gradually refined. Emotion regulation evolves with the maturation of the automatic nervous system. Cortical self-regulation is accomplished with effortful control as the cortex matures. Social attachment is a developmental milestone and, as has been emphasized, is facilitated by release of oxytocin and vasopressin during infancy. Imaginative role-play is important in the emergence of the social self, for moral development, and in the mastery of social developmental tasks. Mastery involves distinct tasks during the three stages of development: infancy, childhood, and adolescence.

## Brain Evolution and Social Neuroscience

Evolutionary neurobiologist Paul MacLean (1990) provided an evolutionary perspective on the development of social behaviors that lead to empathy and the capacity for altruism. He suggested that the emergence of the capacity to "look with feeling" links the emotional and visual brain. MacLean (1985) traced the origins of family to the evolutionary transition from reptiles to mammals. Reptiles follow daily routines and show territorial defense. They establish a home base but do not show mother–infant attachment. An analysis of reptilian behavior suggests that basic territorial patterns, including attachment to place, not parent, are essential to their species survival. MacLean (1985) suggested that in the evolutionary transition from reptiles to mammals, several changes take place that facilitate mother–infant contact and interpersonal bonding. Among the most important evolutionary steps is the establishment of audiovocal contact when separated, with maternal responsiveness to the infant's separation call. Reptiles do not hear the separation call because they do not have ossicles bones in the inner ear.

Hearing the infant's separation call is a new step in mammalian evolution. Two small bones of the jaw joint of the earlier mammal-like reptiles, the articular and the quadrate bones, evolved to become the malleus (hammer) and incus (anvil) bones (Romer, 1966). The evolution of the ossicles in the inner ear created an auditory system allowing the cry of the newborn to be heard. Concurrently, the descent of the larynx into a new position is of evolutionary significance because it allows vocalization and the production of the separation cry.

Three linked evolutionary events underlie social attachment and the establishment of social skills: audiovocal contact (the separation call) between the mother and infant; nursing (the milk let-down reflex elicited by the separation call); and the emergence of play behavior in apes and humans, allowing the practice of social skills. These evolutionary advances allow mother–infant contact to be maintained vocally, allow feeding in a secure setting, and facilitate interpersonal learning by social rehearsal. This learning first begins with imitation and then leads to play that facilitates social learning.

According to MacLean (1990), the brain regions involved in these evolutionary advances are the limbic system, the striatal complex, and the cingulate cortex. "Looking with feeling" requires a further evolutionary adaptation that links the visual system with the prefrontal cortex and the limbic or emotional brain, thus providing a neuroethological basis for empathy. Awareness of the feelings of others within the family is a prerequisite to develop a sense of concern for others besides oneself. Ultimately, awareness of others' feelings leads to responsibility for planning for the future of members of a family (MacLean, 1990). Dawkins (1989) proposes that a unique quality of humans is the "capacity for genuine, disinterested [non-selfish] altruism" (p. 200). He notes that humans potentially have the power to defy the selfish genes of their birth using conscious foresight to imagine their future.

## Social Bonding, Altruism, and Empathy

In mammals, the social bond is established through reciprocal behavioral synchrony between parent and infant. Mutual aid is a critical factor in evolution (Kropotkin, 1989). Early attachment behavior is the basis of mutual aid within the family. Studies in neuroethology make clear that within the neo-Darwinian framework, the emphasis is on fitness. Within the fitness framework, traditionally it has been difficult to account for altruism because adaptive fitness emphasizes the production of progeny, the "selfish gene hypothesis." As one moves from insects to humans, the number of progeny produced decreases substantially. Sociobiology regards altruistic care as aimed at survival of the young and continuation of one's own genes. Simon (1990) proposed that the neo-Darwinian emphasis on fitness accounts only for reciprocal altruism—behavior that is usually reciprocated—which has no meaningful net effect on fitness. However, he noted that being receptive to social influence (docility) may be selected too and that it also contributes to fitness. The cost of receptivity may be the loss of an individual for the maintenance of group fitness if sociability is selected in evolution. Importantly, the selection for cooperativeness of individuals in groups may have as its outcome the production of some individuals who are altruistically self-sacrificing. This occurs most often in kinship group selection, altruism within the family. Such sacrifice, both within kinship and more broadly, may save the group from threat and contribute to species survival, even though certain individuals are lost.

In evolution, adaptability for a species is ultimately selected at the level of the group. Altruism is an important aspect of this selection process. Yet, these views on group and kin selection are controversial in sociobiology, in which it is questioned that if all selection is at the gene level and genes propagate themselves at other genes' expense, what is the selective advantage of behavior that leads to others' genes surviving at the expense of one's own (Wilson, 1975/2000). The genetic roots for receptivity to social influence continue to be studied. Donald (1991) proposes that consideration of altruism in humans must include not only the genetics but also the culture. Such study includes the emergence of advanced representational abilities and memory systems in humans that provide the cognitive capacity to understand another person's perspective (theory of mind) as well as empathy.

## The Origins of Sociability

The ontogeny of individual development becomes progressively more important as one moves up the phylogenetic tree and the number of offspring produced decreases. The study of individual development leads to the study of the relationships in human and animal behavior. In evaluating the origins of behavior, we consider not only features that are uniquely present in humans but also their phylogenetic origins. Through identifying the roots of these behaviors, animal studies of social behavior can be utilized to shed light on human problems. However, there are risks of cross-species generalization, so caution is needed when comparisons are made.

Eibl-Eibesfeldt (1979) suggests that several steps may have been necessary for the evolution of social behaviors. Perhaps the earliest form is seen in the congregation of fish into swarms for protection against predators. Because physical proximity is necessary for fertilization, the emergence of social behaviors may begin initially with physical contact, as in some deep-sea fishes when the male adheres to the female. The next step in bonding occurs when there is a behavioral fixation on the sex partner. Initially, proximity may be to a specific location and later a compatible partner. The presence of that specific partner may become necessary for certain behaviors to occur. This has been reported in songbirds, in which duet singing may only be satiated in the partner's presence, or the triumph ceremony of the Greylag geese, which occurs only in the presence of a partner (Eibl-Eibesfeldt, 1979). In the evolution of mammals, pair bonding requires partner proximity and compatibility.

The evolution of contact and bonding in young mammals involves nursing, the separation call, and play (MacLean, 1985). Parental care is a turning point in behavioral evolution. The next turning point is individual bonding between mother and infant. Here, parents and young seek one another's proximity and will defend the bond between them against any intervention; strangers will be ignored. A repertoire of infant signals lead to an innate social response from the mother and a reciprocal response from the young. Mothers respond to distress or isolation calls, and olfactory cues are important to recognize their young. In some species, bonding occurs during a brief "sensitive developmental period." For example, mother goats that remain with their kids for only the first 5 min after birth and then are separated from one another for 1 hr will respond when the kid is returned. However, if they are separated immediately after birth and reunited 1 hr after birth, the kid is treated as a stranger. The peptide oxytocin is believed to be a mediator of this brief "sensitive period" (Eibl-Eibesfeldt, 1979).

Parental care and mutual aid provide the origins of social behaviors. In humans, a decisive evolutionary event is the establishment of mother–infant bonding. Sexuality, territorial defense, and fear of predators, although important, are not adequate as pre-adaptations for the development of social behaviors. The intensity of early mother–infant bonding was investigated by Harlow and colleagues, who studied orphaned rhesus monkeys reared with surrogate mothers (Harlow & Zimmermann, 1959). They found that breaking the attachment bond through early separation led to behavioral symptoms that were similar to those described in hospitalized infants and children separated from their parents (Bowlby, 1969; Robertson, 1958; Spitz, 1946). Suomi and Harlow (1972) subsequently studied the social rehabilitation of isolate-reared monkeys.

They found that the basis of affectionate attachment is contact comfort with the parent, who acts as a secure base. When infant rhesus macaques are isolated from their mothers, they show phases of agitation, protest, withdrawal, despair, and detachment similar to the response of human infants. Moreover, in monkeys with early separation, the effects of isolation from the mother and the infant's responses to the environment depend on characteristics of a mother-surrogate (Mason & Capitanio, 1988), mother–infant feedback (Hinde, 1983), food availability, and the social setting.

The degree of behavioral disruption produced by social isolation is proportional to the age when the isolation occurs and its duration. Isolation from birth has greater effects than isolation after having had some mother or peer-aged contact. Six months of isolation has greater impact than 3 months of isolation. If the monkey is isolated for 12 months, complete re-socialization with the mother is essentially impossible. However, monkeys isolated for shorter periods of time can be rehabilitated, making them difficult to distinguish from their socially reared counterparts. Still, rehabilitated monkeys do not develop fully socially sufficient strategies when challenged by competing for resources with others. They do not appear to accurately understand social relationships, nor do they respond appropriately to social cues (Anderson & Mason, 1978). With severe isolation, both infant monkeys and infant humans show self-hugging, self-sucking, and self-biting. In addition, they show stereotypical movements such as rocking, and they react to others with inappropriate fear and aggression. Rhesus monkey mothers that had been reared socially isolated failed to show normal mothering behavior and neglected their infants (Kraemer, 1985).

Physiologically, there is failure to thrive in isolated infant rhesus infants, which become immunologically compromised. Moreover, anatomical and neurochemical changes have been demonstrated in the brains of monkeys that were socially isolated for the first 9 months of life. These socially isolated monkeys throughout their development exhibited persistent stereotyped movements, self-directed behaviors, and maladaptive psychosocial behavior (Sackett, 1972). When autopsied as adults, the socially isolated monkeys had substantial alterations in the chemoarchitecture of the striatum. Neuronal cell bodies and processes immunoreactive for substance P (SP) and enkephalin were depleted markedly in the striosome and matrix regions of the caudate nucleus and putamen; the average density of SP-immunoreactive neurons was reduced 58% relative to control monkeys. Calbindin and tyrosine hydroxylase immunoreactivities were diminished in the matrix of caudate and putamen of the isolated monkeys (Martin et al., 1991).

In human studies, Spitz's (1946) classic paper on anaclitic depression demonstrated the effects of early sensory and social deprivation on human infant development. Spitz found not only failure to thrive socially in sensory-deprived infants but also an increase in infant mortality. Subsequently, Bowlby (1973, 1988) used an ethological approach to investigate the establishment of the social bond between mother and infant. Bowlby examined neurobiological origins of separation and studied the severity of the psychological distress that children experience when separated from their mothers. His work in children drew on ethological studies of bonding in birds and mammals, in which strong bonds between parents and offspring are observed. Bowlby concluded that attachment and bonding have evolved as universal protective mechanisms for the young.

Bowlby (1988) proposed that mother–infant bonds (a) have basic survival functions; (b) can be understood by assuming a homeostatic cybernetic system with a biological basis in each partner maintaining close relationship during development; (c) are followed by working models of mother–infant relationship at the level of the mind, of one's self, of others, and a pattern of interaction between them; and (d) suggest *pathways* of developmental progression rather than specific phases of fixation during development or of regression in times of stress. The way these bonds form from child to parent and parent to child has major developmental consequences in later life.

## Romania's Abandoned Children

The consequences of early social deprivation have been most extensively studied in the follow-up of Romania's abandoned children (Nelson et al., 2014). In 1989, the fall of the Ceausescu regime in Romania resulted in the discovery in that country of approximately 700 overcrowded, impoverished institutions for children abandoned by their parents as a result of Ceausescu's ban of birth control. Children were deprived of socially responsive care, social engagement with caregivers, infant stimulation, and psychological support. The Bucharest Early Intervention Project was conducted to investigate foster care as an alternative to institutionalization for these children. Children were randomly assigned to a foster home specifically established for the study or remained in the institutions. Throughout the study, children were systematically examined for their physical growth, cognitive development, brain development, and social behavior. A third comparison group of children were enrolled, who were raised by their birth families. The institutionalized children enrolled in the study were found to be cognitively impaired with lower IQ scores. They were diagnosed with severe social and emotional disorders and showed differences in brain development. The earlier the placement in foster care, the better the cognitive, social, and behavioral outcomes. Among all the domains studied in these children, the greatest impairment was in social and emotional behavior. Most striking were deficits in social attachment behaviors. These deficits resulted from significant absence of social interactions with caregivers within the institutions. Deprivation occurred in the earliest years of life and impacted connectivity of brain regions involved in the emergence of typical social behaviors (Debnath et al., 2020; Wade et al., 2019).

Experience-expectant environmental experiences were missing in their early lives. Typically, infants exposed to experience-expectant social contact developed close relationships with adults and tight social bonds. Social behavior deficits were evident for both externalizing and internalizing behaviors in the institutionalized children. There was socially inappropriate engagement with adults. In the fifth edition of the *Diagnostic and Statistical Manual of Mental Disorders* (American Psychiatric Association, 2013), the diagnostic term *disinhibited social engagement disorder* was introduced to describe children who have experienced severe social neglect. The disorder is characterized by indiscriminate sociability and disinhibited social behaviors. The children also show reduced or absent reticence in approaching unfamiliar objects. Other diagnoses in the Romanian children were internalizing behavior disorders, social withdrawal, and excessive anxiety. Children who were the most severely maternally deprived were unable to establish deep emotional relationships despite adoption into warm and nurturing families.

## Neuroception: Autonomic Self-Regulation
## of Social Behavior

The newborn is dependent on the mother and the caregiver to meet basic needs for protection, warmth, and nutrition. During development, the neural regulation of the autonomic nervous system is established through social engagement. In response to the environment, through the senses, the nervous system continually monitors whether people or situations are safe, dangerous, or life-threatening. The term *neuroception* describes how neural circuits make determinations of safety. Neuroceptive mechanisms determine whether an infant coos at a caregiver or cries at a stranger or when a toddler eagerly embraces a parent or turns away from a stranger. Whether a child perceives a safe environment or a dangerous one engages the autonomic nervous system and leads to prosocial engagement or defensive behaviors. Although a child may not be aware of danger at a cognitive level, at a neurophysiological level, the autonomic nervous system responds. Perceived risk initiates a sequence of neural and neuroendocrine responses that facilitate adaptive responses. Neuroceptive awareness helps us understand why children may immediately recoil from unfamiliar people or eagerly join a friend in play.

What are the neurobiological mechanisms underlying social engagement in one situation and social withdrawal in another? How does one switch from defensive withdrawal back to social engagement? The autonomic nervous system assesses risk. If the environment is deemed safe, defensive strategies such as flight, flee, and psychological dissociation are inhibited. Over the course of human evolution, the autonomic nervous system has evolved to facilitate social engagement when one feels safe. If one senses danger, the autonomic nervous system adaptively responds to threat. Only in a safe environment is it adaptive to inhibit psychological defensive systems and show positive social responsiveness and engagement. When the autonomic nervous system detects safety, metabolism adjusts, breathing slows, heart rate regularizes, and one relaxes. When danger is detected, the fight-or-flight response axis is activated, resulting in increased metabolism, increased heart rate, and cortisol release. The stress response is mediated by the sympathetic nervous system and the hypothalamic–pituitary axis. A neuroception of safety prevents the physiologic fight-or-flight stress response. In contrast, when the stress is overwhelming, the despair response with physiologic shutdown, dissociation, a drop in blood pressure and heart rate, and respiratory apnea ensues.

Figure 10.1 shows how the nervous system responds to environmental challenges in these situations: safety, danger, and overwhelming threat. fMRI studies have identified neural structures that correlate with detecting risk. When safe, specific brain networks are activated that detect positive facial expressions such as smiling and vocal behavior such as neonatal cooing that facilitate a sense of trustworthiness. For example, specific brain networks in the temporal lobe are activated when one hears a familiar voice or sees a familiar face.

## Evolution of the Autonomic Nervous System

The nervous system has evolved so that human can express emotions, communicate with one another, and regulate their behavioral states. The polyvagal autonomic nervous

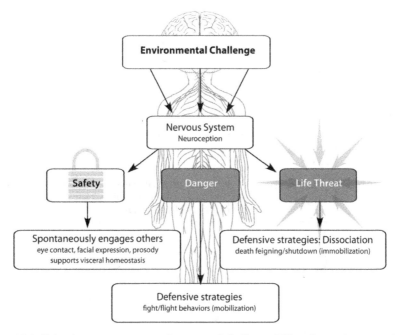

**Figure 10.1** Behavior responses to environmental challenge. When the environment is deemed to be safe, the person spontaneously engages others. When it is deemed dangerous, the stress response is excited. When it is deemed to be life-threatening, there is dissociation metabolic shutdown.

From Porges (2004); redrawn by Tim Phelps (2021).

system model proposed by Stephen Porges posits that neural regulation of the autonomic nervous system has evolved phylogenetically in three major stages to cope with overwhelming threat or danger and to recognize safe setting. Each of these is associated with a different behavioral strategy (Porges, 2001, 2004). The evolution of these responses to challenge is shown in Figure 10.1. The first stage in autonomic nervous system evolution involves the primitive unmyelinated visceral vagal nerve. When the animal faces overwhelming threat, metabolic activity is decreased and the animal may feign death, whereas humans may psychologically dissociate. Behaviorally, freeze when a threat is overwhelming and becomes immobilized by fear. The second evolutionary stage is characterized by the development of the sympathetic nervous system. When faced with threat, metabolic output increases, the unmyelinated visceral vagus is inhibited, and mobilization behaviors are initiated to fight back or to flee from danger. The final stage, social communication and self-caring, is facilitated by neural regions innervated by myelination of the vagal nerve. The myelinated vagal nerve regulates heart rate and cardiac output to facilitate social engagement. These stages are shown in Table 10.1.

Figure 10.2 shows that the myelinated vagal nerve is linked to cranial nerves that regulate social engagement. These cranial nerves (V, VII, IX, X, and XI) regulate social contact through facial expression and adaptive social vocalization. The cranial nerves regulate facial expression, turn the head toward the listener, tighten the stapedius muscle in the inner ear to hear speech sound clearly, and regulate breathing and heart rate to be more attentive.

**Table 10.1** Polyvagal Theory: Phylogenetic Stages of Neural Control

| Stage | Autonomic Nervous System Component | Behavioral Function | Lower Motor Neurons |
|---|---|---|---|
| I | Unmyelinated vagus (dorsal vagal complex) | Immobilization (death feigning, passive avoidance); dissociation and adaptive failure | Dorsal motor nucleus of the vagus |
| II | Sympathetic–adrenal system (sympathetic nervous system) | Mobilization (active avoidance) | Spinal cord |
| III | Myelinated vagus (ventral vagal complex) | Social communication, self-soothing and calming, inhibit sympathetic–adrenal influences | Nucleus ambiguous |

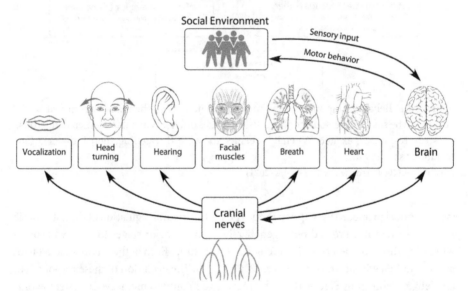

**Figure 10.2** The role of cranial nerves in social engagement. The social engagement system involves both somatic and visceral components. Somatic nerve pathways regulate the striatal muscles of the face and head involved in head turning, listening, hearing, and vocalizing. The visceral component involves the myelinated vagus that regulates the heart and bronchi in the lungs.

From Porges (2001); redrawn by Tim Phelps (2021).

In summary, as the autonomic nervous system evolved, it was integrated with other physiological systems that respond to stress. These include the cerebral cortex, the hypothalamic–pituitary axis, the neuropeptides oxytocin and vasopressin, and the immune system.

## Early Development of the Autonomic Nervous System

Developmental changes in neural pathways that regulate autonomic function take place in the third trimester of pregnancy and continue through infancy. The neural pathways that regulate autonomic state offer a platform to support emerging abilities of the infant to engage with people and objects in a changing environment. Both social interactive and associated behaviors can be understood in the context of autonomic nervous system maturation during early development. Maturational changes in the autonomic nervous system mediate dynamic engagement with the social environment. Social separation and isolation of infants disrupt the capacity to regulate their psychologic state and impact both mental and physical health. This includes delays in cognition, physical growth, and motor development. Lack of social support can have disastrous effects on human development, as illustrated in studies of Romanian orphans (Nelson et al., 2014). For these orphans, functional and structural changes in the brain involved the orbital frontal gyrus, infralimbic prefrontal cortex, medial temporal structures (amygdala and hippocampus), and left uncinate fasciculus (Chugani et al., 2001; Eluvathingal et al., 2006). In a typical expectable social environment, the autonomic nervous system prepares the infant for social engagement and behavior. As these neuronal mechanisms mature and facilitate self-regulation, the infant's dependence on others in the regulation of physiological states diminishes, moving from basic needs (safety, warmth, and food) to prosocial engagement.

The heavily myelinated vagus circuit facilitates early social engagement. If social safety is not achieved, the other two autonomic circuits essential to survival are activated when one is threatened. These older defensive survival circuits appear first in brain development; the prosocial myelinated vagus system develops last and is most vulnerable to stressful experiences. The human infant at birth does not have a completely functioning vagal system. There is an increase in the number of myelinated vagal fibers from 24 weeks of gestation that continues throughout the adolescent years, with the greatest increase in myelinated fibers occurring between 30 weeks of gestation and approximately 6 months postpartum (Sachis et al., 1982; Figure 10.3). In contrast, the number of unmyelinated fibers remains constant.

Preterm infants, who are born before 30 weeks of gestational age, are compromised because of the lack of a functioning myelinated vagus nerve. Consequently, an infant born before 30 weeks has a limited capacity to regulate visceral state and is solely dependent on the sympathetic nervous system and the phylogenetically older myelinated vagus to address regulatory needs (Porges & Furman, 2011). The premature infant's

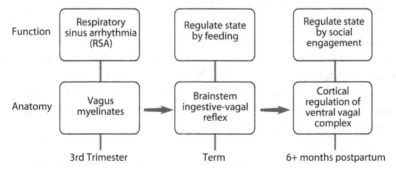

**Figure 10.3** The developmental timeline for myelination of the vagus nerve from the last trimester of pregnancy, at term, and through the first months of life. The figure illustrates the role of the myelination vagus in the cortical regulation of early social engagement.
From Porges and Furman (2011); redrawn by Tim Phelps (2021).

compromised physiological adaptation when coping with distress may lead to dangerous risks for hypotension (low blood pressure) and lower oxygen saturation, which result from episodic bradycardia (low heart rate) and apneic episodes (cessation of breathing). With the maturation of the myelinated vagus in the final months of typical gestation, rapid adaptive shifts in autonomic states becomes possible by birth. At this time in development, vagal tone regularizes heart rate and facilitates self-regulated calmness through the tonic myelinated vagal effects on the primary cardiac pacemaker, the sinoatrial node. Vagal regulation produces a heart rate much lower than the intrinsic rate of the cardiac pacemaker alone. Thus, vagal activity acts as a brake that limits how rapidly the heart can beat, leading to physiological calming (Porges & Furman, 2011).

The state of functioning of the vagal brake can be quantified by measuring respiratory sinus arrhythmia (RSA). RSA is a naturally occurring heart rhythm that oscillates at approximately the frequency of spontaneous breathing and represents the beat-to-beat heart rate variability. Essentially, RSA is a biomarker that allows quantification of heart rate when the individual is stressed. RSA can be accurately measured in premature infants, full-term infants, and children in socially supportive or stressful situations (Bazhenova et al., 2001). Thus, RSA is an indicator of the functional activity of the myelinated vagal nerve. The efficacy of RSA reactivity depends on the number of myelinated vagal fibers as well as the ratio of myelinated to unmyelinated vagal fibers. In the preterm infant, the maturation of RSA parallels the maturation of myelinated vagal fibers, with an increase in RSA from 32 to 37 weeks of gestational age coincident with the increased vagal myelination as shown in Doussard-Roosevelt et al. (1997).

A parent–infant intervention that uses skin-to-skin contact between the mother and the preterm infant enhances the development of RSA. This intervention, known as kangaroo care, is a widely practiced method of infant care, especially for those born prematurely. The naked or partially dressed infant is held against the bare skin of a parent, typically the mother, every day. It is a well-documented means to care for and stabilize low-birth-weight or premature infants. Kangaroo care maintains infant body temperature, enhances positive RSA, and facilitates neurodevelopmental maturation. The *Family Nurture Intervention* (FNI) has been introduced for treating high-risk preterm infants in the neonatal intensive care unit (Porges et al., 2019). FNI is a comprehensive approach to facilitate autonomic regulation in preterm infants.

In a controlled study, preterm infants born between 26 and 34 weeks of gestation received either standard care or standard care plus FNI. RSA was used to quantify myelinated vagal effects on the sinoatrial node as the outcome measure at 35 and 41 weeks of pregnancy, with heart rate and RSA quantified with electrocardiogram. Across these two time points, the infants receiving FNI showed greater RSA, indicating greater vagal efficiency. This finding is consistent with FNI enhancing autonomic self-regulation and greater maturation of cardiac functioning. It is a demonstrably effective means to optimize postnatal development in infants born prematurely. Building upon kangaroo care, FNI begins while the infant is still in an incubator in the nursery.

The first step in FNI is maternal engagement with the infant, designated as "calming sessions" in which the mother communicates with the infant for an hour or more until both are calm. The mother reaches into the incubator to allow a firm sensation of touching the infant and is instructed to speak to the infant expressing their feelings about the infant's fragile condition while making eye contact with the infant. These sessions are conducted 6 hr per week (Welch, 2016; Welch et al., 2013). When the infant is stabilized enough to be taken from the incubator, the calming sessions involve skin-to-skin or non–skin-to-skin holding in a supportive emotional environment. Eye contact with the infant is initiated. Sessions are held an average of 3.5 times per week for an average of 6 weeks. A nurturance specialist regularly conducts meetings with parents to emphasize the importance of calming sessions.

Research studies confirm that FNI enhances maternal sensitivity. This intervention also is documented in neuroimaging studies to increase functional brain connectivity using EEG coherence methodology, especially in the frontal brain regions (Myers et al., 2015). The family nurturance calming cycle therapy facilitates later parent–infant attachment. Oxytocin levels in mother and infant have been shown to be co-regulated by emotional connection and are disrupted by the failure to make emotional connection. This autonomic co-conditioning learning can facilitate change from a negative physiologic state to a positive. Oxytocin plays an important role in emotional behavior and may result in behavioral change through anti-inflammatory gut–brain stem signaling (Welch & Ludwig, 2017). With RSA as a biomarker, FNI accelerated maturation of autonomic nervous system control in preterm infants. By continuous engagement of the social engagement system, cranial nerves (nerves V, VII, IX, and X) involved in the regulation of striatal muscles of the face, head, and special visceral afferents are activated, leading to social engagement and state regulation through myelinated vagal pathways.

Studies of the maturation of the autonomic state and FNI are important because preterm infants are at increased risk for medical problems, attention deficits, language deficits, perturbed executive functioning, anxiety, depression, and impaired cognition (Brydges et al., 2018). When introduced in the neonatal intensive care unit, FNI has been reported to improve social-relatedness, attention, and neurodevelopmental outcome at 18 months of age in a randomized control study (Welch et al., 2015).

## Social Engagement System and the Vagus Nerve

The vagal nerve that controls the parasympathetic nervous system is the longest of the cranial nerves. It "wanders" widely through the body communicating motor and sensory impulses to all bodily organs. As the cerebral cortex develops, it gains greater direct and indirect control over the brain stem (corticobulbar pathways). Indirect control (corticoreticular) is via neural pathways that have their source in the motor cortex and terminate in the nuclei of the myelinated motor fibers that are in the brain stem. Vagal pathways are embedded in five cranial nerves (V, VII, VIII, X, and XI). These cranial nerves extend to control muscles of the face, head and neck, heart, and pulmonary bronchi. The myelinated vagus nerve facilitates the social engagement system through its extensive innervations. It controls social gaze and gesture by regulating the eyelids through the orbicularis oculi muscle. It controls emotional expression through innervation of the muscles of facial expression. It facilitates listening and extracts human voice from background noise through innervation of the middle ear muscles. It initiates sucking and ingestion of food by innervation of the facial muscle of mastication. It facilitates vocalizing, swallowing, and breathing through innervation of the larynx (vocalizing) and pharynx (swallowing and breathing). It facilitates social orientation, social gestures, and social reciprocity in conversation through innervation of muscles involved in head turning and tilting. Active together, all these muscles make possible our capacity to observe the facial expressions of others and our capacity to detect changes in emotional prosody (the patterns of intonation and stress in the rhythm of speech/ sound). Thus, the vagal nerve makes possible the actions that we make to socially engage others. Importantly, the development of the myelinated vagal nerve establishes the facial recognition/heart connection, which links social engagement with autonomic regulation of the heart and results in the emergence of adaptive social behavior. For newborns and young infants, the social engagement system sets the stage for later social bonding and the emergence of reciprocal social behavior. The myelinated vagal nerve is not the only mediator of autonomic state or heart rate; these are also influenced by the sympathetic nervous system. Table 10.1 shows the phylogenetic stages of autonomic neural control, relation to behavioral function, and brain regions involved.

The evolutionarily oldest component of the autonomic nervous system is made up of unmyelinated vagal nerve fibers that originate from the dorsal motor nuclei of the vagus and begin its development in utero. It first appears at 9 weeks of gestation in the brain stem. Subdivisions are detectable by 13 weeks and are clearly demarcated by 23 weeks of gestation. By 28–30 weeks, the myelinated vagal system is largely mature, although there are changes in its length and size postnatally. With maturation of the autonomic nervous system, the source nuclei in the brain shift from the dorsal motor nucleus, the source of the cranial nerves, where the unmyelinated vagal pathways originate, to the nucleus ambiguous in the medulla oblongata in the brain stem, as noted in Table 10.1.

Inhibitory control of the heart involves input to the sinoatrial node. The unmyelinated vagus is linked to the dorsal vagal complex, which includes the nucleus of the solitary tract and the interneuronal communication between this tract and the dorsal motor nucleus of the vagus. The dorsal vagal complex has inhibitory influence on the heart and bronchi. Its activity is triggered by perceived loss of oxygen (hypoxia), and it is functional in the hypoxic human fetus. The dorsal vagal complex facilitates the tone of the gut and digestion, but when overactive, it may increase gastric acid secretion and produce ulcers.

The sympathetic nervous system emerges in utero along with the parasympathetic nervous system. The sympathetic nervous system follows the segmentation of the spinal cord. The cell bodies of the preganglionic sympathetic motor neurons are located in the lateral horn of the spinal cord. The sympathetic nervous system increases heart rate through release of norepinephrine at the sinoatrial node. It increases contractility of the heart by its effect on the beta receptors on the ventricle's myocardium. The adrenal secretion of cortisol is integrated with the sympathetic nervous system for mobilization when faced with threatening situations. Cortisol release increases sympathetic activation with the release of catecholamines. Cortisol secretion both facilitates mobilization and maintains it.

In summary, infants and children are continuously regulating their responses to stress, which are adaptive to a constantly changing environment, sometimes safe and at other times dangerous. Our early psychological development is facilitated by how well our caregivers help us modulate our biological perception of the environment. Although the myelinated vagus' role in the infant's social engagement system is dominant, all three autonomic systems are adaptive because they have evolved to facilitate our sense of safety and respond to threat.

## Oxytocin and Vasopressin and Social Behavior

Oxytocin and vasopressin are peptides synthesized in the paraventricular and supra-optic nuclei of the hypothalamus. Oxytocin and vasopressin release is strongly related to the perception of environmental safety. The central effects and systemic effects of these peptides differ. The central release of oxytocin regulates the output of the dorsal motor nucleus of the unmyelinated vagus with an anti-stress effect (Carter, 1998). Peripheral systemic release of oxytocin facilitates uterine contractions at delivery of a newborn and breast milk ejection. The central release of vasopressin modulates afferent feedback from the viscera and changes set points for vagal reflexes, including the baroreceptor re-flex, which is sensitive to changes in blood pressure. Raising the baroreceptor set point leads to increased cardiac output. The fight-or-flight response is potentiated following sympathetic excitation of the heart. In summary, central release of oxytocin modulates parasympathetic vagal nerve processes, and central release of vasopressin modulates sympathetic nervous system function.

Figure 10.4 illustrates the role of the autonomic nervous system to adapt social en-gagement in a safe environment and to engage survival responses in dangerous and life-threatening ones. When faced with threat, neural and neuroendocrine systems respond in a predictable order and rapidly reorganize to varying environmental challenges in a flexible manner that regulates physiological state, behavior, and adaptation.

## Socialization in Infancy (Birth to 18 Months)

Although the infant visually engages the world for the first time at birth, the infant has already acquired some socially relevant information in utero. A newborn infant prefers the mother's voice at birth (DeCasper & Fifer, 1980). Within 1 hr after birth, an infant can track a moving face-like image better than a non-face image. Although visual acuity at birth is 10–30 times poorer than that of adults, in their first 3 days of life, newborns recognize the orientation of the face, preferring upright faces rather than upside-down faces (Cassia et al., 2004). Within the first 3 days of life, infants show preference for their mother rather than a stranger. The earliest face recognition of the mother is reported to depend on the capacity to link the mother's face to the mother's voice, which became fa-miliar prenatally (Sai, 2005). Neural correlation of face processing was documented by fMRI in 2-month-old infants (Tzourio-Mazoyer et al., 2002). The same brain regions in-volved in adult face processing are used in infants. Damage to this fusiform face region of the brain in the first day of life impairs the infant's facial recognition. The fusiform face area gradually increases in size and is three times larger in adults than in a compar-ative group of young children.

## Interactional or Behavioral Synchrony

Assessment of early mother–child interactions is essential to understand social de-velopment. Studies of infant responses to static faces document the infant's prefer-ence to attend to the mother's and other familiar family caregivers' faces. *Interactional*

(a)

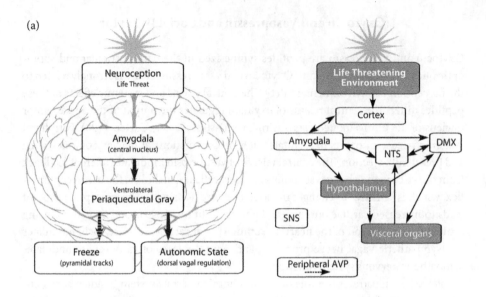

Inhibitory pathways ----------------
Excitatory pathways ————————

(b)

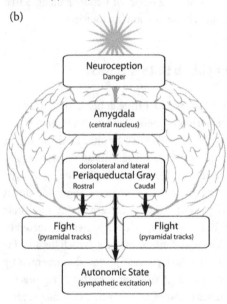

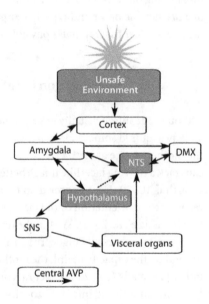

Inhibitory pathways ----------------
Excitatory pathways ————————

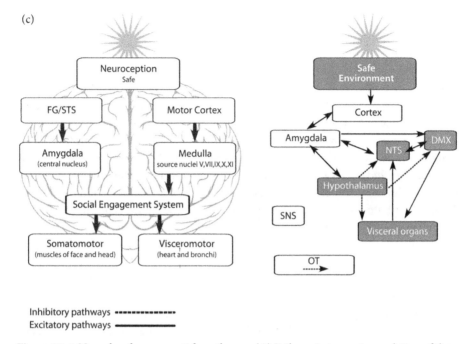

Inhibitory pathways ▪▪▪▪▪▪▪▪▪▪▪▪▪▪
Excitatory pathways ▬▬▬▬▬▬▬

**Figure 10.4** Neural and neuropeptide pathways. (A) Failure. Autonomic regulation of the dorsal vagal complex in extreme life-threatening situations. The amygdala stimulates the periaqueductal gray as it does in dangerous situations. In danger, the sympathetic nervous system facilitates an adaptive fight-or-flight response. When stress is overwhelming and fight or flight is not an option, one is immobilized by fear, freezes, or dissociates. The dorsal vagal motor complex sends surges to the visceral organs. In panel B, the amygdala stimulates the stress hormone, cortisol, released from the hypothalamus that sends inhibitory signals to the visceral organs and excitatory stimulation from the dorsal motor complex to visceral organs. The dorsal motor signals are potentiated by the release of systemic vasopressin. Systemic release of vasopressin further triggers dorsal motor vagal output. It does so by stimulating visceral afferents through the nucleus tractus solitarius and area postrema. Overall, defense and avoidance behaviors have a vagal component expressed through the dorsal vagal complex.

(B) Danger. When responding to danger is adaptive, central vasopressin pathways change the set point of vagal reflexes through vasopressin's communication between the the hypothalamus and both the nucleus solitarius and area postrema. Sympathetic nervous system activation facilitates mobilization and increases blood pressure via the baroreceptors to take action.

(C) Safety. Oxytocin is released centrally to the sensory and motor portions of the dorsal vagal complex in the brain and systematically to the visceral organs. Through this mechanism, oxytocin facilitates social sensitivity and a calming anti-stress state. There is a sense of safety. The left panel shows the inhibition of the amygdala and the activity of cranial nerves V, VII, IX, X, and XI, whose effect is to build social reciprocity through empathetic listening, calm breathing, and stimulation and a slowing of the heart rate. As the myelinated vagal brake is applied, the right panel shows that oxytocin (anti-stress effects) dynamically moderates the autonomic nervous system dorsal vagal complex in dangerous situations. Oxytocin's effects on the vagal pathway allow increased levels of oxytocin and food digestion to support adaptation to a challenging environment. AVP, ; DMX, ; NTS, nucleus tractus solitarius; OT, oxytocin; SNS, sympathetic nervous system.

From Porges (2001); redrawn by Tim Phelps (2021).

*synchrony*, a key feature in mother–infant interactions, refers to dynamic mutual, reciprocal, rhythmic, and harmonious interpersonal interactions (Leclère et al., 2014). Synchronized reciprocal interaction occurs in real time with shared affect between the mother and infant. Successful mother–infant biobehavioral synchrony in typically developing children leads to positive developmental outcomes. The interactive engagement between mother and infant is a single bidirectional dynamic relational dyadic unit. The infant may influence the caregiver and vice versa. The flow between rhythm (balanced exchange) and synchrony (dynamic and reciprocal adaptation of the time-based structure of behavior) of exchanges has been investigated. Elements of biobehavioral synchrony include verbal and nonverbal communication and emotional responses (facial display, gestures, gaze behaviors, and vocalizations). Biobehavioral synchrony incorporates both infant and mother's responsivity to one another and engages mutual emotional capacity to respond.

Affective bonding and selective and enduring social attachment involve genetic, autonomic, neurohormonal, epigenetic, behavioral, and mental engagement (Feldman, 2012). Precursors of biobehavioral synchrony can be observed in the first hours after birth; infants are biologically ready to engage in coordinated social interaction with their mothers. Engagement begins with maternal gaze at the infant's face, a warm smile, and an affectionate touch. Social engagement is enhanced by the release of oxytocin, which facilitates physiological and behavioral readiness of social conduct (Meyer-Lindenberg et al., 2011). Oxytocin receptors are located in brain regions involved in socialization, including the amygdala, hippocampus, striatum, suprachiasmatic nucleus, and brain stem. Research strategies include (a) use of global interaction rating scales, (b) use of biobehavioral synchrony scales, and (c) micro-coded time-series analyses of social interactions.

Global interaction scales include dyadic items. These scales include the Coding Interactive Behavior scale (Black & Logan, 1995), Qualitative Ratings for Parent–Child Interaction (Owen et al., 1996), Coding System for Mother–Child Interactions (Healey et al., 2010), and Parent–Child Interaction Feeding and Teaching scales (Keefe et al., 1996). These global scales measure the quality of dyadic interactions but not biobehavioral synchrony per se. Dedicated synchrony scales are also global but differ because the core focus is on biobehavioral synchrony, and they do not include subscores of each partner's behavior. For example, the Bernieri scale (Bernieri et al., 1988) and the Synchrony Global Coding System (Skuban et al., 2006) consider synchrony globally. They use the coder's perceptions and judgments of synchrony. These judgments are coded using specific definitions of the items chosen. Assessor's coded video sessions score lists behaviors observed along with time sampling for an overall score. The third approach uses micro-coded time-series analysis analyzed statistically. For example, rating includes use frequency counts of both infant and maternal behaviors. Coders use a list of agreed upon behaviors and divide mother–infant observations into units of time for scoring.

The mean duration of synchrony has been studied by examining the onset, end time, and duration of vocalization and silence between them, as well as their pitch and loudness. This has been studied with American, French, and East Asian mother–infant pairs. A study of duration used the spectrogram with visual representation of voice and sound frequency to examine interactional synchrony; the coordination between mother and infant vocalization was also examined. The greatest overlap in vocalization between mother and infant was in East Asian mothers, who also had the highest ratio of non-verbal to verbal interaction (Gratier, 2003).

## Interactional Synchrony in the First Year of Life

Newborns sporadically scan the environment visually. Mothers engage their infant by responding to the infant's gaze. Thus, continuity is established between the infant's internal state (visual scanning) and maternal behavior. Mothers provide vocal and tactile stimulation targeting the infant's alert visual scanning to make meaningful contact. Infant alertness to the mother gradually increases as a function of maternal targeted coordination with infant gaze. The extent of this maternal behavior attention to the infant predicts infant–mother synchrony and infant–father synchrony at age 3 months. It correlates with both cognitive and neural behavioral development in the first 3 months of life (Feldman & Eidelman, 2007). By age 3 months, infants join in face-to-face interactions with the parent and respond with visual facial and vocal responses to maternal social cues. Before they begin to walk, an infant's main engagement with the world is through back-and-forth social exchanges important for the development of the social brain. Social exchanges include simultaneous social gaze, joint vocalizing with a parent, coordinated arousal level and linked parental affectionate touch, and infant social gaze (Feldman & Eidelman, 2004). For example, an infant's babble modulates affective involvement with the parent. As the infant shifts from lack of social interest to attentive gaze, the mother responds seconds later with a parallel shift from being quietly attentive to positive emotional attention directed toward the infant (Feldman et al., 2007). When such coordination is nonmatched between them, the mismatch is typically repaired in the next few seconds.

During the second 6 months of life, interactive synchrony substantially increases. Social gaze and co-vocalization diminish, but shared attention directed toward objects substantially increases while the time to responsivity to social cues decreases. By the end of the first year of life, infants begin using words and social gestures. Thus, human interactional synchrony in the first year initiates and coordinates complex social behaviors and focused expression by the emerging "person." This early behavioral synchrony lays the foundation for a person's capacity to engage in intimate interpersonal relationships throughout one's lifetime.

Figure 10.5 summarizes parent–infant synchrony through early pregnancy to the end of infancy in humans. From the first trimester until birth, the release of oxytocin and vasopressin initiates the maternal behavior. By the third trimester, the cardiac pacemaker and biological clock prepare the infant for coordinated activity after birth. At birth, the newborn and mother social cues will lead to enduring social bonds. By 3 months postnatally, parents are actively involved in synchronous interactions with their infant. By 9 months of age, there are shorter lag times to synchrony as infant and parent jointly explore objects. After the first year, symbolic play begins with increases in the nonverbal component of relational engagement. At a verbal level, relations between symbolic representation are observed.

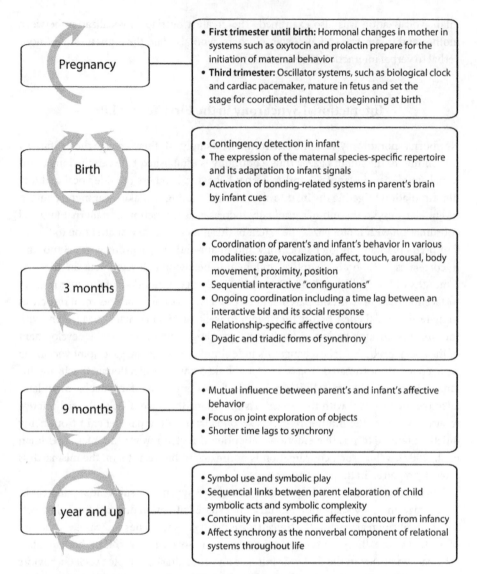

**Figure 10.5** Synchrony across the period from early pregnancy to the end of infancy (he polyvagal theory: phylogenetic substrates of a social nervous sand the emergence of physiological oscillators in the fetus during pregnancy prepare for coordinated interactions at birth. The organization of discrete social behavior into synchronous interactions begins at approximately age 3 months and undergoes reorganization at approximately age 9 months. From age 1 year onward, social interactions between close partners contain two parallel levels: a nonverbal level, marked by sequential relations between the partners' social behaviors, and a verbal level, in which sequential relations between symbolic expressions of the interacting partners are observed.

From Feldman (2007); redrawn by Tim Phelps (2021).

## Biological Correlates of Parent–Infant Synchrony

Synchrony has neurophysiological correlates during early mother–infant interactions. These are evident in vagal tone, cortisol levels, and skin conduction studies. Vagal tone, measured by RSA, plays an essential role in the regulation of social interaction, behavior, attention, and emotion. The infant's cardiac rhythms and biological clock provide the physiological foundation for social rhythms. The cardiac pacemaker controls heart rhythm, and the biological clock organizes the sleep–wake cycle. The biological maturation of these oscillators results in the regulation of arousal. Internal states shift within each of us in real time—for example, awareness of hunger and drowsiness.

These rhythms were assessed weekly from mid-pregnancy to full term in a study involving three preterm and full-term infants (Feldman, 2006). In this study, a developmental trajectory of the cardiac and biological oscillators was predictive of mother-infant synchrony at age 3 months (Feldman, 2006). The author confirms that these oscillators provide a basis for interactional synchrony. Further confirmation comes from a study of 122 mothers and infants that examined interactional synchrony. In this study, the mother interacted with the infant for 3 min, then maintained a still nonexpressive face, and then positively re-engaged. In instances in which there was high interactional synchrony during the initial 3 min of full play with the infant, the mother and infant's heart rates became synchronized such that an increase or decrease in the mother's heart rhythm was attained within less than 1 s. The mother's focused attention to the infant's social cues regulates the infant's heart rhythm. Repeated experiences such as these are internalized, establishing a sense of security that facilitates infant attachment (Feldman et al., 2007). Vagal tone is another indicator. Increased vagal tone leads to a reduction in heart rate variability and is a biological marker for the capacity to regulate emotions. In the study of the 122 mother–infant pairs, infants who showed more social engagement, measured by RSA, showed a positive response to maternal touch (Feldman et al., 2007).

## Role of Oxytocin and Vasopressin in Social Bonding

The neuropeptide oxytocin plays a preparatory role in the interaction of mother–infant behavior, the first step in mother–infant bonding. In a longitudinal study, oxytocin was measured in 62 women during the first trimester of pregnancy, the last trimester of pregnancy, and the first month after birth. Mothers with high levels of oxytocin in early pregnancy maintained high levels of oxytocin into late pregnancy and during the first postpartum month. Mothers with the highest oxytocin levels were able to facilitate mother–infant interactional synchrony better than those with low levels of oxytocin in the first trimester. Moreover, mothers with the highest oxytocin levels reported more pleasurable and vivid thoughts about their infants (Feldman et al., 2007). Thus, oxytocin prepares new mothers to initiate social engagement and facilitate maternal–infant bonding.

Oxytocin originated from an ancestral peptide, vasotocin, that is present across vertebrate and invertebrate species. Oxytocin and vasopressin have been evolutionarily conserved for more than 60 million years. Throughout this evolutionary history, they have played an essential role in adaptation to changing environments (Feldman et al., 2016). Oxytocin and vasopressin work together and are integrated into an adaptive system, the oxytocin–vasopressin pathway. Vasopressin, evolutionarily older, supports individual survival and is important in defensive aggression. Oxytocin facilitates social behavior and is involved in parenting, empathy, and stress management. Variants of the oxytocin receptor correlate with social sensitivity. Mothers who engage in more interactional synchrony with their infants demonstrate more coherent activations of the amygdala and nucleus accumbens to stimuli from their infants. These regional activations correlate with maternal plasma oxytocin (Atzil et al., 2011). Interactional synchrony is shown between mothers' and fathers' behavioral and physiological responsiveness to infant cues. In 6-month-old infants, maternal and paternal oxytocin correlated with interactional synchrony between parents (Geary, 2000).

An fMRI study examined whether mothers and fathers would synchronize their brain responses to cues from their own infant. Videotapes of mother–infant and father–infant interactions and of infant engaged in solidarity play were used as fMRI stimuli. Comparisons were made between own-infant and a video of an unfamiliar infant. Mothers and fathers synchronized brain activations in regions involved in social cognition, theory of mind, and empathy. Mothers showed greater activation in limbic brain regions, and fathers showed greater activation in social cognitive cortical brain regions. These findings correlated with oxytocin and vasopressin associated with male and female bonding (Atzil et al., 2012).

Early synchronous parent–infant interaction is important in shaping the development of the social brain. In a longitudinal study, the brain response was measured in 45 parents, who were caregivers to their infants. Their interactions with their infants were measured, and prenatal oxytocin was assayed (Abraham et al., 2016). Network connectivity was computed in three resting-state brain networks in the prenatal brain: core limbic (emotional brain) network, embodied stimulation network, and cortical (mentalizing) network. Preschool child competency in emotional regulation was subsequently measured and correlated. Integration of the parent's subcortical (limbic) and cortical (mentalizing) networks with the infant's networks predicted social outcomes in preschool children. Parent–infant synchrony mediated links between the connection of parental networks and preschool cognitive/emotional self-regulation. Parents' limbic network connectivity predicted oxytocin levels in preschool children, which were moderated by parents' oxytocin levels. This study demonstrates how parent–infant engagement potentially has a long-term impact on children's social and emotion regulation.

The integration of oxytocin with parent–infant synchrony can shape the expression of social reciprocity. A 3-year study of 160 mothers and fathers and their first-born children measured oxytocin levels in parents at postpartum months 1 and 6 (Feldman et al., 2013). Parent–infant interactions were videotaped and micro-coded. Genetic variants of the oxytocin receptor were measured at age 3 years. The children's total salivary oxytocin was measured during interaction with the mother, father, and a best friend. Parental oxytocin, stable over the 3 years, correlated with the low-risk oxytocin receptor CD38 allele and predicted child oxytocin levels. Social reciprocity of the child with a friend was correlated with the child's oxytocin levels and with mother–child reciprocity but not with father–child reciprocity. In this study, behavioral experiences within the parent–child bond were found to shape children's social affirmation and social behavior across attachment relationships.

## Neuroimaging Studies of Synchrony

An fMRI study examined parental responses to photographs of their own infants compared to unknown infants. Parents who were engaged in synchronous interactions with their infants demonstrated greater activation in the anterior cingulate cortex, superior temporal gyrus, thalamus, and midbrain; subcortical brain regions correlated with parenting, empathy, and emotion regulation (Swain, 2008).

Interactional synchrony also has been studied using ERPs. In these studies, the stimulus is locked to electrophysiological recordings. In one ERP study (Feldman, 2007b), 6-month-old infants observed pictures of their mothers' faces with neutral, sad, and angry expressions. Next, mother–infant interactions were videotaped, and interactional synchrony was assessed. In infants whose mothers were depressed, minimal interactional synchrony was detected. For infants shown their mother's angry face, the ERP response was increased. Interactional synchrony is dependent on a time-keeping mechanism that maintains a positive mood, social orientation, and attention to moment-to-moment microlevel shifts in social relational behavior. In summary, interactional synchrony has been examined across multiple physiological and neuroendocrine systems, confirming its importance in social bonding.

## Synchrony and Development

During development, human interactional synchrony involves behavior; autonomic nervous system activation; and hormones, primarily oxytocin and vasopressin. Synchrony is important for the development of the social brain and facilitates social attachment throughout the life cycle. Interactional synchrony underpins mother–infant physiologic attachment by coordinating parent and infant heart rhythm coupling behavior to the key nodes in the social brain. Biobehavioral interactional synchrony is evident among close friends through behavioral reciprocity, romantic partners as they coordinate loving gaze and emotional arousal, and in groups of people working closely together. Biobehavioral synchrony at each of these levels is illustrated in Figure 10.6.

Figure 10.6 illustrates the coupling of partner physiology and behavior in mother- and father-specific parent–infant engagement, with romantic partners, among close friends, and when strangers form groups to solve problems. For each of these groups, Figure 10.6 shows biobehavioral interactional synchrony in each of the four affiliative constellations: parental, romantic, friendship, and strangers. Four elements of behavioral synchrony (behavioral interactional synchrony, heart rate coupling, endocrine, and roles of oxytocin and cortisol) and brain-to-brain synchrony alpha and gamma oscillations are shown (Kinreich et al., 2017). The mastery of behavioral interactional synchrony in social attachment is correlated with developmental outcomes. For example, mother–infant interactional synchrony at 3 and 9 months predicted

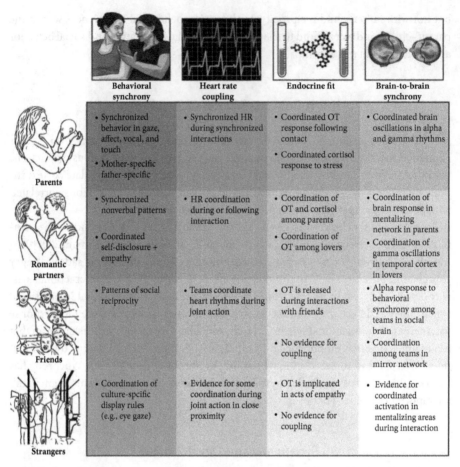

| | Behavioral synchrony | Heart rate coupling | Endocrine fit | Brain-to-brain synchrony |
|---|---|---|---|---|
| **Parents** | • Synchronized behavior in gaze, affect, vocal, and touch<br>• Mother-specific father-specific | • Synchronized HR during synchronized interactions | • Coordinated OT response following contact<br>• Coordinated cortisol response to stress | • Coordinated brain oscillations in alpha and gamma rhythms |
| **Romantic partners** | • Synchronized nonverbal patterns<br>• Coordinated self-disclosure + empathy | • HR coordination during or following interaction | • Coordination of OT and cortisol among parents<br>• Coordination of OT among lovers | • Coordination of brain response in mentalizing network in parents<br>• Coordination of gamma oscillations in temporal cortex in lovers |
| **Friends** | • Patterns of social reciprocity | • Teams coordinate heart rhythms during joint action | • OT is released during interactions with friends<br>• No evidence for coupling | • Alpha response to behavioral synchrony among teams in social brain<br>• Coordination among teams in mirror network |
| **Strangers** | • Coordination of culture-spcific display rules (e.g., eye gaze) | • Evidence for some coordination during joint action in close proximity | • OT is implicated in acts of empathy<br>• No evidence for coupling | • Evidence for coordinated activation in mentalizing areas during interaction |

**Figure 10.6** Behavioral synchrony in human attachments at different stages in the life cycle. Behavioral synchrony is characterized by partners' physiological and behavioral attunement during social engagement. In humans, four stages of affiliative bonding are shown: parental, romantic, friendship, and with strangers. Behavioral synchrony is illustrated behaviorally, physiologically, hormonally, and through coordinated activation between the brains of the partners. HR, heart rate; OT, oxytocin.

From Feldman (2017); redrawn by Tim Phelps (2021).

self-regulation at 2, 3, and 6 years, IQ measurement at 2 and 4 years, the depth of play at 3 years, and the use of words that reflect internal feelings. Maternal interactional synchrony at 3 months correlated with security of social attachment at 1 year and fewer behavioral difficulties at age 2 years. Interactional synchrony predicts school adjustment at kindergarten (Harrist et al., 1994). Finally, a 10-year follow-up study from 3 to 13 years supports the importance of interactional synchrony in facilitating the capacity for empathy and better adjustment in adolescence (Feldman et al., 2007).

Measuring interactional synchrony is also important in predicting risk. Premature infants who find it difficult to sustain social contact show reduced interactional synchrony (Feldman et al., 2007). In toddlers, lack of synchrony is related to temperamental problems and more internalizing behavior problems. Children are sensitive to synchronous parental behaviors—for example, synchronous turn-taking. Mother and father dyads and father–child interactions may differ. Depressed mothers show flat affect and decreased maternal behaviors so that moments of shared gaze are uncommon and patterning of shared engagement is disrupted. Males of depressed mothers are more vulnerable than females of depressed mothers (Weinberg et al., 2006). Although anxious mothers engage in smiling and vocalizing, they are less sensitive to the infant's emotional state. High and low interactional synchrony is predictive of secure or insecure attachment states affecting the quality of maternal representations in the attachment relationship (Crandell et al., 1997; Isabella & Belsky, 1991; Isabella et al., 1989).

In summary, interactional synchrony is not all or none. It is best to think of these as dynamic interpersonal interactions. They involve socially engaging, approaching and moving away from synchrony, and returning (Harrist & Waugh, 2002). In child development, interactional synchrony is unequivocally an important factor in attachment, interpersonal cognitive development, and behavioral development (Feldman et al., 2007).

# References

Abraham, E., Hendler, T., Zagoory-Sharon, O., & Feldman, R. (2016). Network integrity of the parental brain in infancy supports the development of children's social competencies. *Social Cognitive and Affective Neuroscience*, *11*(11), 1707–1718.

American Psychiatric Association. (2013). *Diagnostic and statistical manual of mental disorders* (5th ed.). American Psychiatric Publishing.

Anderson, C. O., & Mason, W. A. (1978). Competitive social strategies in groups of deprived and experienced rhesus monkeys. *Developmental Psychobiology*, *11*(4), 289–299.

Atzil, S., Hendler, T., & Feldman, R. (2011). Specifying the neurobiological basis of human attachment: Brain, hormones, and behavior in synchronous and intrusive mothers. *Neuropsychopharmacology*, *36*(13), 2603–2615.

Atzil, S., Hendler, T., Zagoory-Sharon, O., Winetraub, Y., & Feldman, R. (2012). Synchrony and specificity in the maternal and the paternal brain: Relations to oxytocin and vasopressin. *Journal of the American Academy of Child & Adolescent Psychiatry*, *51*(8), 798–811.

Bazhenova, O. V., Plonskaia, O., & Porges, S. W. (2001). Vagal reactivity and affective adjustment in infants during interaction challenges. *Child Development*, *72*(5), 1314–1326.

Bernieri, F. J., Reznick, J. S., & Rosenthal, R. (1988). Synchrony, pseudosynchrony, and dissynchrony: Measuring the entrainment process in mother–infant interactions. *Journal of Personality and Social Psychology*, *54*(2), 243–253.

Black, B., & Logan, A. (1995). Links between communication patterns in mother–child, father–child, and child–peer interactions and children's social status. *Child Development*, *66*(1), 255–271.

Bowlby, J. (1969). *Attachment*. Basic Books.

Bowlby, J. (1973). *Attachment and loss: Separation, anxiety and anger* (Vol. 2). Plimlico.

Bowlby, J. (1988). Developmental psychiatry comes of age. *American Journal of Psychiatry*, *145*(1), 1–10.

Brydges, C. R., Landes, J. K., Reid, C. L., Campbell, C., French, N., & Anderson, M. (2018). Cognitive outcomes in children and adolescents born very preterm: A meta-analysis. *Developmental Medicine & Child Neurology*, *60*(5), 452–468.

Carter, C. S. (1998). Neuroendocrine perspectives on social attachment and love. *Psychoneuroendocrinology*, *23*(8), 779–818.

Cassia, V. M., Turati, C., & Simion, F. (2004). Can a nonspecific bias toward top-heavy patterns explain newborns' face preference? *Psychological Science*, *15*(6), 379–383.

Chugani, H. T., Behen, M. E., Muzik, O., Juhász, C., Nagy, F., & Chugani, D. C. (2001). Local brain functional activity following early deprivation: A study of postinstitutionalized Romanian orphans. *NeuroImage, 14*(6), 1290–1301.

Crandell, L. E., Fitzgerald, H. E., & Whipple, E. E. (1997). Dyadic synchrony in parent–child interactions: A link with maternal representations of attachment relationships. *Infant Mental Health Journal, 18*(3), 247–264.

Dawkins, R. (1989). *The selfish gene.* Oxford University Press.

Debnath, R., Tang, A., Zeanah, C. H., Nelson, C. A., & Fox, N. A. (2020). The long-term effects of institutional rearing, foster care intervention and disruptions in care on brain electrical activity in adolescence. *Developmental Science, 23*(1), e12872.

DeCasper, A. J., & Fifer, W. P. (1980). Of human bonding: Newborns prefer their mothers' voices. *Science, 208*(4448), 1174–1176.

De Haan, M., & Gunnar, M. R. (Eds.). (2009). *Handbook of developmental social neuroscience.* Guilford.

Donald, M. (1991). *Origins of the modern mind: Three stages in the evolution of culture and cognition.* Harvard University Press.

Doussard-Roosevelt, J. A., Porges, S. W., Scanlon, J. W., Alemi, B., & Scanlon, K. B. (1997). Vagal regulation of heart rate in the prediction of developmental outcome for very low birth weight preterm infants. *Child Development, 68*(2), 173–186.

Eibl-Eibesfeldt, I. (1979). Human ethology: Concepts and implications for the sciences of man. *Behavioral and Brain Sciences, 2*(1), 1–26.

Eluvathingal, T. J., Chugani, H. T., Behen, M. E., Juhász, C., Muzik, O., Maqbool, M., Chugani, D. C., & Makki, M. (2006). Abnormal brain connectivity in children after early severe socioemotional deprivation: A diffusion tensor imaging study. *Pediatrics, 117*(6), 2093–2100.

Feldman, R. (2006). From biological rhythms to social rhythms: Physiological precursors of mother–infant synchrony. *Developmental Psychology, 42*(1), 175–188.

Feldman, R. (2007a). Parent–infant synchrony and the construction of shared timing: Physiological precursors, developmental outcomes, and risk conditions. *Journal of Child Psychology and Psychiatry, 48*(3–4), 329–354.

Feldman, R. (2007b). Parent–infant synchrony: Biological foundations and developmental outcomes. *Current Directions in Psychological Science, 16*(6), 340–345.

Feldman, R. (2007c). Mother–infant synchrony and the development of moral orientation in childhood and adolescence: Direct and indirect mechanisms of developmental continuity. *American Journal of Orthopsychiatry, 77*(4), 582–597.

Feldman, R. (2012). Parent–infant synchrony: A biobehavioral model of mutual influences in the formation of affiliative bonds. *Monographs of the Society for Research in Child Development, 77*(2), 42–51.

Feldman, R., & Eidelman, A. I. (2004). Parent–infant synchrony and the social–emotional development of triplets. *Developmental Psychology, 40*(6), 1133–1147.

Feldman, R., & Eidelman, A. I. (2007). Maternal postpartum behavior and the emergence of infant–mother and infant–father synchrony in preterm and full-term infants: The role of neonatal vagal tone. *Developmental Psychobiology, 49*(3), 290–302.

Feldman, R., Gordon, I., Influs, M., Gutbir, T., & Ebstein, R. P. (2013). Parental oxytocin and early caregiving jointly shape children's oxytocin response and social reciprocity. *Neuropsychopharmacology: Official Publication of the American College of Neuropsychopharmacology, 38*(7), 1154–1162.

Feldman, R., Monakhov, M., Pratt, M., & Ebstein, R. P. (2016). Oxytocin pathway genes: Evolutionary ancient system impacting on human affiliation, sociality, and psychopathology. *Biological Psychiatry, 79*(3), 174–184.

Feldman, R., Weller, A., Zagoory-Sharon, O., & Levine, A. (2007). Evidence for a neuroendocrinological foundation of human affiliation: Plasma oxytocin levels across pregnancy and the postpartum period predict mother–infant bonding. *Psychological Science, 18*(11), 965–970.

Geary, D. C. (2000). Evolution and proximate expression of human paternal investment. *Psychological Bulletin, 126*(1), 55–77.

Gratier, M. (2003). Expressive timing and interactional synchrony between mothers and infants: Cultural similarities, cultural differences, and the immigration experience. *Cognitive Development, 18*(4), 533–554.

Harlow, H. F., & Zimmermann, R. R. (1959). Affectional responses in the infant monkey. *Science, 130*(3373), 421–432.

Harrist, A. W., Pettit, G. S., Dodge, K. A., & Bates, J. E. (1994). Dyadic synchrony in mother–child interaction: Relation with children's subsequent kindergarten adjustment. *Family Relations, 43*(4), 417–424.

Harrist, A. W., & Waugh, R. M. (2002). Dyadic synchrony: Its structure and function in children's development. *Developmental Review, 22*(4), 555–592.

Healey, D. M., Gopin, C. B., Grossman, B. R., Campbell, S. B., & Halperin, J. M. (2010). Mother-child dyadic synchrony is associated with better functioning in hyperactive/inattentive pre-school children. *Journal of Child Psychology and Psychiatry, 51*(9), 1058–1066.

Hinde, R. A. (1983). Feedback in the mother–infant relationship. In R. A. Hinde (Ed.), *Primate social relationships: An integrated approach* (pp. 70–73). Blackwell.

Isabella, R. A., & Belsky, J. (1991). Interactional synchrony and the origins of infant–mother attachment: A replication study. *Child Development, 62*(2), 373–384.

Isabella, R. A., Belsky, J., & von Eye, A. (1989). Origins of infant–mother attachment: An examination of interactional synchrony during the infant's first year. *Developmental Psychology, 25*(1), 12–21.

Kanner, L. (1942). Exoneration of the feebleminded. *American Journal of Psychiatry, 99*, 17–22.

Keefe, M. R., Kotzer, A. M., Froese-Fretz, A., & Curtin, M. (1996). A longitudinal comparison of irritable and nonirritable infants. *Nursing Research, 45*(1), 4–9.

Kinreich, S., Djalovski, A., Kraus, L., Louzoun, Y., & Feldman, R. (2017). Brain-to-brain synchrony during naturalistic social interactions. *Scientific Reports, 7*(1), 1–12.

Kraemer, G. W. (1985). Effects of differences in early social experience on primate neurobiological–behavioral development. In M. Reite (Ed.), *The psychobiology of attachment and separation* (pp. 135–161). Academic Press.

Kropotkin, P. I. (1989). *Mutual aid: A factor in evolution.* Black Rose.

Leclère, C., Viaux, S., Avril, M., Achard, C., Chetouani, M., Missonnier, S., & Cohen, D. (2014). Why synchrony matters during mother–child interactions: A systematic review. *PLoS One, 9*(12), e113571.

MacLean, P. D. (1985). Brain evolution relating to family, play, and the separation call. *Archives of General Psychiatry, 42*(4), 405–417.

MacLean, P. D. (1990). *The triune brain in evolution: Role in paleocerebral functions.* Springer.

Martin, L. J., Spicer, D. M., Lewis, M. H., Gluck, J. P., & Cork, L. C. (1991). Social deprivation of infant rhesus monkeys alters the chemoarchitecture of the brain: I. Subcortical regions. *Journal of Neuroscience, 11*(11), 3344–3358.

Mason, W. A., & Capitanio, J. P. (1988). Formation and expression of filial attachment in rhesus monkeys raised with living and inanimate mother substitutes. *Developmental Psychobiology, 21*(5), 401–430.

Meyer-Lindenberg, A., Domes, G., Kirsch, P., & Heinrichs, M. (2011). Oxytocin and vasopressin in the human brain: Social neuropeptides for translational medicine. *Nature Reviews Neuroscience, 12*(9), 524–538.

Myers, M. M., Grieve, P. G., Stark, R. I., Isler, J. R., Hofer, M. A., Yang, J., Ludwig, R. J., & Welch, M. G. (2015). Family Nurture Intervention in preterm infants alters frontal cortical functional connectivity assessed by EEG coherence. *Acta Paediatrica, 104*(7), 670–677.

Nelson, C. A., Fox, N. A., & Zeanah, C. H. (2014). *Romania's abandoned children: Deprivation, brain development, and the struggle for recovery.* Harvard University Press.

Owen, M. T., Barfoot, B., Vaughn, A., Domingue, G., & Ware, A. M. (1996). *54-month parent-child structured interaction qualitative rating scales.* NICHD Study of Early Child Care Research Consortium.

Porges, S. W. (2001). The polyvagal theory: Phylogenetic substrates of a social nervous system. *International Journal of Psychophysiology, 42*(2), 123–146.

Porges, S. W. (2004). Neuroception: A subconscious system for detecting threats and safety. *Zero to Three, 24*(5), 19–24.

Porges, S. W., Davila, M. I., Lewis, G. F., Kolacz, J., Okonmah-Obazee, S., Hane, A. A., Kwon, K. Y., Ludwig, R. J., Myers, M. M., & Welch, M. G. (2019). Autonomic regulation of preterm infants is enhanced by Family Nurture Intervention. *Developmental Psychobiology, 61*(6), 942–952.

Porges, S. W., & Furman, S. A. (2011). The early development of the autonomic nervous system provides a neural platform for social behaviour: A polyvagal perspective. *Infant and Child Development, 20*(1), 106–118.

Robertson, J. (1958). *Young children in hospital.* Tavistock.

Romer, A. S. (1966). *Vertebrate paleontology.* University of Chicago Press.

Sachis, P. N., Armstrong, D. L., Becker, L. E., & Bryan, A. C. (1982). Myelination of the human vagus nerve from 24 weeks postconceptional age to adolescence. *Journal of Neuropathology & Experimental Neurology, 41*(4), 466–472.

Sackett, G. P. (1972). *Isolation rearing in monkeys: Diffuse and specific effects on later behavior* (Animal models of human behavior No. 198, pp. 61–110). Colloques Internationaux du Centre National de la Recherche Scientifique.

Sai, F. Z. (2005). The role of the mother's voice in developing mother's face preference: Evidence for intermodal perception at birth. *Infant and Child Development, 14*(1), 29–50.

Simon, H. A. (1990). A mechanism for social selection and successful altruism. *Science, 250*(4988), 1665–1668.

Skuban, E. M., Shaw, D. S., Gardner, F., Supplee, L. H., & Nichols, S. R. (2006). The correlates of dyadic synchrony in high-risk, low-income toddler boys. *Infant Behavior and Development, 29*(3), 423–434.

Spitz, R. A. (1946). Anaclitic depression: An inquiry into the genesis of psychiatric conditions in early childhood. *Psychoanalytic Study of the Child, 2,* 313–342.

Suomi, S. J., & Harlow, H. F. (1972). Social rehabilitation of isolate-reared monkeys. *Developmental Psychology, 6*(3), 487–496.

Swain, J. E. (2008). Baby stimuli and the parent brain: Functional neuroimaging of the neural substrates of parent–infant attachment. *Psychiatry, 5*(8), 28–36.

Tzourio-Mazoyer, N., De Schonen, S., Crivello, F., Reutter, B., Aujard, Y., & Mazoyer, B. (2002). Neural correlates of woman face processing by 2-month-old infants. *NeuroImage, 15*(2), 454–461.

Wade, M., Fox, N. A., Zeanah, C. H., & Nelson, C. A., 3rd. (2019). Long-term effects of institutional rearing, foster care, and brain activity on memory and executive functioning. *Proceedings of the National Academy of Sciences of the USA, 116*(5), 1808–1813.

Ward, J. (2016). *The student's guide to social neuroscience.* Psychology Press.

Weinberg, K. M., Olson, K. L., Beeghly, M., & Tronick, E. Z. (2006). Making up is hard to do, especially for mothers with high levels of depressive symptoms and their infant sons. *Journal of Child Psychology and Psychiatry, 47*(7), 670–683.

Welch, M. G. (2016). Calming cycle theory: The role of visceral/autonomic learning in early mother and infant/child behaviour and development. *Acta Paediatrica, 105*(11), 1266–1274.

Welch, M. G., Firestein, M. R., Austin, J., Hane, A. A., Stark, R. I., Hofer, M. A., Garland, M., Glickstein, S., Brunelli, S., Ludwig, R., & Myers, M. M. (2015). Family nurture intervention in the neonatal intensive care unit improves social-relatedness, attention, and neurodevelopment of preterm infants at 18 months in a randomized controlled trial. *Journal of Child Psychology and Psychiatry, 56*(11), 1202–1211.

Welch, M. G., Hofer, M. A., Stark, R. I., Andrews, H. F., Austin, J., Glickstein, S. B., Ludwig, R. J., Myers, M. M., & FNI Trial Group. (2013). Randomized controlled trial of Family Nurture Intervention in the NICU: Assessments of length of stay, feasibility and safety. *BMC Pediatrics, 13*(1), Article 148.

Welch, M. G., & Ludwig, R. J. (2017). Calming cycle theory and the co-regulation of oxytocin. *Psychodynamic Psychiatry, 45*(4), 519–540.

Wilson, E. O. (2000). *Sociobiology: The new synthesis.* Harvard University Press. (Original work published 1975)

# 11

# Attachment Security Disorders

Attachment theory has important implications not only for typically developing children but also for children with neurodevelopmental disorders. Attachment relationships, secure and insecure, influence adaptation in neurodevelopmental disorders by interacting with other risk factors. When attachment is secure, it reduces risk; when it is insecure, it may increase vulnerability to stressors. The strength of Bolwby's formulation of attachment is that it is based on research across many species, not just humans (Bowlby, 1982; see also Ainsworth & Bowlby, 1991). Thus, it is based in evolutionary biology.

In his original proposal, Bowlby (1982) emphasized that attachment is not the whole of social relations; however, it is of particular importance to children with neurodevelopmental disorders. For them, we need to use attachment security paradigms, particularly the Strange Situation procedure, for the development of internal working models (DeKlyen & Greenberg, 2008; Rutter et al., 2009; van IJzendoorn et al., 2007) about the applicability of the disorganized attachment category to people with neurodevelopmental disorders and the use of the term "attachment other" in reference to children raised in institutions with limited social engagement and physical stimulation. In institutional settings, caregiving can be seriously disrupted so that attachment is so atypical that there is diagnosable attachment disorder. Also in institutional settings, there may be no reliable caregiver to whom the infant can become attached. This chapter discusses both the impact of severe early deprivation on attachment in typically developing children and attachment issues in those with neurodevelopmental disorders.

## Stress-Related Reactive Attachment Disorders and Disinhibited Social Engagement Disorder

Concerns for institutionalized children led to investigation of the effects of severe maternal deprivation on child development after World War II. These studies revealed that disrupted attachment led to the diagnosis of reactive attachment disorder, a diagnosis included in the third edition of the *Diagnostic and Statistical Manual of Mental Disorders* (DSM-III; American Psychiatric Association [APA], 1980). Reactive attachment disorder was defined as a pervasive disturbance in relationships that occurred before age 10 months with "failure to thrive." In DSM-IV (APA, 1994), two subgroups were introduced: emotionally withdrawn/inhibited and indiscriminately social/inhibited. In the category "trauma and stress-related disorders," the age was changed to 5 years or younger, and "failure to thrive" was dropped as a criterion. In DSM-5 (APA, 2013), the disorder types are distinct. The first is an inhibited form with characteristic fear, social withdrawal, hypervigilance, and ambivalence; and the second is a disinhibited type diagnosed when the infant is indiscriminately friendly and shows very limited evidence of a specific attachment. In both classifications, documentation of pathologic care is required.

Although disturbed attachment is apparent, these diagnoses are not consistent with attachment theory models in typically developing children because their severity is beyond the category of "insecure attachment" (Zeanah, 1996). In these clinical diagnoses, the criteria are focused on general social behavior rather than on the relationship with a specific primary caregiver or caregivers. Based on experience with such severe deprivation, the alternative terms "non-attachment" or "disordered attachment" and "disruption in attachments" have been proposed (Zeanah & Boris, 2000). Children in the non-attachment category, who had no specified attachment figure, may exhibit indiscriminate sociability or might fail to seek out or respond to caregiver support gestures as shown by typically developing children. A child with the non-attachment diagnosis must have a mental age of at least 10 months to distinguish it from substantial cognitive deficits or an autism spectrum disorder (ASD) diagnosis. Zeanah and Boris' second category, disordered attachment, proposes a "selective" but disturbed attachment. This is indicated by the child's extreme inhibition and compulsive compliance. The third category, disruption of attachment, includes children whose attachment to a primary caregiver was disrupted by loss of a caregiver with grieving.

In DSM-5, reactive attachment disorder refers to emotionally withdrawal, inhibited behavior. The second and new diagnostic category, disinhibited social engagement disorder, is not the result of disinhibited attachment to a specific caregiver but, rather, a general failure to inhibit behavior and recognize social boundaries. It is a behavioral pattern that results from very deficient early caregiving, but these diagnoses do not preclude the capacity to form secure attachment with a supportive and caring adult. In DSM-5, both reactive attachment disorder and disinhibited social engagement disorder are categorized in the broader category "trauma and stressor-related disorder" along with post-traumatic stress disorder, acute stress disorder, and adjustment disorder.

## Reactive Attachment Disorder

Children diagnosed with reactive attachment disorder are emotionally inhibited and rarely seek comfort when distressed, and they show minimal response to efforts to comfort them. There is an absence of organized attachment. They may be hypervigilant and ambivalent to emotional approach without bursts of unexplained irritability, fear, or sadness. Often, due to frequent changes in foster care homes or institutional care, these children have experienced social neglect of being comforted and receiving affectionate care. The diagnosis is made most often between 9 months and before 5 years of age. The diagnosis is typically not made after age 5 years. This disorder often co-occurs with cognitive and language development delay. It is relatively rare in clinical settings. Among children who are severely neglected, this diagnosis is relatively uncommon, occurring in approximately 10% of such children (APA, 2013, p. 266). Treatment of DSM-5 attachment disorders is focused on remedial nurturant foster care. In a randomized control study that examined the effects of foster care in children from Romanian institutions who were severely neglected, inhibited reactive attachment disorder was commonly diagnosed before foster care placement. In one study, 24 out of 56 children demonstrated markedly inhibited reactive attachment disorder before foster care. After foster care, only 1 child met diagnostic criteria for severe inhibited type. Overall, there was a clear benefit from foster care (Rutter et al., 2007).

## Disinhibited Social Engagement Disorder

Children with disinhibited social engagement disorder respond quite differently to strangers than do those with reactive attachment disorder. Rather than being inhibited, they will readily go off with a stranger. They show limited differentiation among adults. They are not reticent or shy with strangers, lack social reserve, and do not hesitate to interact with unfamiliar adults. They do not check with an adult caregiver, walking away even when the setting is not familiar to them. Their verbal and/or physical contact with strangers is culturally inappropriate. There is a history of social neglect and deprivation of basic emotional care in the early months of life. If in foster care, they have changed homes frequently. The developmental age required to make a diagnosis is at least 9 months. The disorder is persistent, lasting more than 12 months. Because of the extent of neglect, the disorder may co-occur with cognitive and language developmental delay. The diagnosis is rare even among groups of children who are severely neglected in institutions or in multiple foster care placements, occurring in approximately 20% of such cases (APA, 2013, p. 269). Typically, neglect occurs in the early months of life. There is no evidence that neglect beginning after age 2 years is associated with this disorder. With early onset, the disorder may persist into preschool and in the middle childhood years. These children tend to be verbally and socially intrusive and attention-seeking. In adolescence, peer relationships are generally inappropriate, leading to indiscriminate social behavior with interpersonal conflicts. Peer relationships tend to be superficial. Some affected children may have co-occurring diagnosis of attention-deficit/hyperactivity disorder (APA, 2013, p. 270).

In the study of English and Romanian adoptees from institutional care (Rutter et al., 2007), the association with early institutional deprivation was still evident at age 11 years, at least 7 years following adoption into nurturant home settings. More than half of children removed from these Romanian institutions demonstrated one or more features of disinhibited social engagement disorder at age 11 years, compared to 8% of children who were adopted to the United Kingdom. Moreover, the disorder was not associated with variations in quality of adoptive homes. These findings show that this is not a disorder characterized by insecure attachment as defined in typically developing children. Instead, it is a disorder essentially characterized by a "failure to develop committed intimate relationships" (Rutter et al., 2009, p. 536).

Overall, in the Romanian studies, reactive attachment disorder was common in children who remained in institutions. Yet, with appropriate supportive foster care, the rate declined and the level could approach that of the typical children who lived in the community where they were raised. Disinhibited social engagement disorder persisted if the affected children remained in institutional care. When children with this disorder were placed in community foster care, they showed limited improvement, with their aberrant behavior largely persisting in the foster care. The inhibited group's improvement was correlated with the quality of caregiving in foster care but less so for the disinhibited group. This suggests there is not a critical developmental period for the inhibited at-tachment group. However, as indicated by the limited improvement in foster care, there apparently is a critical period—a developmental window—for the disinhibited group (Rutter et al., 2009).

## Attachment in Children with Neurodevelopmental Disorders

Evaluation of attachment in children with neurodevelopmental disabilities must take into account the parental sensitivity to and acceptance of their child despite their disabilities. Mental health and social functioning result from early life experiences with an attachment relationship with emotionally engaged parents and other involved caregivers. When attachments are disrupted, both mental and physical health suffer, forcing children to rely on rudimentary survival skills to cope. Most early research on attachment security focused on typically developing children. However, during ap-proximately the past 20 years, attachment research has increasingly addressed children with neurodevelopmental disorders, particularly those with intellectual developmental disorders (IDDs) and ASD. The attachment behavior is flexible and responsive to envi-ronmental input as children learn to perceive and respond to social cues emotionally and activate social attachment and behavioral strategies to regulate emotion through seeking contact with trusted, familiar caregivers. Caregivers support emotional co-regulation by comforting and consolidating, making sense of how emotions can be regulated, and providing help and support (Schuengel et al., 2013). When an infant's or child's parent-directed attachment behaviors are rejected or met with anxiety or hos-tility by the caregiver, the effect is detrimental to child self-esteem and mental health.

In behavioral science, attachment behavior can be broadly understood as behavior directed toward a caregiver to seek, maintain proximity, and find affection. Attachment can be examined developmentally as the pattern of seeking and maintaining prox-imity to establish relationships that lead to internal representations or internal working models of those relationships to rely on when distressed. For children with IDDs, there are differences in the rate, form, and patterning of attachment behaviors. Attention to the roles of both the parent and the child is important because it has long been acknowl-edged that cognition plays an integral role in the formation of an attachment relation-ship. For example, intelligence is an important element in establishing attachment needs for proximity. Cognition is key to establishing internal working models that are not simply memories of past experiences but are active constructs that can be restructured in response to environmental, affective, and necessary cognitive challenges.

Among children with an IDD, there are differences in affective responses, which for some may be blunted or delayed, making it difficult for the caregiver to interpret them. Children with an IDD may be withdrawn or lethargic, irritable, or show stereotypies or challenging behaviors (aggression and self-injury). Sensitive responsiveness of caregivers to such behaviors may modify them. For example, parental scaffolding, taking the child step-by-step when coping with a difficult task, may reduce disruptive behaviors and lead to better social skills. Combined maternal sensitivity and structuring facilitates attachment security despite low cognitive functioning (Feniger-Schaal &

Joels, 2018). Parental scaffolding in the context of attachment can facilitate emotional regulation and enhance social development when there is behavioral difficulty (Baker et al., 2007). Scaffolding facilitates a child's effort for self-control by guiding the child's learning by providing or withdrawing emotional support to enhance self-regulation. Contingent scaffolding provides support when the child needs to inhibit reflexive and automatic emotional reactions. The goal is to encourage the child to be more deliberate and reflective in selecting appropriate behaviors to achieve a task.

## Attachment Relationships

Children and adults with IDD may show attachment behaviors toward professional caregivers in daycare and residential care (De Schipper & Schuengel, 2010). Infants and children adapt their attachment in response to their caregivers. Typically developing children develop internal working models of relationships that stabilize over time. Internal working models are demonstrated in attentiveness to relationships, in emotional responses, and in behavior when interacting with caregivers, especially when stressed. These responses are calibrated by the caregiver's sensitive response to emotional needs of the child (Ainsworth et al., 1978).

The Strange Situation Procedure has been used in studies of infants with developmental disorders. Studies of children with Down syndrome find that those children are less likely to signal their attachment needs. They are less likely to approach their mothers and also less likely to make physical contact with their mothers on reunion. Despite this, children with Down syndrome can engage in the Strange Situation procedure. Although their distress when separated is muted compared to that of typically developing children, the organization of their response to separation is similar. Despite caution in interpreting Strange Situation findings, many children with Down syndrome can be classified as securely attached. The first large-scale study of children with Down syndrome using the Strange Situation procedure was carried out by Vaughn et al. (1994). In this study, 138 Down syndrome children aged 14–54 months were enrolled from three different cohorts. Forty-eight percent of children with Down syndrome were classified as secure compared to 60% in a comparison group of typically developing children aged 12–24 months. A fourth group of children were unclassifiable; some may have been disorganized. Another study enrolled 53 children with Down syndrome and employed the Strange Situation procedure (Atkinson et al., 1999). Atkinson et al. found that 40% were classified as secure at age 26 months, and 48% were classified as secure at age 42 months. They reported a similar proportion were unclassifiable (it was unclear if these were insecure or lacked secure base behavior). Two percent were classified as having disorganized attachment at age 26 months and 12.5% at age 42 months.

A third study examined 30 infants with Down syndrome using the Strange Situation procedure at ages 19 and 27 months (Ganiban et al., 2000). Ganiban et al. found that 43% were securely attached at age 19 months and 53% at age 27 months. Overall, they concluded that between 12 and 24 months of developmental age, attachment is consolidated in Down syndrome, with an organization of Strange Situation responses similar to that of typically developing children. Secure attachment was found to be the normative pattern in Down syndrome, as it is in typically developing children.

However, it cannot be automatically assumed that findings in Down syndrome apply to children with other etiologies with IDDs. The development of children with Down syndrome has been reported to be similar to that of other children with IDDs if IQ level is taken into account. However, others propose that children with Down syndrome have higher levels of adaptive behavioral skills and more sociable personalities (Hodapp, 2002). Using the Strange Situation procedure, 40 children with Down syndrome were compared to children with IDD of unknown etiology ranging in age from 2½ to 5½ years. Forty percent were found to be secure, 35% insecure organized, and 25% insecure disorganized (Feniger-Schaal et al., 2012). The rate of attachment insecurity was higher than that in typically developing children.

## Disorganized Attachment and Intellectual Developmental Disorder

Use of the term disorganized attachment requires further scrutiny when applied to neurodevelopmental disorders in children who have not been neglected, physically abused, or sexually abused (Rutter et al., 2009). In the Strange Situation procedure, the term disorganized is used when the child seems to lack observable goals, has limited social interactions, explores the environment less than typically developing children, and displays disrupted behavior. When used in typically developing children, disorganized children have typically experienced psychological neglect or abuse and may appear dazed and confused (Atkinson et al., 1999). There also may be stereotypic behavior, odd posturing, freezing, and apprehensive approach behavior toward the parent. Main and colleagues (2005) found that many disorganized infants become organized by age 6 years. However, most showed insecurity on the Adult Attachment Inventory when followed into adult life. Another long-term study concurred with these findings (Sroufe et al., 2005). Disorganized attachment may represent a frightened response to threatening parental behavior or a response to unresolved loss. Parents of children with IDDs may react with strong emotions, despair, and confusion as they grieve the loss of an expected child (Blacher, 1984). This may differ from children in institutions who have been physically and socially deprived before placement in nurturant homes (Vorria et al., 2006). Grieving parents may be psychologically unavailable to the infant and display behavior that is frightening to the infant, resulting in disorganized attachment (Granqvist et al., 2017). In children with IDDs, rather than responding to experienced threat or loss, disorganized attachment may reflect cognitive deficits that lead to difficulty in emotion regulation. In ASD, disorganization results from deficits in social understanding rather than issues of neglect, abuse, or parental sensitivity. Compared to typically developing children, those with IDDs have higher rates of insecure and unclassified forms of attachment.

## Mental Representations of Attachment Relationships

The development of attachment in an infant requires sufficient cognitive attainments, including object permanence, discrimination in learning, selective attention, and memory acquired by the end of the first year of life in typically developing children. These cognitive attainments will emerge in children with an IDD later in life. In studies of Down syndrome, Cicchetti and Serafica (1981) demonstrated that these children developed attachments to their mother like typically developing children but at a later chronological age as their cognitive capacity advanced. Thus, these results with Down syndrome support the *similar sequence* view of development in children with IDD (Zigler, 1967). Also, differences are noted in the quality of attachment in lower and higher functioning children with Down syndrome; the lower functioning children were less likely to be securely attached (Atkinson et al., 1999). Finally, cognitive delays along with social and emotional problems with IDD may impact biobehavioral synchrony with the parent.

As discussed above, mother–infant biobehavioral synchrony is important in establishing secure attachment. The security of attachment can be measured in the reunion response following mother–child separation in both typically developing children and those with atypical development. As cognition develops, the closeness of the attachment relationship proceeds with the establishment of internal cognitive working models of relationships. Such internal working models influence how the relationship is expressed by children as they become increasingly independent. During development, the working models of strategies used in early attachment with parents are extended to new relationships. Mental representations are an essential component of relationships in social situations, especially attachment relationships.

In adulthood, the attachment interview draws on memories of early life to categorize attachment-related information, examining the coherence of recall for clear, secure, positive, loving relationships or negative ones with caregiver or incoherence of recall. Incoherent recall may result from ambivalence, over-idealization, dismissal of the value of early relationships, or lack of recall for attachment-related events. Recall may be incoherent, too, if there is a preoccupation with anger or overwhelmingly negative memories or unresolved reactions to childhood loss or abuse. There are no published reports of the Adult Attachment Interview used in people with an IDD. Deficits in attention, working memory, and verbal capacity in adults make it difficult for the interviewer to distinguish between incoherent recall due to such developmental deficits in establishing working models of relationships (Larson et al., 2011).

An alternative to the Adult Attachment Interview is the picture-based Adult Attachment Projective Picture System designed to use with people who have an IDD (George & West, 2011). This is a shorter inventory than the Adult Attachment Interview and does not involve accessing autobiographical memory. The pictures focus on revealing a person's interpersonal expectations of others. The assessment examines defensive responses within the stories prompted by the pictures. The test has also been modified for use with people with mild IDD to allow coding and classification of their attachment status. George and West (2011) found a strong correspondence with recalled case histories. This approach can assess attachment state of mind (internal working models), focusing as it does on expectations in adults with IDD (Gallichan & George, 2014). Studies such as these provide a means to evaluate attachment status as a risk factor in people with an IDD.

The following rating scales have been developed to assess attachment in people with IDDs (Box 11.1): the Adult Attachment Projective Picture System, the Self-Report Assessment of Attachment Security, the Secure Base Safe Haven Observation, and the Manchester Attachment Scale–Third party observational measure. The first two of these rely on self-report by people with an IDD who can respond verbally. The first

---

**Box 11.1  Attachment Measures**

---

- Adult Attachment Projective Picture System (Gallichan & George, 2018)
  - Looking at and telling a story about each of seven pictures (one is a neutral picture)
  - Coding as secure, dismissive, insecure, or undescribed
- Self-Report Assessment of Attachment Security (Smith & McCarthy, 1996)
  - Verbal self-report of comfort-seeking when stressed
  - Behavior
  - Grammatically simplified questioning
  - Multiple choice
- Secure Base Safe Haven Observation (SBSHO)
  - Caregiver interview for moderate to severe intellectual developmental disorder
  - 20-item list of observations rated on a 7-point Likert scale
  - Higher scores rated at secure attachment
  - Developed from the attachment Q-Sort
- Manchester Attachment Scale–Third party observational measure (MAST; Penketh et al., 2014)
  - Caregiver interview adults
  - 16-item scale
  - Rated on a 4-point Likert scale
  - Total score summary of item scores
  - Based on Q-sort methods
  - Seeks comfort when distressed
  - Accepts attention from others
  - Seeks to maintain social contact
  - Includes emotional rating scale

---

is a self-report measure, and the second is a picture-guided interview. The other two are based on caregiver reports of interactions and behavior, and they may be used with adults who are more severely cognitively impaired. All four of these are based on shifting clinical focus away from examination of external behavior, particularly noncognitive operant behavior approaches, to focus the person's personal thoughts and feelings.

The Adult Attachment Projective Picture System has been examined for interrater reliability and face validity in a pilot study in relation to secure, dismissing, preoccupied, and unresolved attachment. The study found reliable interrater reliability and stability over time (Gallichan & George, 2018).

### The Self-Report Assessment of Attachment Security

Reliability for the Self-Report Assessment of Attachment Security was determined in subjects aged 20–54 years through a repeated measurement at 10 weeks (Smith &

McCarthy, 1996). Construct validity was examined by analysis of this measure with re-lated measures of self-esteem and of personal independence in the social setting. Both males and females were examined. One-third of the subjects had Down syndrome, but ASD was excluded. All subjects were living at home with their families. Participants were asked how they would respond to negative emotion with three options: tell someone, keep your feelings to yourself, or show feelings in an uncontrolled way (yell, self-injury, and tantrum). Smith and McCarthy reported 41% would confide feelings to others and were deemed secure. Test–retest reliability was 90%. Subjects must use verbal communication to effectively be assessed. Concurrent measures of attachment are needed to confirm validity (Fletcher et al., 2016).

## The Secure Base Safe Haven Observation

The Secure Base Safe Haven observational scale was developed from the attachment Q-sort (Waters, 1995) and adapted for use along with additional items that reflect attach-ment behavior in people with IDD when stressed. Behaviors selected include looking to the caregiver when stressed, responding to comfort by caregiver, using the caregiver for comfort, returning to the caregiver for support when stressed by others, and greeting the caregiver on entry to a group (De Schipper & Schuengel, 2010; Schuengel et all., 2010). It was designed specifically for people with moderate to severe IDD, who may have limited language, low cognition, and limited experiences; it does not examine their thoughts.

## The Manchester Attachment Scale

The Manchester Attachment Scale (Penketh et al., 2014) utilized Q-sort methodology to reach consensus on the security of attachment in people with IDD. The caregiver rates behaviors including active solicitation of caregiver comfort when distressed, accept-ance of the caregiver also supporting others, and effort to maintain social interaction with the caregiver. The internal consistency, reliability, and validity of the Manchester Attachment Scale have been examined, focusing on test–retest reliability and face, con-current, and predictive validity for secure attachment behavior. With regard to emo-tional rating, the Manchester Attachment Scale was found to be reliable over time and to have concurrent validity. Like the Secure Base Safe Haven Observation, it does not obtain verbal reports about the perspective of the person being assessed.

In summary, a combination of measures, a tool kit, for clinical research staff and clinicians is required to assess secure attachment in subjects with a varying degree of in-tellectual disability. These people range in intelligence from mildly to severely affected, have varying degrees of receptive and expressive language ability, and may have associ-ated physical handicaps. The tool kit used might include a self-report interview such as the Self-Report Assessment of Attachment Security and observational measures such as the Secure Base Safe Haven Observation or the Manchester Attachment Scale, along with assessment of self-esteem and emotional well-being. These ratings are best used as a part of a case formulation in determining a treatment plan.

## The Adult Attachment Projective Picture System

The Adult Attachment Projective Picture System is the subject of ongoing re-search to facilitate its adoption in clinical practice. The early development of attachment relationships with caregivers is important to subsequent emotional development. Bowlby (1982) proposed that experiences of relationships influence patterns of thinking, leading to internal mental representations of relationships with the emergence of a sense of self-worth. If a child feels inadequate or incompetent when seeking adult approval, this can lead to negative internal self-mental representations. When lovingly experienced, mental representations lead to positive self-worth. Internal working models of relationships have been examined empirically. For example, reaction time has been examined in people with secure and insecure attachment based on the Adult Attachment Projective Picture System (Wichmann et al., 2016). The examiners sought to determine whether reaction time differed with respect to a person's attachment representation. The measurement of reaction time drew upon experimental research with the implicit (nondeclarative) association task, which examines automatic cognitive processing in the evaluation of the self and others in social cognition research. It assesses the complexity of the underlying mental processes: The more complex the cognitive processing, the longer the reaction time response to specific details of past interpersonal experiences and associated feelings.

Internal working models include expectations about the self and others. Importantly, they involve nondeclarative but not declarative memory, functioning outside conscious awareness. They guide attention to memory and interpretation of past attachment experiences. In one study, subjects were asked to accept or reject statements about secure and insecure attachment categories (Wichmann et al., 2016). Pictures from the Adult Attachment Projective Picture System were presented accompanied by sentences representing different patterns of attachment. The assessment focused on how long it took for the subjects to decide—that is, to accept or reject the description. The authors hypothesized that people with a secure attachment would accept secure descriptors faster. For example, those with a high attachment security index would promptly reject insecure prototype descriptors. The authors found that lower attachment security index scores were associated with prompt acceptance of insecure sentences and rejection of secure ones. Thus, the reaction time test used a narrative attachment measure to capture implicit (nondeclarative) automatic aspects of attachment. The study's hypothesis was confirmed: The use of reaction time in the measurement of attachment security in this paradigm was validated.

The Adult Attachment Projective Picture System uses a standard set of line drawings depicting solitude, separation, illness, threat, and death. The standard warm-up begins with neutral pictures (two children playing ball) as an introduction. The participant is asked to tell a story about what is happening in the picture that led up to the scene depicted. Then they are asked to describe what the characters are thinking or feeling and what happens next. The attachment situations are then introduced. The participants are told there are no right or wrong answers. Sessions are tape-recorded for analysis (Gallichan & George, 2018). Four standard adult attachment groups are identified: secure/flexibility integrated, dismissive, preoccupied, and unresolved. The pilot study showed good validity.

## The Attachment Bond

The attachment bond refers to the depth of affective investment in an enduring relationship over time with a particular person. When separated from this person, there is an intense desire for renewed contact. Attachment is not simply reliance on a friend when in need of some support but, rather, a deeper relationship with a sense of loss when separated from them. When apart, distress is substantial, especially if separation is prolonged. Separation distress and bereavement after loss are complicated when attachment is insecure. People with insecure avoidant attachment tend to hide their feelings of loss, complicating the provision of support from others. For people with IDD, bereavement is complicated because there is considerable individual variation in their understanding of the concept of death (McEvoy et al., 2012).

Complicated grief is an important issue following parental loss in people with mild to moderate IDD. In one study, one-third of adults in the mild to moderate range of IDD who lost a parent showed as least 10 or more clinical symptoms of complicated grief (Dodd et al., 2008). An important concern, too, is the bereavement response to separation when professional caregivers in school settings or group homes are rotated to other jobs, especially if there is high staff turnover. Frequent staff turnover affects their mental health, social functioning, and behavior (Buntinx, 2008). People with an IDD bond to long-term staff, which is often not fully appreciated. When staff change is anticipated, considerable preparation is needed to address issues of loss in people with an IDD.

## Coping with Stress and Attachment

People with an IDD are more vulnerable to stress and are less effective in coping with stress. Their attachment relationships assume importance in coping with stress, especially through secure attachment with caregivers who provide a secure base. Because they have a higher prevalence of insecure or disorganized attachment, people with an IDD are at greater risk for developing behavioral problems. A stress attachment model is a useful framework to examine development mechanisms that lead to behavioral problems (Janssen et al., 2002).

Institutional support staff play a major role, as do parents, as attachment figures in modulating dysregulated behavior when people with IDD are emotionally stressed. In one report, 156 young participants (70% male; median age, 9 years) in a group care setting diagnosed with mild to moderate IDD were studied. Two members of the classroom support staff completed the Secure Base Safe Haven Observation checklist. In addition, challenging behaviors (e.g., aggression and self-injury) were assessed using the Aberrant Behavior Checklist. Those with more secure attachment were less irritable, less lethargic, and showed fewer stereotypic behaviors. Developmental age and co-occurring ASD were taken into account in this assessment. Adaptation was facilitated by the integration of relationships with the support staff, which reduces stress and affects the regulation of challenging behavior (De Schipper & Schuengel, 2010).

## Parenting Children with a Neurodevelopmental Disorder

Parents play a critical role in the socioemotional development of their children. In a study of parents' perspectives on child–parent attachment, semistructured interviews were carried out with 54 parents regarding their child's socioemotional behavior and attachment status using the attachment framework method. Parents described their perceptions of conditions needed to establish a secure relationship for children diagnosed with severe or profound IDD. The children ranged in age from 15 months to 7 years. The parents reported clear preferences about how they regulated their child's stress. However, children did differ in the extent that they used their parents' support to explore new environments. Parents stated that, overall, the attachment relationship with their child was positive yet challenging. The parents served as a safe haven for their children and, to a lesser extent, a secure base. This study illustrates the importance of serious discussion with parents about the challenges they face in building a secure attachment with their child (Vandesande et al., 2019). Moreover, this study reveals how invested parents are in their children, regardless of cognitive level. Maternal as well as paternal sensitivity to their child's limit-setting and scaffolding were found to be important.

## Maternal Sensitivity and Attachment

How can we account for the higher rate of insecure attachment in children with an IDD diagnosis? There are challenges in applying the classical Strange Situation procedure to these children. One issue is how these children respond to stress, and another is how and when the behavioral system involved in response to distress is evolved by infant–parent separation. Children with Down syndrome do demonstrate clear awareness of separation, although their responses at reunion are more difficult to interpret. The Strange Situation procedure is validated in numerous studies in typically developing children in the first year of life based on sensitivity of the mother to the infant's signals and that child's attachment. Accurate reading of the infant's signals by the mother is constantly correlated with secure infant attachment in studies of both children with IDD (Feniger-Schaal et al., 2012) and children with ASD (many with co-occurring disorders) (Koren-Karie et al., 2009).

Maternal sensitivity is a major factor in individual differences in attachment classification. When children with Down syndrome were studied over a 2-year period under varying conditions, classification status was related to maternal sensitivity. Mothers of secure children were rated as more sensitive than those rated as insecure (Atkinson et al., 1999). In another study using the attachment behavior Q-sort rather than the Strange Situation procedure with toddlers with neurodevelopmental disorders, secure attachment status was positively correlated with maternal sensitivity (Moran et al., 1992). Still, the percentage of children found to be insecurely attached is higher in those with IDD compared to typically developing children. For children with neurodevelopmental disorders, maternal structuring (scaffolding) is essential in addition to maternal sensitivity. The adult attachment status of the mother is important as well (Feniger-Schaal & Joels, 2018). Both maternal structuring and adult attachment status have been examined in typically developing children (Bretherton, 2000). Maternal structuring refers to the degree to which the parent appropriately guides (scaffolds) and monitors the child's activity, both of which correlate positively with secure attachment (Biringen et al., 2014).

Children with limited communication skills and cognitive deficits have a lower capacity to cope with rejection or frightening behavior toward them linked to the lack of parental resolution of loss (Bernier & Meins, 2008). Studies of the interaction between mothers and children with IDDs recognize the tendency for parents to be didactic and directive (Hauser-Cram et al., 2012). Attachment quality is linked to combined maternal sensitivity and structuring. In a study of 40 preschool children (aged 26–75 months) with nonspecific IDD diagnoses and a mean developmental age of 23 months, both maternal sensitivity and maternal structure were examined. Both were deemed important in secure attachment. Forty percent of the children were securely attached, in contrast to 60–70% of typically developing children. Correlations were significant for maternal sensitivity and structure but not for the extent of cognitive disability (Feniger-Schaal & Joels, 2018). A child with a neurodevelopmental disability disrupts typical caregiving behavior by a parent, requiring greater structure (Marvin & Pianta, 1996).

Overall, for children with IDD, a secure attachment relationship may paradoxically be even more important in facilitating socioemotional development than in typically developing children. Parenting a child with IDD is difficult and is associated with parental distress. Therefore, it is important that parents of children who have neurodevelopmental disabilities be provided with the support that they need to enhance their capacity to cope with their children's disability. Both parental sensitivity and limit-setting must take into account the parent's mental representation of their child that builds on their ability to "see things from the children's point of view." The parents must come to terms with the child's diagnosis and cognitive limitations, and they must work through the consequent emotional conflicts. The extent of insight and resolution affects caregiving behavior.

Parents of children with IDDs are at risk for burnout from the demands of child care and experiencing a sense of helplessness that may lead to depression (Feniger-Schaal et al., 2012). The divorce rate is higher than that of couples with typically developing children (Gath, 1977). There may be negative effects in the child's siblings as a result of the demands for care of the child with a developmental disability, as well as financial stressors (Hannah & Midlarsky, 1999). Yet, longitudinal studies find that although parents are stressed initially, over time, the negative impact may decrease through mastery of caregiving requirements (Barnett et al., 2006). Counterintuitively, having a child with a developmental disability may have positive effects on the family. For example, children with a Down syndrome sibling have been shown to demonstrate more empathy and kindness toward that sibling and assist in caregiving more than siblings in a comparison group of typically developing children (Cuskelly & Gunn, 2003). Finally, some parents of a child with intellectual disability do not experience severe stress and respond differently to it. Overall, there are both positive and negative effects of having a child with an IDD.

## Parental Insightfulness and Resolution of Diagnosis

Commitment to caregiving is facilitated by a caregiving behavioral system. This system organizes caregiving around mental representations of the child, which shape caregiving behavior and guide sensitive responding to the child (George & Solomon, 1999). Parental insightfulness and parents' emotional resolution over the children's diagnosis are essential to forming parents' mental representations of their children (Oppenheim & Koren-Karie, 2002). Sensitive parenting is characterized by parental capacity to see things from the child's point of view—their insightfulness. Assessment of insightfulness involves observation of the child and parent in several different contexts recorded in video vignettes, which serve as the basis of the parental interview. Parental interviews focus on their perceptions of the child's thoughts and feelings as their own. They are asked what they believe the child was thinking and feeling and how they felt in the video segments while watching it with the interviewer. The interviews are transcribed, rated on 10 indices, and classified into four groups: (a) positive insightfulness, (b) one-sided, (c) disengaged, and (d) mixed. The last three reflect a lack of insight (Oppenheim & Koren-Karie, 2002). The 10 indices are insight into child's motives, openness of child, complexity in description of child, maintenance of focus on child, richness of description of child, coherence of thought in interview, acceptance of child, expressions of angry feelings, worry about the child, and sees child as a separate person. There are three main components of parental insight: (a) consideration of the motivation of the child's behavior, (b) maintaining an emotionally complex view of the child as a person, and (c) being open to new and unexpected information from the child. All three are basic to interpreting the child's emotional signals and responding appropriately to them to enhance emotion regulation and feelings of security.

In the interview, positive and negative aspects of the child as a whole person are discussed in a nonjudgmental manner. Openness is key rather than a preconceived view of who the child is as a person. Insightful parents are open to unexpected behaviors. This generally requires the parent to reflect openly on themself. In studies of typically developing children, maternal insight is positively correlated with secure attachment (Koren-Karie et al., 2002). When maternal insightfulness was measured in preschool children referred to a clinic for emotional and behavioral problems, children whose behavior improved were those whose mothers showed improvement in their insightfulness toward their children (Oppenheim et al., 2004). Moreover, maternal insightfulness has been shown to be important for security of attachment in children with IDDs, just as with typically developing children (Feniger-Schaal et al., 2019). In the study by Feniger-Schaal et al., the mother's representation of their child's inner world, their insightfulness, was found to be linked to sensitive behavior toward the child. Thirty-eight mothers and their children with nonspecific IDD, aged 2½–5½ years, were included. Forty-one percent of the mothers were judged positively insightful, whereas 39% were judged emotionally disengaged. Positive mothers showed higher levels of sensitive behavior based on videotaped emotional availability indices. The insightfulness-sensitivity finding was not associated with developmental level of the child.

## Resolution of the Child's Diagnosis

The capacity for seeing the child's point of view requires acknowledgment and acceptance of the child's diagnosis and developmental level. Parental resolution not only is important for parental mental health and well-being but also has implications for the child's development (Marvin & Pianta, 1996). Resolution is important because failure to resolve negatively impacts parental capacity to respond sensitively to the child.

To examine the relationship of emotional resolution to the disability and maternal sensitivity, 40 children aged 2½–5½ years were recruited (25 boys and 15 girls) with nonsyndromic IDD (mean mental age, 26 months). The mothers completed the Reaction to Diagnosis Interview. There was 100% interaction reliability on the resolved/unresolved classification among raters. Maternal sensitivity was assessed using the emotionally availability indices. Mother–child interactions were examined in the three videotaped play sessions and scored by blind scorers. Mothers who were resigned to their child's disability showed greater maternal sensitivity in two of the three play episodes. The association held for the child's responsiveness and involvement with the mother, controlling for the child's behavior toward the mother or severity of the disability (Feniger-Schaal & Oppenheim, 2013). Emotional resolution is defined as the acceptance of the disability that leads to reorientation, refocusing of attention, effective problem-solving behaviors, and moving on in life. The parent acknowledges the child's developmental level, conflict is resolved with benefits to parental mental health.

Better understanding of the benefits of insightfulness and emotional resolution has led to interventions both in individuals and in groups. Barnett and colleagues (2003) developed a group intervention program to facilitate parental adaptation through updating or rebuilding mental representations of the child in keeping with the diagnosis. The focus was on an accurate perception of the child's abilities and limitations to enhance positive development. Other interventions enhance capacity for insightfulness, helping parents to understand the roots of a child's behavior and inner experience. These focused interventions are complemented by psychoeducational support, marriage and family therapy, respite care (short breaks), and mindfulness-based stress reduction procedures (Dykens, 2015). The goals for intervention are to enhance the child's feeling of security and of being understood. Emotional experiences such as these enhance development of children with IDDs to maximize their potential (Feniger-Schaal et al., 2012).

## Attachment in Autism Spectrum Disorder

Most studies of attachment in children with ASD find evidence of attachment behaviors in these children despite their impairments in reciprocal social interactions, social awareness, and restricted or repetitive patterns of thought and behavior. In a meta-analysis of 16 studies on attachment in children with ASD that included 10 studies with data on attachment security ($N = 287$), child–parent attachment was reviewed. In 4 of these studies using the Strange Situation procedure, 53% of the children were found to be securely attached, although less so than a typically developing comparison group. This difference from typically developing children was not present in samples of children with ASD with higher cognitive ability. However, children with co-occurring IDD and ASD were at greater risk of insecure attachment. The authors concluded that attachment security is compatible with ASD and can be assessed in young children using the Strange Situation procedure (Rutgers et al., 2004). However, children with strictly defined ASD with more severe deficits in reciprocal social interactions were less securely attached and less responsive to caregivers.

The construction of internal working models of attachment is more difficult for children with combined IDD and ASD. These children demonstrate the most difficulties with behaviors that require the interdependence of a working memory model of the self and the others (Rogers et al., 1993; Yirmiya & Sigman, 2001). Although the impairment in emotional understanding and interpersonal responsiveness may benefit and be attenuated in higher functioning people with ASD by using compensatory cognitive strategies, such strategies do not compensate for their interpersonal deficits (Dissanayake & Sigman, 2000; Sivaratnam et al., 2015). Young children with ASD preferentially respond to their caregivers compared to a stranger. They spend more time directing social behavior and do seek close proximity to caregivers. However, issues remain because the Strange Situation procedure is based on the assumption that the child can attach meaning to the parent's departure to assess secure attachment, which is less evident in ASD.

Central coherence theory has been applied to ASD. *Central coherence* refers to the ability to "see the big picture" and to "put things in context." People with ASD have weak central coherence. As a group, they focus on details and not on the whole situation. In a study of central coherence, not only those with ASD but also parents and brothers of boys with ASD were tested on four measures of central coherence. Overall, the fathers showed piecemeal processing across the four tests. These findings support weak cognitive coherence as cognitive style (Happé et al., 2001), which is more prevalent in first-degree relatives of ASD probands (Landa et al., 1992).

Impaired central coherence in children with ASD impacts how they make sense of the world around them and their relationships. Their mental development and social understanding affect the construction of an internal working model of the attachment relationship. Cognitive level also must be considered in studies of internal working models of people with ASD. Lower functioning children may have weaker central coherence and greater difficulty constructing internal working models. In a study of 2- and 3-year-old children with ASD, separation and reunion were examined in both mothers and fathers using the Strange Situation Procedure. Children were found to have differences in their relationships with mothers and fathers, especially with regard to how the fathers interacted with the children. Compared with mothers, fathers received fewer prosocial behaviors from the child. Children showed more affect when reunited with mothers than with fathers (Grzadzinski et al., 2014).

Disorganized/disoriented attachment has also been examined in children with ASD (Capps et al., 1994). Disorganized behaviors may be inherent in ASD, especially with central coherence. Significantly more psychologic stress reactivity, measured by heart rate variability, has been reported in disorganized children with ASD compared to those who are not disorganized (Willemsen-Swinkels et al., 2000). This physiological measure allows disorganization to be studied in lower functioning and higher functioning children with ASD.

Maternal sensitivity is typically reported to facilitate secure attachment. When mothers of children with ASD were classified according to their attachment security, those who were securely attached demonstrated greater sensitivity to their children than those classified as insecurely attached (Capps et al., 1994). In another study, children were diagnosed with ASD at age 4 years. Two years before the diagnosis, attachment status was assessed with the Strange Situation procedure. Using the Emotional Availability Scale, parental sensitivity was measured along with child involvement in free play. Because ASD has high heritability, parents were assessed for their differences in social sensitivity compared to a control group of parents. Were these parents less sensitive to their children's needs because they potentially fell on the broader autism phenotype with inborn social impairment themselves? The authors also examined whether children with ASD showed disorganized attachment. Finally, they examined whether parental sensitivity predicts attachment security for children with ASD as those without this diagnosis? Fifty-five children (35 boys and 20 girls) with a mean age of 28.4 months had been enrolled at the time of earlier Strange Situation assessment (van IJzendoorn et al., 2007). The authors found that the parents of children with ASD did not significantly differ from parents of children with IDD or typically developing children. Social involvement of children with an ASD was significantly lower than that of the group without ASD. Furthermore, children with ASD scored lower on the Attachment Security Scale than did children without ASD. Within the group of children with ASD, the lower scores on the Autism Diagnostic Observation Schedule significantly correlated with attachment security when controlling for developmental level. Children with ASD with more autistic symptoms were less securely attached. Finally, parental attachment security score did *not* correlate with the child's attachment security score for children with ASD, in contrast to typically developing children, for whom there is a correlation. For ASD, disorganized attachment was not explained by parental sensitivity to the child.

In ASD, the emergence of secure working models of attachment may never be achieved because working models require the capacity to appreciate the perspectives of another person. In ASD, the typical attachment behaviors, such as proximity seeking, might serve a different function than for attachment in neurotypical children. In ASD, seeking a secure base may refer to proximity to a familiar situation—that is, to a familiar person, not necessarily a specific person or a familiar object. Proximity may function to maintain sameness and avoid the overload of unfamiliar disturbing stimuli. Thus, proximity seeking would not necessarily be dependent on differences in parenting sensibility as much as the severity of the inborn deficits in social awareness and social communication. In addition, the extent of neurobiological compromise in ASD is an important factor in the assessment of disorganized attachment rather than parental influences such as unresolved loss or traumatic experience.

Children with ASD are unable to compensate for the biological constraints in social communication characteristic of the disorder. Individual differences in attachment in children with ASD are largely dependent on underlying neurobiology—for example, preservation of contact with someone to help cope with sensory overload. Essentially, the social deficits in ASD challenge the application of attachment theory to this diagnosis. Importantly, attachment, and particularly biobehavioral synchrony, is an issue for parents of children with ASD. Parents must attempt to decipher their children's emotional signals because the children do not express emotions explicitly. Parents must cope with the child's anxious response to interference with the child's preferred stereotypical routines. In some instances, parents who meet criteria for the broad autism phenotype may themselves display reduced capabilities for social interaction. Typically, parents of children with ASD employ more control strategies with their children than do parents of neurotypical children.

## Issues in Therapeutic Intervention in Autism Spectrum Disorder

Early intervention is critical for children with an ASD diagnosis. The earlier the intervention, the better the long-term outcome. However, once the autistic social communication deficit, perseveration of sameness, and repetitive stereotypical behavior become established, effective interventions may be more difficult. Autistic behaviors typically become manifest in the middle to end of the second year of life. ASD symptoms are not readily apparent in the first year of life, especially in the first 6 months. The high-risk autism sibling study provided an opportunity to initiate intervention very early. Approximately one in five younger siblings of ASD probands develop symptoms of ASD with varying degrees of severity (Landa et al., 2013; Ozonoff et al., 2011). Findings in high-risk sibling studies likely generalize to families with only one child diagnosed with ASD. There is evidence in favor of pursuing the earliest interventions in siblings of children with known ASD. Younger siblings in families in which there is already an older sibling with ASD have been shown to demonstrate improved cognitive performance relative to families with a single child with ASD (Dissanayake et al., 2019).

Studies have been undertaken to determine whether there is an identifiable autistic prodrome in the first year of life in order to initiate intervention in the first months of life. Screening is focusing on delayed motor and language skills, reduced social gesturing, impaired patterns of eye gaze, and repetitive behaviors (French & Kennedy, 2018; Shen & Piven, 2017). Siblings of ASD probands at high risk for ASD evaluated from 6 weeks after birth onward have been found to demonstrate reduced attentiveness to their parent, less affective signals to socially engage, limited coordination of communication, and less use of communicative gestures (Wan et al., 2019). There are similar findings in children who were later diagnosed with ASD in the Avon Longitudinal Study of Parents and Children (Bolton et al., 2012). Nevertheless, there are concerns about specificity of these findings in the early months of life because it is not possible to distinguish ASD children with these behavioral signs observed in the first 6 months of life from children who may later manifest neurodevelopmental disorders. However, when these behavioral features are combined with brain imaging in infants later diagnosed with ASD, the prospects for presymptomatic improvement increase (Shen & Piven, 2017).

The identification of a biological marker for ASD in the first months of life is important because there is significant neural plasticity during the first year, as evidenced by the doubling of brain size during this year. Brain regions develop within particular "time windows" known as critical periods. Brain connectivity at 6 months was examined with fMRI in a prospective study of 59 infants at high risk for ASD (baby siblings) because of an affected sib. Findings of aberrant connectivity positively correlated with subsequent ASD diagnosis at age 24 months (Emerson et al., 2017). Similar differences between ASD infants and neurotypical infants have also been identified using electroencephalography and event-related potentials (Shen & Piven, 2017). Despite these promising imaging findings, there is considerable heterogeneity in ASD with later onset of symptoms in some children, comorbid disorders, and the instability of symptoms.

Overall, combining identified biomarkers such as these along with a systematic clinical assessment is essential to detect ASD reliably early because it is a polygenic syndrome with variable phenotypic expression and other co-occurring psychiatric diagnoses.

Earlier preemptive interventions have been called for by the International Society for Autism to be initiated before 6 months of life when there is maximal brain neuroplasticity. Douglas (2019) has proposed a comprehensive neuroprotective care model targeting the first 100 days of life for infants identified to be at high risk due to a parent having ASD or for infants with an older sibling with ASD. The intervention begins with anticipatory guidance in the antenatal period and both educational and clinical support throughout the first 12 months of life. This approach provided better outcomes in low-weight premature infants when care was initiated in the neonatal intensive care unit (Als, 2009; Altimier & Phillips, 2016). The neuroprotective intervention emphasizes the importance of early motor and sensory development. Ameliorating chronic hyperarousal of the sympathetic nervous system and hypothalamic–pituitary axis and disrupted parent–infant attachment with the ASD infant may reduce the impact of intrinsic developmental vulnerabilities (Douglas, 2019; Feldman, 2007).

## Hypersociability

Autism spectrum disorder is associated with deficits in social behavior and restricted social attachments. Indiscriminate friendliness is the opposite trait of hypersociability. It is characteristic of the genetic disorder Williams–Beuren syndrome (WBS) and the attachment disorder resulting from extreme deprivation characterized by indiscriminate social approach. Thus, both genetic and environmental factors are associated with pathological hypersociability in both humans and animal models (Toth, 2019). Sociability follows a normal statistical distribution in the general population (St. Pourcain et al., 2013). Deficits in social interactions are typically found in people with both anxiety disorders and ASD (Trull & Widiger, 2013). Twin and family studies in humans and genetic mapping in rodents indicate that high and low sociability are partially heritable (Ebstein et al., 2010). In twin studies, heritability genes contributed to 50% of the variance reported for self-reported measures of altruism, empathy, and nurturance. Using the Social Responsibility Questionnaire, Rushton (2004) compared 174 monozygotic twin to 148 dizygotic twins and found that 42% of the variance was due to genes, 23% to a common environment, and the rest to an unshared environment. Overall, sociability is a polygenic trait involving the interaction of multiple genes, each making small contributions. However, single nucleotide polymorphisms (SNPs) of the oxytocin receptor are linked to the extent of sociability. Oxytocin increases the salience and reinforcement of social stimuli. As noted above, allelic variants of the oxytocin receptor impact prosocial temperament and hypothalamic function (Tost et al., 2010).

In a study that included 1,830 Asian subjects, those with a greater number of G alleles at OXTR 53576 exhibited greater empathy (Chen et al., 2011). In the meta-analysis involving more than 6,000 subjects, the finding was confirmed in both Europeans and Asians (Gong et al., 2017). A study involving Caucasian and non-Caucasian infants found that the A allele of OXTR 2254298 was associated with attachment security in non-Caucasian infants. Those with the A allele were four times more likely to have a secure attachment than those without it (Chen et al., 2011).

Unlike their ancestors, wolves, dogs spontaneously initiate social contact with humans. WBS is characterized by delayed development, cognitive impairment, behavioral abnormalities, and hypersociability, and it results from a deletion of approximately 1.5 mB containing 28 genes on HSA 7q11.23 (vonHoldt et al., 2017). vonHoldt et al. hypothesized that genes located within the WBS deletion might account for the appearance of high sociability in the evolution of dogs. They identified two sites—structural variants of the GTF21 and GTF21RD1 genes—on canine chromosome 6, homologous to sites in the WBS region, that are robustly associated with hypersociability in dogs.

## Pathological Hypersociability in Genetic Conditions

Hypersociability is viewed as a developmental abnormality linked to the amygdala. The amygdala link either increases reward or reduces aversion and is located in the ventral tegmental area–nucleus accumbens pathway. In WBS, there is a reduced amygdala response to fearful facial expressions and increased reactivity to positive social stimuli in fMRI studies, which may underlie social disinhibition in WBS (Haas et al., 2009). Genes in the WBS deletion region are linked to social behavior, with loss of function in the QTF21 SNP13229433 AA genotype associated with lower social anxiety and reduced amygdala activation to threat. The genetic disposition to sociability in WBS and its age of onset were examined in a study comparing 64 children with WBS, 31 with Down syndrome, and 27 typically developing children, who ranged in age from 1 to 12 years. Parents rated their children using the Salk Institute Sociability Questionnaire. Hypersociability was apparent in very young children with WBS, who exceeded children with Down syndrome in every age group in expressing global sociability and approach behavior to strangers (Doyle et al., 2004).

The deleted chromosomal region in WBS includes more than 25 genes. Most cases of WBS have the full deletion, but there are examples of deletion of single genes in this region. For example, a single gene deletion in the region results in supravalvular aortic stenosis and cutis laxa with no cognitive or behavioral problems. Other deleted genes in the WBS region are associated with visual–spatial construction deficits. In one case of WBS, there was a deletion of all genes except GTF21. The affected individual, unlike most cases with WBS, did not exhibit hypersocial behaviors (Dai et al., 2009). This result combined with previous data from small deletions suggest the gene GTF2IRD1 is associated with WBS visual–spacial construction deficits and that GTF2I may contribute to WBS social behaviors, including increased gaze and attention to strangers. However, the fact that there is genetic variability (rather than a hemizygous deletion) in GTF21 in healthy, typically developing people does support the role of GTF21 in social behavior. The polymorphism rs13227433AA, an SNP in GTF21, has been associated with low social anxiety and increased social communication capacity similar to that found in WBS (Doyle et al., 2004). Hypersociability in WBS is accompanied by poor understanding of the dynamics of social engagement, facial expressions, and body language. Unlike ASD, in which there is a gaze aversion, people with WBS have an intense penetrating gaze when approaching strangers. Throughout their lives, people with WBS require social support in everyday life (Toth, 2019).

Both people with WBS and those previously institutionalized, who were socially deprived, exhibit heightened amygdala responses to strangers (Olsavsky et al., 2013). Neurobiologically, it is important to link hypersociability genes and environment to neuronal functioning. Multiple neuronal mechanisms may be involved when the genetic etiology in WBS is considered. Abnormality at the neuronal level may eventually help in understanding neuronal network abnormalities involved in hypersocial behavior (Toth, 2019).

# References

Ainsworth, M. D. S., Blehar, M. C., Waters, E., & Wall, S. (1978). *Patterns of attachment: A psychological study of the strange situation.* Hillsdale, N.J.: Lawrence Erlbaum.

Ainsworth, M. S., & Bowlby, J. (1991). An ethological approach to personality development. *American Psychologist, 46*(4), 333–341.

Als, H. (2009). Newborn Individualized Developmental Care and Assessment Program (NIDCAP): New frontier for neonatal and perinatal medicine. *Journal of Neonatal–Perinatal Medicine, 2*(3), 135–147.

Altimier, L., & Phillips, R. (2016). The neonatal integrative developmental care model: Advanced clinical applications of the seven core measures for neuroprotective family-centered developmental care. *Newborn and Infant Nursing Reviews, 16*(4), 230–244.

American Psychiatric Association. (1980). *Diagnostic and statistical manual of mental disorders* (3rd ed.).

American Psychiatric Association. (1994). *Diagnostic and statistical manual of mental disorders* (4th ed.).

American Psychiatric Association. (2013). *Diagnostic and statistical manual of mental disorders* (5th ed.). American Psychiatric Publishing.

Atkinson, L., Chisholm, V. C., Scott, B., Goldberg, S., Vaughn, B. E., Blackwell, J., Dickens, S., & Tam, F. (1999). Maternal sensitivity, child functional level, and attachment in Down syndrome. *Monographs of the Society for Research in Child Development, 64*(3), 45–66.

Baker, J. K., Fenning, R. M., Crnic, K. A., Baker, B. L., & Blacher, J. (2007). Prediction of social skills in 6-year-old children with and without developmental delays: Contributions of early regulation and maternal scaffolding. *American Journal of Mental Retardation, 112*(5), 375–391.

Barnett, D., Clements, M., Kaplan-Estrin, M., & Fialka, J. (2003). Building new dreams: Supporting parents' adaptation to their child with special needs. *Infants & Young Children, 16*(3), 184–200.

Barnett, D., Clements, M., Kaplan-Estrin, M., McCaskill, J. W., Hunt, K. H., Butler, C. M., Schram, J. L., & Janisse, H. C. (2006). Maternal resolution of child diagnosis: Stability and relations with child attachment across the toddler to preschooler transition. *Journal of Family Psychology, 20*(1), 100–107.

Bernier, A., & Meins, E. (2008). A threshold approach to understanding the origins of attachment disorganization. *Developmental Psychology, 44*(4), 969–982.

Biringen, Z., Derscheid, D., Vliegen, N., Closson, L., & Easterbrooks, M. A. (2014). Emotional availability (EA): Theoretical background, empirical research using the EA Scales, and clinical applications. *Developmental Review, 34*(2), 114–167.

Blacher, J. (1984). Sequential stages of parental adjustment to the birth of a child with handicaps: Fact or artifact. *Mental Retardation, 22*(2), 55–68.

Bolton, P. F., Golding, J., Emond, A., & Steer, C. D. (2012). Autism spectrum disorder and autistic traits in the Avon Longitudinal Study of Parents and Children: Precursors and early signs. *Journal of the American Academy of Child & Adolescent Psychiatry, 51*(3), 249–260.

Bowlby, J. (1982). *Attachment and Loss: Vol. 1. Attachment* (2nd ed.). Basic Books.

Bretherton, I. (2000). Emotional availability: An attachment perspective. *Attachment & Human Development, 2*(2), 233–241.

Buntinx, W. (2008). The logic of relations and the logic of management. *Journal of Intellectual Disability Research, 52*(7), 588–597.

Capps, L., Sigman, M., & Mundy, P. (1994). Attachment security in children with autism. *Development and Psychopathology, 6*(2), 249–261.

Chen, F. S., Barth, M., Johnson, S. L., Gotlib, I. H., & Johnson, S. C. (2011). Oxytocin receptor (*OXTR*) polymorphisms and attachment in human infants. *Frontiers in Psychology, 2*, Article 200.

Cicchetti, D., & Serafica, F. C. (1981). Interplay among behavioral systems: Illustrations from the study of attachment, affiliation, and wariness in young children with Down's syndrome. *Developmental Psychology, 17*(1), 36–49.

Cuskelly, M., & Gunn, P. (2003). Sibling relationships of children with Down syndrome: Perspectives of mothers, fathers, and siblings. *American Journal of Mental Retardation, 108*(4), 234–244.

Dai, L., Bellugi, U., Chen, X. N., Pulst-Korenberg, A. M., Järvinen-Pasley, A., Tirosh-Wagner, T., Eis, P. S., Graham, J., Mills, D., Searcy, Y., & Korenberg, J. R. (2009). Is it Williams syndrome? *GTF21* implicated in sociability and *GTF21RD1* in visual–spatial construction revealed by high resolution arrays. *American Journal of Medical Genetics A, 149*, 302–314.

DeKlyen, M., & Greenberg, M. T. (2008). Attachment and psychopathology in childhood. In J. Cassidy & P. R. Shaver (Eds.), Handbook of attachment: Theory, research, and clinical applications (pp. 637–665). Guilford.

De Schipper, J. C., & Schuengel, C. (2010). Attachment behaviour towards support staff in young people with intellectual disabilities: Associations with challenging behaviour. *Journal of Intellectual Disability Research, 54*(7), 584–596.

Dissanayake, C., Searles, J., Barbaro, J., Sadka, N., & Lawson, L. P. (2019). Cognitive and behavioral differences in toddlers with autism spectrum disorder from multiplex and simplex families. *Autism Research, 12*(4), 682–693.

Dissanayake, C., & Sigman, M. (2000). Attachment and emotional responsiveness in children with autism. International Review of Research in Mental Retardation, *23*, 239–266.

Dodd, P., Guerin, S., McEvoy, J., Buckley, S., Tyrrell, J., & Hillery, J. (2008). A study of complicated grief symptoms in people with intellectual disabilities. *Journal of Intellectual Disability Research, 52*(5), 415–425.

Douglas, P. S. (2019). Pre-emptive intervention for autism spectrum disorder: Theoretical foundations and clinical translation. *Frontiers in Integrative Neuroscience, 13*, Article 66.

Doyle, T. F., Bellugi, U., Korenberg, J. R., & Graham, J. (2004). "Everybody in the world is my friend": Hypersociability in young children with Williams syndrome. *American Journal of Medical Genetics Part A, 124*(3), 263–273.

Dykens, E. M. (2015). Family adjustment and interventions in neurodevelopmental disorders. *Current Opinion in Psychiatry, 28*(2), 121–126.

Ebstein, R. P., Israel, S., Chew, S. H., Zhong, S., & Knafo, A. (2010). Genetics of human social behavior. *Neuron, 65*(6), 831–844.

Emerson, R. W., Adams, C., Nishino, T., Hazlett, H. C., Wolff, J. J., Zwaigenbaum, L., Constantino, J., Shen, M., Swanson, M., Elison, J., Kandala, S., Estes, A., Botteron, K., Collins, L., Dager, S., Evans, A., Gerig, G., Gu, H., McKinstry, R., . . . Piven, J. (2017). Functional neuroimaging of high-risk 6-month-old infants predicts a diagnosis of autism at 24 months of age. *Science Translational Medicine, 9*(393), eaag2882.

Feldman, R. (2007). Parent–infant synchrony and the construction of shared timing; Physiological precursors, developmental outcomes, and risk conditions. *Journal of Child Psychology and Psychiatry, 48*(3–4), 329–354.

Feniger-Schaal, R., & Joels, T. (2018). Attachment quality of children with ID and its link to maternal sensitivity and structuring. *Research in Developmental Disabilities, 76*, 56–64.

Feniger-Schaal, R., & Oppenheim, D. (2013). Resolution of the diagnosis and maternal sensitivity among mothers of children with intellectual disability. *Research in Developmental Disabilities, 34*(1), 306–313.

Feniger-Schaal, R., Oppenheim, D., & Koren-Karie, N. (2019). Parenting children with intellectual disability: Linking maternal insightfulness to sensitivity. *Journal of Intellectual Disability Research, 63*(10), 1285–1289.

Feniger-Schaal, R., Oppenheim, D., Koren-Karie, N., & Yirmiya, N. (2012). Parenting and intellectual disability: An attachment perspective. In J. A. Burack, R. M. Hodapp, G. Iarocci, & E. Zigler (Eds.), *The Oxford handbook of intellectual disability and development* (pp. 334–348). Oxford University Press.

Fletcher, H. K., Flood, A., & Hare, D. J. (2016). *Attachment in intellectual and developmental disability: A clinician's guide to practice and research.* Wiley.

French, L., & Kennedy, E. M. (2018). Annual research review: Early intervention for infants and young children with, or at-risk of, autism spectrum disorder: A systematic review. *Journal of Child Psychology and Psychiatry, 59*(4), 444–456.

Gallichan, D. J., & George, C. (2014). Assessing attachment status in adults with intellectual disabilities: The potential of the Adult Attachment Projective Picture System. *Advances in Mental Health and Intellectual Disabilities, 8*(2), 103–119.

Gallichan, D. J., & George, C. (2018). The Adult Attachment Projective Picture System: A pilot study of inter-rater reliability and face validity with adults with intellectual disabilities. *Advances in Mental Health and Intellectual* Disabilities, *12*(2), 57–66.

Ganiban, J., Barnett, D., & Cicchetti, D. (2000). Negative reactivity and attachment: Down syndrome's contribution to the attachment–temperament debate. *Development and Psychopathology, 12*(1), 1–21.

Gath, A. (1977). The impact of an abnormal child upon the parents. *British Journal of Psychiatry, 130*(4), 405–410.

George, C., & Solomon, J. (1999). Attachment and caregiving: The caregiving behavioral system. In J. Cassidy & P. R. Shaver (Eds.), Handbook of attachment: Theory, research, and clinical applications (pp. 649–670). Guilford.

George, C., & West, M. (2011). The Adult Attachment Projective Picture System: Integrating attachment into clinical assessment. *Journal of Personality Assessment, 93*(5), 407–416.

Gong, P., Fan, H., Liu, J., Yang, X., Zhang, K., & Zhou, X. (2017). Revisiting the impact of OXTR rs53576 on empathy: A population-based study and a meta-analysis. *Psychoneuroendocrinology, 80*, 131–136.

Granqvist, P., Sroufe, L. A., Dozier, M., Hesse, E., Steele, M., van IJzendoorn, M., Solomon, J., Schuengel, C., Fearon, P., Bakermans-Kranenburg, M., Steele, H., Cassidy, J., Carlson, E., Madigan, S., Jacobvitz, D., Foster, S., Behrens, K., Rifkin-Graboi, A., Gribneau, N., . . . Duschinsky, R. (2017). Disorganized attachment in infancy: A review of the phenomenon and its implications for clinicians and policy-makers. *Attachment & Human Development, 19*(6), 534–558.

Grzadzinski, R. L., Luyster, R., Spencer, A. G., & Lord, C. (2014). Attachment in young children with autism spectrum disorders: An examination of separation and reunion behaviors with both mothers and fathers. *Autism, 18*(2), 85–96.

Haas, B. W., Mills, D., Yam, A., Hoeft, F., Bellugi, U., & Reiss, A. (2009). Genetic influences on sociability: Heightened amygdala reactivity and event-related responses to positive social stimuli in Williams syndrome. *Journal of Neuroscience, 29*(4), 1132–1139.

Hannah, M. E., & Midlarsky, E. (1999). Competence and adjustment of siblings of children with mental retardation. *American Journal of Mental Retardation, 104*(1), 22–37.

Happé, F., Frith, U., & Briskman, J. (2001). Exploring the cognitive phenotype of autism: Weak "central coherence" in parents and siblings of children with autism: I. Experimental tests. *Journal of Child Psychology and Psychiatry and Allied Disciplines, 42*(3), 299–307.

Hauser-Cram, P., Howell-Moneta, A., & Young, J. M. (2012). Dyadic interaction between mothers and children with Down syndrome or Williams syndrome: Empirical evidence and emerging agendas. In J. A. Burack, R. M. Hodapp, G. Iarocci, & E. Zigler (Eds.), *The Oxford handbook of intellectual disability and development* (pp. 318–333). Oxford University Press.

Hodapp, R. M. (2002). *Parenting children with mental retardation.* In M. H. Bornstein (Ed.), *Handbook of parenting: Children and parenting* (pp. 355–381). Erlbaum.

Janssen, C. G. C., Schuengel, C., & Stolk, J. (2002). Understanding challenging behaviour in people with severe and profound intellectual disability: A stress-attachment model. *Journal of Intellectual Disability Research, 46*(6), 445–453.

Koren-Karie, N., Oppenheim, D., Dolev, S., Sher, E., & Etzion-Carasso, A. (2002). Mothers' insightfulness regarding their infants' internal experience: Relations with maternal sensitivity and infant attachment. *Developmental Psychology, 38*(4), 534–542.

Koren-Karie, N., Oppenheim, D., Dolev, S., & Yirmiya, N. (2009). Mothers of securely attached children with autism spectrum disorder are more sensitive than mothers of insecurely attached children. *Journal of Child Psychology and Psychiatry, 50*(5), 643–650.

Landa, R. J., Gross, A. L., Stuart, E. A., & Faherty, A. (2013). Developmental trajectories in children with and without autism spectrum disorders: The first 3 years. *Child Development, 84*(2), 429–442.

Landa, R., Piven, J., Wzorek, M. M., Gayle, J. O., Chase, G. A., & Folstein, S. E. (1992). Social language use in parents of autistic individuals. *Psychological Medicine, 22*(1), 245–254.

Larson, F. V., Alim, N., & Tsakanikos, E. (2011). Attachment style and mental health in adults with intellectual disability: Self-reports and reports by carers. *Advances in Mental Health and Intellectual Disabilities, 5*(3), 15–23.

Main, M., Hesse, E., & Kaplan, N. (2005). Predictability of attachment behavior and representational processes at 1, 6, and 19 years of age: The Berkeley Longitudinal Study. In K. E. Grossmann, K. Grossmann, & E. Waters (Eds.), *Attachment from infancy to adulthood: The major longitudinal studies* (pp. 245–304). Guilford.

Marvin, R. S., & Pianta, R. C. (1996). Mothers' reactions to their child's diagnosis: Relations with security of attachment. *Journal of Clinical Child Psychology, 25*(4), 436–445.

McEvoy, J., MacHale, R., & Tierney, E. (2012). Concept of death and perceptions of bereavement in adults with intellectual disabilities. *Journal of Intellectual Disability Research, 56*(2), 191–203.

Moran, G., Pederson, D. R., Pettit, P., & Krupka, A. (1992). Maternal sensitivity and infant–mother attachment in a developmentally delayed sample. *Infant Behavior and Development, 15*(4), 427–442.

Olsavsky, A. K., Telzer, E. H., Shapiro, M., Humphreys, K. L., Flannery, J., Goff, B., & Tottenham, N. (2013). Indiscriminate amygdala response to mothers and strangers after early maternal deprivation. *Biological Psychiatry, 74*(11), 853–860.

Oppenheim, D., Goldsmith, D., & Koren-Karie, N. (2004). Maternal insightfulness and preschoolers' emotion and behavior problems: Reciprocal influences in a therapeutic preschool program. *Infant Mental Health Journal, 25*(4), 352–367.

Oppenheim, D., & Koren-Karie, N. (2002). Mothers' insightfulness regarding their children's internal worlds: The capacity underlying secure child–mother relationships. *Infant Mental Health Journal, 23*(6), 593–605.

Ozonoff, S., Young, G. S., Carter, A., Messinger, D., Yirmiya, N., Zwaigenbaum, L., Bryson, S., Carver, L., Constantino, J., Dobkins, K., Hutman, T., Iverson, J., Landa, R., Rogers, S., Sigman, M., & Stone, W. (2011). Recurrence risk for autism spectrum disorders: A Baby Siblings Research Consortium study. *Pediatrics, 128*(3), e488–e495.

Penketh, V., Hare, D. J., Flood, A., & Walker, S. (2014). Attachment in adults with intellectual disabilities: Preliminary investigation of the psychometric properties of the Manchester Attachment Scale-Third party observational measure. *Journal of Applied Research in Intellectual Disabilities, 27*(5), 458–470.

Rogers, S. J., Ozonoff, S., & Maslin-Cole, C. (1993). Developmental aspects of attachment behavior in young children with pervasive developmental disorders. *Journal of the American Academy of Child & Adolescent Psychiatry, 32*(6), 1274–1282.

Rushton, J. P. (2004). Genetic and environmental contributions to pro-social attitudes: A twin study of social responsibility. *Proceedings of the Royal Society of London Series B: Biological Sciences, 271*(1557), 2583–2585.

Rutgers, A. H., Bakermans-Kranenburg, M. J., van IJzendoorn, M. H., & van Berckelaer-Onnes, I. A. (2004). Autism and attachment: A meta-analytic review. *Journal of Child Psychology and Psychiatry, 45*(6), 1123–1134.

Rutter, M., Kreppner, J., Croft, C., Murin, M., Colvert, E., Beckett, C., Castle, J., & Sonuga-Barke, E. (2007). Early adolescent outcomes of institutionally deprived and non-deprived adoptees: III. Quasi-autism. *Journal of Child Psychology and Psychiatry*, *48*(12), 1200–1207.

Rutter, M., Kreppner, J., & Sonuga-Barke, E. (2009). Emanuel Miller Lecture: Attachment insecurity, disinhibited attachment, and attachment disorders: Where do research findings leave the concepts? *Journal of Child Psychology and Psychiatry*, *50*(5), 529–543.

Schuengel, C., De Schipper, J. C., Sterkenburg, P. S., & Kef, S. (2013). Attachment, intellectual disabilities and mental health: Research, assessment and intervention. *Journal of Applied Research in Intellectual Disabilities*, *26*(1), 34–46.

Schuengel, C., Kef, S., Damen, S., & Worm, M. (2010). "People who need people": Attachment and professional caregiving. *Journal of Intellectual Disability Research*, *54*, 38–47.

Shen, M. D., & Piven, J. (2017). Brain and behavior development in autism from birth through infancy. *Dialogues in Clinical Neuroscience*, *19*(4), 325–333.

Sivaratnam, C. S., Newman, L. K., Tonge, B. J., & Rinehart, N. J. (2015). Attachment and emotion processing in children with autism spectrum disorders: Neurobiological, neuroendocrine, and neurocognitive considerations. *Review Journal of Autism and Developmental Disorders*, *2*(2), 222–242.

Smith, P., & McCarthy, G. (1996). The development of a semi-structured interview to investigate the attachment-related experiences of adults with learning disabilities. *British Journal of Learning Disabilities*, *24*(4), 154–160.

Sroufe, L. A., Egeland, B., Carlson, E. A., & Collins, W. A. (2005). *The development of the person: The Minnesota Study of Risk and Adaptation from Birth to Adulthood*. Guilford.

St. Pourcain, B., Whitehouse, A. O., Ang, W. Q., Warrington, N. M., Glessner, J. T., Wang, K., Timpson, N., Evans, D., Kemp, J., Ring, S., McArdle, W. L., Golding, J., Hakonarson, H., Pennell, C., & Smith, G. (2013). Common variation contributes to the genetic architecture of social communication traits. *Molecular Autism*, *4*(1), Article 34.

Tost, H., Kolachana, B., Hakimi, S., Lemaitre, H., Verchinski, B. A., Mattay, V. S., Weinberger, D. R., & Meyer–Lindenberg, A. (2010). A common allele in the oxytocin receptor gene (OXTR) impacts prosocial temperament and human hypothalamic–limbic structure and function. *Proceedings of the National Academy of Sciences of the USA*, *107*(31), 13936–13941.

Toth, M. (2019). The other side of the coin: Hypersociability. *Genes, Brain and Behavior*, *18*(1), e12512.

Trull, T. J., & Widiger, T. A. (2013). Dimensional models of personality: The five-factor model and the DSM-5. *Dialogues in Clinical Neuroscience*, *15*(2), 135–146.

Vandesande, S., Bosmans, G., & Maes, B. (2019). Can I be your safe haven and secure base? A parental perspective on parent–child attachment in young children with a severe or profound intellectual disability. *Research in Developmental Disabilities*, *93*, 103452.

van IJzendoorn, M. H., Rutgers, A. H., Bakermans-Kranenburg, M. J., Swinkels, S. H., van Daalen, E., Dietz, C., Naber, F., Buitelaar, J., & van Engeland, H. (2007). Parental sensitivity and attachment in children with autism spectrum disorder: Comparison with children with mental retardation, with language delays, and with typical development. *Child Development*, *78*(2), 597–608.

Vaughn, B. E., Goldberg, S., Atkinson, L., Marcovitch, S., MacGregor, D., & Seifer, R. (1994). Quality of toddler–mother attachment in children with Down syndrome: Limits to interpretation of strange situation behavior. *Child Development*, *65*(1), 95–108.

vonHoldt, B. M., Shuldiner, E., Koch, I. J., Kartzinel, R. Y., & Hogan, A. (2017). Structural variants in genes associated with human Williams–Beuren syndrome underlie stereotypical hypersociability in domestic dogs. *Science Advances*, *3*, e1700398.

Vorria, P., Papaligoura, Z., Sarafidou, J., Kopakaki, M., Dunn, J., van IJzendoorn, M. H., & Kontopoulou, A. (2006). The development of adopted children after institutional care: A follow-up study. *Journal of Child Psychology and Psychiatry*, *47*(12), 1246–1253.

Wan, M. W., Green, J., & Scott, J. (2019). A systematic review of parent–infant interaction in infants at risk of autism. *Autism*, *23*(4), 811–820.

Waters, E. (1995). Appendix A: The attachment Q-set (Version 3.0). *Monographs of the Society for Research in Child Development, 60*(2–3), 234–246.

Wichmann, T., Buchheim, A., Menning, H., Schenk, I., George, C., & Pokorny, D. (2016). A reaction time experiment on adult attachment: The development of a measure for neurophysiological settings. *Frontiers in Human Neuroscience, 10*, Article 548.

Willemsen-Swinkels, S. H., Bakermans-Kranenburg, M. J., Buitelaar, J. K., van IJzendoorn, M. H., & Engeland, H. V. (2000). Insecure and disorganised attachment in children with a pervasive developmental disorder: Relationship with social interaction and heart rate. *Journal of Child Psychology and Psychiatry, 41*(6), 759–767.

Yirmiya, C., & Sigman, M. (2001). Attachment autism. In J. Richer & S. Coates (Eds.), *Autism: Putting together the pieces.* Kingsley.

Zeanah, C. H. (1996). Beyond insecurity: A reconceptualization of attachment disorders of infancy. *Journal of Consulting and Clinical Psychology, 64*(1), 42–52.

Zeanah, C. H., Jr., & Boris, N. W. (2000). Disturbances and disorders of attachment in early childhood. In C. H. Zeanah, Jr. (Ed.), Handbook of infant mental health (pp. 353–368). Guilford.

Zigler, E. (1967). Familial mental retardation: A continuing dilemma. *Science, 155*(3760), 292–298.

# 12
# Emergence of the Self

The social self was first proposed by William James (1890) and later emphasized by others (Cooley, 1902; Baldwin, 1895, 1906, 1911; Mead, 1934) to introduce the study of the self to empirical psychology. In psychiatry, the focus on self-development arose independently in the early psychodynamic object relations schools. Object relations theorists, like social psychologists, emphasized that the self emerges from relations with others, particularly from the early mother–infant relationship (Winnicott, 1958). Bowlby (1969, 1973, 1980) expanded the early object relations approaches by developing an ethological model and subsequently incorporated research on internal representation, information processing, and memory formation into his model. Moreover, Bowlby emphasized the need to study healthy as well as disturbed children. He proposed that children construct "internal working models" of self and parent that derive from the infant–parent interaction. An "internal working model" may allow the infant to predict the parent's behavior. Developmental psychologists and cognitive psychologists have extended Bowlby's hypothesis beyond the attachment context of models of parental behavior to consider internal working models of the self. These psychologists suggest that attachment theory can be extended to expand our understanding of the concept of the social self. They emphasize script formation as an important element in the emergence of the social self (Bretherton, 1991).

This chapter reviews the history of the social self in attachment theory, the executive "I" and its internal working models, the development of a sense of self, the development of a theory of mind, the self in developmental disorders, and the neurobiological framework of self as object.

## History

### Social Psychology

In classical psychological studies of the self, the self is considered both as object and as subject. In considering the social nature of the self, the unity of the self as well as the ideal or potential self are considered. The empirical self (as object) includes the body self and its possessions, the social self and its self-recognition, and the ethical self. Because the social self is derived from social experience, there are many social selves. In these analyses, *self-worth* is derived from the difference between the actual self and the potential self toward which one strives. Mead (1934) thought that the integration of the social selves occurs with the construction of a model of the self that considers how it is viewed by others.

From a developmental perspective, Mead (1934) suggests that children learn to take the role of others in pretend play by acting out individual adult attitudes as well as societal attitudes. In this way, the child may incorporate social roles and integrate the multiple selves originating in dyadic relationships with their parents into a unified self. The result is an understanding of self and others in relationship to oneself as the child learns to construct models of both self and parent.

Baldwin (1906) initially proposed that self and other are mutually interdependent. He suggested that developmentally, children know others by their behavior and by their effects on them. The next milestone in the establishment of the self is the realization that others have bodies and experience them just as one experiences one's own body. An awareness of having similar experiences to others may lead to the eventual consolidation of prosocial feelings (i.e., caring for others, fairness, and the emergence of empathy). Children begin to understand others by focusing on their selfhood and, through imitation, may form internal representations of others as well as of themselves. In this way, patterns of behavior come to be understood through interactions with others.

Individual differences in relationships develop out of readjusting old experiential schemata with new ones. As relationships with others are assimilated and new learning from parents is accommodated, an ethical self forms as limits on social freedom are acknowledged. The active intervention of caregivers and other adults is crucial to the development of the ethical self. The ethical self is projected onto others whom the child expects to demonstrate behavior in conformity with their new social understanding. For example, children object to an adult ignoring rules and expect others to conform to the same rules that they have learned. In essence, Baldwin suggested that children acquire a sense of self through construction, impute subjectivity to others, expand their experience through imitation of others, and assimilate new experiences to the objective self (me) or to internal representations (self-schemata) (Bretherton, 1991). Baldwin emphasized social reciprocity and feedback in the development of individual differences as well as in the establishment of the group self. He addressed the representational processes that underlie the sense of self.

## Object Relations Schools

In classical social psychology, the emphasis is on general processes of social development rather than on a specific individual. However, the object relations school of psychoanalysis has placed its emphasis on the healthy versus pathological social development of the individual. Harry S. Sullivan (interpersonal theory) and Donald Winnicott are representative of these views; both emphasize individual differences in the development of the social self.

Sullivan (1953), the primary exponent of the interpersonal school, focused on individual differences in development through his emphasis on anxious caregiving. He suggested that the infant identifies the anxious caregiver as the "bad mother" and the sensitive caregiver as the "good mother," thereby incorporating two separate personifications or schemata of self-experience. These personifications are created in periods of integrated caregiving experience with the "real" mother—not as a living person but, rather, as "an elaborate organization" of the infant's mothering experience. It is the process of being cared for that is integrated. Subsequently, separate generalized good and bad person functions come to be differentiated and may be elaborated into representations of specific persons as good or bad. Later, in the first year, personifications of the self are created as "good me" and "bad me" depending on whether the parenting experiences were anxious ones or not. In addition, Sullivan proposes "not me" experiences, which are so intensely anxious that they are not personified in awareness as "me" at all. In development, personifications of "me" and "mother" become part of the self. Sullivan suggests that the self-system protects itself through "security operations" (defense mechanisms or coping strategies) that repress "bad me" and "not me" experiences, yet defense mechanisms interfere with the integration of ongoing new experiences. Sullivan states that security operations "interfere with observation and analysis" of new experiences. He emphasizes that different forms of interpersonal relatedness are present at different times in the life cycle—with parents, best friends (chums), and marital or intimate partners. However, during these relationships "me–you" patterns emerge that may be maladaptive schemata of the self or other. Moreover, these early dysfunctional relationships may negatively influence later relationships.

Winnicott (1958, 1965), an important representative of the object relations school, emphasized the quality of mother–infant relationships for the establishment of the self. He described an unintegrated infant who, through the psychological "holding environment" provided by the emotionally attuned parent, eventually develops the psychological organization of a person. The parent is critical for this task of "self-integration." Winnicott proposed a biological state in the early weeks after delivery (referred to as "primary maternal preoccupation") when the mother is physiologically sensitive to the infant's cry and biologically prone to be synchronized to the infant's needs. Moreover, by being continually available, she allows a sense of infantile omnipotence (competence) to develop. By also being nonintrusive, yet psychologically attuned to when the infant needs her, she provides the continuity that establishes the basis for the subsequent "capacity for aloneness" in later life. Winnicott considered the capacity for aloneness to be central to the integration of a stable self. This continual attunement by the mother allows the infant the ease and security to become attuned to their own bodily rhythms, processes, and urges.

Once infantile omnipotence or competence (Bretherton, 1991) is fully established, the infant must learn that this sense of omnipotence is not complete. Winnicott (1965) suggests this understanding is realized gradually as the mother's responses decrease, and she reduces her attunement to the child's signals, moods, and needs. Such graduated failures in availability may have adaptive significance and play an essential role in the infant's self-differentiation, but they may also induce experiences of anger toward a mother, who is no longer perfectly responsive. Now the mother's task is to show that she will not retaliate despite the infant's negative feelings of anger. By her consistency, she shows that she is not harmed by the infant's anger and, by being resilient, can survive the infant's destructive negative affect (anger). Although no longer perfectly attuned, a "good enough mother" remains sufficiently responsive to maintain support for a healthy self in the growing child.

## Attachment Theory: The Social Self

In attachment theory, as in the approaches of Sullivan and Winnicott, the infant is thought to be prepared to engage in social interactions from birth. Moreover, in attachment theory, maternal responsiveness is essential for the development of the self, and actual mother–child transactions are reflected in mental representations of the self and mother. In addition, subsequent patterns of relating between them are built on earlier ones. Bowlby (1969), an attachment theorist, places substantial emphasis on the emergence of the healthy self. In doing so, he proposed that the individual constructs "internal working models" to interact with the physical and personal world. These working models aid in perceiving and interpreting events, predicting the future, and devising new plans. An internal working model suggests dynamic mental structures that an individual may use to devise strategies for action. The model or the models are essentially a small-scale construction of external reality that includes the potential for future actions. Although not fully accurate or perhaps not very detailed, the relational structure of working models is consistent with the reality that they represent, for example, spatial, temporal, and causal relations. A working model, in a sense, is a description of the internal world that is created to represent the external world from stores of memories and earlier perceptions. These are representations of the self and others as internalized complexes of experienced relationships. Such formulations are similar to earlier theories. Sullivan (1953) had spoken of "personifications of mother and me" and "me–you patterns." Psychoanalysts such as Sandler and Sandler (1978) write of "interactions between self and object representations that make unconscious dialogs possible." Kernberg (1976) describes self–object affective units that are "positively or negatively toned interaction schemata that become a basis of self and object representations." Conceptually, the working model offers advantages over static terms, such as "internal object" and "object representation."

Bowlby (1969) postulated that internal working models of self and attachment figures grow out of actual patterns of infant–caregiver transactions and emerge around the end of the first year of life when the infant has reached the developmental phase of object permanence and has begun to acquire language. Because of their origins in transactional patterns, these working models are established in close complementarity and, taken together, may represent the relationship. Such models of the self must be understood in the context of the relationships within which they emerged and are developing. A nurturant relationship with parents may construct a working model of the self as competent and loved; if the attachment figures are rejecting, however, a complementary internal working model of the self as untrustworthy may form. When emotional support is insufficient but not rejecting, the child may potentially form working models of the world as dangerous and perceive the self as weak and helpless. In order to adapt to change and guide the interpretation of interpersonal transactions with the caregiver, working models of the self must be continuously deconstructed and reconstructed to accommodate changes that take place over development. With increasing competence and more highly developed thought processes, the child and caregiver respond differently to one another. This leads to greater complexity in content of both the child's and the parent's internal working models. In this process, internal working models of the self as competent and accepted may be maintained as the parent continues to be encouraging and supportive of autonomy, thus retaining the child's affective stability over time.

Although they do change over time, internal working models do not remain in continuous flux (Bretherton, 1991). Ways of acting and thinking that are initially deliberately chosen tend to become less accessible to awareness as automatic processing occurs when they enter long-term memory. Consequently, young people may focus their attention on unfamiliar or new situations. However, stability is achieved in relation to the interpersonal world with the risk of excessive simplification and possible distortions as models are generalized. Adaptations in working models must follow when new experiences do not fit the corresponding internal working models and previous adaptations are not adequate. In such situations, an individual may cling to outdated working models and use processes Bowlby (1980) referred to as "defensive exclusion." This may take place when two incompatible interpersonal choices come into consciousness, and one is chosen while the other is monitored outside awareness. That such processing occurs has been demonstrated in dichotic listening experiments, in which incompatible messages are presented to both ears but the subject normally hears "only one message."

Defensive exclusion is most likely to occur in response to conflicting messages that produce psychic pain—for example, if the parent continually ridicules the child's security seeking but the child reinterprets this rejection as motivated by parental love or in other ways denies negative feelings toward the parent. In these circumstances, the child may defensively exclude from awareness the working model of the "bad" unloving parent but retain in consciousness access to the "good" loving parent. Idealized models of unconditionally loving and of completely rejecting parents generally do not correspond to reality and often become maladaptive. The confusion that may ensue may lead an individual to attempt to operate with two or more conflicting working models of the same attachment figure and two or more conflicting models of the self. Models acquired earlier in life that are out of awareness may conflict with more recent but incompatible, contemporary working models. In later life, through identification with their parents, children may adopt the same patterns of behavior toward their own children that they experienced during their childhood. In this way, patterns of interaction may be transmitted from one generation to the next. Bowlby (1973, p. 323) suggests that social transmission through the medium of family microculture is no less important than inheritance through the medium of genes.

Bretherton (1988, 1991) reports that findings from observational studies of parent–infant or parent–toddler attachments and from attachment-related interviews involving the use of storytelling with preschoolers, kindergarten children, and adults are consistent with Bowlby's (1973) formulations. In observational studies, when children's attachment or autonomy signals are ignored or misread, the development of open communication between parent and child is affected (Ainsworth et al., 1974; Blehar et al., 1977).

Children who are securely attached are able to discuss attachment relationships without insisting that they or their attachment figures are perfect. However, insecure-avoidant children and adults tend to defend themselves against interpersonal closeness by restrictiveness when they discuss attachment relationships. They tend to be aloof and may have a strong tendency to idealize parents or themselves when making global judgments and are unable to find adequate examples of adaptation in their autobio-graphical memory (Main, 1990). Such memories may be absent or contradictory.

Before the infant is born, parents have internal working models of themselves as caregivers and working models of the unborn infant (Zeanah et al., 1985). These antic-ipatory working models may be influenced by the parents' own experiences in child-hood; however, later relationship experiences certainly play a role in establishing these models. When encountering the real infant, anticipatory working models are imposed on the new relationship. To be adaptive, these must fit the temperament and needs of the new infant or child. If the parents' anticipatory working models are coherent, well-organized, and accessible to awareness without much defensive exclusion, the ad-aptation may take place smoothly. However, if parental internal working models are poorly organized and subject to extensive defensive exclusion, the parent may read the infant's cues selectively and may not be able to take the infant's perspective or recog-nize the infant's goals and respond to them empathetically (Ainsworth et al., 1974). When infants' or children's signals are not appropriately recognized, their own devel-oping working models may become distorted and inflexible. Moreover, if the infant is developmentally disabled or handicapped, a discrepancy between the parents' working model of a child and the child's presentation may require that the parents grieve the loss of the expected normal child in order to accept the infant that they have.

## Developments in Attachment Research

Current attachment research focuses on issues of multiple attachments, the outcome of secure and insecure attachment, and the developing complexity of working models with age. The infant and child have multiple attachments and multiple social selves. Different attachment relationships call for different responses so that the quality of an infant's re-lationship to the mother or to the father may vary. Main and Weston (1981) evaluated infants with their father and with their mother at 12 and 18 months. Concordant se-cure and insecure patterns of attachment with both parents were not demonstrated. Main et al. (1985) investigated the child's representation of attachment at age 6 years in response to a family picture and to a projective test about separation. These authors found that responses were highly predictable from the early pattern of attachment with the mother but not with the father, suggesting that the principal attachment figure may be more influential than another in the construction of a working model of the self. In the Main and Weston (1981) study, it is suggested that models of the self in some circumstances may be averaged so that when the relationship to both parents is inse-cure, later outcome may be less favorable. Models of the self might be intermediate if the relationship to one parent is insecure and the relationship to the other is secure.

Other areas of ongoing research deal with the later outcome of insecure and secure attachment. Developmental progression in the differentiation and integration of the self in secure individuals has been studied extensively in specific age groups (Bretherton, 1987) and cross-culturally (K. E. Grossmann & Grossmann, 1990). Children with the secure pattern tend to develop competence in their explorations of the world. Children with insecure attachment may lack confidence that support will be available and may not seek out a caregiver when stressed (insecure-avoidant pattern) or may be uncertain of the caregiver's availability and show separation anxiety symptoms (insecure-ambivalent pattern). A fourth group has been described by Main and colleagues (Main & Hesse, 1990; Main & Solomon, 1986) as the "insecure-disorganized" attachment pattern. These are children who are fearful of their caregiver. They are unable to use their caregiver as a secure base and are inhibited in their exploration of the world.

To investigate long-term psychological functioning, Jacobsen et al.(1993) have extended attachment studies beyond infancy and early childhood, focusing on the relationship between children's attachment representations and their cognitive functioning in middle childhood and adolescence. At age 7 years, 85 children were classified as securely or insecurely attached based on their discussion of a story that involved parental separation. The authors found three of the attachment groups: secure, insecure-avoidant, and insecure-disorganized. After controlling for the child's IQ and for attentional problems, these three groups were compared at ages 7, 9, 12, 15, and 17 years using Piagetian tasks that assessed concrete and formal reasoning. Children with an insecure-disorganized representation showed the lowest scores on the deductive reasoning tasks at each of the age periods. This finding indicates that children with an insecure-disorganized attachment may be specifically disadvantaged in their subsequent cognitive functioning. Their negative self-concept and fears of their caregivers, along with possible doubts about their own abilities, may interfere with their deductive reasoning. The children with a secure attachment scored significantly better on the cognitive functioning tasks. These findings support a possible link between internal representations of attachment and long-term psychologic functioning, suggesting that attachment security may facilitate children's cognitive functioning. Alternatively, impaired deductive reasoning may predispose for insecure-disorganized attachment.

Another area that is being investigated relates to the construction of a potential or ideal self in adulthood. Main et al. (1985) studied secure-autonomous adults who had insecure childhoods. They found that the parents' attitude toward attachment, in general, most strongly predicted child security and not necessarily the security or insecurity of the parents' own early relationships. Others (K. Grossmann et al., 1988) suggest that children are more secure if parents consciously express the desire that their own parents had been more supportive of them. Finally, it is clinically useful to discuss representations of the self and other as "inner persons" who may engage in imaginary interactions. Research in this area may benefit from recent studies of mental representation, which emphasize the capacity for inter-subjectivity.

## Cognitive, Structural, and Motivational Approaches to the Self

Object relations and attachment theories provide approaches to the social self. In summary, object relations theorists locate the self in social interactions and specify internalization of self-relevant information as a central developmental process. This involves the incorporation of affective, behavioral, and cognitive information that is communicated by significant adults in the mechanisms of changes in the self over time. Attachment theorists link the emergence and the quality of working models of the self to early and current experiences with caretakers. In these formulations, the responsivity and sensitivity of caregivers are the primary social interactive processes, leading to the individual's sense of self in relationship to others.

A second group of theorists approach the self through cognitive understanding. Cognitive approaches for understanding the self emphasize knowledge, beliefs, theories, and schema to describe what is known about oneself. As the self develops, it acquires and organizes this knowledge. This leads to structural approaches to the self that stress the ways such self-knowledge is organized, as in Piaget's description of the developmental progression of children's moral understanding. Others study organizational changes in the content of children's and adolescents' responses to the question, "Who am I?" and evaluate shifts in the thematic content of their answers. Structural theorists emphasize age-related changes in thematic content and complexity of self-knowledge. Those who study information processing use computer metaphors to describe how information about the self is processed.

A third group of self-theorists emphasize motivationally based conceptions of the self (Connell & Wellborn, 1991). Motivational approaches emphasize how self-related cognition and affect develop. In some instances, self-worth or self-esteem is taken as an organizational construct (Sroufe & Waters, 1977). Self-worth is hypothesized to relate to perceived confidence and to attributions of success and failure. On the other hand, psychodynamic theorists emphasize fundamental biological drives and identification processes in establishing self-esteem. Here, a sense of self emerges from a dynamic relationship between the constraints of the external world and instinctual drives. Others, such as Erikson (1950), emphasize identity formation through the mastery of a series of psychosocial crises. McClelland (1985) points to power, achievement, and affiliation as distinct entities that are relevant to the development of the self. For motivational theorists, emotional processes and psychological needs are central in shaping the self. Thus, self-actualization (Maslow, 1970), self-determination (Deci, 1980), and competence (White, 1959) are essential.

Connell and Wellborn (1991) integrate the various models of the self by proposing a model with the following characteristics: (a) There are fundamental psychological needs for competence, autonomy, and relatedness; (b) the self-system processes emerge from the interaction of psychological needs in social contexts; (c) aspects of social context most relevant to meeting psychological needs are the provision of structure, autonomy, support, and involvement; and (d) the inter- and intra-individual variations in the self-system processes lead to various patterns of action. In their model, the developing person is an active partner in the construction of the self-system from early life, and the self-system itself is viewed as a set of appraisal processes in which the individual evaluates their status in a particular context with respect to the psychological needs mentioned (i.e., competence, autonomy, and relatedness). Their model provides a motivational perspective of the developing person. The need for competence involves the production of desired outcomes; the need for autonomy leads to the experience of choice in initiating, maintaining, and regulating activity along with the experience of there being a connection between one's actions and personal goals. Relatedness refers to the need to feel securely connected to the social environment and to experience oneself as worthy of respect and love. Competence requires having the capacity to act effectively. Autonomy involves self-regulation and acknowledgment of what is important to the self.

## The Executive "I" and Internal Working Models

When considering the self, a distinction is drawn between the self as an agent, "knower," or the "I" from the self as the object of knowledge or the "me." William James (1890) first presented this analysis of the self, which has continued to be instrumental in defining the self since his original proposal. The self has been viewed by some as having a central role in personality development but by others as a source of confusion and complication. The disagreement largely is the result of failing to distinguish between the self as object and the self as agent. There has been little disagreement about the value of studying the self as object because people have views about themselves that influence their feelings and behavior. With regard to the self as object, it is possible to conduct research using self-report procedures to measure people's views about themselves, which are treated as objective data. However, the self as agent cannot be measured; it is a theoretical construct.

Epstein (1991) suggested that there are two conceptual systems that contain selves as objects—a rational system and an experiential one. In the rational system, the views people hold about themselves can be readily reported. The experiential self consists of cognitions that come from emotionally significant experiences, of which the person may or may not be currently aware. An individual may, on verbal self-report, identify themselves as self-accepting and confident yet show through their nonverbal behavior evidence of low self-esteem through avoidance of eye contact, defensive aggression, and excessive bravado. On the other hand, the self as agent may be defined as an individual's self-theory, which contains descriptive beliefs and motivational beliefs or beliefs about the outcome of self-initiated action.

This chapter emphasizes the interdependence between the "I" as "knower" and the "me" as representation or working model of the self. The dual nature of the self is not emphasized by Sullivan, Winnicott, or Bowlby, yet Epstein's rational and experiential selves must both be considered in assessment of both the child and the adult.

The relationship between the "I," as the executive operating system, and the "me," as the internal working model of the self or self-representation, deserves consideration. Johnson-Laird (1983) suggested that consciousness is our experience of our individual executive system. Using a computer model, he suggests that the executive or operating system is capable of monitoring and processing input from many lower level processes in sequence. Rather than operating serially, the lower level processes are thought to operate in parallel, and the operating system has access to the output of these parallel systems but not to their internal working. The operating system gives higher level commands to the lower level processing systems, which produce specific actions.

Bretherton (1991) suggested that the executive system is more than a "knower" because it is a meta-system that sets priorities among inputs from various lower level processes, which can send conflicting commands. In Johnson-Laird's (1983) model, the lower level processes maintain some autonomy, so there is "relative will power" based on the degree to which the operating system or the "I" can carry out its decisions. Executive plans may be disrupted by motivational systems that regulate survival behavior, including escape, attachment, and aggression. These are emergency signals that generally represent emotional responses of the body and the mind. Such cognitive–affective links are essential to adaptive functions. Maladaptive behavior may occur when the executive system is overwhelmed by the lower level systems or when it overcontrols them, such as when survival signals are received. In each of these instances, incoming information is not appropriately processed.

In this model, the executive system would consult internal working models of the world and particularly those of the self-system. If the working models are not adequate for adaptation or dissociated from one another, the executive system, or "I," cannot properly forecast and make interpretations to guide effective action. This model suggests that the correlation and interrelationship between the "I" and the "me" require investigation into both secure and insecure relationships. One might consider that if attachment relationships are secure, the "I" and "me" will function well in relation to one another, but if attachment is insecure, then the integration of "I" and "me" may be disturbed.

The "I"–"me" relationship must also be considered in terms of social transmission of working models from the parent to the infant. The infant's executive operating system, or "I," is not developed and not well-coordinated, so internal working models may exist only at a sensorimotor level. As a result, the infant must rely on the adult to regulate external events to develop. Those who function as auxiliary "I"'s to whom an infant is attached require integrated "I"–"me" systems to facilitate the infant's internal organization of "I" and "me." This formulation suggests that better understanding of the relationship of "I" and "me" throughout development is essential for understanding the establishment of the social self.

## The Development of a Sense of Self

The self and its counterpart, the sense of other, are universal phenomena that crucially influence all social experiences. Self-awareness is fundamentally used in psychology from a developmental perspective. From birth, infants have a complex sense of their bodies as different from others (Rochat, 2003). During development, several senses of self-emerge. Stern (1985) described these as the sense of self that is a single, distinct integrated body—that is, an agent of actions, an experiencer of feelings, an establisher of intentions, a developer of plans, a transposer of experience into language, and a communicator who shares personal knowledge with another. Stern emphasized that some senses of the self-exist prior to self-awareness and language. Among these are the senses of agency, physical cohesion, continuity in time, and possibly having intentions in mind. Through self-reflection and with the development of language, these preverbal existential senses of the self begin to reveal their own ongoing existence and are transformed into new experiences. If the sense of self begins before verbalization, then rather than searching for a time the sense of self begins, it is more productive to describe developmental continuities and changes. With regard to a preverbal self, Stern refers to "non-self-reflexive awareness" that arises on the occasion of an infant's actions or mental processes. It may begin as the organizing subjective experience that will later be verbally referenced as the self. With the emergence of self, there is a sense of continuity, affective contact, intersubjectivity, creating organization out of disorganization, and transmitting meaning from one individual to another.

According to Stern (1985), infants experience a sense of the emerging self from birth as they become aware of biologically based self-organizing processes. Consequently, the infant is selectively responsive to social events in the external environment. From 2 to 6 months, infants are thought to consolidate a sense of a core self as a separate, cohesive physical unit, with the beginnings of agency, affectivity, and continuity in time. During these early periods, there is no autistic-like phase of development, nor is there a symbiotic-like phase. The infant is actively involved in organizing and making sense of the environment and contacts with others.

From approximately 7 to 15 months, the sense of a subjective self is formed. Now the infant is devoted to seeking and creating intersubjective union with another. This process involves an awareness that one's subjective life, consisting of the mind's contents and the qualities of one's feelings, may be shared. This subjective self is emerging concurrently with the time when attachment and separation are beginning to take place. The subjective self is followed by the establishment of the verbal self, which forms after 18 months. The verbal self does not replace the emerging self, core self, or subjective self; rather, these senses of self remain fully functional throughout life and continue to grow.

Stern (1985) suggested that affective experiences enter the intersubjective domain through a phenomenon called "affective attunement." The sharing of affective states is the most essential aspect of intersubjective relatedness. In affective attunement, contact is established between parent and infant not by imitation but, rather, through a kind of cross-modal matching. The modality of expression used by the parent to match the infant's behavior differs from that used by the infant. For example, the duration and intensity of an infant's vocalization may be matched by the mother's body movements, or the infant's movements may be mirrored by the mother's voice. For example, a boy bangs his hand on a soft toy and sets up a steady rhythm; his mother begins to vocalize with the rise and fall of his hand in attunement. In affective attunement, what is matched is not another's behavior specifically but, rather, an aspect of the behavior that reflects the other person's feeling state, so what is matched is the feeling state rather than external behavior. As a result, there are matching expressions of an inner state. These expressions may differ in their form, but in some sense, they exist as manifestations of a single and recognizable internal state. Such contact uses metaphor as behaviors are jointly expressed by parent and infant. The quality of feeling of a shared affective state is thus demonstrated through affective attunement (Stern, 1985). Infants begin to behave differently to familiar and strange adults by approximately age 7–9 months. Wariness of an unfamiliar peer compared to a familiar one typically develops between 10 and 12 months of age (Cowie et al., 2015). Developmental landmarks are attributed to specific ages. At age 6–9 months, infants discriminate between the approach of a child and that of an adult. Height, movement, voice, and appearance are cues.

It is during the second year of life that the infant's language begins to emerge and the process of senses of self and others takes on new meaning. With language, there is different and distinct personal word knowledge because language allows the creation of shared meanings. As language continues to emerge, the child begins to construct a narrative of their own life. At approximately age 15–18 months, children begin to represent things in their minds in such a way that symbolic representation occurs. Symbolic play and language allow a child to refer to themselves as an external or objective entity. Now communication may take place about things and persons who are not present. Verbal levels such as "baby," "mommy," and "daddy" are expressed at age 18–24 months.

The infant develops the capacity to perform delayed imitations in that the representation of an original act is remembered as performed by someone else and the infant executes their own imitation of what was observed. In a sense, two versions are adjusted—that observed and that accomplished. A psychological relationship develops to motivate delayed imitation. Representation of the self as an objective entity occurs and may be observed from the outside as well as felt subjectively from the inside. After age 18 months, infants develop an objective sense of self, which is evidenced by their behavior before a mirror, their use of names and pronouns for self-designation, acts of empathy, and the development of a core gender identity (Stern, 1985). For example, after age 18 months, an infant with a colored rouge marker on his nose will point to himself rather than to his reflection, as is the case for younger infants. The infant touches his own face when he looks in the mirror rather than pointing to the reflection he sees in the mirror (Fernyhough, 2010). Stern referred to this as the "objective self," whereas Lewis and Brooks-Gunn (1979) use the term "categorical self." At approximately the same time, the pronouns "I," "me," and "mine" are used to refer to the self. They use words such as "want," "see," and "look" to refer to internal states of perception or emotions. Empathetic acts may also be evidence of the emergence of self. To act empathetically, it is necessary to imagine the self as an object that may be experienced by another in the objectified other's subjective state.

With the establishment of a verbal self, language finally brings about the ability to narrate one's own life story. Narrative involves a different mode of thought from problem-solving. To narrate, one must consider persons who act as agents with intentions and goals that are presented in a sequence, giving the narrative a beginning, a middle, and an end. Narratives are constructed or co-constructed with parents and begin to form an autobiographical history. In the development of a verbal self, the categorical or objective self labels and identifies, and the narrated self creates a story from elements that describe the self in action, such as agency, intentions, and goals.

## The Development of a Theory of Mind

Human infants are prepared from birth to engage in social interactions with a caregiver. Infants understand self and other in the development of a theory of mind as they begin to anticipate others' intentions. Bretherton (1991) described the following phases: (a) interfacing of minds (preverbal stage, 9–14 months), (b) interfacing minds through language (the early verbal phase), (c) interfacing minds through language (transition to early childhood), and (d) understanding mind (the preschool years and beyond).

Studies of infant memory have documented that cued recall of motor activity is possible as early as age 3 months (Rovee-Collier & Fagan, 1981). Based on a better understanding of infant memory, Stern (1985) hypothesized that infants may register their daily interactional sequences with a parent as generalized episodes that store "small, coherent chunks of lived experience, including not only actions but also sensations, goals and effects of self and other in a temporal–physical–causal relationship." He referred to these generalized structures in memory as representations of interactions that have been generalized as the sensorimotor interaction schema. Stern suggested that such schemata are accessed in memory when a familiar self–other episode occurs. Developmentally, the idea of sensorimotor interaction schema is supported through research studies that show older infants can anticipate another person's behavior in context. For example, Izard (1978) found that 8-month-old infants showed fear when their arm was being prepared for an injection and subsequently refused to interact with the nurse who gave the injection. Moreover, infants at this age show an anticipatory smile during peek-a-boo games before a parent or playmate reappears from behind a cloth as they appear and disappear. There is an early landmark of person permanence indicating an internal representation with continuity in space and time (Cowie et al., 2015).

## Interfacing of Minds (Age 9–14 Months)

Closely related to person permanence is the establishment of object permanence, there is a transition from reliance on sensorimotor interactional schemata to working models, or representational schemata. Between ages 6 and 9 months, infants respond to an adult's negative facial–vocal displays with crying or frowning, but after 9 months they seem to understand that the adult partner's emotional expression may provide information about external events. At approximately age 9 months, infants come to understand that intentions and affective states may be shared. At 9 months, infants may reliably follow their mother's line of visual regard. Before 9 months, this "shared reference" is only intermittently seen. The ability to understand communication about a joint topic is then evident. At this age, infants' affective, vocal, and gestural communications attract and direct others' attention to topics of mutual interest. Concurrently, infants begin to understand others' communications to them as messages. This advance suggests that by the end of the first year of life, infants have acquired an early "theory of mind" or ability to impute mental states to the self and others. One mind now can be interfaced with another through conventional comprehensible signals. Maternal affect attunement may be the caregiver's response to these changes in the infant's psychological understanding. Stern (1985) suggested that these cross-modal experiences of attunement focus the infant's attention on psychological, rather than behavioral, sharing of experience. Individual differences in affect attunement may be important factors in the development of individual differences in a working model of the self. A mother may under-attune or over-attune to certain infant behaviors. This poorly coordinated responding may undermine an infant's ability to attend to their own inner states. Findings on parent–infant communication and secure and insecure attachment relationships corroborate Stern's suggestion that exaggerated attunement may be detrimental. Overstimulating mothers may be engaged in over-attunement, and mothers of insecure-avoidant infants may be non-attuned to distress signals (Escher-Graeub & Grossmann, 1983).

## Interfacing Minds Through Language (Early Verbal)

Attention-seeking and other communicative symbols deriving from the preverbal stage help establish initial infant–parent contact. However, the emergence of single words into gestural messages leads to a more precise interface between parent and child. Once the child has gained object names and relational words, the capacity for intentional intersubjectivity becomes more apparent. A 2-year-old uses two types of words differentially such that if parent and child had established a focus of joint attention, the child comments on the action component with a relational word (Greenfield & Smith, 1976). If a joint topic of attention has not been established, the object is labeled first. By the middle of the second year, simple conversations about absent objects and people are possible. Moreover, by age 18 months, some toddlers are able to label internal states if given an appropriate context. Their first references are to hunger, pain, disgust, and moral approval (Bretherton et al., 1981). This labeling ability, along with the use of perspective-shifting pronouns ("you" and "I"), develops rapidly during the third year of life. Empathy toward distressed others, the use of dolls as active partners in symbolic play, and self-recognition in the mirror also are occurring at this time. The shift that occurs may represent a gradual transition from an implicit to an explicit theory of mind. The establishment of language may also result in some contradiction for children because verbal explanations to them may be simplified too much and may be at variance with the child's own interpretation. At the beginning of language, verbal working models, which are available to conscious reflection, and nonverbal working models may be in conflict.

## Interfacing Minds Through Language
### (Transition to Early Childhood)

During the second year of life, children begin to entertain a more explicit theory of mind. This conclusion was based originally on data recorded from mothers who listed their children's utterances about internal states in everyday context (Bretherton & Beeghly, 1982). By age 28 months, a majority of 30 infants in the study had a vocabulary that allowed the discussion of internal states and were able to talk about perceptions, sensations, and volition. Approximately two-thirds of the sample identified some emotions. The use of terms for moral judgment and utterances about cognitive processes become more common after age 30 months (Shatz et al., 1983). Children in the middle of the second year of life sometimes made causal statements about internal states—for example, "Grandma mad; I wrote on wall." Causal statements reported by Bretherton and Beeghly (1982) included utterances about events or actions that precede a particular emotional state, utterances about negative states that act as motivators or causes for later behavior, and utterances that explain an emotion in terms of another related mental state. Moreover, 2- and 3-year-olds may be able to impute emotions and intentions to themselves, dolls, and playmates during make-believe play (Bretherton et al., 1986).

Wellman (1988) suggested that the term "theory of mind" is appropriate to describe 2½-year-old toddlers' talk about internal states. He suggested several criteria must be met to demonstrate an explicit theory of mind: (a) basic categories for defining reality exist, (b) these basic categories are organized into a coherent system of interrelationships, and (c) a causal attributional framework of human behavior has been acquired by the individual. Some children at age 28 months are able to distinguish real from non-real (e.g., "It's not real; it's only pretend") and to define one mental state in terms of another, appearing unhappy and being sad and talking about the consequences of emotional states such as happiness and anger. Therefore, children at this age quite frequently do distinguish between reality and internal states, in keeping with the theory of mind model.

## Understanding Mind: Preschool Years and Beyond

Children can be more formally interviewed regarding mind by age 3 years. Three-year-olds could distinguish between concrete objects and imagined objects. When asked about absent objects in contrast to "pictures in your head" (Estes et al., 1989), 3-, 4-, and 5-year-old children gave different reasons for not being able to touch a real but absent object (i.e., because "it's not there") or an imagined object (because "it's not real"). Therefore, young children have categories for distinguishing mental and non-mental phenomena. Three-year-olds do define mental states in terms of other mental states— for example, "People can't see my imagination." Moreover, they use a causal explanatory framework and give causes for several positive and negative emotions. Consequently, 3-year-olds do demonstrate a theory of mind (other's emotions, desires, and beliefs). In addition, they tend to think of intentions as causes of behavior. As they grow older, children have different conceptions of mind such that younger children think of mind as a container that holds information. By age 4 years, reasoning about cognitions and feelings is more in keeping with an implicit theory of mind as a processor that interprets information. Differences between 3-year-olds' and 4- and 5-year-olds' conceptions of mind are evident in their responses to false belief tasks. For example, in the theory of mind tasks, 4-year-olds who have looked inside a matchbox filled with candy can correctly predict that another child, who does not know the secret of the candy being there, would wrongly guess that it contained matches. Three-year-olds, in contrast, are incapable of imputing false beliefs. The 3-year-old says the other child will guess correctly. Moreover, 4- and 5-year-olds can impute knowledge to others that they do not possess.

Older preschool children can grasp that their truth is not necessarily another's truth. Four- and 5-year-olds also can understand that two children who receive the same gift may feel differently about it (Gove & Keating, 1979). However, although young infants have mental models, they cannot manipulate them out of context. When preschoolers can rearrange the components of mental models and create alternative realities in "pretend" or anticipate the future, they have reached the level of representation. By age 4 years, an additional capacity, meta-representation, may emerge. Older preschool children do not just manipulate alternative models of events; they can also construct mental models of belief states about events. This is meta-representation because they manipulate mental models of mental models.

After approximately age 7 years, the capacity for meta-representation becomes further developed. Now children think not only about what others believe or think but also about what others think about them (Cowie et al., 2015). To do this requires an ability to manipulate a mental model of two individuals' belief states as they relate to each other. The capacity for meta-representation may be necessary for a child to understand another's deceptive intentions in games that involve hiding and guessing, their ability

to understand second-order false beliefs (Perner & Wimmer, 1985), and their awareness that others as well as the self can be deliberately fooled about what is felt about the
self. At age 7 years, children can feel a different emotion (meta-representations) and
can reflect on that understanding. The meta-representational ability becomes further
enhanced in dealing with abstractions during adolescence.

## The Self in Developmental Disorders

The establishment of the self is influenced by general cognitive limitations and
disordered development in specific domains, such as the phonologic, visuospatial, and
sociocognitive ones. Both executive and non-executive functions may be disturbed
in the developmental disorders. Attachment and stranger anxiety may be delayed in
intellectual developmental disorders, language disorders can adversely influence the
development of working models, visuospatial disturbance can influence the establishment of the body self, and theory of mind disturbances can be apparent in autistic disorder. Parental discrepant working models of the expected normal child may reduce the
parents' capacity to become attuned and limit the emergence of an adaptive self-system.

Cicchetti et al. (1990) noted the dearth of experimental studies on the development of
the self during the transition from infancy to early childhood in children with developmental disorders and in children who have been abused. They studied the development
and coherence of the self-system in children with Down syndrome and in maltreated
children. In the first instance, biological factors assume primary importance; in the
second, environmental factors (parent–child interactions) are primary. These authors
found that during play, children with Down syndrome showed similar, but delayed,
sequences in their conceptions of self and other compared to nonhandicapped children.
Children with Down syndrome, who utilized play to represent self and other in hypothetical situations, were the most cognitively mature. Nonlinguistic representations
of the self were more advanced than linguistic representations. In contrast, maltreated
children showed poor-quality internal working models about themselves and in their
relationship to attachment figures. Deviations in self system processes were found in
visual self-recognition, linguistic representations of the self and others, and perceived
self-competence. Studies such as this highlight the importance of investigating children
with developmental disorders to understand the emergence of the self system and to
provide guidelines for treatment.

## Neurobiological Framework of Self as Object

Self-representation is essential to mental functions. Traditionally, greater emphasis has
been placed on the self as subject; however, the self is considered both as subject and as
object, including the body self. William James (1890) referred to "me" and "I." The "me"
is the self as object, and "I" is the self as agent. The "me" is made up of a physical, social,
and spiritual self. The self as object can be studied from the perspective of psychology,
embodied cognition, and social neuroscience. Using these perspectives, a neural framework of the self is proposed (Sui & Gu, 2017). A neural framework of the self is drawn

from interaction between a brain core self-network centered in the medial prefrontal cortex; a cognitive control network involving the dorsolateral prefrontal cortex and posterior superior temporal sulcus; and a salience network that involves the insula, striation, and amygdala. Imaging studies show activation of the medial prefrontal cortex for objects that are "mine" (Kim & Johnson, 2014). Self-processing involves the integration of perceptual, cognitive, and affective processes (Northoff, 2011), referred to as the integration of self (Sui & Humphreys, 2015). A key feature of the medial prefrontal cortex is to reflect representations of ourselves with the posterior superior sulcus linked to self–other processing and sensory integration.

Bodily signals have been thoroughly examined in selfhood. Proprioceptive and physiological signals (e.g., heart rate) are essential to conscious awareness of feelings and self "as object" (Gu et al., 2013; Niedenthal, 2007). Importantly, interoception—awareness of physiological responses in the body—correlates with emotion awareness (Critchley et al., 2004; Zaki, 2012). Interoception involves an extensive group of brain regions, including the thalamus, brain stem, hypothalamus, amygdala, insula, and somatomotor areas (Critchley et al., 2004). Our awareness of emotions and feelings is derived through interoceptive inferences about internal body states (Sui & Gu, 2017). Interoceptive inference of self-process is demonstrated in autism spectrum disorder (ASD; Gu et al., 2015). Studies of interoception are consistent with the proposal of an "embodied self," similar to William James' (1884) proposal of a "material me" and embodied cognition proposal (Seth, 2013).

Theory of mind, the ability to infer others' feelings and beliefs, has been investigated with regard to the self, the neurobiological basis of self-awareness, and theory of mind, as well as awareness of others. Self-awareness can be measured by recognition of one's own face compared to faces of others. For theory of mind, false belief tasks are used to identify neural correlates. A meta-analysis of functional magnetic resonance imaging studies of self-face recognition and false belief tests revealed that for distinct face recognition, the brain regions activated are right superior temporal gyrus, right inferior frontal gyrus/anterior cingulate, and inferior parietal lobe. The brain areas involved in false belief are the medial prefrontal cortex, bilateral temporoparietal junction, precuneus, and bilateral middle temporal gyrus. There are overlaps of superior temporal gyrus and ventral areas of the medial prefrontal cortex. van Veluw et al. (2014) confirmed that self-recognition and awareness of others engaged separate, distinct neural pathways, with some overlap of higher order prefrontal cortex when these processes combined. These findings comport with the results of studies in ASD. Compared to typically developing children, those diagnosed with ASD exhibit reduced activation of the medial prefrontal cortex during theory of mind processing, consistent with children with ASD having a core deficit in knowing about others' mental state. Thus, the medial prefrontal cortex is involved in reasoning about others' minds with ongoing evaluation of others' intentions (O'Nions et al, 2014).

Neural activation of the insula is linked to the feeling of disgust with one's self and observing disgust in others (Wicker et al., 2003). The insula–anterior cingulate cortex network is activated in perceiving one's own pain and in perceiving others' pain (Lamm et al., 2011). The amygdala also responds to self and other's emotions (Lamm et al., 2011). Thus, the self and other are linked in both cognitive and affective domains. A neural framework of the self as object views the self as emergent through interactions of brain networks. These interactions link the core self, cognitive control, and salience processing. They characterize how cognitive representation and emotional responsiveness relate to the self. In this framework, there is a gradient in self-related processing: The dorsal medial prefrontal cortex is more engaged with other related judgments, and the ventromedial prefrontal cortex is involved in internal self-processing linking it to social attention and cognitive control. The neural framework of the self is pertinent to developmental neuropsychiatric disorders in regard to self-processing (Sui & Gu, 2017).

# References

Ainsworth, M. D. S., Bell, S. M., & Stayton, D. F. (1974). Infant–mother attachment and social development. In M. P. Richards (Ed.), *The introduction of the child into a social world* (pp. 99–135). Cambridge University Press.

Baldwin, J. M. (1895). *Mental development of the child and the race: Methods and processes.* Macmillan.

Baldwin, J. M. (1906). *Social and ethical interpretations in mental development* (4th ed.). Macmillan.

Baldwin, J. M. (1911). *The individual and society: Or, psychology and sociology.* Badger.

Blehar, M. C., Lieberman, A. F., & Ainsworth, M. D. S. (1977). Early face-to-face interaction and its relation to later infant–mother attachment. *Child Development, 48,* 182–194.

Bowlby, J. (1969). *Attachment and loss: Vol. 1. Attachment.* Basic Books.

Bowlby, J. (1973). *Attachment and loss: Vol. 2. Separation.* Basic Books.

Bowlby, J. (1980). *Attachment and loss: Vol. 3. Loss, sadness and depression.* Basic Books.

Bretherton, I. (1987). New perspectives on attachment relations: Security, communication, and internal working models. In J. Osofsky (Ed.), *Handbook of infant development* (pp. 1061–1110). Wiley.

Bretherton, I. (1988). Open communication and internal working models: Their role in the development of attachment relationships. *Nebraska Symposium on Motivation, 36,* 57–113.

Bretherton, I. (1991). Pouring new wine into old bottles: The social self as internal working model. In M. R. Gunnar & L. A. Sroufe (Eds.), *Self processes and development* (pp. 1–41). Erlbaum.

Bretherton, I., & Beeghly, M. (1982). Talking about internal states: The acquisition of an explicit theory of mind. *Developmental Psychology, 18*(6), 906–921.

Bretherton, I., Fritz, J., Zahn-Waxler, C., & Ridgeway, D. (1986). Learning to talk about emotions: A functionalist perspective. *Child Development, 57,* 529–548.

Bretherton, I., McNew, S., & Beeghly-Smith, M. (1981). Early person knowledge as expressed in verbal and gestural communication: When do infants acquire a "theory of mind"? In M. E. Lamb & L. R. Sherrod (Eds.), *Infant social cognition* (pp. 333–373). Erlbaum.

Cicchetti, D., Beeghly, M., Carlson, V., & Toth, S. (1990). The emergence of the self in atypical populations. In D. Cicchetti & M. Beeghly (Eds.), *The self in transition* (pp. 309–344). University of Chicago Press.

Connell, J. P., & Wellborn, J. G. (1991). Competence, autonomy, and relatedness: A motivational analysis of self-esteem processes. In M. R. Gunnar & L. A. Sroufe (Eds.), *Self processes and development* (pp. 43–77). Erlbaum.

Cooley, C. H. (1902). *Human nature and the social order.* Scribner's.

Cowie, H. A., Smith, P. K., & Blades, M. (2015). *Understanding children's development (6th ed.).* Wiley.

Critchley, H. D., Wiens, S., Rotshtein, P., Öhman, A., & Dolan, R. J. (2004). Neural systems supporting interoceptive awareness. *Nature Neuroscience, 7*(2), 189–195.

Deci, E. L. (1980). *The psychology of self-determination.* Heath.

Epstein, S. (1991). Cognitive–experiential self theory: Implications for developmental psychology. In M. R. Gunnar & L. A. Sroufe (Eds.), *Self processes and development* (pp. 79–123). Erlbaum.

Erikson, E. (1950). *Childhood and society*. Norton.

Escher-Graeub, D., & Grossmann, K. E. (1983). Bindungssicherheit im zweiten Lebensjahr-die Regensburger Querschnittuntersuchung [Attachment security in the second year of life: The Regensburg cross-sectional study] [Research report]. University of Regensburg.

Estes, D., Wellman, H. M., & Wooley, J. D. (1989). Children's understanding of mental phenomena. *Advances in Child Development and Behavior, 22*, 41–87.

Fernyhough, C. (2010). *The baby in the mirror: A child's world from birth to three*. Granta Books.

Gove, F. L., & Keating, D. (1979). Empathic role-taking precursors. *Developmental Psychology, 1515*(6), 594–600.

Greenfield, P. M., & Smith, J. H. (1976). *The structure of communication in early development*. Academic Press.

Grossmann, K., Fremmer-Bombik, E., Rudolph, J., & Grossmann, K. E. (1988). Maternal attachment representations as related to patterns of infant–mother attachment and maternal care during the first year. In R. A. Hinde & J. Stevenson-Hinde (Eds.), *Relationships within families: Mutual influences* (pp. 241–260). Oxford University Press.

Grossmann, K. E., & Grossmann, K. (1990). The wider concept of attachment in cross-cultural research. *Human Development, 33*(1), 31–47.

Gu, X., Eilam-Stock, T., Zhou, T., Anagnostou, E., Kolevzon, A., Soorya, L., Hof, R., Friston, K., & Fan, J. (2015). Autonomic and brain responses associated with empathy deficits in autism spectrum disorder. *Human Brain Mapping, 36*(9), 3323–3338.

Gu, X., Hof, P. R., Friston, K. J., & Fan, J. (2013). Anterior insular cortex and emotional awareness. *Journal of Comparative Neurology, 521*(15), 3371–3388.

Izard, C. E. (1978). Emotions as motivations: An evolutionary–developmental perspective. *Nebraska Symposium on Motivation, 26*, 163–200.

Jacobsen, T., Edelstein, W., & Hofmann, V. (1993). Children's representations of attachment as related to later cognitive functioning. Poster presented at the 40th Annual Meeting of the American Academy of Child and Adolescent Psychiatry, October, 1993, San Antonio, TX.

James, W. (1890). *The Principles of Psychology, Vol. 1*. Henry Holt, New York.

James, W. (1884). What is an emotion? *Mind, 9*, 188–205.

Johnson-Laird, P. N. (1983). *Mental models: Towards a cognitive science of language, inference, and consciousness* (No. 6). Harvard University Press, Cambridge, MA.

Kernberg, O. (1976). *Object relations theory and clinical psychoanalysis*. Aronson, New York.

Kim, K., & Johnson, M. K. (2014). Extended self: Spontaneous activation of medial prefrontal cortex by objects that are "mine". *Social Cognitive and Affective Neuroscience, 9*(7), 1006–1012.

Lamm, C., Decety, J., & Singer, T. (2011). Meta-analytic evidence for common and distinct neural networks associated with directly experienced pain and empathy for pain. *Neuroimage, 54*(3), 2492–2502.

Lewis, M., & Brooks-Gunn, J. (1979). *Social cognition and the acquisition of self*. Plenum Press, New York.

Main, M. (1990). *A typology of human attachment organization with discourse, drawings, and interviews*. Cambridge University Press, New York.

Main, M., Kaplan, K., & Cassidy, J. (1985). Security in infancy, childhood and adulthood: A move to the level of representation. In I. Bretherton and E. Waters (Eds.), *Growing points of attachment theory and research, Monographs of the Society for Research in Child Development*, 50:66–104.

Main, M., & Solomon, J. (1986). Discovery of an insecure-disorganized/disoriented attachment pattern: Procedures, findings and implications for the classification of behavior. In M. Yogman & T. B. Brazelton (Eds.), *Affective development in infancy* (pp. 95–124). Ablex, Norwood, NJ.

Main, M., & Weston, D. (1981). The quality of the toddler's relationship to mother and father: Related to conflict behavior and the readiness to establish new relationships. *Child Development, 52*, 834–840.

Main, M., & Hesse, E. (1990). Parents' unresolved traumatic experiences are related to infant disorganized attachment status: Is frightening and/or frightened parental behavior the linking mechanism? In M. Greenberg, D. Cicchetti, & M. Cummings (Eds.), *Attachment in the pre-school years* (pp. 161–182). University of Chicago Press, Chicago.

Maslow, A. H. (1970). *Motivation and personality*, 2nd ed. Harper & Row, New York.

McClelland, D. C. (1985). *Human motivation*. Scott, Foresman, Dallas, TX.

Mead, G. H. (1934). *Mind, self and society*. University of Chicago Press, Chicago.

Niedenthal, P. M. (2007). Embodying emotion. *Science, 316*(5827), 1002–1005.

Northoff, G. (2011). Self and brain: What is self-related processing?. *Trends in Cognitive Sciences, 15*(5), 186–187.

O'Nions, E., Sebastian, C. L., McCrory, E., Chantiluke, K., Happe, F., & Viding, E. (2014). Neural bases of Theory of Mind in children with autism spectrum disorders and children with conduct problems and callous-unemotional traits. *Developmental Science, 17*(5), 786–796.

Perner, J., & Wimmer, H. (1985). "John thinks that Mary thinks that . . . " attribution of second-order beliefs by 5-to 10-year-old children. *Journal of Experimental Child Psychology, 39*(3), 437–471.

Rochat, P. (2003). Five levels of self-awareness as they unfold early in life. *Consciousness and Cognition, 12*(4), 717–731.

Rovee-Collier, C. K., & Fagen, J. W. (1981). The retrieval of memory in early infancy. *Advances in Infancy Research.*

Sandler, I., & Sandler, A. (1978). The development of object relationships and affects. *Journal of Psycho-Analysis, 59*, 285–296.

Seth, A. K. (2013). Interoceptive inference, emotion, and the embodied self. *Trends in Cognitive Sciences, 17*(11), 565–573.

Shatz, M., Wellman, H. M., & Silber, S. (1983). The acquisition of mental verbs: A systematic investigation of the first reference to mental state. *Cognition, 14*(3), 301–321.

Sroufe, L. A., & Waters, E. (1977). Attachment as an organizational construct. *Child Development, 48*, 1184–1199.

Stern, D. N. (1985). *The interpersonal world of the infant*. Basic Books, New York.

Sui, J., & Humphreys, G. W. (2015). The integrative self: How self-reference integrates perception and memory. *Trends in Cognitive Sciences, 19*(12), 719–728.

Sui, J., & Gu, X. (2017). Self as object: Emerging trends in self research. *Trends in Neurosciences, 40*(11), 643–653.

Sullivan, H. S. (1953). *The interpersonal theory of psychiatry*. W. W. Norton, New York.

van Veluw, S. J., & Chance, S. A. (2014). Differentiating between self and others: An ALE meta-analysis of fMRI studies of self-recognition and theory of mind. *Brain Imaging and Behavior, 8*(1), 24–38.

Wellman, H. M. (1988). First steps in the child's theorizing about the mind. In J. Astington, P. Harris, & D. Olson (Eds.), *Developing theories of mind* (pp. 64–92). Cambridge University Press, New York.

White, R. W. (1959). Motivation reconsidered: The concept of competence. *Psychological Review, 66*(5), 297–333.

Wicker, B., Keysers, C., Plailly, J., Royet, J. P., Gallese, V., & Rizzolatti, G. (2003). Both of us disgusted in My insula: The common neural basis of seeing and feeling disgust. *Neuron, 40*(3), 655–664.

Winnicott, D. W. (1958). *From pediatrics to psychoanalysis*. Hogarth Press, London.

Winnicott, D. W. (1965). *The maturational processes and the facilitating environment: Studies in the theory of emotional development*. International Universities Press, New York.

Zaki, J., Davis, J. I., & Ochsner, K. N. (2012). Overlapping activity in anterior insula during interoception and emotional experience. *Neuroimage, 62*(1), 493–499.

Zeanah, C. H., Keener, M. A., Stewart, L., & Anders, T. F. (1985). Prenatal perception of infant personality: A preliminary investigation. *Journal of the American Academy of Child Psychiatry, 24*(2), 204–210.

# 13
# Temperament

Temperament is defined as constitutionally based individual differences in reactivity and self-regulation (Posner & Rothbart, 2018; Rothbart, 2011). Temperament describes the initial state from which personality develops and is essential to understanding the origins of personality development. The infant's brain is not a blank slate at birth to be shaped by parenting; children differ from infancy and afterwards in their temperament. Neurobiologically, temperament links individual differences in behavior to underlying neural networks. Temperament and personality describe different phenomena and different processes (Rutter, 1987).

Developmental considerations are of considerable importance in assessing temperament. From a developmental standpoint, questions that must be addressed include "How does temperament develop?" and "How much of an infant's behavior can be designated as temperament?" These questions are important for infant and child social and cognitive development. How much temperament contributes to their development depends on the developmental course of the temperamental dimensions themselves. Temperament is the "how" of behavior, whereas personality is the "what." The personality emerges as temperament and experience come together as the child becomes aware of their self, others, and their relationship to the social world. Personality incorporates personal values, attitudes, beliefs, and coping strategies following an individual's development trajectory (Rothbart, 2007).

In this chapter, the roles of temperament and personality in socioemotional development are reviewed from a developmental perspective. The chapter includes a historical introduction to temperament and a review of various definitions of temperament. It addresses the effects of temperament on others, the neurobiology of temperament, temperament and cognition, and the assessment of temperament in children with developmental disabilities.

## History

Awareness of temperament and personality emerged in early civilizations. In China, the Confucian thinker Mencius (372–298 BCE) proposed four features of the ideal personality: benevolence (*ren*), righteousness (*yi*), proper conduct (*li*), and wisdom (*zhi*). Mencius believed these attributes were inborn qualities of humans. People have feelings of commiseration, a sense of shame, and a sense of right and wrong. Mencius believed that education and socialization in childhood and adolescence were essential to facilitate an innate goodness (Chen & Schmidt, 2015). Other concepts of temperament are rooted in ancient attempts to link personal characteristics with physiologic processes. More than 2,000 years ago, the Greek physician Hippocrates (470–370 BCE) described the importance of four elements in nature: earth, air, fire, and water. He also taught that health was maintained by the balance of four bodily fluids called "humors": blood, phlegm, yellow bile, and black bile derived from the heart, liver, spleen, and head. Subsequently, both Galen (130–200 CE) and Vindician (fourth century CE) have been credited with elaborating on this theory and proposing that there were four personality styles, each reflecting a characteristic humor: the sanguine (sociable cheerful) buoyant type; the phlegmatic (calm, rational) type; the choleric (aggressive, ambitious) type; and the melancholic (sad, despairing) type (Chen & Schmidt, 2015). Each of these represented the excess of a humor. Galen indicated that individual differences in the strength of these features defined one's temperament. Galen discussed temperament in young children (Rothbart, 1989) and stated that "the starting point of my entire discourse is the knowledge of the differences which can be seen in little children and which reveal the faculties of the soul. Some are very sluggish, others violent . . . shameless, or shy." He went on to suggest that if their souls were interchangeable, they would be expected to act in similar ways from their earliest days; but because there are behavioral differences, "the nature of the soul is not the same for all" (Diamond, 1974, p. 604). Subsequently, an aberration or eccentricity of personality was attributed to a humor.

The fourfold humoral approach to temperament continued throughout the Middle Ages and Renaissance, when the literature defined a "humor character" as one in which one passion predominated. Richard Burton (1621) provided a comprehensive overview of this concept in *The Anatomy of Melancholy*, which was still being discussed by Emmanuel Kant in 1798. In medicine, the theory of humors lost currency in the 19th century with Virchow's theory of cellular pathology. By 1903, William Wundt had changed the emphasis from typologies of temperament to dimensions of individual variability. He proposed temperamental dimensions of feelings and addressed the strength and speed of change of feeling. Ebbinghaus proposed the dimensions of optimism–pessimism and emotionality (Eysenck & Eysenck, 1987). In the 20th century, the Russians, exemplified by Pavlov, focused on properties of the nervous system (i.e., strong or weak) in response to environmental stimuli and related these to temperament. The British began to derive temperamental factors from self-report measures. Webb (1915) used factor analysis to assess emotionality, activity, and self-qualities. These earlier views have been replaced by modern theories and perspectives based on research findings (Chen & Schmidt, 2015).

## Definitions of Temperament

The word "temperament" originates from the Latin *temperamentum*, meaning "a mixture of the bodily humors," from *temperare*, "to mingle in due proportion" (Rothbart, 1989). Definitions of temperament have been proposed by a number of authors (Campos et al., 1983; Goldsmith et al., 1987). Those suggested by Thomas and Chess (1977), Rothbart (1981), and Kagan (1997) are representative and are emphasized in this chapter.

### Thomas and Chess

The modern study of child temperament was initiated by Thomas, Chess, and colleagues (1963) in their New York Longitudinal Study. Their focus on temperament emphasizes individual differences in development; the child is viewed as an active agent who shapes their responses to the environment. Their focus is on socioemotional aspects of development rather than cognitive aspects (Rutter, 1987). Temperament has a neurobiological basis that includes genetic influences. Thomas and Chess (1977) conceptualized temperament as the stylistic component of behavior. They described it as the "how" of behavior (style), rather than the "why" of behavior (motivation) or the "what" of behavior (type of performance or ability). They proposed that although a group of individuals, children or adults, could have the same motivation to perform a task and have similar levels of ability to carry it out, they may differ in their performance because of temperamental features. These include their intensity of activity, mood, adaptability in carrying out the task, persistence, and distractibility. Each of these characteristics is a component of temperament. For these authors, temperament is an independent psychological attribute that is not secondary to other attributes, such as cognition, arousal, motivation, or emotionality. However, temperament does reciprocally interact with other attributes. Consequently, a child with temperamentally low persistence could stick to a particular task with greater persistence if highly motivated.

Thomas and Chess differentiated temperament from motivations, abilities, and personality. Temperament is expressed as a response to external stimuli, opportunities, demands, and expectations. The social context may intensify or minimize the expression of temperamental features. The influence of temperament is bidirectional in that the response to a particular environmental influence can be affected by the child's temperament. In addition, a child's temperament will influence judgments, attitudes, and behaviors of significant individuals toward the child. These authors organized their observations into nine temperament dimensions. Defined in infancy, these are clustered to form three main temperamental groups: (a) easy, (b) difficult, and (c) slow warm-up dimensions that are stable over time. They noted patterns of individuality in infant reactivity that included the sleep–wake cycle, eating behavior, and response to external stimuli. The nine dimensions of temperament were identified from interviews with parents. These are activity level, approach/withdrawal, intensity, threshold, adaptability, rhythmicity, mood, attention span, persistence, and distractibility. Thomas and Chess (1977) emphasized parent–child interactions and proposed the phrase "goodness of fit" between parent and child in discussing how infant temperament and that of the parents were similar or not similar. Thus, developmental outcomes tended to be positive when a match exists between an infant's temperament and parental temperament and parenting style. However, if there is a mismatch between infant temperament and parenting behavior or parental expectations, the child is at greater risk for behavioral problems. They advised parents and teachers to recognize temperamental differences in a child's capacity to adapt to environmental and interpersonal challenges.

## Rothbart

Rothbart (1981) defined temperament as relatively stable, primarily biologically based, individual differences in reactivity and self-regulation using the terms surgency, negative activity, and effortful control to describe its components. Temperament refers to individual differences in emotional, motor, and attentional reactivity and self-regulation. These are assessed with regard to threshold, latency, intensity, recovery, and rise times.

Self-regulation refers to attention, approach, avoidance, and inhibition, which serve to modulate (i.e., to enhance or inhibit) reactivity. Temperament is observed behaviorally as individual differences in patterns of emotionality, activity, and attention. From a phenomenological standpoint, it is experienced by the individual as feelings of energy, interest, and affectivity. Rothbart has examined activity level, smiling and laughter, fear, distress at limitations (frustration), soothability, and duration of orienting as temperamental variables.

Temperament is observed in human infants and in nonhuman animals. Temperamental dispositions may form the bases for the developing personality. Across species, approach and withdrawal behaviors vary according to the intensity of stimuli required to involve reactivity. Rothbart proposes that children differ in their reactivity to sensory stimuli, especially to novel and intense stimulation. Reactivity is measured by latency to respond, response intensity, and duration of the response physiologically and behaviorally. The extent of reactivity affects an infant's capacity to sustain physiological homeostasis. Children also differ in their ability to respond to reactivity by self-soothing—that is, to regulate their reactivity. This capacity to self-regulate matures during development, with individual differences among children. Rothbart emphasizes that attention is an essential feature. There is a relationship between temperament during development and the neural circuitry of attention based on self-regulation and a dynamic maturation of temperamental features with experience (Posner & Rothbart, 2018). Mastery in self-regulation is gained with the capacity to modulate the timing and intensity of an individual's reactivity. Maturation of attention strategies results in increased effortful control (Rueda, 2012).

As the infant matures, the attention network develops greater voluntary attentional control. With greater effortful control of temperament, an infant can more easily resolve conflict, shift cognitive state, and adapt their responses more readily and more appropriately. This leads to great capacity to inhibit responses, emotions, and thoughts. Brain regions involved in supporting this network are the areas of the anterior midfrontal lobe that includes the anterior cingulate cortex, the dorsolateral ventral, and orbitofrontal cortex. In addition, the anterior cingulate engages the amygdala in emotion control. More broadly, attention facilitates internal feeling, word choice, and environmental location (Rothbart, 2011).

In the study of temperament, Rothbart's focus on reactivity and capacity to self-regulate differs from the focus of Chess and Thomas on nine temperamental dimensions. Rothbart re-examined these dimensions in her description of the structure of temperament and its relationship to personality development, adaptability to the environment, social development, and developmental psychopathology (Rothbart, 2011).

Chess and Thomas (1977) established that infants' reaction patterns were established by age 3–6 months from their parents, who reported infants' reactions to everyday situations such as feeding, bathing, and playing. For example, the parent was asked how the infant reacted when first offered cereals to eat. Did the infant eagerly like the food or dislike it by spitting it out? Reactivity was recorded into what became the nine categorical dimensions that they established: activity level, rhythmicity (regularity and predictability of times when hungry, sleepy, etc.), approach versus withdrawal, negative or positive reactions to a new persons, object or situation, adaptability to changes in directions from caregiver, threshold (intensity of stimulation needed to get the child to respond), intensity (energy level of the child's reaction), mood (pleasant response contrasted with unpleasant one), distractibility, and attention span/persistence (i.e., attention to an activity and continuation with it despite frustration).

The temperamental dimensions mentioned earlier categorized as easy, slow to warm up, or difficult were based on five of the nine dimensions. For example, difficult children tend to withdraw from novelty, have predominant negative mood, show problems in adapting to change, and show irregular rhythm and intense responses. Easy children are high on approach to novelty, show positive mood and adaptability, are highly regular in their responses, and show low intensity. Finally, children who are slow to warm up are initially withdrawn and low in the intensity of their reactivity; they gradually adapt to change. Studies of temperament are a way to recognize the child's individuality as a person distinct from the parent's expectations. When parents fully appreciate their child's individuality, the child's growth is facilitated.

Chess and Thomas (1989) used these dimensions for counseling parents on how to cope with a child with a difficult temperament that deviated from the parents' temperament. Positive goodness of fit was accomplished "when the child's capabilities, motivations, and temperament are adequate to master the demands, expectations, and opportunities of the environment" offered by the parent. For example, a family focused on community activity such as sports might welcome an active and fearless infant. Another family, in which quiet, sedate, and self-controlled behavior is valued, may not. There may be poor goodness of fit when parents are extroverted and the infant is introverted and cautious. Therefore, parents who adapt to their infant's temperamental features show a "good fit," but if they disapprove of the infant's temperamental features, it is a "poor fit." A good fit is typically a good temperamental match; however, a good fit may occur when there are different temperaments between child and parent. For example, an extroverted child may be valued by parents who are temperamentally shy. Moreover, as children develop, a temperamental trait might be viewed as adaptive in infancy but problematic when the child is older. For example, an easily distracted, easy to soothe infant might be a reasonable fit in infancy but later recognized with attention deficit disorder at school age (Rothbart, 2011).

Rothbart and colleagues have refined temperament models. They find a lack of consistency among the nine originally proposed by Chess and Thomas. Rothbart's group found that intensity, threshold for reactivity, adaptability, and rhythmicity are not consistently homogeneous across situations and responses. Rothbart's studies indicated that temperament is not a style as proposed earlier, leading her group to take a more neurobiological perspective (Rothbart, 2011). Moreover, they found inconsistency on the mood dimension as well. Identifying positive mood at one pole and negative mood at the other did not allow for a child to be high on both emotional poles. Their findings on the mood dimensions affect the approach–avoidance dimension. The Chess and Thomas study focused on either approaching or avoiding novel stimuli or situations.

Rothbart and colleagues found that positive emotions were linked to approach and activity level, leading them to propose a separate dimension of positive emotionality termed "surgency." Surgency is defined as a trait of emotional reactivity linked to high levels of positive affect, cheerfulness, spontaneity, and sociability. The surgency scale includes positive anticipation of pleasurable activity, positive vocalization, enjoyment, smiling and laughter, perceptual sensitivity, and increasing motor activity with pleasure. They proposed a second and separate negative reactivity scale, which includes expressions of sadness, extent of low mood with object loss, and general low mood. Negative emotional reactivity is expressed when limits are placed on one's preferred activity, leading to frustration and anger. Fear is another element of negative reactivity and is expressed as being startled or distressed with sudden changes in ongoing stimulation. Finally, negative reactivity is related to the rate of recovery or capacity to calm down when distressed. Rothbart and colleagues' third scale is the orienting/regulation scale. It includes the extent of enjoyment exhibited during low levels of stimulation, addressing emotional expression when playing quietly, the extent of enjoyment in being touched or hugged, and the capacity to be soothed when distressed.

Kagan and colleagues have carried out longitudinal studies of stability of individual differences in one temperament type—"behavioral inhibition" (Kagan et al., 1987, 2007). Kagan et al. identified individual differences in reactivity to novelty in infants in the early part of the first year of life as a temperament feature; these infants are motorically overactive but exhibit distress to novelty with inhibited and shy behavior. Of the infants studied, 15–20% showed this highly reactive temperament. They were recognized to have both behavioral and physiological reactivity to novelty.

Toddlers that Kagan identified were particularly cautious and vigilant when facing unfamiliar environmental contexts. This wariness that persisted from infancy into childhood and adolescence is a core feature of the personality trait of neuroticism. These infants and children differed in that they were not just on an extreme of the temperamental continuum but also were distinct. Kagan documented a physiologic pattern of high autonomic reactivity, an elevation in stress hormone levels, heightened startle, and avoidant or freezing behavior. Both rodent and nonhuman primate studies of threat conditioning are consistent with Kagan's findings in infants (Kenwood & Kalin, 2021). Moreover, Kagan's model is pertinent to understanding the origin of human anxiety disorders (Fox & Walker, 2015).

## Temperament in Nonhuman Animals

The temperamental dimensions reported in infants and preschool children are similar to reports of temperament in nonhuman animals. Panksepp (2004) reviewed reactivity to danger (fear), reaction to obstacles to preferred activity (frustration), and seeking reward (approach) as evidence of stable emotional systems operating in nonhuman. Temperament studies in nonhuman primates use methods similar to those used in humans. These include coded observations of animals as they socially engage, completion of questionnaires by animal caretakers, and observations made the laboratory where the response to stimulation is measured.

There is evidence of continuity of temperament in nonhuman primates to humans. Assessment of reactivity to environmental stimulation allows study within species and comparisons between them. Temperament studied in rhesus monkeys reveal broad temperamental features of hostile, fearful, and socially positive behavior (in play). A study of captive gorillas found four factors: extraverted (sociable, playful, and curious), dominant (aggressive and irritable), fearful (apprehensive and tense), and understanding (affiliative and nurturant) (Rothbart, 2011). Studies in chimpanzees have identified traits: submissiveness (element of fear) versus dominance or aggressiveness, agreeableness, negative emotionality, openness, dependability, and impulsiveness with low aggression (King & Figueredo, 1997). Thus, research findings show substantial overlap in human and chimpanzee temperament. In both humans and chimpanzees, the five-factor model of temperament is pertinent. Personality dimensions shared with nonhuman primates include surgency, fearfulness, irritability/aggressiveness, capacity for affiliation (affection and feeling of closeness to others), general emotionality/distress proneness, and openness (perceptual sensitivity) (Rothbart, 2011). In addition, studies of chimpanzees find individual differences in effortful control that are not reported in other nonhuman primates (Gosling & John, 1999). Humans, of course, differ from chimpanzees due to our advanced cognitive development, highly developed language, and self-construct.

Just as temperamental models proposed by Rothbart and others have been examined in nonhuman primates, the behavioral inhibition model proposed by Kagan has been as well. In children, behavioral inhibition is characterized by withdrawal in the presence of strangers when faced with novel situations. Later in development in humans, behavioral inhibition is associated with increased risk for anxiety, depression, and restricted social behavior. Chun and Capitanio (2016) examined behavioral inhibition in rhesus monkeys. In this study, rhesus monkeys that showed evidence of behavioral inhibition in infancy in response to separation were compared to non-inhibited peers, which were not separated. During their juvenile years, their behavior was examined in response to relocation, human intruder challenge, and a naturalistic outdoor corral. In young adulthood (age 4 years), data were collected in outdoor field corrals to measure the adult social consequences of behavioral inhibition, including sex, dominance rank, and number of available kin. The behaviorally inhibited juvenile monkeys maintained their prior behavioral differences when relocated and when challenged with a human intruder, exhibiting a greater emotionality compared to non-inhibited control animals. Anxious behavior in juvenile rhesus monkeys included scratching, yawning, clasping, and vocalizations. The behaviorally inhibited juveniles showed greater anxiety with relocation, spending more time hanging on the edge of the cage; with the human intruder, there were fewer affiliative co-vocalizations and more clasping. As young adults, behaviorally inhibited monkeys spent more time hanging on the edge of their cages than engaging with peers: time alone as a juvenile correlated with time alone as an adult. However, other measures of anxiety did not persist into adulthood.

Whereas there was a positive correlation between juvenile and young adult nonsocial behavior for non-inhibited animals, this correlation was not observed in the behaviorally inhibited monkeys. The difference between the groups for juvenile and adult nonsocial behavior may be related to differential susceptibility to the environment (biological sensitivity to context models) (Ellis et al., 2011). Certain individuals may be more susceptible to both positive and negative aspects of the environment, with some behaviorally inhibited animals continuing the pattern of being nonsocial as adults, whereas others did not. This might be accounted for by differences in maternal care, social group dynamics, etc. The non-inhibited group showed greater variation in juvenile nonsocial behavior, but there was a correlation between the juvenile and adult nonsocial duration, suggesting that this group may be less susceptible to the environment (Chun & Capitanio, 2016). In young adulthood (age 4 years), behaviorally inhibited monkeys spent less time alone, whereas they spent more time grooming as juveniles. This observation indicates that higher quality social interaction at a younger age may mitigate the social consequences of behavioral inhibition and may be pertinent to behavioral inhibition in humans (Chun & Capitanio, 2016). These findings in rhesus monkeys are consistent with the human literature indicating that some children become less inhibited when their parents make a focused effort to help them (Davis & Panksepp, 2011; Gartstein et al., 2013).

There is a cognitive and neural basis for individual differences in developmental risk and resilience. Behavioral inhibition has been considered in the context of two kinds of information processing. The first is an early autonomic response to novelty, attention bias to threat, and incentive processing. The second is controlled attention—that is, the capacity for attention shifting and inhibitory control. If the first of these remains robust and stable, the risk for adult social anxiety disorder is increased. The second approach is consistent with Rothbart's focus on effortful control, attention shifting, conflict management, and response monitoring (Rothbart et al., 2007). Effective inhibitory control facilitates emotion regulation. Interventions emphasize enhancing attention flexibility and attention shifting (Henderson et al., 2015). These interventions have sought to mimic day-to-day challenges that are found with children with heightened behavioral inhibition (Guyer et al., 2014). Thus, when attention is drawn to potential threatening situations, how quickly can children with behavioral inhibition process the threat and effectively respond to it in their social environments? Interventions are being developed to facilitate mastery of such challenges.

As children who are behaviorally inhibited mature, they are at risk for anxiety, depression, loneliness, and negative self-esteem (Kagan et al., 2007). Adolescents with increased behavioral inhibition as toddlers have higher levels of social anxiety. A meta-analysis of behavioral inhibition found a moderate effect size for later anxiety disorders (Clauss & Blackford, 2012). Moreover, large longitudinal studies show convergent evidence that children who are shy–inhibited and highly reactive are at risk for developing internalized social emotional difficulties. These include social anxiety in adolescence and adulthood. A subset of children with stable behavioral inhibition from infancy through middle childhood are at greater risk. These children have higher levels of negative activity and reduced competence in executive control in regulating emotional reactions, rendering them more vulnerable to anxiety disorders (Lonigan & Vasey, 2009).

Temperament influences anxiety in several ways. First, temperament may predispose to developing anxiety disorders when interacting with environmental stressors—that is, the diathesis–stress model. A diathesis is an individual's predisposition to a psychological disorder, which can be precipitated by significant stress. Second, temperament through pathoplasticity may influence the course of an anxiety disorder although not its root cause. Third, according to the complication model, temperamental features that facilitate anxiety may emerge as a complication of developing an anxiety disorder. Thus, an anxious child's avoidance and parental and other adults' protective responses to the child's anxiety symptoms may increase the physiological response to anxiety. Fourth, with the continuity model, temperament and anxiety disorders are viewed as reflecting the same underlying processes (Vasey et al., 2014).

Cognitive error monitoring is implicated as moderating the risk between temperament and anxiety symptoms (Fox & Walker, 2015). Cognitive error monitoring is assessed using the Erikson flanker task. The participant's task is to press a button to indicate the direction of an arrow in the middle of a computer screen. The arrow is "flanked" by arrows in the same or a different direction. During the performance of the task, brain electrical activity is recorded with an electroencephalogram (EEG) and is synchronized to the participant's button pressing. When the subject makes an error, an event-related potential is generated called the error-related negativity. Error monitoring is measured by the response times for the trials following an error and compared to response times following correct trials. If inaccurate performance is a significant concern for subject, slower responding occurs in the trial following the error. The individual performance is paired with measurement of error-related negativity. The neural pattern that is associated with cognitive monitoring appears 50 and 150 ms after the response after error commission. Cognitive error monitoring is increased in people with anxiety disorders. When adolescents with high behavioral inhibition were compared to adolescents low on childhood behavioral inhibition, error-related negativity was found to moderate the relationship between early behavioral inhibition and later anxiety disorders (McDermott et al., 2009). Similarly, children with behavioral inhibition documented in infancy were examined for error-related negativity and anxiety symptoms at age 9 years (Lahat et al., 2014). Children with a history of behavioral inhibition in infancy had elevated error-related negativity and higher levels of anxiety.

In another study, behavioral inhibition was assessed at ages 2 and 3 years ($N = 268$) (Buzzell et al., 2017) and then reassessed at age 12 years. EEG was recorded while carrying out the Erikson flanker task under two conditions. In one condition, the children believed that they were being observed by peers, and in another condition they believed that they were not being observed by peers. Using this procedure, isolated changes in error monitoring (error-related negativity) and behavior (post-error reaction time slowing) as a function of social circumstance could be examined. Behavioral inhibition in infancy predicted social-specific error-related negativity increases and social anxiety symptoms in adolescents. Findings in this study extend previous research linking behavioral inhibition, social anxiety, and error monitoring to a social context. When the participant believed a peer was observing, error preoccupation as indicated by error-related negativity negative potential was increased. Future research needs to extend these findings to other social situations such as the family context.

## Temperament Throughout Infant Development

The core of infant temperament in early infancy is linked to proneness to stress in environmental encounters and the capacity for soothability. By age 2 or 3 months, positive affect, approach and surgency, frustration, cuddling, and affiliation are apparent. As these dimensions emerge, they impact the child's interactions with others and their physical environment. For example, one infant might be physically active but quiet when in contact with the mother, moving their hand to their mouth to self-sooth. This infant continually cries when bathed but quickly self-soothes when swaddled. Another child may be more variable in emotionality, often crying and rarely bringing their hand to their mouth to self-sooth.

The Brazelton Neonatal Behavioral Assessment Scale (Brazelton, 1978) includes four common temperamental factors: (a) orientation primarily to visual stimuli when quietly alert; (b) irritability, tension, and activity; (c) soothability; and (d) overall susceptibility to distress. Those more attentive and more oriented to the outside environment are less likely to become distressed. Each of these four factors shows continuity with later development. During infancy, children develop strategies for self-soothing, finding help and comfort with others, gaining reward, and avoiding harm to varying degrees related to individual differences in temperament. Effortful control, an important component of temperament, is more gradually developing into the toddler and preschool years.

Temperamental features are involved in coping behaviors. Negative emotionality is linked to avoidant strategies, positive emotionality to active coping, and attention regulation to more effective coping. The components of temperament change as children develop and mature. Specifically, self-regulation of effortful control continues to develop during preschool and early school years into adulthood. Proneness to distress can be modified by experience. The emerging personality is influenced by life experiences overall and experiences with specific people. What is stable and what is most changeable in individual temperament (Rothbart, 2011)? Stability and change are linked to a balance among systems of temperament, coping strategies, and response to life events. Overall, broad temperamental traits are moderately stable over time and linked to personality traits. Still, there are developmental paths to personality that are influenced by both temperament and an individual's thoughts and cognition.

As temperament develops, new systems of organization emerge with maturation. Beyond childhood, levels of stability increase throughout adolescence and adulthood into middle age. In the Swedish Uppsala Longitudinal Study, from infancy to age 21 years, some temperamental features remained stable—for example, reactivity from infancy into adulthood (Bohlen & Hagekill, 2009). Reactivity also predicts neuroticism as well as internalizing and externalizing problems. Activity and sociability (surgency) at age 20–48 months predicted lower neuroticism and higher extroversion at age 21 years. Shyness at age 20–48 months predicted higher internalization at age 21 years (Rothbart, 2011). Extraversion (surgency) and fearful inhibition (introversion) show stability, as do spontaneity and reserve social inhibition. Another stable dimension from age 3 or 4 years onward is the capacity to delay gratification, a feature of effortful control.

A New Zealand study involving 1,000 subjects aged 3–26 years found that child temperament after the emergence of effortful control offers a basis for the developing personality (Caspi et al., 2003). Undercontrolled 3-year-old children, who were high in surgency and negative emotionality but low in attention control, showed more neurotic traits at age 26 years. Confidence and surgency in childhood were associated with confidence and lack of fearfulness in adulthood. Inhibited and reserved children remained high on fearfulness into adulthood. Inhibited children reported lack of social support as adults, suggesting their temperament impacts how others respond. Despite the evidence of stability, temperament may change with development primarily by an increase in self-regulatory capacity as children grow older.

## Temperament and Adult Personality Factors

The number of factors identified from personality measures ranges from three to seven; however, the most common number of factors identified is the five basic broad factors in personality, known as the five-factor model of personality (McCrae & Costa, 1987). The five-factor model comprises the following factors and their facets:

1. Extraversion with facets of warmth, gregariousness, assertiveness, activity, excitement seeking, and positive emotionality
2. Agreeableness with facets of trust, straightforwardness, altruism, modesty, and tender mindedness
3. Conscientiousness with facets of competence, order, self-discipline, dutifulness, deliberation, and achievement striving
4. Neuroticism with facets of anxiety, anger, hostility, depression, self-consciousness, impulsiveness, and vulnerability
5. Openness to experience with facets of fantasy, aesthetics, and openness to feelings, actions, ideas, and values

As shown in Table 13.1, temperament and personality factors are highly related, supporting the view that the five-factor personality model is based on individual differences. The continuity of the five-factor structure in nonhuman primates and in humans across cultures supports the view that the five-factor model is essentially based on the most fundamental temperament findings (Rothbart, 2011). Temperament research places greatest emphasis on attention and emotion, whereas personality research tends to focus on social factors (McCrae et al., 2000). The differences in approach are complementary. Studying personality traits is important in socialization. Both temperament and personality approaches are studied to identify the underlying genetics and neurobiology (Posner & Rothbart, 2018; Rothbart, 2011; Rothbart et al., 2007).

How do the five personality factors develop from core temperamental features? It is proposed that extraversion develops from surgency; conscientiousness from inhibitory executive attention systems involved in effortful control and personal choices in following societal rules; neuroticism from both aggressive and non-aggressive negative affect (primarily non-aggressive affect); awareness from temperamental low aggressive negative affect and strong affiliativeness; and openness from temperamental perceptual sensitivity. Finally, internalizing negative affectivity, related to temperamental fear, should be distinguished from externalizing negative affectivity/stimulation seeking that are linked to temperamental anger (Victor et al., 2016). Early temperament and attachment have been studied as predictors of the five-factor model of personality (Hagekull & Bohlin, 2003).

In a Swedish study of 85 middle-class children, both the Strange Situation assessment and combined maternal and paternal temperament ratings at age 20 months were used to predict personality rating and emotional negativity by mothers and teachers when the children were aged 8 or 9 years. The personality factor of extraversion (surgency) was best correlated with infant measures and predicted by both temperament and attachment security. Attachment security also predicted neuroticism and openness.

**Table 13.1** Adults Temperament and Personality Scales

| Adult Temperament Questionnaire[a] | Five-Factor Model[b] |
| --- | --- |
| Non-aggressive negative affect | Neuroticism |
|   Fear |   Anxiety, anger, hostility, depression, self- |
|   Sadness |   consciousness, impulsiveness, vulnerability |
| Effortful control | Conscientiousness |
|   Activation control |   Competence, order, dutifulness, achievement, |
|   Attentional control |   striving, self-discipline, deliberation |
| Extraversion/surgency | Extraversion |
|   Sociability |   Warmth, gregariousness, assertiveness, |
|   High-intensity pleasure |   activity, excitement seeking, positive emotions |
|   Positive affect | |
| Orienting sensitivity | Openness to experience |
|   General perceptual sensitivity |   Fantasy, aesthetics, feelings, actions, ideas, |
|   Affective perceptual sensitivity |   values |
|   Associative sensitivity | |
| Affiliation | Agreeableness |
|   Emotional empathy |   Trust, straightforwardness, altruism, |
|   Empathetic guilt |   compliance, modesty, tender-mindedness |
| Aggressive negative affect | |
|   Frustration | |
|   Social anger | |

[a]From Evans and Rothbart (2007).
[b]From Costa and McCrae (1992).

Measures of approach, anxiety systems, and internal working models are foundational to the five-factor personality model.

Historically, the field of personality psychology has focused on personality differences among adults, whereas temperament is typically studied in infants and children. Although temperamental and personality traits have been thought to be relatively stable, a development perspective challenges this viewpoint. Development is essential in examining individual differences. In regard to a developmental perspective, genes are differentially expressed during development, and these experiences may have a modifying effect for these traits. Increasingly, the focus in neuroscience is on identifying common neural networks that may underlie human capabilities and individual differences. Thus, a developmental approach examines how infant temperament influences child and adult personality. The joint study of temperament and personality is valuable for examining how genes and experience shape the development of neuronal networks.

Interest in the joint study of temperament and personality led to the development of the Child Temperament and Personality Questionnaire. This questionnaire was developed through a factor analysis performed on a total sample of 915 children approximately age 7 years. Five factors were identified in the combined measure of child temperament and personality. The first is externalizing negative affect/

sensation seeking, which includes factors of self-centered, noncompliance/aggression and manipulative, anger/irritability, assertiveness, and impulsivity. The second is social extraversion, which includes factors of gregariousness/sociability, warmth, positive emotion, soothabilty, and activity. The first two factors differentiate extraversion into two forms, one less socialized and the other more socialized. The third is internalizing negative activity with facets of fear/worry, self-consciousness, shyness, dependency, and distractibility. The fourth is consciousness, which has subscales of order, diligence, inhibitory control, self-discipline, attentional focusing, and distractibility. The fifth factor, openness to experience, has four subscales: aesthetics/creativity, openness to ideas, intellect/quick to learn, and temperamental perceptual sensitivity. The combined scale differs from the five-factor personality model by splitting extroversion into sociable extroversion and externalizing negative affectivity/stimulation seeking, the externalizing negative affectivity factor. Agreeableness at the positive pole is part of social extroversion. At the negative pole, it is part of the externalizing negative affectivity factor.

In summary, the five factors include differentiated negative affect factors (internalizing and externalizing), social extraversion, consciousness, and openness (Victor et al., 2016). Viewed developmentally within extraversion, the combined model suggests that infant extraversion/surgency may branch into two trajectories from infancy. In the first social extroversion, children exhibit gregariousness, sociability, warmth, and soothability. In the second, they show externalizing negative affectivity, temperamental excitement, anger/irritability, impulsiveness, self-centeredness, noncompliance, and manipulative behavior. Internalizing negative affectivity includes fear/worry, self-consciousness, shyness, and distractibility. Development outcomes may differ based on the balance of fear and anger/irritability that may depend on the extent of socialization. Inhibitory control and attention-focusing aspects of executive control are increasingly developed between ages 2 and 7 years. Linking consciousness to the temperamental features of executive attention and mastery, motivation may facilitate the development of consciousness. Temperamental perceptual sensitivity is linked developmentally to openness, making it a key component of openness. Victor et al. propose that integrated temperament and personality measures will facilitate differentiated measurement of individual differences.

Temperamental features may be linked to psychopathology by providing a description of developing problematic behavior. The child's experience and personal developmental understanding of events influence their development. This is particularly true for negative affectivity, expressions of fear and internalizing emotions, and anger and externalizing emotions. Surgency and excessive exuberance with anger and aggression can lead to problematic behavior. The link of strong affiliations may lead to low mood and depression. Personality disorders may emerge from interpersonal relations and temperament among the dependent, avoidant, paranoid, and antisocial personality traits.

Effortful control is a key factor in the prevention of problem behaviors and their persistence. Effortful control is important to school success, social skill development, and active coping. It is sensitive to parental influence and environment experiences, especially in the preschool years when the greatest development of executive control is taking place. Attention is an important element in effortful control. Individual differences in orienting are important in anxiety disorders, in which an anxious person may find it difficult to orient away from a negative attentional focus. Attention deficit disorder is an example of problems in executive control. Effortful control is essential to the prevention of behavior problems and, once established, in correcting them.

In conclusion, the structure of adult personality maps into temperamental dimensions of affiliation, perceptional sensitivity, surgency, fear, frustration, and effortful control, among others. This indicates that much of personality may derive from the neurobiological base core of temperament. Moreover, dimensions of temperament relate to behavioral problems and disorders of self-regulation, with similarities in child and adult. As children develop, they find coping strategies to avoid situations that trigger negative emotions and seek socialization as they progressively master developmental tasks. As development proceeds, toddlers and preschool children establish cognitive understanding about themselves and others, and they have specific expectations, hopes, and also anxieties in adapting. Some children, influenced by temperament, develop defensive attitudes, whereas others remain more fully engaged and less fearful. Thus, temperamental dispositions are transferred into cognitive features of personality, finding adaptive meaning in their lives.

There is a continuous interface between temperament reactivity and personal self-regulation to life challenges. During infancy, temperamental dispositions are generally reactive, involving negative emotions. Overall, self-regulation is increasingly mastered over time. Still, some temperamental features, such as self-soothing, are characteristic of some infants. Children develop the capacity to balance their urges to act with the choice to hesitate and reflect before acting. The development of effortful control in the preschool years increasingly facilitates such choices. Finally, temperament plays a role in the development of competences and social skills, both facilitated by emerging language skills and greater understanding about the world and themselves. Despite aspects of temperament that are relatively resistant to change, emerging cognitive and emotional self-understanding allows the child to be more open to positive emotions and affiliation with others. In this way, temperament provides the tools to master their limitations and lead productive and satisfying lives (Rothbart, 2011).

Research has been conducted on temperament leading to the development of a common language to describe it and to find greater correlations. Ongoing longitudinal studies that use multiple measures of temperament and personality are increasingly focusing on the contributions of both genes and life experiences to developmental outcomes. Research is also ongoing into the continuities as well as discontinuities in temperament development. Advances in neuroscientific studies of brain function and temperament are contributing to our understanding of the basic individual differences in temperament. Respecting those individual differences allows us to value the uniqueness and meaning of the lives of us all.

## Genetics, Temperament, and Personality

There are individual constitutional (biological) differences in temperament that have been examined in twin studies, inbred nonhuman animal species, and studies involving molecular genetics. Twin and adoption studies have been used to examine the behavioral genetics of child temperament (Saudino, 2005). These studies show the importance of nonshared environmental influences on temperament, genetic continuity, and environmental changes throughout development. Although behavioral dimensions vary in the models, all temperament features and emotionality are consistent among them. The most commonly used measures of temperament are the Colorado Child Temperament Inventory and the Children's Behavior Questionnaire. Twin studies offer strong evidence of genetic influences in temperament, consistently showing that monozygotic co-twins have greater similarity than dizygotic twins across temperament measures including emotionality, activity, shyness, sociability, adaptivity, and positive negative affect (Saudino, 2005). Soothabilty and rhythmicity, originally proposed dimensions, show little genetic influence. Monozygotic twins correlations are moderate, indicating substantial similarity. Dizygotic twins show less than half the monozygotic correlations and often show very few (Plomin et al., 1993). Thus, the concordance for dizygotic twins is essentially similar to that of two randomly paired children, and some dizygotic twins have opposing temperaments. Moreover, adoption and twin studies using objectively assessed temperament yield similar estimates of heritability (Braungart et al., 1992). Regarding behavioral inhibition, monozygotic twins showed stronger interclass correlations of inhibited and fearful behavior to unfamiliar stimuli than dizygotic twins and non-twin siblings (Dilalla et al., 1994).

Overall, genes may account for 40–50% of the variability in temperament for measures using the Big five personality factor dimensions in adults. The Big Five personality factor dimensions have corresponding temperamental factors: extraversion (surgency), agreeableness (affliction vs. anger and frustration), neuroticism (negative emotionality), consciousness (effort and control), and openness (orienting sensitivity). In adult studies of twins raised together or raised separately, the traits for monozygotic twins raised apart were high and similar to those for identical twins raised together. The heritability estimate is approximately 50% (Tellegen et al., 1988). In the study by Tellegen et al., correlations for twins raised apart were substantial for the temperamental dimension of negative emotionality (pertinent to stress response, sense of well-being, control, low risk-taking, and aggression). For positive emotionality, the monozygotic and dizygotic twins raised together were more similar than those raised apart. Moreover, a review of six studies of behavioral genetics in children demonstrated substantial heritability of temperament (Goldsmith et al., 1997). Similar to adults, there was evidence of family influence on positive emotionality and approach. Supportive evidence was found for both genetic and shared family influences in Rothbart's Children's Behavior Questionnaire on effortful control, indicating the importance of family influence. Thus, heritability of personality traits may not always be 50%. There are also gene–environmental interactions that lead to correlation of personality and parenting (Krueger et al., 2008).

In addition to the authors of the three approaches previously discussed, several other authors have contributed to research in temperament. Goldsmith and Campos (1986) define temperament as individual differences in the probability of experiencing and expressing the primary emotions and general arousal. Their definition is confined to the behavioral level because they believe temperament is most meaningful in a social context. Kagan et al. (1987) add a further element to temperament—that of behavioral inhibition to the unfamiliar.

## Overview of Temperament

Overall, temperament is viewed as a relatively small number of simple, nonmotivational, noncognitive, stylistic features (Rutter, 1987). Emotionality, activity, and sociability are generally agreed to be aspects of temperament. Each of these characteristics may have neurobiological correlates. The key definitional requirement is to clarify how to separate temperament from other aspects of personality. For example, emotional reactivity is a temperamental characteristic that shows how a child will respond to a new situation, but a specific fear is predictive of behavior only in limited situations. Negative mood may be a temperamental feature, but helplessness and depression are not, consistent with the focus on temperament as the style of interaction. In this way, nonmotivational and noncognitive factors, and noncomplex behavioral tendencies, are taken into account. Using the same line of thinking, activity level is an aspect of temperament, but suspiciousness and obsessiveness are not.

The general consensus is that temperament refers to a group of related traits and not just to a single trait. The designation "temperament" may be analogous to the term "cognition" in that temperament, like cognition, refers to several phenomena (e.g., activity, emotionality, and sociability), whereas cognition includes attention, memory, comprehension, and problem-solving. Viewing temperament as a group of related traits results in definitions that describe a class of temperamental features which may be described in structural terms or in functional terms. Structural approaches come largely from adult personality research, whereas functional thinking is applied to the internal regulatory roles of temperament. The importance of temperament in regulating social behavior has its roots in clinical research, developmental behavioral genetics, and developmental psychology.

Because of changes with maturation, the issue of temperament being modifiable must be considered. Still, it may be that the core features of temperament show continuity but that the expression of temperament is modifiable over time. If so, temperamental traits can have a dynamic quality. This modifiability, the dynamic changes, might be expressed genetically. The expression of genes would be one substrate for dynamic regulation of temperament during the life span.

Temperamental qualities such as sociability and shyness are generally considered to be dimensional. Kagan et al. (1987) asked whether some temperamental features could better be dealt with in terms of physiobehavioral patterns that are qualitatively distinct. These authors treated temperamental constructs as categories of children instead of assuming a continuous dimension such as sociability. They suggest that their work on inhibition or lack of inhibition to the unfamiliar illustrates the value of this approach (Kagan et al., 1989). Differences among investigators who study temperament reflect different boundaries for defining temperament. Thus, their criteria for the qualities that make up behavioral style, for the relationship of temperament to emotional behavior, for stability of temperament over time, and for the inheritance of temperament vary among them.

In summary, several issues regarding temperament can be said to be established. First, individual children differ from one another in important ways, which can be assessed. These include activity level, autonomic and emotional reactivity, behavioral inhibition in social situations, and sociability (Goldsmith et al., 1987). Second, these differences are important with regard to later development and risk of developing a psychiatric disorder. Interview measurements of temperament predict emotional and behavioral disorders later in development for both high-risk and normal populations (Graham et al., 1973; Kagan et al., 1987; Maziade, Côté, et al., 1989; Maziade, Thivierge, et al., 1989; McCall, 1986; Rutter et al., 1964; Wolkind & De Salis, 1982). For example, questionnaire studies demonstrate an association of difficult temperament with an increased rate of sleep disturbance, colic, and accidents (Bates, 1980; Carey, 1985). In addition, Dunn and Kendrick (1982) demonstrated an increased rate of emotional disturbance in a follow-up study of the impact of the birth of a sibling on a child's behavior. Rutter (1978) demonstrated that temperamental features reported by parents subsequently predicted behavioral disturbances in school 1 year later. Therefore, temperament has been shown to predict behavior at a later date and in new and different social contexts.

Another area of outcome research concerns sex differences in temperament that may arise in early development. How does temperament affect outcome in boys and girls? For example, girls may be at less risk for negative outcomes until entry into adolescence. Temperament exerts its effects through transactions with others and in combination with other risk or protective factors. Regarding outcome, most research has focused on maladjustment, but temperament is also important in successful adjustment. This was demonstrated in Werner and Smith's (1982) population study on the island of Kauai, Hawaii, which discussed the positive influence of an outgoing positive and social temperament in disadvantaged children. The study of protective factors in children's development (Garmezy, 1985; Garmezy et al., 1984) emphasizes temperament as an important feature. Outcome studies of this type emphasize competence rather than psychopathology.

## Effects of Temperament on Others

Children's temperament influences the way others respond to them. For example, Lee and Bates (1985) demonstrated that temperamentally difficult infants had more confrontations with their mothers. Rutter (1978) showed that children with aversive temperament were more likely to be targeted for criticism by their parents. Children with negative mood, a feature of temperament, had greater likelihood of having mothers who were irritable and teachers who seemed to react hostilely. Although the effects do tend to be reciprocal, Stevenson-Hinde and Hinde (1986) found that the effect is greater for that of the child on the adult rather than the reverse.

## Temperament and Neurobiology

The relationship of temperament to neurobiological processes has been suggested by several authors. This approach to viewing neurobiology has been studied more commonly by adult personality theorists. Cloninger (1986) suggested that among the personality dimensions, certain characteristics, such as harm avoidance, are related to high serotonin activity; novelty seeking, low baseline dopaminergic activity, and reward dependence to low basal noradrenergic activity. However, Kagan et al.'s (1987) studies of behavioral inhibition to the unfamiliar relate this characteristic to a low threshold of responsiveness in the limbic and hypothalamic structures, changes in autonomic reactivity, and changes in cortisol levels. Although the reasons for lower thresholds in the limbic sites are not clear, and probably complex, one factor that is likely to contribute is tonically higher levels of central norepinephrine or a higher density of norepinephrine receptors (Kagan et al., 1989). Kagan et al. suggested that the actualization of inhibited behavior may require some form of chronic environmental stress that interacts with the temperamental disposition—a diathesis–stress hypothesis.

## Temperament and Cognition

Whether temperament, the style of responding, is fully independent of cognitive processes has been considered by Prior (1992). One cannot assume there is a period when behavior is not influenced by cognition. For example, when considering self-regulation, behavioral inhibition requires cognitive mediation. Furthermore, cognition influences approach, withdrawal, and sociability. Martin (1989) reviewed studies that investigated the relationship between temperament, particularly adaptability and persistence, and IQ. One longitudinal study (Maziade et al., 1987) found difficult temperament linked to IQ, yet these studies still support the independence of temperament and cognitive factors in very young children. Overall, the interaction between temperament and cognition is increasingly important as the child grows older.

Some temperamental factors may be mediated more by cognition than others. Emotionality is likely to influence cognition because affect may be primary in directing or guiding behavior. Similarly, the feedback between emotionality and cognition must be considered when studying behavioral outcomes. Sociability may have nontemperamental characteristics because it is learned through repeated experiences along with cognitive re-evaluation (Chess & Thomas, 1989). However, individuals do seek out environments that match their temperamental traits, and there is an active role in sustaining temperamental characteristics through environmental feedback. As Scarr and McCartney (1983) have noted, "The genotype determines responsiveness of the person" to the environment. Parental approval and disapproval of temperamental expressions influence these "innate" predispositions, so the child learns to modify their interpersonal behavior (Scarr & McCartney, 1983).

Children do indeed adapt their reactions to who and what is involved in their conflicts. Furthermore, when children fail to develop flexible cognitive scripts, their behavior may become stereotyped. Maladaptive behavior with extreme aggression is an example. Therefore, it is difficult to think of temperament as occurring without cognition or being independent of cognition. Temperament and cognition work in parallel and modify one another. Developmental ideas about schemas and internal working models and cognitive scripts are important in thinking about temperament. Culturally based schemas also contribute to cultural differences in temperament. In the future, cognitive scripts may be found to play a role in modifying temperament and provide conceptual bridges between temperament and personality. These scripts are thought to emerge and become elaborated over time throughout development. The interface of temperament as innate, biologically influenced, and genetically determined, its shaping by environmental experience, and subsequent cognitive interpretation of experience and modification of behavior lead to a broader view of temperament. It is particularly important in developmental disabilities to understand the relationship between temperament and cognition.

## Temperament and Attachment

The constructs of temperament and attachment have been examined with regard to similarities and differences. Does temperament contribute to overall attachment security or influence the specific category of attachment? Although the type of secure or insecure attachment formed with the parent's temperament does not alone determine if a child is securely or insecurely attached (Mangelsdorf & Frosch, 1999), certain temperamental dimensions, such as negative emotionality, can influence the child's behavior in the Strange Situation procedure. Negative emotionality may be associated with proneness to distress during separations. However, this temperamental dimension does not predict overall attachment security. Potentially, a cluster of temperament traits rather than one alone may have correlation rather than a single feature. Examining clusters of temperamental traits may be of value to understand individual differences within attachment categories. Addressing constellations of temperamental features illustrates the value of a transactional approach when considering early social–emotional development. Potentially, temperament and attachment may interact in social–emotional development. Thus, goodness of fit between an infant and parent may predict the security of attachment. Moreover, the effect of infant temperament on infant–caregiver attachment may be indirect and moderated by maternal personality and social support. Overall, temperament and attachment are distinct constructs.

## Assessment of Temperament in Children with Disabilities

The assessment of temperament using behavior ratings is essential in personality research (Carey, 1983; Dunn & Kendrick, 1980; McDevitt & Carey, 1978). Refinement of methodology to study temperament in children with disabilities and those without disabilities is under way with a life span developmental approach. However, temperament has been difficult to evaluate because its measurement is not the assessment of a specific observable and discrete behavior but, rather, the assessment of a pattern of behaviors typically seen in interactions with others. Temperament ratings require that others rate the child's behavior so that biases in an individual's perceptions of a child's behavior or their attributions about the child do not influence their rating. Moreover, temperament measures may encompass both objective and subjective factors.

For behavior rating, the situation used to observe the child's behavior must be clearly defined by the rater. The behavior observed indicates not only personal traits but also a situation-specific reaction to the setting. Because testing usually occurs in a social context, the elicitation of temperament features depends on the properties of that social context. The context includes temperament characteristics in the observer or the person interacting with the child and their past history of interactions together (Dodge, 1980).

For evolutionary purposes, temperament traits have been regarded as aspects of behavior that are pervasive over situations and consistent over time, once bias and behavioral attributions by others have been excluded. The assessor must keep in mind that some behavior traits are only present in specific situations. For example, although emotional reactivity shows heritability and stability over time, it is reliably measured only in stressful situations. This is the case even though temperament is ordinarily considered to be pervasive across all situations.

Kagan et al. (1987) reported that behavioral manifestations of the same trait may change over the course of development. For example, behavioral inhibition may be expressed in an infant who is seeking close proximity to the mother, but in the school-age child, that same trait of behavioral inhibition may be expressed as caution in approaching new tasks. In addition, the elicitation of inhibition requires that the task must be meaningful to the child. Behavioral variation occurring with progressive development makes it unlikely that a predisposition would be expressed in the same way throughout childhood.

## Temperament and Personality

Although in younger children temperament can effectively be viewed as a nonplanned style of responding, it is most likely a pure construct only in very young children, whose behavior is less specifically guided by cognitive processes. When cognitive processes become involved, then the more comprehensive term "personality" must be considered, although temperament does endure, for the most part, as stable behavioral dispositions. Similar language is used by personality theorists and temperament researchers in dealing with older children, particularly for factors such as emotionality and sociability. In school-age children, it is more difficult to differentiate these factors.

## Temperament and Developmental Disabilities

Few studies of temperament in children with neurodevelopmental disorders have been published. Studies of temperament are important in predicting adjustment in children with developmental disabilities, particularly in transactional interactions with others. Specific studies have been conducted in children with Down syndrome (Fidler et al., 2006; Gunn et al., 1983; Zickler et al., 1998), fragile X syndrome (Low Kapalu & Gartstein, 2016; Tonnsen et al., 2019), mild disabilities (Van Tassel, 1984), mixed disabilities, and in children who are neurologically impaired (Heffernan et al., 1982). Moreover, temperament has been investigated in physically handicapped infants during interactions with their mothers (Greenberg & Field, 1982), in developmentally delayed preschool children (Marcovitch et al., 1987), in older children with intellectual developmental disorder (IDD) (Chess & Korn, 1970), and in blind children (Fraiberg, 1974). Few specific discrepancies were noted when comparing the handicapped/developmentally delayed children to neurotypical population samples. Still, brain damage may increase the risk of interpersonal difficulties. Studies of temperament and adjustment for hearing-impaired children (Prior et al., 1988) show that interpersonal relationships have a multivariate nature. In these studies, it has generally been reported that temperament is not a risk factor. However, temperament, in combination with other biological, environmental, and interpersonal variables, may have a significant effect. Knowledge of a handicapped child's temperament and how it matches with the family and social environment may be helpful in reducing conflict for families. Family factors that mediate outcome include psychological functioning, marital adjustment, child-rearing attitudes and practices, social support, and social stress.

A focus on Down syndrome was initiated because children with this disorder represent the largest homogeneous group of developmentally disabled children who may be studied from birth through infancy and into the school-age years (Cicchetti & Sroufe, 1978). However, most developmentally delayed children comprise a heterogeneous population and differ from the Down syndrome group. Therefore, conclusions should be focused on the specific developmental disorder. In children with Down syndrome, as previously demonstrated in normally developing children, there is a shift toward easier temperament with increasing age. Older children with Down syndrome have been rated as being temperamentally easier than neurotypical peers, although during their infancy they were rated as more difficult (Rothbart & Hanson, 1983).

The Early Infant Temperament Questionnaire was completed by 32 families whose infants were diagnosed with Down syndrome at age 1–4 months. Infants with Down syndrome were rated as more active, less intense, and more distractible than neurotypically developing infants. The authors consider unique features to Down syndrome but conclude that these children were more alike than different from aged-matched peers (Zickler et al., 1998).

Because older children with Down syndrome may be temperamentally "easy" and infants with Down syndrome may be temperamentally "difficult," generalization is of limited utility to understand individual children. In one study, a toddler temperament questionnaire was used with mothers of 15 children with Down syndrome who had been evaluated using the Corey Temperament Questionnaire 2 years earlier. Infants originally showing difficult temperament were rated as easier at follow-up. Noting that these scales are potentially biased by a mother's perception, the changes in rating may also reflect reduced maternal anxiety as the mother became more engaged with her child. There is sufficient temperament variation among developmentally delayed children and among those with Down syndrome, in particular, that generalizations cannot be substituted for individual assessments.

In a study of temperament and behavior problems in children with Down syndrome, 24 individuals at 12, 30, and 45 months of age were examined along with a matched control group of 33 children with mixed etiologies for their developmental disabilities. Both the Infant Temperament Questionnaire and behavioral scales (Bayley Scale of Infant Development and Achenbach Child Behavior Checklist) were used. The study reported that internalizing behavioral problems became apparent later in development than in the comparison group with mixed etiologies. Temperament ratings at age 12 months were a stronger predictor of maladaptive behavior at age 45 months. This trajectory of early development of maladaptive behavior has implications for earlier intervention in young children with Down syndrome (Fidler et al., 2006).

Studies of temperament in fragile X syndrome have been carried out in both the premutation (55–200 repeats) and the full syndrome (≥200 repeats). The premutation (1:209 females and 1:430 males) is associated with attention problems, anxiety, and autism-like social behaviors but not IDD. The less common fragile X syndrome (1:4,000) is associated with IDD and more severe behavioral disturbances. Temperament, measured with the Infant Behavior Questionnaire, was assessed in 22 infants with the premutation, 24 with the full fragile X syndrome, and 24 controls (Gartstein & Rothbart, 2003). Temperament in infants with the premutation was rated as showing similarity to that of infants with typical development; however, there was a trend toward suppressed negative affect as found in the full form. Those diagnosed with the full fragile X syndrome were different from control subjects in domains of negative affect and surgency. These findings indicate that *FMR1* gene mutations are associated with atypical temperament that can be identified in early infancy. The negative affect domain was demonstrated with sadness and distress in response to environmental challenges. Infants with fragile X syndrome in the surgency domain were rated as less active, less likely to seek novelty, less vocal with reduced positive affect, and exhibiting less smiling and less laughter. However, preschool and older affected children, who develop attention deficit disorder, show higher levels of surgency (Tonnsen et al., 2019).

Temperament differences have also been examined in 3- to 7-year-old boys with fragile X syndrome (Low Kapalu & Gartstein, 2016). Twenty-six boys were recruited from a national fragile X syndrome center along with 26 controls. Like the infants, boys with fragile X syndrome overall exhibited less surgency/extraversion and effortful control in comparison to controls. Moreover, they displayed significantly greater activity and shyness and less focused attention, inhibitory control, soothability, and high-intensity pleasure than the comparison group. There was a significant interaction between age and diagnosis (fragile X syndrome vs. control group) in negative affectivity. These findings are consistent with attention and effortful control findings in adolescents with fragile X syndrome.

Using temperament measures in children with disabilities is important because knowing a child's temperament can aid both the parent and the clinician in understanding a particular child. The goal is to guide interventions to encourage positive parent–child interaction. Carey and McDevitt (1980) focused on the hyperactive child and proposed that problems in behavior and learning should be understood in terms of a profile that includes the child's temperament. This approach may also be applied to children with other handicapping conditions. Although there is limited literature that addresses the clinical utility of temperament in establishing interventions with developmentally delayed children, there are data available on parental stress. Relative to populations of normally developing children, children with developmental handicaps are perceived by parents as a greater source of stress than children without handicaps.

## Future Research

Future research with developmentally disabled persons should include the development of a normative database of temperament and personality traits for specific disabled populations, improved documentation of developmental changes over time, clarification of the relationship of temperament factors to social interactions, and the use of parental stress indices to provide clinicians with temperament data (Goldberg & Marcovitch, 1989). With better understanding of the impact of temperament on the developmentally disabled, temperament data might be incorporated into a standard assessment profile. The standardization of assessment of temperament will benefit additional study of personality and personality traits in the developmental disorders.

# References

Bates, J. E. (1980). The concept of difficult temperament. *Merrill–Palmer Quarterly of Behavior and Development, 26*(4), 299–319.

Braungart, J. M., Plomin, R., DeFries, J. C., & Fulker, D. W. (1992). Genetic influence on tester-rated infant temperament as assessed by Bayley's Infant Behavior Record: Nonadoptive and adoptive siblings and twins. *Developmental Psychology, 28*(1), 40–47.

Brazelton, T. B. (1978). The Brazelton Neonatal Behavior Assessment Scale: Introduction. *Monographs of the Society for Research in Child Development, 43*(5–6), 1–13.

Burton, R. (1621). *The anatomy of melancholy.* Oxford University Press.

Buzzell, G. A., Troller-Renfree, S. V., Barker, T. V., Bowman, L. C., Chronis-Tuscano, A., Henderson, H. A., Kagan, J., Pine, D., & Fox, N. A. (2017). A neurobehavioral mechanism linking behaviorally inhibited temperament and later adolescent social anxiety. *Journal of the American Academy of Child & Adolescent Psychiatry, 56*(12), 1097–1105.

Campos, J. J., Barrett, K. C., Lamb, M. E., Goldsmith, H. H., & Stenberg, C. (1983). Socioemotional development. In M. M. Haith & J. J. Campos (Eds.), *Handbook of child psychology: Vol. 2. Infancy and developmental psychobiology* (pp. 783–915). Wiley.

Carey, W. B. (1983). Clinical assessment of behavioral style or temperament. In M. D. Levine, W. B. Carey, A. C. Crocker, & R. T. Gross (Eds.), *Developmental–behavioral pediatrics* (pp. 922–926). Saunders.

Carey, W. B. (1985). Clinical use of temperament data in pediatrics. *Journal of Developmental and Behavioral Pediatrics, 6*, 137–142.

Carey, W. B., & McDevitt, S. C. (1980). Minimal brain dysfunction and hyperkinesis: A clinical viewpoint. *American Journal of Diseases of Children, 134*(10), 926–929.

Caspi, A., Harrington, H., Milne, B., Amell, J. W., Theodore, R. F., & Moffitt, T. E. (2003). Children's behavioral styles at age 3 are linked to their adult personality traits at age 26. *Journal of Personality, 71*(4), 495–514.

Chen, X., & Schmidt, L. A. (2015). Temperament and personality. In M. E. Lamb & R. M. Lerner (Eds.), *Handbook of child psychology and developmental science* (pp. 152–200). Wiley.

Chess, S., & Korn, S. (1970). Temperament and behavior disorders in mentally retarded children. *Archives of General Psychiatry, 23*(2), 122–130.

Chess, S., & Thomas, A. (1989). Issues in the clinical application of temperament. In G. A. Kohnstamm, J. E. Bates, & M. K. Rothbart (Eds.), *Temperament in childhood* (pp. 337–386). Wiley.

Chun, K., & Capitanio, J. P. (2016). Developmental consequences of behavioral inhibition: A model in rhesus monkeys (*Macaca mulatta*). *Developmental Science, 19*(6), 1035–1048.

Cicchetti, D., & Sroufe, L. A. (1978). An organizational view of affect: Illustration from the study of Down's syndrome infants. In M. Lewis & L. Rosenblum (Eds.), *The development of affect* (pp. 309–350). Plenum.

Clauss, J. A., & Blackford, J. U. (2012). Behavioral inhibition and risk for developing social anxiety disorder: A meta-analytic study. *Journal of the American Academy of Child & Adolescent Psychiatry, 51*(10), 1066–1075.

Cloninger, C. R. (1986). A unified biosocial theory of personality and its role in the development of anxiety states. *Psychiatric Developments, 3*(2), 167–226.

Costa, P. T., Jr., & McCrae, R. R. (1992). The five-factor model of personality and its relevance to personality disorders. *Journal of Personality Disorders, 6*(4), 343–359.

Davis, K. L., & Panksepp, J. (2011). The brain's emotional foundations of human personality and the Affective Neuroscience Personality Scales. *Neuroscience & Biobehavioral Reviews, 35*(9), 1946–1958.

Diamond, S. E. (1974). *The roots of psychology: A sourcebook in the history of ideas.* Basic Books.

Dilalla, L. F., Kagan, J., & Reznick, J. S. (1994). Genetic etiology of behavioral inhibition among 2-year-old children. *Infant Behavior and Development, 17*(4), 405–412.

Dodge, K. A. (1980). Social cognition and children's aggressive behavior. *Child Development, 51,* 162–172.

Dunn, J., & Kendrick, C. (1980). Studying temperament and parent–child interaction: Comparison of interview and direct observation. *Developmental Medicine & Child Neurology, 22*(4), 484–496.

Dunn, J., & Kendrick, C. (1982). Temperamental differences, family relationships, and young children's response to change within the family. In R. Porter & G. M. Collins (Eds.), *Temperamental differences in infants and young children* (pp. 87–120). Ciba Foundation.

Ellis, B. J., Boyce, W. T., Belsky, J., Bakermans-Kranenburg, M. J., & Van IJzendoorn, M. H. (2011). Differential susceptibility to the environment: An evolutionary–neurodevelopmental theory. *Development and Psychopathology, 23*(1), 7–28.

Evans, D. E., & Rothbart, M. K. (2007). Developing a model for adult temperament. *Journal of Research in Personality, 41*(4), 868–888.

Eysenck, H. J., & Eysenck, M. W. (1987). *Personality and individual differences.* Plenum Press.

Fidler, D., Most, D., Booth-LaForce, C., & Kelly, J. (2006). Temperament and behaviour problems in young children with Down syndrome at 12, 30, and 45 months. *Down Syndrome Research and Practice, 10*(1), 23–29.

Fox, N. A., & Walker, O. L. (2015). Temperament: Individual differences in reactivity and regulation as antecedent to personality. *Rutter's Child and Adolescent Psychiatry, 6,* 93–104.

Fraiberg, S. (1974). Blind infants and their mothers: An examination of the sign system. In M. Lewis & L. Rosenblum (Eds.), *The effect of the infant on its caregiver.* Wiley.

Garmezy, N. (1985). Stress-resilient children: The search for protective factors. In J. E. Stevenson (Ed.), *Recent research in developmental psychopathology* (pp. 213–233). Pergamon.

Garmezy, N. Masten, A. S., & Tellegen, A. (1984). The study of stress and competence in children: A building block for developmental psychopathology. *Child Development, 55,* 87–111.

Gartstein, M. A., Bridgett, D. J., Young, B. N., Panksepp, J., & Power, T. (2013). Origins of effortful control: Infant and parent contributions. *Infancy, 18*(2), 149–183.

Gartstein, M. A., & Rothbart, M. K. (2003). Studying infant temperament via the revised Infant Behavior Questionnaire. *Infant Behavior and Development, 26*(1), 64–86.

Goldberg, S., & Marcovitch, S. (1989). Temperament in developmentally disabled children. In G. A. Kohnstamm, J. E. Bates, & M. K. Rothbart (Eds.), *Temperament in childhood* (pp. 398–404). Wiley.

Goldsmith, H. H., Buss, K. A., & Lemery, K. S. (1997). Toddler and childhood temperament: Expanded content, stronger genetic evidence, new evidence for the importance of environment. *Developmental Psychology, 33*(6), 891–905.

Goldsmith, H. H., Buss, A. H., Plomin, R., Rothbart, M. K., Thomas, A., Chess, S., Hinde, R. A., & McCall, R. B. (1987). Roundtable: What is temperament? Four approaches. *Child Development, 58*(2), 505–529.

Goldsmith, H. H., & Campos, J. J. (1986). Fundamental issues in the study of early temperament: The Denver Twin Temperament Study. *Advances in Developmental Psychology, 4,* 231–283.

Gosling, S. D., & John, O. P. (1999). Personality dimensions in nonhuman animals: A cross-species review. *Current Directions in Psychological Science, 8*(3), 69–75.

Graham, P., Rutter, M., & George, S. (1973). Temperamental characteristics as predictors of behavior disorders in children. *American Journal of Orthopsychiatry, 43,* 328–339.

Greenberg, R., & Field, T. (1982). Temperament ratings of handicapped infants during classroom, mother, and teacher interactions. *Journal of Pediatric Psychology, 7*(4), 387–405.

Gunn, P., Berry, P., & Andrews, R. J. (1983). The temperament of Down's syndrome toddlers: A research note. *Journal of Child Psychology and Psychiatry, 24*(4), 601–605.

Guyer, A. E., Benson, B., Choate, V. R., Bar-Haim, Y., Perez-Edgar, K., Jarcho, J. M., Pine, D. S., Ernst, M., Fox, N. A., & Nelson, E. E. (2014). Lasting associations between early-childhood temperament and late-adolescent reward-circuitry response to peer feedback. *Development and Psychopathology, 26*(1), 229–243.

Hagekull, B., & Bohlin, G. (2003). Early temperament and attachment as predictors of the Five Factor Model of personality. *Attachment & Human Development, 5*(1), 2–18.

Heffernan, L., William Black, F., & Poche, P. (1982). Temperament patterns in young neurologically impaired children. *Journal of Pediatric Psychology, 7*(4), 415–423.

Henderson, H. A., Pine, D. S., & Fox, N. A. (2015). Behavioral inhibition and developmental risk: A dual-processing perspective. *Neuropsychopharmacology, 40*(1), 207–224.

Kagan, J. (1997). Temperament and the reactions to unfamiliarity. *Child Development, 68*(1), 139–143.

Kagan, J., Reznick, J. S., & Snidman, N. (1987). The physiology and psychology of behavioral inhibition in children. *Child Development, 58*(6), 1459–1473.

Kagan, J., Reznick, J. S., & Snidman, N. (1989). Issues in the study of temperament. In G. A. Kohnstamm, J. E. Bates, & M. K. Rothbart (Eds.), *Temperament in childhood* (pp. 133–144). Wiley.

Kagan, J., Snidman, N., Kahn, V., Towsley, S., Steinberg, L., & Fox, N. A. (2007). The preservation of two infant temperaments into adolescence. *Monographs of the Society for Research in Child Development, 72,* 19–30.

Kenwood, M. M., & Kalin, N. H. (2021) Nonhuman primate models to explore mechanisms underlying early-life temperamental anxiety. *Biological Psychiatry, 89*(7), 659–671.

King, J. E., & Figueredo, A. J. (1997). The five-factor model plus dominance in chimpanzee personality. *Journal of Research in Personality, 31*(2), 257–271.

Krueger, R. F., South, S., Johnson, W., & Iacono, W. (2008). The heritability of personality is not always 50%: Gene–environment interactions and correlations between personality and parenting. *Journal of Personality, 76*(6), 1485–1522.

Lahat, A., Lamm, C., Chronis-Tuscano, A., Pine, D. S., Henderson, H. A., & Fox, N. A. (2014). Early behavioral inhibition and increased error monitoring predict later social phobia symptoms in childhood. *Journal of the American Academy of Child & Adolescent Psychiatry, 53*(4), 447–455.

Lee, C. L., & Bates, J. E. (1985). Mother–child interaction at age two years and perceived difficult temperament. *Child Development, 56,* 1314–1325.

Lonigan, C. J., & Vasey, M. W. (2009). Negative affectivity, effortful control, and attention to threat-relevant stimuli. *Journal of Abnormal Child Psychology, 37*(3), 387–399.

Low Kapalu, C. M., & Gartstein, M. A. (2016). Boys with fragile X syndrome: Investigating temperament in early childhood. *Journal of Intellectual Disability Research, 60*(9), 891–900.

Mangelsdorf, S. C., & Frosch, C. A. (1999). Temperament and attachment: One construct or two? *Advances in Child Development and Behavior, 27,* 181–220.

Marcovitch, S., Goldberg, S., Lojkasek, M., & MacGregor, D. (1987). The concept of difficult temperament in the developmentally disabled preschool child. *Journal of Applied Developmental Psychology, 8*(2):151–164.

Martin, R. (1989). Activity level, distractibility and persistence: Critical characteristics in early schooling. In G. A. Kohnstamm, J. E. Bates, & M. K. Rothbart (Eds.), *Temperament in childhood* (pp. 451–462). Wiley.

Maziade, M., Côté, R., Bernier, H., Boutin, P., & Thivierge, J. (1989). Significance of extreme temperament in infancy for clinical status in preschool years: I. Value of extreme temperament at 4–8 months for predicting diagnosis at 4-7 years. *British Journal of Psychiatry, 154*(4), 535–543.

Maziade, M., Côté, R., Boutin, P., Bernier, H., & Thivierge, J. (1987). Temperament and intellectual development: A longitudinal study from infancy to four years. *American Journal of Psychiatry, 144*(2), 144–150.

Maziade, M., Thivierge, J., Côté, R., Boutin, P., & Bernier, H. (1989). Significance of extreme temperament in infancy for clinical status in preschool years: II. Patterns of temperament change and implications for the appearance of disorders. *British Journal of Psychiatry, 154*(4), 544–551.

McCall, R. B. (1986). Issues of stability and continuity in temperament research. In R. Plomin & J. Dunn (Eds.), *The study of temperament: Changes, continuities, and challenges* (pp. 13–26). Psychology Press.

McCrae, R. R., & Costa, P. T. (1987). Validation of the five-factor model of personality across instruments and observers. *Journal of Personality and Social Psychology, 52*(1), 81–90.

McCrae, R. R., Costa, P. T., Jr., Ostendorf, F., Angleitner, A., Hřebíčková, M., Avia, M. D., Sanz, J., Sanchez-Bernardos, M. L., Kusdil, M. E., Woodfield, R., Saunders, P. R., & Smith, P. B. (2000). Nature over nurture: Temperament, personality, and life span development. *Journal of Personality and Social Psychology, 78*(1), 173–186.

McDermott, J. M., Perez-Edgar, K., Henderson, H. A., Chronis-Tuscano, A., Pine, D. S., & Fox, N. A. (2009). A history of childhood behavioral inhibition and enhanced response monitoring in adolescence are linked to clinical anxiety. *Biological Psychiatry, 65*(5), 445–448.

McDevitt, S. C., & Carey, W. B. (1978). The measurement of temperament in 3–7 year old children. *Journal of Child Psychology and Psychiatry, 19*(3), 245–253.

Panksepp, J. (2004). *Affective neuroscience: The foundations of human and animal emotions.* Oxford University Press.

Plomin, R., Emde, R. N., Braungart, J. M., Campos, J., Corley, R., Fulker, D., Kagan, J., Reznick, J. S., Robinson, J., & Zahn-Waxler, C. (1993). Genetic change and continuity from fourteen to twenty months: The MacArthur Longitudinal Twin Study. *Child Development, 64*(5), 1354–1376.

Posner, M. I., & Rothbart, M. K. (2018). Temperament and brain networks of attention. *Philosophical Transactions of the Royal Society B: Biological Sciences, 373*(1744), 20170254.

Prior, M. (1992). Childhood temperament. *Journal of Child Psychology and Psychiatry, 33,* 249–279.

Prior, M. Glazner, J., Sanson, A., & Debelle, G. (1988). Temperament and behavioural adjustment in hearing impaired children. *Journal of Child Psychology and Psychiatry, 29,* 209–216.

Rothbart, M. K. (1981). Measurement of temperament in infancy. *Child Development, 52*(2), 569–578.

Rothbart, M. K. (1989). Biological processes in temperament. In G. A. Kohnstamm, J. E. Bates, & M. J. Rothbart (Eds.), *Temperament in childhood* (pp. 77–110). Wiley.

Rothbart, M. K. (2007). Temperament, development, and personality. *Current Directions in Psychological Science, 16*(4), 207–212.

Rothbart, M. K. (2011). *Becoming who we are: Temperament and personality in development.* Guilford.

Rothbart, M. K., & Hanson, M. J. (1983). A caregiver report comparison of temperamental characteristics of Down syndrome and normal infants. *Developmental Psychology, 19*(5), 766–769.

Rothbart, M. K., Sheese, B. E., & Posner, M. I. (2007). Executive attention and effortful control: Linking temperament, brain networks, and genes. *Child Development Perspectives, 1*(1), 2–7.

Rueda, M. (2012). Effortful control. In M. Zentner & R. L. Shiner (Eds.), *Handbook of temperament* (pp. 145–167). Guilford.

Rutter, M. (1978). Surveys to answer questions. In P. Graham (Ed.), *Epidemiological approaches in child psychiatry.* Academic Press.

Rutter, M. (1987). Temperament, personality and personality disorder. *British Journal of Psychiatry, 150*(4), 443–458.

Rutter, M., Birch, H., Thomas, A., & Chess, S. (1964). Temperament characteristics in infancy and the later development of behavior disorders. *British Journal of Psychiatry, 110,* 651–661.

Saudino, K. J. (2005). Behavioral genetics and child temperament. *Journal of Developmental and Behavioral Pediatrics, 26*(3), 214–223.

Scarr, S., & McCartney, K. (1983). How people make their own environments: A theory of genotype environment effects. *Child Development, 54,* 424–435.

Stevenson-Hinde, J., & Hinde, R. A. (1986). Changes in associations between characteristics. In R. Plomin & J. Dunn (Eds.), *The study of temperament: Changes, continuities and challenges*. Erlbaum.

Tellegen, A., Lykken, D. T., Bouchard, T. J., Wilcox, K. J., Segal, N. L., & Rich, S. (1988). Personality similarity in twins reared apart and together. *Journal of Personality and Social Psychology*, *54*(6), 1031–1039.

Thomas, A., & Chess, S. (1977). *Temperament and development*. Brunner/Mazel.

Thomas, A., & Chess, S. (1986). *Temperament in clinical practice*. Guilford.

Thomas, A., Chess, S., Birch, H., Hertzig, M., & Korn, S. (1963). *Behavioral individuality in early childhood*. New York University Press.

Tonnsen, B. L., Wheeler, A. C., Hamrick, L. R., & Roberts, J. E. (2019). Infant temperament in the FMR 1 premutation and fragile X syndrome. *Journal of Clinical Child & Adolescent Psychology*, *48*(3), 412–422.

Van Tassel, E. (1984). Temperament characteristics of mildly developmentally delayed infants. *Developmental and Behavioral Pediatrics*, *5*, 11–14.

Vasey, M. W., Bosmans, G., & Ollendick, T. H. (2014). The developmental psychopathology of anxiety. In M. Lewis & K. D. Rudolph (Eds.), *Handbook of developmental psychopathology* (pp. 543–560). Springer.

Victor, J. B., Rothbart, M. K., Baker, S. R., & Tackett, J. L. (2016). Temperamental components of the developing personality. In U. Kumar (Ed.), *The Wiley handbook of personality assessment* (pp. 44–58). Wiley.

Webb, E. (1915). Character and intelligence. *British Journal of Psychology Monographs Supplements*, No. 3.

Werner, E. E., & Smith, R. S. (1982). *Vulnerable but invincible: A study of resilient children*. McGraw-Hill.

Wolkind, S. N., & De Salis, W. (1982). Infant temperament, maternal mental stage and child behavioural problems. *Ciba Foundation Symposium*, *89*, 221–239.

Wundt, W. (1903). *Grundzuge der physiologischen Psychologie* (5th ed., Vol. 3). Engelmann.

Zickler, C. F., Morrow, J. D., & Bull, M. J. (1998). Infants with Down syndrome: A look at temperament. *Journal of Pediatric Health Care*, *12*(3), 111–117.

# PART IV
# NEURODEVELOPMENTAL DISORDERS

# 14

# Intellectual Developmental Disorder

How to best define and classify intellectual deficits in the classification of mental disorders has been a long-standing debate. Historically, Esquirol (1845) referred to intellectual deficits overall as conditions of incomplete mental development based on known (or unknown) biological or environmental causes, indicating that it is a neurodevelopmental disorder. Over the past centuries, the diagnostic terminology has changed at least 10 times. Moreover, because people with intellectual deficits are often undervalued in society, terms for describing them have been used disparagingly, leading to stigmatization. Throughout the years, the terms moron, imbecile, and idiot were replaced in classification by "mental deficiency," "mental handicap," and "mental retardation" as less pejorative terminology. With continuing efforts to deal with the social meaning of diagnostic labels for disabling conditions, these terms, too, by focusing on deficiencies, became pejorative. Thus, we currently use the more neutral term intellectual developmental disorder (IDD). From a neurodevelopmental perspective, IDD is a failure of cognitive progression with onset in infancy. It is classified in the fifth edition of the *Diagnostic and Statistical Manual of Mental Disorders* (DSM-5; American Psychiatric Association [APA], 2013) under the general category neurodevelopmental disorders. There are concurrent deficits in adaptive reasoning, adaptive behaviors, and functioning in academic and social domains in DSM-5, the focus of which is on mental disorders. For the American Association on Intellectual and Developmental Disabilities (AAIDD), the focus of which is on disability and functional deficits, greater emphasis is placed on identification of needed supports (Schalock, 2011; Schalock et al., 2021).

This chapter uses the term *intellectual developmental disorder* in keeping with the diagnostic terms used in the DSM-5 and the 11th revision of the *International Statistical Classification of Diseases and Related Health Problems* (ICD-11; World Health Organization [WHO], 2018). IDD is not a static condition but, rather, a dynamic one, which has multiple etiologies that must be considered in treatment planning. It is not a disease or an illness in itself but, rather, has heterogeneous etiologies. In IDD, thinking is not characteristically disordered, and perception is not distorted unless there is a concurrent mental disorder. This heterogeneous group of conditions ranges from genetic and metabolic disorders to functional changes following trauma to the nervous system at birth or later in development. Because of its heterogeneity, each case must be considered independently according to whether there is an associated syndrome (e.g., Down syndrome) or an associated etiology (e.g., head trauma). There is no single cause, mechanism, clinical course, or prognosis.

Persons with an IDD can suffer from a full range of mental disorders. In fact, the occurrence of an associated mental disorder is three or four times greater than in the general population. Furthermore, persons with an IDD are at greater risk for exploitation and physical or sexual abuse. Because adaptive functioning is, by definition, impaired, social stressors are particularly problematic. However, in protective social environments in which adequate support is available, their impairments may not be obvious; this is particularly true of persons with mild involvement.

This chapter reviews the history, diagnosis and classification, epidemiology, etiology, developmental issues, genetics, psychiatric assessment, psychopathology, and treatment of IDD. Public law and the right to education and legal competency are also discussed.

## History

Historically, the earliest reference to IDD is in the Egyptian Papyrus of Thebes (1552 BCE) (Bryan, 1930). Despite recognition since antiquity, there is little evidence of early medical interest in IDD. Religious references in the various traditions suggest people with IDD be treated with kindness. Despite these admonishments, humane education is a recent development. In Greek and Roman cultures, infanticide was practiced, and trephining has been used in Europe and Central and South America as an intervention, presumably to release or remove evil spirits. People diagnosed with an IDD may have become slaves in some cultures or chosen for court jesters. Throughout history, attitudes varied from humane concern to ostracism and abuse. In some countries, persons with IDD were viewed as harmless innocents who were allowed to wander at will. Henry II of England showed a more enlightened view and promulgated legislation to provide for their protection, making them wards of the king.

It was not until approximately the end of the 18th century that a rising respect for the individual, which provided the impetus for the French and American Revolutions, began to address the rights not only of slaves, mentally ill people, the blind, and the deaf but also those with IDD (Kanner, 1964). Early interventionists such as Jean-Marc-Gaspard Itard, against the better judgment of the experts of the time, spent 5 years (1801—1806) trying to teach Victor, the wild boy of Aveyron (Lane, 1976). Although Victor did not achieve normalization, the methods Itard developed were recognized as highly meritorious by the French Academy of Sciences, which closely followed his interventions. Subsequently, an organized effort to educate persons with IDD began in Switzerland and eventually spread to other areas of Europe and to the United States. Interest in IDD at the time was stimulated by new, more hopeful ideas about development inspired by the philosophy of Rousseau, the encyclopedists, and Pestalozzi. Itard's subsequent work in an institution for deaf-mutes encouraged Edouard Séguin to devote himself to the investigation and treatment of persons with IDD. Itard was influenced not only by his teachers but also by his religious orientation. He was "striving for a social application of the principles of the gospel, for the most rapid evolution of the lowest and poorest by all means and institutions, mostly by free education" (Kanner, 1960).

Like Itard, Séguin began to work individually with a boy with intellectual deficits and, based on his success, began working with more children at the Hospice for Incurables (Kanner, 1960). By 1844, Séguin was acknowledged by a commission of the Paris Academy of Sciences, and his achievements were documented in his classical textbook (Séguin, 1846). He reported that his training of persons with an IDD embraced "the muscular, imitative, nervous, and reflective functions." Later, Séguin came to the

United States, where he contacted Samuel Gridley Howe, who was instrumental in establishing interventions for people with IDD. Séguin's (1866) textbook, *Idiocy and Its Treatment by the Physiological Method*, advocated building an institution as an instrument for the treatment setting for children who were too severely disordered in intellectual development to profit from normal classroom instruction. In 1876, Séguin was selected as the first president of the Medical Officers of American Institutes for Idiotic and Feeble-Minded Persons, which is now the American Association on Intellectual and Developmental Disabilities.

The first medical periodical devoted to IDD, *Observations on Cretinism*, was published in 1850. Wilhelm Griesinger (1876) stated that although every cretin is developmentally impaired, every person with an IDD is not a cretin. In doing so, he insisted that IDD is a comprehensive category (meta category) and not a single entity (Salvador-Carulla et al., 2011). The general trend at that time was to make no distinctions among the various types of IDD. Amentia or idiocy was thought to be a homogeneous category, and both "idiocy" and "insanity" were regarded as interchangeable entities. Subsequently, a breakthrough was made in distinguishing the heterogeneous nature of IDD by John L. H. Down in his classical paper, *Observations on an Ethnic Classification of Idiots* (Down, 1866).

With the recognition that IDD was not a homogeneous category, a new interest developed in classification. However, Down was initially misled by the physical appearance of the individuals he examined. In the hope of absolving parents of self-blame by emphasizing a constitutional basis, he developed an ethnic classification, suggesting the various forms of IDD represented regressions to earlier racial forms. He subsequently abandoned this idea and proposed that the best classification is one based on etiology. He recognized three major groups: (a) congenital, which included microcephalic, macrocephalic, hydrocephalic, epileptic, and paralytic; (b) developmental, with a vulnerability to mental breakdown during a developmental crisis; and (c) accidental (caused by injury or illness). Subsequently, William Weatherspoon Ireland (1877), in his textbook *On Idiocy and Imbecility*, suggested 10 subdivisions: genetic (congenital), microcephalic, epileptic, eclamptic, hydrocephalic, paralytic, traumatic, inflammatory, cretinism, and idiocy by deprivation. The way was prepared to differentiate specific conditions that differed in both pathology and etiology but were characterized by intellectual deficits. Later, tuberous sclerosis was identified by Desire-Maglione Bourneville (1880), and many degenerative diseases were recognized, such as Tay–Sachs disease. These findings established the view that IDD is caused by brain pathology and is incurable. Thus began an era of searching for more clearly defined disorders, which were commonly named after their discoverers. It was an era in which syndromes were recognized, but medicine had little to offer therapeutically. The only amelioration that was offered was provided by educators. The recognition of brain pathology raised questions about the possibility of any medical habilitation.

With the discovery of intelligence testing and the establishment of an interest in eugenics, interest turned to the heredity of disorders of intellectual development. Psychometric tests were developed in France by two physicians, Alfred Binet and Theodore Simon, in 1904. They viewed their test as a way to identify children for specialized education. However, when they were introduced in the United States in 1908 by Henry Goddard, these tests were used specifically to diagnose IDD. The testing of large numbers of individuals at various ages was carried out in the United States. Intelligence quotients (IQs), which resulted from the tests, were considered to be an accurate measure of intelligence. Intelligence was thought to be a constant feature that reflected a permanent and inherent level of mental ability. Because the tests were considered objective and scientific, they gradually replaced the individualized clinical evaluation. The tests were used in correctional institutions, where drug abusers, prostitutes, and others showing antisocial behavior commonly tested in the mild range of IDD. Some considered IDD to be the source of their antisocial behavior rather than considering fully the relationship of socially maladaptive behavior to neglect, poverty, and mistreatment.

Following the discovery of Gregor Mendel's principles of genetic inheritance, books such as Goddard's (1912) *The Kallikak Family* sought to document that IDD and antisocial behavior were genetically rather than socially transmitted. Goddard's description of the Kallikak family pictured persons with IDD as menaces to society and a source of criminality, drug abuse, and the genetic source of children with an IDD. Subsequently, the eugenics movement embraced the idea that persons with mild disorders of intellectual development were a danger to society due to their "moral imbecility," indiscriminate sexual behavior, and excessive procreation. The eugenics movement suggested their indiscriminate sexual behavior would lead to an increase in persons with an IDD, resulting in an increasingly delinquent population. Eugenic considerations led to a movement to place persons with an IDD in institutions and to sterilize them. As a result of such views, the size of the institutionalized population increased, as did the numbers admitted with emotional and behavior disorders.

The first preventive intervention for IDD occurred when Ivar Asbjörn Følling (1888–1973) in 1934 recognized that phenylketonuria (PKU) was a metabolic disturbance that could be reversed by dietary restrictions. The recognition of a biochemically based syndrome led to the establishment of IDD research as a legitimate focus in the biological sciences. The medical profession began to more carefully attempt to to identify the etiology of IDD syndromes (Kanner, 1967).

Following World War II, change in community attitudes re-emphasized the possibility of remediation, analogous to what had taken place a century and a half before when Itard initiated the first remedial education program. This impetus for improved remediation developed from the response of parents to the needs of their children. In the 1950s, parent groups were organized in the United States and other countries, culminating in the establishment of the National Association for Retarded Children in the United States. An advisory board drawn from representatives of the various specialties, who might work for the study of prevention and care of IDD, was established. This new thrust was most clearly demonstrated by U.S. President John F. Kennedy (February 5, 1963). In his congressional message on mental illness and IDD, he called for "a national program to combat intellectual developmental disorder." This national program brought medicine, education, psychology, sociology, genetics, and other specialties that are pertinent to the needs of children who have IDD together into special centers affiliated with universities to provide intervention. Through research centers for IDD that were federally funded, research began to grow. Finally, academic medicine had become fully involved with other specialties, community organizations, and parent groups to study the etiology of neurodevelopmental syndromes, establish therapeutic interventions, and develop habilitation and prevention programs.

Neuropsychiatrists were frequently superintendents of the early institutions for persons with IDD. Later, child guidance clinics were involved in preventive care. However, with the expansion of psychoanalytic schools in the United States after World War II, psychiatric involvement with IDD declined as verbal, psychodynamically oriented therapy became the primary mode of treatment. Because of their cognitive deficiencies, persons with IDD were unable to benefit from a traditional psychoanalytic approach that was verbal, conceptual, and insight oriented. Advances in neuroscience, developmental psychology, developmental psychopathology, phenomenology as well as classification, family history, behavior, and drug treatments have led to a new perspective in psychiatry and a renewed commitment to persons with IDD. Recognition of the role of experience in brain development and a better understanding of the natural history of specific IDD syndromes have led to participation of psychiatrists with other professionals in the habilitation of individuals with IDD.

## Diagnosis and Classification

Intellectual developmental disorder is defined in the DSM-5, ICD-11, and by the AAIDD (Schalock et al., 2021). Although all of these definitions include standardized measurement of intelligence and adaptive functioning, each provides a different emphasis, so it is important to be familiar with each of them. In applying the definitions, keep in mind that specific adaptive abilities often coexist with strengths in other adaptive skills or personal capabilities; therefore, adaptive strengths must be carefully considered.

WHO, unlike the USA, has two classifications: the *International Classification of Diseases* (ICD) and the *International Classification of Functioning* (ICF). The DSM-5 definition of IDD, following the ICD, focuses on health conditions and makes clear that it is a classification of mental disorders. ICD-11 uses the diagnostic term *disorders of intellectual development*, and following the ICD, DSM-5 uses the designation *intellectual developmental disorder*. The ICF focuses on human functioning. The AAIDD, rather than emphasizing an underlying person-centered neurobiological deficit, focuses on the social interface between a person and the environment.

The AAIDD states that without adequate environmental supports, the degree of functional disability can worsen. The differences in DSM-5 and AAIDD classification systems reflect the importance of having two systems, as does the WHO, to address both the mental disorder (DSM-5) and the importance of providing supports (AAIDD) to enhance functioning. Both DSM-5 and the AAIDD require intellectual deficit measures based on individualized standardized testing, deficits in adaptive functioning, and skills in cognitive, practical, and social domains with onset in the developmental period.

DSM-5 is the official classification for mental disorders in the United States, and by international agreement, it shares diagnostic codes with the ICD. For DSM-5, there was liaison with the WHO ICD-11 committee to ensure harmonization of the two classifications. The ICD-11 committee at the time that DSM-5 was being finalized used the term *intellectual developmental disorder* (the newest draft uses *disorders of intellectual development*). To harmonize the naming and to make clear that the DSM-5 definition was on disorder, the final naming agreed upon in DSM-5 is *intellectual disability (intellectual developmental disorder)*. The term *intellectual developmental disorder* in parentheses is listed to make clear that the DSM-5 focus is on disorder and not the disability construct preferred by the AAIDD and the ICF. Moreover, the term *intellectual disability* is used in the scientific literature in the United States for both the disorder construct and the disability construct. In DSM-5, severity is not based on IQ score but, rather, on the severity of the adaptive functioning impairments in conceptual, social, and practical domains.

DSM-5 states that the use of a battery of neuropsychological tests that measure discrete intellectual functions, such as verbal comprehension, executive functions, and memory, provides a better description of a person's overall cognitive abilities than an IQ test alone. As noted in the explanatory text to DSM-5, "In some instances if adaptive deficits are severe, then one can meet criteria based on those adaptive deficits even if the IQ is in the 70s" (APA, 2013, p. 37).

The third criterion is onset of deficits in the developmental period, which means that the deficits in adaptive functioning are recognized in early life and persist throughout life. Intellectual disability (ID) is not simply a developmental delay but, rather, a long-term chronic disorder of functioning. Thus, any assessment of adaptive functioning must take into account early developmental history and make reference to school records, testing, and reports.

Finally, individuals with IDD are at increased risk of co-occurring mental disorders that further impair their adaptive functioning. These diagnoses occur in up to one-third of cases with IDD in published studies and include the full range of psychiatric disorders, such as attention deficit disorder, schizophrenia, major depression, and bipolar disorder. The co-occurrence of mental disorders further impacts adaptive functioning (Harris, 2014).

## Adoption of the Deviation IQ Method

The first widely used intelligence test was devised in France by Binet and Simon in the first decade of the 20th century. Goddard and Terman express the results as a measure of mental age (MA). This was determined by establishing mean scores for all subjects in a standardization sample. The tested individual is compared to a norm table, and their MA is established identifying the comparable age mean. Thus, if a 15-year-old subject scored at the mean level of a 10-year-old, they would have a chronological age (CA) of 15 years and an MA of 10 years.

## DSM-5

### Diagnostic Features

In DSM-5, the essential features of IDD are deficits in general mental abilities (Criterion A) and impairment in everyday adaptive functioning, in comparison to an individual's age, gender, and socioculturally matched peers (Criterion B). Onset is during the developmental period (Criterion C). In DSM-5, the diagnosis of IDD is based on both clinical assessment and standardized testing of intellectual functions, along with standardized neuropsychological tests.

Importantly, in DSM-5, the emphasis changed, putting greater weight on adaptive functioning and less emphasis on the IQ number. The new conceptualization of IDD draws attention to a range of neuropsychiatric syndromes, each of which has early onset with cognitive impairments and deficits in learning and adaptive functioning. Because intelligence is made up of distinct but related processes, individuals with the same IQ level may have different cognitive profiles (Bertelli et al., 2014, 2018; Greenspan, 2017; Greenspan, Harris, et al., 2015; Greenspan & Woods, 2014; Harris & Greenspan, 2016; Haydt et al., 2013). Moreover, the range of intellectual deficits requires that neuropsychological tests be used to measure mental functions such as executive functioning and spatial cognition.

Included among intellectual functions listed in Criterion A are those that involve reasoning, problem-solving, planning, abstract thinking, judgment, learning from instruction and experience, and practical understanding (Evans, 2008; Gottfredson, 1997; Harris, 2006; King & Kitchner, 2002; Margolis, 1987; Schalock, 2011; WHO, 2011). Critical components assessed on testing include verbal comprehension, working memory, perceptual reasoning, quantitative reasoning, abstract thought, and cognitive efficacy. Importantly, intellectual functioning must be measured using individually administered and psychometrically valid, comprehensive, and culturally appropriate tests of intelligence. Individuals with IDD have scores of approximately 2 standard deviations (SDs) or more below the population mean. Because the IQ score represents a range, a margin for measurement error (generally ±5 points) is included. Therefore, on tests with an SD of 15 and a mean of 100, this yields a score with a range of 65–75 (70 ± 5). Clinical training and judgment are needed to interpret test results and assess actual intellectual performance.

Still, IQ test scores are approximations of conceptual functioning. They may be insufficient to assess reasoning in real-life situations and the mastery of practical tasks (Bertelli et al., 2018; Flanagan & McGrew, 1997; Harris, 2006; Harris & Greenspan, 2016; Schalock, 2011; Yalon-Chamovitz & Greenspan, 2005). An individual with an IQ score above 70 may have severe adaptive behavior problems in social judgment, social understanding, and other areas of adaptive functioning so that their actual social functioning is comparable to that of individuals with a lower IQ score. Consequently, clinical judgment is needed for interpreting the results of IQ tests.

Practice effects (learning from a repeated testing) may affect IQ test scores. Moreover, the IQ number must be adjusted when test scores are updated and renamed. The "Flynn effect" refers to the need to readjust scores by up to 3 points to account for out-of-date test norms. Current data support a model of intelligence made up of distinct but related processes, as noted above. Individuals with the same IQ level may have different cognitive profiles (Bertelli et al., 2014, 2018; Greenspan, 2017; Greenspan, Harris, et al., 2015; Greenspan & Woods, 2014; Harris & Greenspan, 2016; Haydt et al., 2014).

The second criterion, deficits in adaptive functioning (Criterion B), refers to how well a person can cognitively meet community standards of personal independence and social responsibility compared to others of similar age and sociocultural background (Tassé et al., 2012). Adaptive functioning is defined in three domains: conceptual, social, and practical. The conceptual (academic) domain includes competence in memory, language, reading, writing, math reasoning, acquisition of practical knowledge, problem-solving, and judgment in novel situations, among others. The social domain includes awareness of others' thoughts, feelings, and experiences; empathy; interpersonal communication skills; friendship abilities; and social judgment; among others. The practical domain includes learning and self-management across life settings, such as personal care, job responsibilities, money management, recreation, self-management of behavior, and school and work task organization, among others. Intellectual capacity, education, motivation, socialization, personality features, vocational opportunity, cultural experience, and coexisting general medical conditions or mental disorders influence adaptive functioning. The second criterion is met when at least one of the three domains of adaptive functioning—conceptual, social, or practical—is impaired so that ongoing support is essential for the person to effectively engage in one or more of these life settings: school, work, home, or the community.

The third criterion, Criterion C, requires onset during the developmental period. It recognizes that intellectual and adaptive deficits must be present during childhood or adolescence (Greenspan, 2016; Harris & Greenspan, 2016; Tassé et al., 2016). Co-occurring disorders that affect communication, language, and/or motor or sensory function may affect test scores. Individual cognitive profiles based on neuropsychological testing as well as cross-battery intellectual assessment (using multiple IQ or other cognitive tests to create a profile) are more useful for understanding intellectual abilities than a single IQ test score (Flanagan & McGrew, 1997; Greenspan, 2017). The rationale for adding cross-battery intellectual assessment is that the use of multiple IQ or cognitive tests, when available, allows the creation of profiles.

## Differential Diagnosis

The diagnosis of IDD should be made whenever Criteria A–C are met. However, diagnosis of IDD should not necessarily be assumed because a person has a particular genetic or medical condition. A genetic syndrome linked to IDD should be noted as a specifier.

### Major and Mild Neurocognitive Disorders
These disorders are not neurodevelopmental but diagnosed in later life and may be degenerative like Alzheimer's disease.

### Communication Disorders and Specific Learning Disorder
These disorders are specific to the communication and learning domains and do not demonstrate deficits in intellectual and adaptive behavior. However, they may co-occur with IDD. Both diagnoses are made if full criteria are met for IDD and a communication disorder or specific learning disorder.

### Autism Spectrum Disorder
Intellectual developmental disorder is not uncommon among individuals with autism spectrum disorder (ASD; Mefford et al., 2012; Moss & Howlin, 2009). However, in ASD, assessment of intellectual ability may be complicated because of social communication

and behavior deficits inherent to ASD. These symptoms often interfere with under-standing and complying with test procedures. Therefore, appropriate assessment of intellectual functioning in ASD is necessary. Measurement is required across the de-velopmental period because IQ scores in ASD can be unstable, particularly in early childhood.

### Co-Occurring Conditions

Co-occurring mental, neurodevelopmental, medical, and physical conditions are fre-quent in people with IDD. The rates of some conditions—for example, mental disorders, cerebral palsy, and epilepsy—are three or four times higher than in the general pop-ulation (Harris, 2006). Moreover, prognosis and outcome of co-occurring diagnoses may be impaired by the presence of IDD. Importantly, assessment procedures may need modifications because of co-occurring disorders such as communication disorders, ASD, and motor, sensory, or other disorders. Recognition of symptoms such as irrita-bility, mood dysregulation, aggression, eating problems, and sleep problems requires reliable informants.

The most frequently co-occurring mental and neurodevelopmental disorders are attention-deficit/hyperactivity disorder (ADHD), depression and bipolar disorders, anxiety disorders, ASD, stereotypic movement disorder (with or without self-injurious behavior), and impulse-control disorders. Major depressive disorder may occur throughout the range of severity of IDD. Self-injurious behavior requires prompt di-agnostic attention and often requires a separate diagnosis of stereotypic movement dis-order. Individuals with IDD, especially those with more severe intellectual disability, may also exhibit aggression and disruptive behaviors, which include harm of others or property destruction.

Individuals with IDD with co-occurring mental disorders are at risk for suicide, although the presentation may be atypical. They think about suicide, make suicide attempts, and may die from them (Dodd et al., 2016; Ludi et al., 2012). Thus, screening for suicidal thoughts is essential in the assessment process. Because of a lack of aware-ness of risk and danger, accidental injury rates are increased (Finlayson et al., 2010).

Health problems are frequent, including obesity. Often, the person cannot verbalize the physical symptoms they are experiencing. Thus, health problems such as appendi-citis may go undiagnosed and untreated (Conrad & Knowlden, 2020; Emerson, Hatton, et al., 2016; Emerson, Robertson, et al., 2016; U.S. Public Health Service, 2001).

## Associated Features Supporting Diagnosis

Intellectual developmental disorder is a heterogeneous condition with multiple causes. There may be associated difficulties with social judgment; assessment of risk; self-management of behavior, emotions, or interpersonal relationships; or motivation in school or work environments. Lack of communication skills may predispose to disrup-tive and aggressive behaviors. Gullibility is often a feature, involving naiveté in social situations and a tendency for being easily led by others (Greenspan et al., 2001, 2011). Gullibility and lack of awareness of risk may result in exploitation by others and possible victimization, fraud, unintentional criminal involvement, false confessions, and risk for physical and sexual abuse. These associated features can be important in criminal cases, including Atkins-type hearings involving the death penalty (Greenspan, 2009; Tassé, 2009).

## Relationship to Other Classifications

ICD-11 uses the term *disorders of intellectual development* to indicate that these are disorders that involve impaired brain functioning early in life. These disorders are described in ICD-11 as a meta-syndrome occurring in the developmental period analogous to dementia or neurocognitive disorder in later life (Reed et al., 2019; Salvador-Carulla & Bertelli, 2008; Salvador-Carulla et al., 2011, 2018; WHO, 2011, 2018). There are four subtypes in ICD-11—mild, moderate, severe, and profound—based on IQ and clinical description. The AAIDD (Schalock et al., 2021) also uses the term *intellectual disability*. The AAIDD's classification is multidimensional rather than categorical, and it is based on the disability construct.

## ICD-11 Definition

The ICD-11 definition is as follows (WHO, 2018):

> Disorders of intellectual development are a group of etiologically diverse conditions originating during the developmental period characterized by significantly below average intellectual functioning and adaptive behavior that are approximately two or more standard deviations below the mean (approximately less than the 2.3rd percentile), based on appropriately normed, individually administered standardized tests. Where appropriately normed and standardized tests are not available, diagnosis of disorders of intellectual development requires greater reliance on clinical judgment based on appropriate assessment of comparable behavioral indicators.

ICD-11 indicates that for these disorders, there are significant limitations in intellectual functioning across various domains, such as perceptual reasoning, working memory, processing speed, and verbal comprehension. Moreover, there is variability in the extent to which any of these psychological domains are affected in an individual. There are significant limitations in adaptive behaviors—a set of conceptual, social, and practical skills performed by people in their everyday lives. Conceptual functioning involves application of knowledge (e.g., reading, writing, calculating, solving problems, and making decisions) and communication. Social skills are utilized in managing interpersonal interactions and relationships. These include social responsibility, capacity to follow rules and obey laws, and avoiding victimization. Practical abilities include self-care, health and safety, occupational skills, recreation activities, the use of money, mobility, and transportation. They also include the practical use of home appliances and technological devices.

The Third Criteria
Onset occurs during the developmental period. Among adults with disorders of intellectual development who come to clinical attention without a previous diagnosis, it is possible to establish developmental onset through the person's history—that is, retrospective diagnosis.

## AAIDD Definition and Development

Although the DSM-5 and ICD-11 definitions are used in standard classifications, the AAIDD definition focuses on the individual's needs and what can be done to improve functioning. The definition and detailed descriptions are provided in the manual *Intellectual disability: Definition, Diagnosis, Classification, and Systems of Support* (Schalock et al., 2021). The AAIDD definition of intellectual developmental disability provides a comprehensive orientation to the person with an intellectual developmental disability but does not specify levels of severity. In contrast, the ICD-11 and DSM-5 approaches maintain the levels of IDD as mild, moderate, severe, and profound. These are based on both IQ level and clinical description in ICD-11. In DSM-5, severity is based on adaptive functions in cognitive, social, and practical domains. It must be emphasized that from a developmental perspective, the inclusion of levels of impairment is helpful. The AAIDD definition is as follows (Schalock et al., 2021):

> Intellectual disability is characterized by significant limitations both in intellectual functioning and in adaptive behavior as expressed in conceptual, social, and practical adaptive skills. This disability originates during the developmental period, which is defined operationally as before the individual attains age 22.

With the exception of increasing the operational age from 18 to 22 years, the AAIDD definition is the same as that in the 11th edition published in 2010. The definition makes the following five assumptions:

1. Limitations in present functioning are considered with the context of the community environment typical of the person's age, peers, and culture.
2. Assessment takes into account culture and linguistic diversity and differences in communication, sensory, motor, and other behaviors.
3. The person's limitations coexist with strengths.
4. The purpose of describing limitations is to develop a profile of support.
5. With personalized supports over an extended period of time, the person's life and functioning generally will improve.

This description emphasizes functional ability and considers the congruence of intellectual and adaptive abilities along with stressors that impact on adaptive functioning. Adaptive ability has been defined as "the effectiveness or degree with which an individual meets the standards of personal independence and social responsibility expected of his age and cultural group" (Grossman, 1983). Because these skills vary with chronological age, the assessment must take age into account. The low intelligence score and limited adaptive ability must occur before age 22 years, the age when adult roles are typically assumed. The age was changed because brain development continues into the 20s, especially in males. It is essential to remember that intellectual disability is not a static condition; the developmental goal is to establish a "best fit match" of the person with environmental supports to maximize adaptive ability.

Appropriate supports are matched to an individual's needs and include supportive individuals and services. Although intellectual disability in those with mild involvement may not be lifelong, supports may be needed for an extended period or, in some instances, throughout life. Improvement in function is expected for the majority, but supports are needed to maintain a basic level of function and to prevent regression.

## Levels of Intellectual Disability (Intellectual Developmental Disorder)

Intellectual developmental disorder is divided into four levels of severity in DSM-5, reflecting the extent of adaptive impairment: mild, moderate, severe, or profound. Adaptive functioning is defined in three domains: conceptual, social, and practical. DSM-5 provides descriptors for the four levels of severity. Depending on severity, the person requires comparable levels of support.

### Mild Intellectual Developmental Disorder

For mildly impaired persons, previously referred to as "in the educable range," problems with the use of language and speech difficulties may limit independence in adult life. This group makes up approximately 85% of those who are classified as persons with mild IDD because children often are not distinguishable from typically developing children in the early months of life but are recognized at school entry. During the preschool years (ages 0–5 years), social and communication skills generally develop, although there may be minimal impairment in sensorimotor function. By their late teens, they may acquire academic skills up to the fifth- or sixth-grade level. During their adult years, persons with mild IDD may develop sufficient social and vocational abilities and only need a minimum of external support. Still, ongoing guidance will be needed during stressful social conditions or economic hardship.

Most individuals with mild IDD appear successful in the community and may live independently or in supervised apartments or group homes. Their developmental achievements allow them to hold conversations and participate in clinical interviews. Their learning difficulties may become evident in academic work. When academic achievement is not required, their problems may be minimal. Yet there may be a noticeable degree of social and emotional immaturity leading to difficulties in coping. There often is an inability to cope with the demands of marriage or child-rearing or to meet specific cultural expectations. For the most part, their behavioral, emotional, and social problems and their need for psychosocial and behavior treatment and support are similar to those of persons with normal intelligence. Brain abnormalities are identifiable in a minority of this group. Associated conditions include ASD, other developmental disorders, epilepsy, conduct disorders, and physical disability.

## Moderate Intellectual Developmental Disorder

The full-scale IQ score can be deceptive because variable cognitive profiles of abilities are common for this group—for example, some individuals may have higher visuospatial skills than language skills. Moreover, some persons with a moderate IDD may be thought to be functioning at a lower level due to motor incoordination, although they can be socially interactive and communicative with appropriate assistance. Language development is variable across those in the moderate range, spanning from the capacity to participate in simple conversations to simple language limited to communication of basic needs. Those who never learn language may understand simple instruction or learn to use sign language to compensate for speech difficulties. There are also limitations in their achievement of self-care and motor skills. School progress is limited, but the higher functioning individual may learn basic skills in reading, writing, and counting. As adults, persons with a moderate IDD may participate in simple, practical work that is carefully structured, but they generally need consistent supervision by others. Completely independent living is rarely achieved in adulthood. Individuals with a moderately IDD make up approximately 10% of the population bearing this diagnosis.

Regarding etiology, brain abnormality can be identified in the majority. Seizure disorder and other neurological and physical disabilities also commonly occur. ASD may be associated, leading to additional problems in social adaptation. Psychiatric diagnosis may be difficult because of their limited language development and often requires the use of other informants. In the past, the term "trainable" was used for persons with a moderate IDD, but it should be avoided because many individuals in this group can benefit from educational programs. Efforts should be made to identify appropriate sheltered workshops, group homes, and supportive employment programs.

## Severe Intellectual Developmental Disorder

Except for the degree of impairment, persons with severe IDD are similar to those with moderate IDD in terms of their clinical picture and presence of brain abnormalities. A significant portion of persons with a severe IDD have marked motor impairment and other associated deficits. During the preschool years, poor motor development and lack of communicative speech are readily recognized. During the school-age years, language may emerge and elementary self-care skills may be taught. Depending on their cognitive ability, basic survival skills may be learned, including sight reading of essential words such as "stop," "man," and "woman." In adulthood, supervision is needed to aid in task performance. Community programs and group homes are frequently needed or, in some cases, specific in-home assistance to families is required. Associated disabilities may require specialized nursing care. Persons with IDD make up 3% or 4% of the IDD population.

## Profound Intellectual Developmental Disorder

Language comprehension and use are generally limited to understanding simple commands and making simple requests. Adaptive function is highly variable, although certain visuospatial skills, such as matching and sorting, may be acquired. With supervision and guidance, the child, and later the adult, may take part in practical tasks and domestic routines. As a result of their various disabilities, a highly structured environment with continual aid and supervision is necessary. Individualized relationships with caregivers are emphasized to facilitate optimal development. Self-care, communication skills, and motor abilities may require training in a structured setting. Living arrangements include small group homes in the community, intermediate care facilities, or living with their families along with day program support.

Brain abnormalities occur in the majority of persons with profound IDD. Neurological and physical disabilities that affect mobility are common, as are associated seizure disorders and visual and hearing impairments. This group constitutes 1% or 2% of those with IDD.

## Global Developmental Delay

This diagnosis is reserved for individuals younger than age 5 years when the clinical severity cannot be reliably assessed during early childhood. This category is diagnosed when an individual fails to meet expected developmental milestones in several areas of intellectual functioning, and it applies to individuals who are unable to undergo systematic assessments of intellectual functioning, including children who are too young to participate in standardized testing. This category requires reassessment after a period of time.

## Unspecified Intellectual Disability (Intellectual Developmental Disorder)

This category is reserved for individuals older than age 5 years when assessment of the degree of intellectual disability (IDD) by means of locally available procedures is rendered difficult or impossible because of associated sensory or physical impairments, as in blindness or prelingual deafness; locomotor disability; or the presence of severe problem behaviors or co-occurring mental disorder. This category should only be used in exceptional circumstances and requires reassessment after a period of time.

## AAIDD Human Functioning

The AAIDD focuses on an integrated model of human functioning, systems of support, and outcomes. Since 1992, the AAIDD has proposed that the intensity of support required should be used for subgrouping. Support needs take into account limitations in adaptive behavior; conceptual, social, and practical skills; and intellectual functioning. The terms intermittent, limited, extensive, and pervasive are used. The extent of limitations of adaptive behavior on conceptual, social, and practical skills is based on a standardized test that results in behavior scores in those adaptive behavior domains. The following terms are used for subgroups: mild (adaptive behavior score of approximately 50–55 to 70–75), moderate (score of approximately 40–45 to 50–55), severe (score of approximately 25–30 to 40–45), and profound (score of approximately <20–25). For the severe and profound levels, standardized tests have a floor score that can be generated (Schalock et al., 2021), so there is considerable variability in these groups.

Importantly, the AAIDD, in grouping the extent of limitations in intellectual functioning, uses the terms mild, moderate, severe, and profound. Grouping is established based on full-scale IQ scores, taking into account the standard error of measurement for each range (e.g., approximately 50–55 to 70–75 for mild). Supports are provided based on the perspective of disability. These perspectives include biomedical, psychoeducational, sociocultural, and social justice. The last perspective refers to societal arrangements and government programs. These focus on social inequality, injustice, discrimination, and denial of rights. Social justice focuses on affirmation of rights, legal counseling, and self-advocacy as needed supports. Biomedical concerns medical and mental health interventions. Psychoeducational supports include counseling, special education, and assistive technology. Sociocultural supports consist of environmental enrichment and environmental accommodation. With these supports, the AAIDD seeks to improve overall functioning with the following outcomes:

1. Intellectual functioning: Improved executive functioning with initiation of behavior inhibitions of competing stimuli, capacity to select task goals, and solve problems
2. Adaptive behavior: Better conceptual use of language, using money, and telling time
3. Social functioning: Better expression of self-esteem with reduced gullibility and to practically demonstrate occupational skills, use of caution in dangerous situations, and follow routines
4. Participation: More involvement and engagement in home and community living and more interactive with family

The overall goal is to structure the patient's life so that the patient is able to use opportunities, make choices, live in the least restrictive environment, have access to lifelong learning, and age at home in place.

## Epidemiology

The prevalence of IDD in the general population is approximately 1%; however, the prevalence rates vary with age. Prevalence of severe intellectual disability is approximately 6 per 1,000 (Einfeld & Emerson, 2008; Roeleveld et al., 1997). Accurate estimates of population prevalence are needed on numbers of persons with an IDD both for planning purposes and to gain better knowledge of the impact of interventions. Therefore, the prevalence and incidence of IDD have been studied extensively, dating back at least to 1811 when Napoleon ordered a census of "cretins" to be made in one of the Swiss cantons (Kanner, 1964). Although little information is available about how these data were used, many surveys have been carried out since that time. In modern studies, there is variability in prevalence estimating from the heterogeneous nature of IDD and variation in the methodology for ascertainment. Because of etiologic heterogeneity, IQ scores do not follow a normal distribution.

How IDD is defined and how the epidemiologic data are collected are critical to interpreting results. Both the prevalence of IDD in the general population and separate prevalence for specific IDD syndromes are required. Screening for IDD in children who have very low birth weight or experience early trauma or illness is critical. Epidemiologic studies must be careful to consider the various terms used for IDD—that is, intellectual disability, mental deficiency, mental handicap, mental subnormality, developmental delay, and learning disability. When reviewing previous studies, the definitions used in case findings must be carefully scrutinized.

At least three approaches have been used in epidemiologic research to define cases: statistical models, pathological models, and social systems models. Currently, the statistical model, which utilizes an IQ score 2 SD below the mean along with an assessment of adaptive function to IDD, is the accepted method. Yet this statistical model implies a continuum of cognitive abilities that does not exist. Variability in cognitive profile and associated conditions that complicate assessment make it necessary to utilize general categories such as mild, moderate, severe, and profound.

The pathological model focuses on specific neurodevelopmental syndromes, such as Down syndrome, or a particular etiology, such as intraventricular hemorrhage. The social systems perspective designates individuals with IDD if they are labeled by a social system, most commonly the school. For these purposes, children are typically not regarded as having an IDD until they start school and will no longer have the diagnosis after they leave school if they are functioning adequately in society and have sufficient physical and social skills to work independently. The most pragmatic definitions are those provided by the statistical model, which considers psychometric scores and adaptive functions criteria, and the pathological model, which emphasizes adaptive functioning.

Despite the various approaches used in epidemiologic studies, there is general consistency in cross national studies of prevalence rates (Einfeld & Emerson, 2008). Overall population prevalence of IDD is approximately 1%. The population in the United States is approximately 331 million (2020), so a 1% prevalence predicts 3.3 million people with IDD. Yet a 3% prevalence has often been chosen, using the statistical approach and basing the diagnosis on an IQ standardized score less than 70. The 3% rate assumes that the mortality of afflicted individuals is similar to that of the general population, that IDD is routinely identified in infancy, and that the diagnosis does not change with increasing age. These assumptions cannot be supported. Because of the multiple etiologies, the survival rate is typical only for those with mild IDD. Moreover, IDD is not always diagnosed in preschool children. Thus, the prevalence may be higher during the school years due to the inclusion of persons with mild IDD. However, their adaptive abilities may improve, so the diagnosis may no longer apply after leaving school. Consequently, the diagnosis of IDD may vary over time and, in this instance, is age related. Prevalence also differs among states, depending on the methods of ascertainment.

Other factors influence prevalence, such as normalization, mainstreaming, and improved interventions, especially for those who have been educationally and socially deprived. The reduction of poverty, improvement in nutrition, and more refined medical diagnoses also influence outcome. Greater availability of genetic counseling and abortion services for high-risk pregnancies are also factors in prevalence, as are dietary/hormonal treatments for inborn errors of metabolism, such as galactosemia and PKU, and endocrine disorders such as congenital hypothyroidism. Improved obstetrical techniques have lowered the incidence of brain damage at birth; however, improvements in care for the very small premature have led to an increased rate of IDD in this population in some instances.

Demographic considerations that influence prevalence include age, sex, socioeconomic level, race, and variations between urban and rural populations (Roeleveld et al., 1997). Regarding age, most surveys show an increase in prevalence from the preschool years (0–4 years) to middle childhood (5–12 years). Because performance expectations are greater in school, milder neurodevelopmental disorders become more apparent. In the mid-teen years, there may also be an apparent increase in rate when increasing demands are imposed by the school system. At this age, adaptive difficulties related to social judgment, and behavioral control may emerge. In young adulthood (22–34 years), prevalence rates generally decrease following the completion of school as people find employment suited to their intellectual capacity. Finally, in older persons, rates decrease as demands from vocational programs are reduced. Because of all these considerations, epidemiologic studies must consider age-specific rates for planning.

The rate of IDD is higher in males than in females because congenital anomalies are more prevalent in boys, as are prematurity, neonatal death, and stillbirth. Another important factor in males is the presence of X-linked intellectual disability IDD. Moreover, due to their greater tendency to show aggressive behavior, boys may come to the attention of authorities more often than girls and may be more likely to be diagnosed. Yet not all studies show an increased prevalence among males, probably because both age and extent of IDD need to be considered. Higher rates among males have been reported in persons with a mild IDD, but the gender difference is less apparent among persons who are severely impaired.

Socioeconomic level is an important consideration as it relates to IDD due to sensory and psychosocial deprivation, leading to the designation "mental impairment due to psychosocial disadvantage" (Grossman, 1983) or "cultural familial intellectual developmental disorder" (Zigler, 1967). Psychosocial factors, including poor living conditions, overcrowding, and lack of educational opportunity, contribute to IDD, particularly in the mild range; however, genetic factors must be taken into account for these cases. For the more severe levels of IDD, clear-cut differences in socioeconomic status are less common. Prevalence rates are reported to be higher among racial minorities, but this is likely linked to socioeconomic level rather than to race. Similarly, differences between urban and rural populations may be influenced by educational, occupational, and cultural opportunities. In some surveys, rates have been reported to be higher in rural areas, whereas in other surveys, they have been reported to be higher in inner-city populations.

Living arrangements vary, with the higher functioning groups tending to live in community residences or with family members. Individuals with moderate IDD are more often placed in foster and group homes, whereas the most severely and profoundly impaired individuals are placed in institutional settings as well as in foster and group home settings. The percentage living with family members and in the communities is inversely related to the degree of intellectual deficit.

In a 35-year follow-up study based on a nationwide population, life expectancy of persons with mild IDD was not reduced compared to the general population, nor did they have poorer life expectancy in their first three decades. With moderate IDD, expected life lost was <20% for all age groups. Prevalence at age older than 40 years was

0.4% (Patja et al., 2000). The life expectancy of persons with IDD is correlated with their level of intellectual functioning and the etiology of the disorder. Yet, life expectancy among persons with IDD is increasing, particularly for those who survive beyond the first year of life. Overall, survival rates show a negative association between severity and survival. Median life expectancies are 74.0, 67.6, and 58.6 years, respectively, for mild, moderate, and severe levels.

## Development and Course

By definition, onset of IDD is during the developmental period. The features at onset depend on the etiology and severity of brain dysfunction. Delayed motor, language, and social milestones may not be recognized within the first 2 years of life among those diagnosed with more severe intellectual disability. Mild levels may not be recognized until school age when difficulty with academic learning becomes apparent (Reschly, 2009). All criteria (including development onset Criterion C) must be fulfilled. Some children younger than age 5 years initially have deficits that meet criteria for global developmental delay.

When IDD is associated with a genetic syndrome, physical appearance (e.g., Down syndrome) may be characteristic. Some genetic syndromes have a *behavioral phenotype*, which refers to specific behaviors that are characteristic of a particular genetic disorder (e.g., Lesch–Nyhan syndrome) (Harris, 2010). When IDD is acquired, onset may be abrupt if following an illness, such as meningitis or encephalitis, or following severe head trauma. When IDD results from a loss of previously acquired cognitive skills, as in severe traumatic brain injury, the diagnoses of both IDD and a neurocognitive disorder should be given.

IDD is typically nonprogressive. However, in certain genetic disorders (e.g., Rett syndrome), there are periods of worsening, followed by stabilization, and in others there is progressive worsening of intellectual function in varying degrees (e.g., Down syndrome and Sanfilippo syndrome) (Wester Oxelgren et al., 2019). Although the disorder is generally lifelong, severity levels may change over time. The clinical course may be influenced by underlying medical or genetic conditions and co-occurring conditions (e.g., hearing or visual impairments and epilepsy). Importantly, early and continuous interventions may improve adaptive functioning throughout childhood and into adulthood. In some instances, these result in significant improvement of intellectual functioning so that the diagnostic criteria of IDD are no longer met.

When assessing infants and young children, it is common practice to delay the diagnosis of IDD until after appropriate intervention is provided. Especially for older children and adults who are higher functioning, the extent of support provided may allow for full participation in all activities of daily living and improved adaptive functioning. However, diagnostic assessments are needed to determine if improved adaptive skills are the result of a stable, generalized new skill acquisition (in which case, the diagnosis of IDD may no longer be appropriate) or whether the improvement results from providing supports and ongoing interventions (in this instance, the diagnosis of IDD may still be appropriate).

## Gender and Diagnosis

Males are more likely than females to be diagnosed with both mild (average male-to-female ratio of 1.6:1) and severe (average male-to-female ratio of 1.2:1) types of IDD (Einfeld & Emerson, 2008). Still, gender ratios vary widely among studies. Sex-linked genetic factors and male vulnerability to brain injury may account for some of the gender differences.

## Epidemiology of Associated Disabilities

Epidemiologic surveys of IDD typically take into account associated physical disability, such as visual impairment, hearing loss, speech and language problems, seizure disorder, and cerebral palsy. For example, among blind persons, 20%–25% also have IDD; the highest rates of visual impairment occur in those who are more severely cognitively impaired. In addition, subtle problems in visual acuity and colorblindness may be missed in persons with an IDD. The rate of visual disability, depending on the level of IDD, has been reported to be 15 times greater than the rate in the general population.

Hearing impairment is identified at three or four times the population prevalence rate and occurs in approximately 10% of persons with IDD. Moreover, hearing problems in older individuals are more common in certain syndromes, such as Down syndrome, in which there is an increased risk of otosclerosis. Like blindness, hearing impairment is also greatest among severely and profoundly cognitively impaired persons, being five- to eightfold greater in person with severe to profound impairment than in the general population. Assessment requires specially targeted diagnostic tests, such as evoked response audiometry, because of the person's unreliability in responding to standard assessment techniques. Of note, speech and language disorders are among the most common disabilities of persons with IDD. The prevalence of speech and language disorders is up to 80% in institutionalized severely and profoundly impaired individuals. In non-institutionalized persons with an IDD, rates for speech problems are triple that of the general population.

Approximately one-third of person with IDD (generally, persons with a severe IDD) in institutional settings have epilepsy. In non-institutionalized groups, the prevalence of seizures is approximately 15%, in comparison to 1.5% for a control group. For severe IDD, the prevalence of seizures is approximately 33%. Rates of speech and language disorders in persons with a mild to moderate IDD group range from 3–6% to 12–18%, depending on the population evaluated.

Static motor encephalopathy or cerebral palsy frequently co-occurs with IDD. Severely impaired persons have a rate of cerebral palsy ranging from 30% to 60%. Certain types of cerebral palsy are more often related to IDD; for example, children with spastic quadriplegia and diplegia have a higher rate than those with the extrapyramidal forms.

## Etiology

The etiology of IDD is classified in several ways based on identifying either a causative agent or a specific mechanism. The AAIDD includes prenatal causes (chromosomal disorders, syndrome disorders, inborn errors of metabolism, developmental disorders of brain formation, and environmental influences), perinatal causes (intrauterine disorders and neonatal disorders), and postnatal causes (head injuries, infections, demyelinating disorders, degenerative disorders, seizure disorders, toxic metabolic disorders, malnutrition, environmental deprivation, and hypoconnection syndrome). More than 500 genetic disorders are linked with IDD. Many known genetic conditions show their primary clinical effects on the brain, and others may lead to secondary effects to the central nervous system.

Some genetic syndromes involve abnormalities that, although occurring in utero, may not be evident until postnatal life. The best known of these include single-gene-related metabolic disorders (e.g., PKU) whose manifestations are not seen at birth until after feeding. It has been estimated that between 30% and 50% of developmental disorders involve some temporal risk factors. Moreover, chromosomal syndromes may increase susceptibility to perinatal trauma; for example, inadequate central respiratory control may increase the risk of hypoxic–ischemic damage.

Advances in biomedical technology have led to the recognition of the neurobiological etiology for many IDD syndromes. Neurobiological factors play a major etiological role in mild IDD and also many causes of borderline intellectual functioning. A variety of biomedical abnormalities, including subtle chromosomal abnormalities, perinatal trauma, and exposure to toxic substances, underlie 30–45% of cases of mild IDD. These findings have led to a re-examination of the etiological role of psychosocial disadvantage and polygenic risk factors.

In two-thirds of cases, the specific cause for IDD can be identified. The more severe the degree of IDD, the higher the likelihood a specific cause will be identified, with an etiology identified for approximately 80% of those with a severe IDD. Moreover, a medical risk factor (perinatal trauma and genetic disorder) can be identified in approximately 40% of those with a mild IDD and approximately 25–30% of those with borderline intellectual functioning.

Multiple etiologies for IDD indicate that there is a complex interaction between genetic predisposition, environmental insults, and developmental vulnerability. Genetic predisposition also includes individual susceptibilities to the influence of environmental agents. Genetic damage is likely when exposure takes place during periods of DNA replication. Multiple environmental factors may be involved that impinge on the developing organism, including nutritional deficiencies that occur in wars and famine and exposure to exogenous toxins, microorganisms, radiation, and psychosocial stressors. The developmental timing of exposure to potentially hazardous environmental agents is a major consideration because the severity of resulting IDD tends to be related to the timing of the insult to the central nervous system. Overall, prenatal factors, which affect the developing fetal brain, are responsible for 55–75% of severe IDD cases but only for 25–40% of mild IDD cases. Exposure of the fetus to the rubella virus during the first trimester of pregnancy may lead to major congenital anomalies, whereas exposure to the same virus later in gestation or during the postnatal period leads to a milder disorder.

The search for an etiological diagnosis is critical because the effects of some progressive developmental disorders may be arrested or sometimes prevented through early diagnosis and treatment. For example, several inborn errors of metabolism (e.g., PKU and galactosemia) with clinical manifestations can be prevented by recognition and dietary management. Accurate diagnosis leads to interventions including genetic counseling, perinatal diagnosis, and the possibly of corrective gene therapy in the future.

## Developmental Issues

In *Diagnosis of Reasoning in the Retarded*, Barbel Inhelder (1968) suggested that arrests in Piaget's cognitive developmental stages (sensorimotor, preoperational, and concrete operational) correspond to profound, severe, moderate, and mild IDD. Although Mary Woodward (1959, 1961) studied severely and profoundly impaired individuals using Piaget's approach, there has been a notable lack of emphasis on a developmental perspective in IDD.

In addition to developmental sequences, developmental rate must also be considered to understand fully the importance of maturational changes that are related to neurological structures. In Down syndrome, the importance of developmental rate is demonstrated by studies that show a gradual decline in IQ with advancing age. During the first 2 years of life, infants with Down syndrome are noted to fall increasingly further behind typically developing peers. This apparent slowing in development may be due to problems in moving qualitatively from one cognitive stage to another. In contrast, in the fragile X syndrome, IQ improvement occurs until the early teens. At that point, mental age tends to plateau; but potentially, there may be a decline in IQ here as well. In fragile X syndrome, endocrine changes associated with puberty influence brain development and cause cognitive impairment on test items requiring abstract reasoning.

Besides these maturational issues, the environment plays an important role in development, although it is unclear which aspects of the environment are most important and which times in development are most crucial (although the early life is most often associated with greater impact). Environmental concerns have led to an emphasis on transactional intervention models that focus on language input and mother–child interaction, with structure in both linguistic and nonlinguistic environments needed to facilitate development. The development of social communication is particularly important. Most studies emphasize mother–child relationships, but in IDD, it is particularly important to emphasize the role of the father. Environmental outcomes that must be monitored include not only intelligence but also the emergence of social competence and the management of aggression. Children with Down syndrome, fragile X syndrome, ASD, or multiple disabilities may differ from one another in their presentations and their reactions to others, and the behaviors of caregivers toward them may also differ.

A developmental approach to IDD emphasizes how development is organized even in those who are disabled. By studying different etiologic groups, there is an opportunity to make comparisons about developmental organization. Children with Down syndrome have reduced affective responses and difficulties in language development but exhibit relatively high levels of social skills, whereas children with ASD may have severe social skills deficits, echolalia, and a different profile of language development.

Behaviors may show relationships across developmental domains. The study of behavior across domains is important for clarifying how various behaviors fit together in development. In the final stage of Piaget's sensorimotor development sequence, one object is used to retrieve another object—a stage that can be demonstrated for children with an IDD and for those with ASD. Symbolic play is important for early language development in some syndromes, such as Down syndrome. Sequential processing deficits in fragile X syndrome cross domains and affect cognitive, linguistic, and adaptive functioning. Knowledge of cross-modal problems can be applied to an intervention program to assist the child in adapting to their specific impairments.

The study of the various etiologies of IDD takes into account the importance of individual impairments rather than simply targeting global differences in intelligence for intervention. Therefore, when asking about delay during an interview, questions should focus on which specific functions are delayed. Adaptive behaviors are best studied based on which behaviors are specific for a given mental age. The Vineland Adaptive Behavior Scales provide a means to assess adaptive functioning and compare adaptive abilities with IQ level.

## Neurodevelopmental Perspective

A developmental perspective focuses on how an individual engages other people and masters environmental challenges. For people with IDD, there may be progressive thresholds for capacity in cognitive problem-solving. A developmental approach should be used to unravel developmental dynamics by focusing on the development of mental processing. Demetriou et al. (2002) combined information processing models, differential psychology, and neo-Piagetian developmental theory and proposed a framework for study by focusing on the emergence and maturation of working memory, executive functioning, and cognitive efficacy in problem-solving.

## Normalization: The Developmental Model

Although IDD is a chronic condition and not curable, habilitation can be substantial. A developmental model of IDD acknowledges the capacity for growth and strives for independent living. The developmental model specifically emphasizes that adaptive behavior may improve with habilitation, which constitutes an important aspect of normalization in intellectual disability. *Normalization* refers to individuals with an IDD being entitled to services that are as culturally normative as possible to help them establish and maintain appropriate personal behavior (Wolfensberger, 1972). Normalization emphasizes that persons with IDD should live in community settings, attend regular schools, and seek competitive employment. Their behavior should be monitored to assist them to reach the standards for typically developing persons at a comparable developmental age. They should be responsible for their behavior, and it should not be assumed that their IDD precludes their ability to take on this responsibility.

In developmentally based normalization programs, communication skills, previous life experience, and any associated physical disorders are considered. Special efforts are needed to normalize communication—for example, teaching sign language and utilizing facilitated communication. The nonverbal person with a physical disability, such as cerebral palsy, and IDD may require a voice synthesizer, communication board, or picture cards to assist in communication. Normalization attempts to provide the opportunity for decision-making and exposure to varied life experiences. Subsequently, Wolfensberger extended his focus on normalization to social role valorization. *Valorization* is defined as the use of culturally valued approaches to establish, enhance, maintain, and/or defend valued social roles for people with IDD, who are undervalued in society. It is intended to address psychological and social devaluation and defend social roles that give meaning to their lives (Thomas & Wolfensberger, 1999; Wolfensberger, 1983).

## Personality Development

Studies of persons with IDD have focused primarily on intellectual and cognitive functioning but sometimes neglected social and personality development. Problems associated with cognitive functioning have often overshadowed needed attention on adaptive and maladaptive personality features because personality variables and personal motivation are essential for predicting social and vocational adjustment. It is behavioral and social deficits that most commonly lead to psychiatric referral.

Personality dysfunction in children and adolescents fosters characteristics such as overdependency, low ideal self-image, limited levels of aspiration, and an outer-directed approach to problem-solving. These personality characteristics may have their origin in adverse psychosocial experiences, including repeated failure and disapproval, leading to doubts about their capability to succeed. Experiences of rejection and the lack of consistent social support can lead to excessive reliance on others for feedback and guidance. Out of a need for recognition by others, they may suppress the desire to become more independent.

Operant behavior modification programs do not address these needs. These programs do not emphasize making choices but, rather, place primary emphasis on contingency management. As a result, the transition after completion of schooling to vocational programs may be difficult. During their adolescent years, parental restrictiveness and overprotection, peer rejection, and continuing low self-confidence often complicate mastery of developmental tasks involved in establishing the self-concept, sexual awareness, and identity. Adolescents with an IDD may view their lives as being less fulfilling than those of their peers because they commonly experience dissatisfaction with their physical appearance and become frustrated by their difficulty in controlling their impulses, emotions, and behavior. These experiences may lead to social isolation, loneliness, and dysphoric mood.

The failure to master developmental tasks is integral to producing maladaptive personality styles in adulthood. As many as one-half of adults with an IDD may have dysfunctional personalities. Although the diagnosis of personality disorder in persons with IDD has been questioned, several personality disorder inventories that have adequate interrater and test–retest reliability have identified dysfunctional personality traits and personality disorders in IDD adolescents and adults. The types of maladaptive personality characteristics most often found with these inventories include affective instability, explosive and disruptive behaviors, and introverted personality patterns. Menolascino (1988) found that among 543 IDD admissions for psychiatric care over a 5-year period, 13% of those aged 16 years or older had a diagnosis of personality disorder; passive–aggressive and antisocial types were the most common. It should also be kept in mind that the presence of a seizure disorder, especially one involving the temporal lobes, may increase the risk for a personality disorder among individuals with an IDD (Torr, 2003).

## Genetics

Prenatal etiologies of IDD include genetic syndromes (e.g., Mendelian inborn errors of metabolism, sequence variations or copy number variants involving one or more genes, and chromosomal disorders; Kaufmann et al., 2008), brain malformations, maternal disease (including placental disease; Michelson et al., 2011), and environmental influences (e.g., alcohol, other drugs, toxins, and teratogens). Perinatal causes include a variety of labor- and delivery-related events leading to neonatal encephalopathy. Postnatal causes include hypoxic–ischemic injury, traumatic brain injury, infections, demyelinating disorders, seizure disorders (e.g., infantile spasms), severe and chronic social deprivation, and toxic metabolic syndromes and intoxications (e.g., lead and mercury) (Harris, 2006).

General intelligence is a human trait that is believed to account for much of the variation in cognitive abilities in genetic studies. Data from twin and family studies are consistent with a high heritability of intelligence. In a genome-wide association study (GWAS) involving nonclinical populations, a substantial proportion of individual differences in human intelligence was due to genetic variation and was consistent with many genes of small effects underlying additive genetic influences on intelligence (Davies et al., 2011; Hill et al., 2019). The longitudinal stability of IQ in typically developing people is well documented, as is its increasing heritability with age. Despite the fact that increased heritability of general cognitive capacity during the transition from childhood to adolescence is clear in typical development, abilities may plateau in adolescence in some syndromes, such as fragile X syndrome (Dykens et al., 1989).

Genetic and neuroimaging studies are essential next steps to understand brain functioning in persons with IDD. In the early 20th century, Charles Spearman, who developed the correlational method and applied it to examine academic achievement, provided evidence that all cognitive tests measure something in common. He referred to this commonality as a general factor in intelligence or *g*. Thus, Spearman's *g* represents the component of individual variance common across tests of mental ability.

Thomson (1919) challenged Spearman's *g* by proposing that there are a large number of biological units ("bonds") present in brains. When an individual attempted to solve mental test items, each of the items sampled a number of these bonds. The extent to which tests overlapped in the bonds that they sampled accounted for their correlation. In modern parlance, his "bonds" might be considered to be distributed neuronal networks. There is recent support for this model, and current research has documented that both Thomson and Spearman's models of intelligence can account for the psychometric patterning of tests' intercorrelations (Barbey, 2018). A central question regarding these models is how neuroscience evidence from brain imaging on human intelligence may inform psychological theory. Does general intelligence reflect a unitary construct (Spearman, 1904) or a broader set of competencies (Thomson, 1919)?

Spearman's two-factor model has been elaborated to include an intermittent level of broad abilities that address the variance shared across similar domains of cognitive ability. The Cattell–Horn–Carroll theory distinguishes between performance on tests measuring prior knowledge and experience (McGrew, 2005). This is known as capitalized intelligence. Capitalized intelligence is distinguished from tests that require adaptive reasoning when faced with novel situations, referred to as fluid intelligence. Together, these broad general factors account for the pattern of hierarchal correlations demonstrated in tests of mental ability. For example, Christoforou et al. (2014) reported that GWAS-based pathway analysis can differentiate between fluid and crystallized intelligence. Barbey (2018) proposed the term "network neuroscience theory of human intelligence" and summarized neuroscientific evidence to explain how general intelligence, $g$, emerges from individual differences in the network architecture of the human brain.

## Neuroimaging

Structural and functional brain imaging studies have documented differences in brain pathways to intelligence contributing to differences in intellect (Deary et al., 2010). Brain imaging research is directed to studying intelligence as a unitary construct (Spearman, 1904) or as a broader set of competencies (Thomson, 1919). This requires careful analysis because a given brain region may support multiple cognitive functions. Conversely, a given cognitive function can be implemented with multiple brain regions. This complexity complicates the use of neuroscience evaluation of local versus distributed representations to understand the nature of cognitive representations of intelligence. Parietofrontal pathway interaction has strong support (Colom et al., 2010; Jung & Haier, 2007). But, overall brain efficiency correlates positively with intelligence.

Studies of an integrative architecture for general intelligence and executive function have been initiated using lesion mapping (Barbey et al., 2012). Barbey et al. confirmed that psychometric $g$ and executive function largely depend on shared neural substrates and on the communication between frontal and parietal cortex. The analysis also revealed other areas that were related to psychometric $g$ and may not be involved with executive function. General intelligence and executive functioning scores shared 76% of the variance, whereas 24% of the variance was unique. Areas related to executive function but not involved with psychometric $g$ were identified within the left anterior frontal pole, consistent with the anterior prefrontal cortex regions involved in the executive control of behavior.

Overall, psychometric intelligence is associated with a distributed network of brain regions that share common anatomical substrates with brain regions involved in verbal comprehension, working memory, perceptual organization, and processing speed. Executive function deficits were associated with a distributed network of left lateralized brain areas, including regions that are necessary for executive control processes. Second-stratum fluid intelligence and working memory have been studied by neuroimaging (Barbey, Colom, Paul, & Grafman, 2014). This approach allows the examination of the functional networks that support adaptive behavior and novel problem-solving. The authors found that the front lateral parietal network, central to human intelligence, is lateralized, with mechanisms for general intelligence being linked to the left hemisphere and fluid intelligence to the right hemisphere.

Barbey, Colom, Paul, Chau, et al. (2014) have studied a distributed neural system for emotional intelligence by lesion mapping. Latent scores for measures of general intelligence and personality predicted latent scores for emotional intelligence. These processes depend on a shared network of frontal, temporal, and parietal brain regions. The results support an integrative framework for understanding the architecture of executive, social, and emotional processes. In addition, this group used similar approaches to study social problem-solving (Barbey, Colom, Paul, Chau, et al., 2014). They found that working memory, processing speed, and emotional intelligence predict individual differences in everyday problem-solving. Tasks included engagement with friends, home management, and information management. Social problem-solving, psychometric intelligence, and emotional intelligence were demonstrated to engage a shared network of frontal, temporal, and parietal regions, including white matter association tracts. The results support there being an integrative framework for understanding social intelligence.

Finally, adaptive reasoning requires cognitive flexibility. Barbey et al. (2013) investigated the neural underpinning of cognitive flexibility by examining mental flexibility. Lesion mapping results further indicated that these convergent processes depend on a shared network of frontal, temporal, and parietal regions, along with white matter association. Unique variance was explained by selective damage within the right superior temporal gyrus. This is a region known to support insight and the recognition of novel semantic relations. All these findings contribute to the neural foundations of adaptive behavior. This full series of neural lesion studies highlights the importance of adaptive reasoning and for extending this approach to people with IDDs.

## Sexuality and Intellectual Disability Disorder

Persons with IDD are commonly stereotyped concerning their sexual behavior. These stereotypes include their being sexually uninhibited, sexually immature with sexual interests that correspond to their mental rather than chronological age, or lacking sexual interests altogether. Yet, indiscriminate sexual behavior is not a characteristic feature in persons with IDD (Medina-Rico et al., 2018). Based on stereotypes about uninhibited or indiscriminate sexual behavior, sterilization of persons with IDD was routinely practiced in the past, and some U.S. states still have such laws. Marriage between persons with an IDD has been prohibited in the past as a means of reducing the incidence of IDD.

Sexual interest is ordinarily associated with the onset of puberty, so delays in puberty in individuals with IDD related to the particular etiology of the disorder will influence sexual interest. Regardless of the age of pubertal onset, the most severely and profoundly impaired individuals often show little interest in sexual activity with others. However, mildly involved and many moderately involved individuals may have normal pubertal development, demonstrate sexual interests, and establish sexual identities. If the expression of sexual interest is prohibited or prevented, inappropriate sexual activity may occur as a reaction. It may sometimes be used as a way to demonstrate self-importance. During adolescence, sexual behavior can also be part of an attempt to gain acceptance from others in a peer group, just as is the case in peer groups of typically developing individuals. To facilitate the development of a normal sexual identity, encouragement of relationships with others and teaching appropriate social skills are prerequisites that should be emphasized before focusing specifically on instruction about sexual activity.

Mildly and moderately impaired adolescents often lack the most basic understanding of sexual anatomy, venereal disease, and contraceptive issues. Persons with IDD, particularly women, are at risk for sexual exploitation. Knowledge of sexuality is often not well established because the usual sources of information—namely sex education in the schools, intimate peer discussions, and relevant reading material—may be limited or unavailable. Family members may be reluctant to review or discuss sexual matters with their children with IDD or young adult family members. Most often, knowledge of sexuality is based on life experience and sexual opportunity and not on systematic education.

It is important to teach family members and educators to not diminish the value of sexuality and to assist in educating persons with IDD about sexual development and sexuality. Importantly, people with IDD are vulnerable and at a greater risk for sexual abuse (Martinello, 2014). There is little difference in sexual interest for adolescents in the mild range compared to typically developing peers. However, boys with IDD have more behavioral problems, such as public masturbation, and in one study 8% of boys with IDD had experienced sexual abuse (Akrami & Davudi, 2014). Women with IDD are found to have less knowledge about contraceptive methods and use them less. More than half of adolescents with IDD did not have sex education, and 46% had never spoken with parents about sex (Isler et al., 2009).

## Psychiatric Assessment

The psychiatric evaluation of persons with mild or moderate IDD includes the same areas that are covered with typically developing individuals, with slight modifications. A comprehensive assessment includes a review of present concerns and symptoms; past and present developmental, medical, psychiatric, social, and family history; patient interview and physical examination; diagnostic formulation; treatment plan; informing conference; and follow-through. Both the patient and the caregivers, who know the patient well, are used as informants. Disorders of interpersonal functioning, communication, emotion, and behavior are included. The interview must take into account the patient's cognitive and adaptive limitations. Interviews frequently need to be more structured, directive, and shorter than those conducted with typically developing patients. After establishing rapport, the interview should provide overt support and social reinforcement so the patient does not react to the interview as a test that they might fail. Care must be taken to avoid leading questions. Finally, interpretation about emotional and behavioral functioning should be presented within the context of the individual's overall developmental level.

The use of standardized assessment instruments and procedures has been introduced to improve the reliability and validity of psychiatric evaluation for persons with IDD. Because of variability in cognitive functioning and the use of multiple informants (physicians, psychologists, educators, and direct care providers), it is difficult to demonstrate reliability and validity for these instruments. Even so, several behavior checklists and semistructured interviews have been developed for use with patients with IDD and other informants (e.g., caregivers). Some instruments focus on making a specific diagnosis; others are used to assess the range and severity of affective and behavioral symptoms.

Among reviewed instruments for assessing emotional and behavior disorders in individuals with IDD, the following behaviors were commonly included, using factor analytic methodology: (a) aggressive, antisocial behavior; (b) withdrawal; (c) stereotypic behavior; (d) hyperactivity; (e) repetitive verbalization; (f) anxious, tense, and fearful; and (g) self-injurious behavior. Rating scales for younger children have also been validated. Although there is no one screening instrument that can be recommended for preschool children, the Reiss Scales for Children's Dual Diagnosis (Reiss & Valenti-Hein, 1990) should be considered for school-age children. For the assessment of broad behavioral dimensions in the age group, the Aberrant Behavior Checklist (ABC) and the Developmentally Delayed Child Behavior Checklist (Einfeld & Tonge, 1995; Hastings et al., 2001) should be considered.

The ABC is an informant-based questionnaire that assesses the severity of 58 maladaptive behaviors. It is most appropriate for individuals with moderate to profound degrees of intellectual disability (IDD). Extensive psychometric analyses have been carried out in several different countries, utilizing subjects of varying ages and IQ levels. Factor analysis identified five factors—irritability, lethargy/social withdrawal, stereotypic behavior, hyperactivity/noncompliance, and inappropriate speech—and the five-factor structure has been cross-validated. The factors have high internal consistency, and the instrument itself possesses good reliability. Internal consistency has been found to be satisfactory, but interrater reliabilities were relatively low (M. Aman et al., 1995; E. Brown et al., 2002; Kaat et al., 2014; Marshburn & Aman, 1992).

The Psychopathology Instrument for Mentally Retarded Adults (PIMRA) (Balboni et al., 2000; Belva & Matson, 2015; Watson et al., 1988) is a 56-item scale with both self-report and informant versions that are designed to assess psychopathology among persons with mild or moderate IDD. The individual items were derived from the symptom lists based on several DSM disorders and organized into seven clinical subscales. The subscales include the following diagnoses: schizophrenia, affective disorder, psychosexual disorder, adjustment disorder, anxiety disorder, somatoform disorder, and personality disorder. Factor analysis yielded two factors for the self-report version (termed "anxiety and social adjustment") and three factors for the informant version (termed "affective, somatoform, and psychosis"). The psychometric properties of the PIMRA have been evaluated (Belva & Matson, 2015). Initial analysis indicated high internal consistencies of the subscales and total scores, and good interrater and test–retest reliabilities. Yet, follow-up analyses by several investigators have raised questions about this instrument's internal consistency and reliability. Other concerns include a low correspondence between the factor structure and the clinically derived scales and the limited number of disorders represented. Despite some shortcomings, the PIMRA is a useful instrument for the assessment of psychopathology in this population.

The Reiss Screen for Maladaptive Behavior (Reiss, 1988) is an informant-based rating scale that assesses the frequency, circumstances, and intensity associated with various symptoms of psychiatric disorders in persons with intellectual disability disorder. The instrument is organized into seven clinical scales: aggressive disorder, psychosis, paranoia, depression (behavioral signs), depression (physical signs), avoidant disorder, and dependent personality disorder. There are six maladaptive behaviors: drug abuse, over-activity, self-injury, sexual behavior, suicidal tendencies, and stealing. Factor analysis yields clinically meaningful results, and its validity has been documented in conjunction with clinical psychiatric diagnosis. Other instruments for which preliminary psychometric analyses are available are the Emotional Disorders Rating Scale for Developmental Disabilities and the Diagnostic Assessment for the Severely Handicapped scale.

Assessment instruments developed for typically developing children and adolescents have also been used to evaluate psychopathology among children and adults with an IDD. These instruments generally have good test–retest reliability yet vary in terms of their interrater reliability, internal consistency, and validity. Among them are the Child Behavior Checklist, the Rutter Behavioral Scales, the Beck Depression Inventory, the Zung Self-Rating Depression Inventory, and the Standardized Assessment of Personality. Continuing investigation is needed to provide information on their applicability to persons with IDD.

## Basic Medical History

A comprehensive medical history and a careful physical examination are essential to discovering the etiology of IDDs. Following the history and physical examination, laboratory and diagnostic studies are chosen based on the clinical findings. Brain imaging is playing an increasingly important role in the evaluation of children and adults with a variety of developmental disorders. These studies provide a noninvasive means to identify structural and, in some instances, functional abnormalities, such as abnormal metabolic activity, in persons with IDD. Computerized transaxial tomography (CTT), magnetic resonance imaging (MRI), single-photon emission computed tomography (SPECT), diffusion tensor imaging (DTI), and positron emission tomography (PET) techniques may be used in the evaluation of IDD, to study structure–function relationships, and to identify surgically correctable brain lesions associated with specific disorders. CTT and MRI may be used to identify congenital malformations and/or brain changes related to infections of the central nervous system. Ventricular enlargement, cyst formation, cerebral asymmetry, neuronal migration disorders (e.g., polygyria, lissencephaly, and schizencephaly), Chiari malformations, agenesis of the corpus callosum, and cerebral calcifications are among the abnormalities that may be demonstrated. CTT is the preferred procedure for the visualization of calcifications, vascular lesions, and some tumors. MRI is superior to CTT for identification of many structural anomalies (e.g., heterotopias), white matter abnormalities (e.g., demyelinating disorders), abnormality of the gray–white matter junction, and masses in the posterior fossa of the brain.

Diagnostic imaging is essential in the treatment of neurocutaneous disorders in which prognosis depends on the number, size, and location of associated neoplasms (e.g., neurofibromas, tubers, hamartomas, angiomas, and malignancies). This is especially important in tuberous sclerosis, where CTT and MRI may reveal tubers, subependymal calcified nodules, cortical hamartomas, and migration defects. The number and size of the tubers may be correlated with the degree of IDD and the severity of seizures. In Sturge–Weber syndrome, MRI is used to detect the extent and distribution of angiomatosis in the meninges, skull, and within the brain, but CTT is best for detecting cortical calcifications.

PET and SPECT scans are being used to localize seizure foci prior to surgery, determine the extent of malignancy of certain neoplasms, identify tubers in tuberous sclerosis, evaluate the extent of intracranial hemorrhages in premature infants, and contribute to the early diagnosis of Huntington's disease and Sturge–Weber syndrome.

In the future, functional imaging should be available to evaluate children with IDD. DTI is used in research to study white matter tracks.

## Psychopathology

### Epidemiology of Mental Illness and Intellectual Developmental Disorder

For much of the past century, IDD and mental illness were regarded as mutually exclusive conditions. Affective and behavioral disturbances manifested by individuals with IDD generally had been regarded as manifestations of maladaptive learning profiles and adverse psychosocial experiences rather than as indications of psychiatric disorder. This view had been shared equally by IDD and mental health professionals. However, mental disorder diagnosis can be made in those who exhibit signs and symptoms pertinent to psychiatric disturbance among individuals within the general population. This early diagnostic bias was an outgrowth of several factors. First, the development of valid and reliable tests of intelligence and adaptive functioning early in the 21st century enabled professionals to clearly distinguish IDD from mental illness for the first time (resulting in more specific and appropriate treatment interventions and remediation). Second, professionals wished to protect individuals with IDD from the stigma associated with the label of mental illness and ensure that their primary condition received appropriate intervention. Third, professionals believed that the presence of cognitive impairment precluded the development of psychological structures and processes necessary for most forms of psychopathology. Fourth, individuals with IDD were considered to be better candidates for educational and behavioral interventions than traditional methods of psychotherapy.

Epidemiologic studies involving community samples indicate that children, adolescents, and adults with developmental disorders are at significant risk for the development of the emotional and behavioral disturbances categorized in DSM-5. Prevalence rates of psychiatric disorder range between approximately 30% and 70% depending on specific assessment procedures, diagnostic criteria, and the degree of IDD manifested by the subjects. This represents a four- to fivefold increase over the prevalence of psychopathology in the general population.

An early study is noteworthy because of the representativeness of its samples and the systematic and reliable nature of its assessment procedures. Rutter et al. (1970) reported that 30–40% of all 9- to 11-year-old children with IDD living on the Isle of Wight manifested a psychiatric disorder—a prevalence several times higher than that found among children of average intelligence.

Epidemiologic studies of mental disorders in persons with IDD are increasing (Munir, 2016). One issue that has influenced prevalence studies is referred to as "diagnostic overshadowing." This term refers to situations in which the presence of IDD is so apparent that the significance of an associated mental disorder is minimized; for example, IDD is given greater importance in the classification than concurrent emotional and behavior disorders. In early pharmacological trials, persons with IDD were generally excluded because the diagnostic criteria for mental disorders were less well-defined in persons with IDD. Those with an IQ less than 70 were typically excluded.

Despite this lack of emphasis, individuals with IDD have an increased vulnerability to emotional and behavioral disorders. Rates of psychiatric disorder are higher in individuals with mild to moderate IDD compared to the general population and are highest in those who test in the severe to profound range of IDD. Their vulnerabilities are primarily related to a reduced capacity to cope with complex social and cognitive demands; difficulty in problem-solving ability, especially in the resolution of conflicts; poor social judgment; and sensorimotor and language disorders that affect communication. Moreover, they may be further handicapped because mental health professionals may be unwilling to provide treatment for them.

Symptomatic forms of mental disorder related to associated brain dysfunction occur at high rates. Schizophrenia has been reported in 2% or 3% of persons with IDD, a prevalence that includes symptomatic forms. Both major depression and bipolar disorder may occur, but prevalence rates vary. Anxiety disorders, obsessive–compulsive disorder, and repetitive behavior disorders and phobias occur at higher rates than in the general population. There is no established evidence that persons with an IDD have greater vulnerability to affective or anxiety disorders.

IDD has been regarded as a risk factor for criminal behavior. Although a disproportionately higher number of adults with IDD are found in correctional facilities, criminal offenders account for only a small fraction of the entire IDD population. Factors to consider are that those with IDD are more likely to be apprehended when they are involved in antisocial behavior and the affected person may lack the life experience to understand what is appropriate community behavior.

Suicidal behavior is not generally emphasized in persons with IDD, but suicides do occur and suicide threats must be taken seriously. Attempts are most likely to occur in individuals with a mild IDD. As is the case with typically developing persons, it is essential to search for an underlying psychiatric diagnosis. In individuals with IDD, particularly with co-occurring mood disorder, presentation may be atypical. They think about suicide, they make suicide attempts, and not infrequently they die (Dodd et al., 2016; Ludi et al., 2012). Those with higher intellectual and adaptive function with immediate past stressors are at a greater risk (Ludi et al., 2012). Therefore, it is important to screen for suicidal thoughts, paying particular attention to changes in the individual's behavior (Ludi et al., 2012). Suicidal behavior and deliberate self-harm must be distinguished from self-injurious behavior, which typically occurs in persons with severe IDD.

In addition to these disorders, alcohol and substance abuse are problems identified in persons with mild IDD. Alcoholism and alcohol misuse are more common problems than substance abuse (Didden et al., 2020). *Substance abuse* refers to problematic and recurrent patterns of substance use that result in significant impairments in day-to-day functioning, including failure to meet responsibilities in work, home, and school. Substance abuse is associated with emotional and behavioral problems, mental illness, and somatic problems. People with IDD, especially those who test in the mild and borderline range, are overrepresented in prisons for the mentally ill and addiction centers. In an adult forensic addiction treatment center, 39% were identified with moderate to borderline cognitive deficits, in contrast to 12–15% in the general population (Luteijn et al., 2017). Although individuals with IDD do have similar risk factors as their peers, they are more vulnerable to the adverse effects of substance abuse (Didden et al., 2020).

Self-injurious behavior is perhaps the most extreme and dangerous form of behavior seen in IDD (National Institutes of Health [NIH], 1990). Self-injury has been reported in 10–70% of institutionalized persons with IDD. The lower the IQ, the higher the prevalence rate. It occurs most often in severely and profoundly impaired individuals and also in younger children who have associated language disabilities, visual impairments, or seizures. In a community sample, the prevalence of self-injury in 2,663 persons with IDD, ASD, or multiply-disabled children and adolescents in a large community metropolitan school district was assessed (Griffin et al., 1987). Sixty-nine cases or 2.6% demonstrated self-injury during the 12-month period of the study; 59% were male and 41% were female. Most individuals in this group (83%) were severely or profoundly cognitively impaired. The mean age of those surveyed was 10 years; and the majority, three-fourths of the group, demonstrated the behavior daily. For those aged 14 years or older, prevalence was lower, perhaps related to community placement for older individuals. The most common symptoms were hand hitting, head hitting, and head banging. Other forms of self-injury included eye gouging, hair pulling, and nail picking, as well as multiple forms of self-injury in one individual.

The pattern of psychopathology seen in severely affected persons with IDD is different than that seen in persons with mild or moderate IDD. A particularly common association with IDD is social impairment. Wing and Gould (1979) conducted an epidemiologic study of children with severe IDD in London and concluded that more than half were socially impaired. Social impairment in children with brain dysfunction consisted of a triad of symptoms encompassing social interaction, nonverbal and verbal communication, and imaginative development, accompanied by an increase in repetitive and stereotyped behaviors. Although some children in Wing and Gould's study met diagnostic criteria for ASD, the majority had less severe social impairments. Of these, three subgroups of social impairment were identified: (a) aloof and indifferent to others; (b) passive acceptance of social approaches; and (c) active, but odd and inappropriate, interactions. In other studies, the prevalence of social impairment has ranged from 25% to 42%. Depending on the population studied, the general prevalence of IDD in individuals with ASD is approximately 55%.

When evaluating individuals with IDD, it is important to keep in mind that they are generally multiply disabled. Some are mobile, and some are nonmobile. Community surveys will frequently demonstrate two or more additional disabilities. These disabilities are not simply additive but, rather, multiplicative in their effects. With regard to psychiatric presentations, persons with an IDD experience the full range of psychiatric disorders; these usually present as maladaptive behavior. The origin of psychopathology is multiply determined. Moreover, the onset of a psychiatric disorder may initially present as an increase in the rate of a previously established maladaptive behavior.

## Spectrum of Psychiatric Disorders

Systematic investigations indicate that the full spectrum of recognized psychiatric disorders can be identified among those with IDD. Chart reviews of clinical diagnoses, however, indicate that psychotic disturbances are overdiagnosed, and anxiety, affective, and personality disorders are underrecognized.

Children and adults with mild to moderate IDD manifest a profile of psychiatric symptoms and disorders similar to what occurs within the typically developed population. Studies using standardized methods of assessment reveal similar rates of ADHD, conduct disorder, anxiety disorders (phobias, obsessive–compulsive disorder, and generalized anxiety), affective disorders, personality disorders, and schizophrenia. Some symptoms occur with particular frequency among community residents, including feelings of social inadequacy, dependency, and sensitivity to criticism (affecting one-fourth to one-half), anxiety (affecting one-third), and aggressive behavior (affecting one-fifth to one-fourth).

Affective disorders (e.g., major depression, bipolar disorder, and dysthymia) occur commonly and are responsible for a significant degree of morbidity. Approximately 2–10% of individuals with IDD manifest serious affective disorders; as many as 50% suffer from dysthymia. Preliminary investigations have reported the successful use of assessment instruments developed for the general population (e.g., the Beck Inventory of Depression, Schedule for Affective Disorders and Schizophrenia, and Children's Depression Inventory). However, studies are needed to confirm adequate reliability and validity with this population. Biological markers have been sought to improve diagnostic accuracy.

Schizophrenia occurs at a rate two or three times higher than that reported among the general population. Although schizophrenia was once a controversial diagnosis in persons with IDD, it is now recognized (H. Aman et al., 2016). Careful studies have documented the presence of such symptoms as hallucinations, delusions, and thought disorder. The expression of these symptoms is generally more concrete and less elaborate than their occurrence in the general population. Comparisons of persons with an IDD and typically developed schizophrenic patients reveal that the former group has an earlier age of onset and a less favorable premorbid history. However, both groups exhibit a very similar profile of psychotic symptoms (e.g., hallucinations, delusions, thought disorder, etc.).

Among those with severe and profound IDD, a somewhat different profile of psychopathology is present. Certain symptoms occur less frequently, primarily because of limitations in cognitive and symbolic processes. These include delusions, hallucinations, referential ideation, obsessions, and guilty ruminations. Other symptoms occur more frequently. For example, stereotyped behaviors, such as finger flicking and hand flapping, are present in 15–50% of individuals; self-injurious behaviors, such as eye gouging and head banging, are present in 10–20%. Several disorders are more common among children and adults with severe to profound IDD, including ASD and related pervasive developmental disorders. As many as 4–8% of children with an IDD meet criteria for ASD, or approximately three to six times the prevalence in the general population. Conversely, approximately 55% of children and adults with ASD meet criteria for IDD.

## Treatment

Treatment for children and adults with an IDD must address the complex interplay of neurobiological and psychosocial factors. A comprehensive interdisciplinary approach is essential, and consideration should be given to the full range of treatments used with typically developing children. In most instances, multiple treatment modalities are needed. The AAIDD (Schalock et al., 2021) multidimensional approach provides guidelines for intervention. Better environmental provision, cognitive and behavioral interventions, individual and family psychotherapy, and psychopharmacology are all applicable approaches. The efficacy of each of these interventions has been demonstrated when appropriately selected and implemented.

## The Environmental Provision

Living conditions, vocational opportunities, and leisure time activities are essential environmental provisions for persons with IDD. It is equally important that they participate by expressing preferences and making personal choices about living conditions, work, and recreational activities. These issues have received increasing attention, and when handled well, they lead to an improved quality of life and a substantial reduction in maladaptive affective and behavioral symptoms. In the case of a child with an IDD, the parent requires particular support in providing for the child's needs. A home program includes increasing access to preferred activities, offering choices regarding household tasks, and scheduling highly preferred tasks and activities immediately following nonpreferred (but essential) ones.

## Educational Interventions/Skill Development

A fundamental challenge in the care and treatment of persons with an IDD is to assist them in finding new ways to interact with others appropriately. Emotional and behavioral disturbances commonly result from a lack of self-monitoring and adaptive control over their inner lives and external environment. Communication deficits, learning difficulty, and limited educational experience often deprive them of the requisite skills needed for personal competence and social responsibility. Therefore, an educationally based program should emphasize social, communication, and vocational skills to reduce maladaptive behavior by improving self-control. Essential elements of such a program include independence training (teaching self-help and leisure skills), communication training (enhancing speech and nonverbal communication—signing, gestures, and picture/word boards), and self-management skill development (teaching strategies for self-monitoring and self-reinforcement).

Social skills training provides concrete instructions; uses observation and modeling of effective behavior; offers reinforcement; and focuses on teaching through simple, observable behaviors. Social skills training emphasizes the enhancement of appropriate interpersonal behavior in a variety of social situations, such as being introduced to another person and properly responding, initiating and participating in social group activities, and learning to interpret and respond appropriately to verbal and nonverbal social cues. Successful social skills programs combine demonstration by instructors, modeling, role-play, social practice, constructive feedback, and positive reinforcement. The training sequence might include initial instruction and practice in a therapeutic environment, followed by practice in natural community settings.

## Behavioral Interventions

Behavioral approaches are the most widely used and best studied treatment interventions for behavioral disturbances in persons with IDD. Although behavioral procedures are based on the principles of learning theory (which posits that maladaptive patterns of behavior are the result of faulty conditioning), they are effective for emotional and behavioral symptoms that result primarily from pathophysiological dysfunction. Behavioral procedures have been developed for improving adaptive behavior, reducing maladaptive behavior, and broadening skill development through direct training and education. Behavioral interventions may be specifically indicated for self-injurious behavior, self-stimulatory behavior, aggressive behavior, and habit training; these interventions are described in Chapter 19.

Behavioral approaches are generally grouped into those designed to enhance adaptive behavior and those designed to suppress maladaptive behavior. Behavior enhancement procedures are preferable because they reduce inappropriate behaviors by teaching adaptive solutions. This is accomplished by reinforcing appropriate behaviors and suppressing maladaptive ones.

Behavior enhancement procedures may be subdivided into several types of differential reinforcement strategies. The most used method for behavioral enhancement is the differential reinforcement of other behavior, in which the individual is rewarded for not exhibiting the target behavior (Lory et al., 2020). If the undesirable behavior does not occur within a specified time interval, positive reinforcement is provided. The time interval for positive reinforcement is determined from the frequency of the target behavior. It should be long enough to require some effort but short enough to promote success. When the procedure is successful, the frequency of target behaviors decreases as the frequency of the more adaptive, competing behaviors (those that are reinforced) increases. For maladaptive behaviors that occur very frequently, differential reinforcement of low rates of behavior may be used. In this procedure, a predetermined frequency of the target behavior (lower than that occurring at baseline) is reinforced. This frequency is progressively lowered until the target behavior is eliminated. Another

procedure, differential reinforcement of incompatible behavior, involves the direct reinforcement of preselected adaptive behaviors that compete with, and eventually replace,
the target behaviors. The competing behaviors are chosen because they are incompatible with the target behaviors (e.g., using one's hand to shake another's hand rather than
to slap another's face). These procedures are based on a careful determination of the
characteristics of the maladaptive behaviors (frequency, duration, intensity, etc.) and
through identification of a variety of motivating reinforcers. Negative reinforcement is
sometimes used to enhance behavior. This procedure involves allowing the individual
to avoid a predetermined punishment by engaging in desirable behavior.

Behavior reduction procedures involve the introduction of unpleasant consequences
immediately following the occurrence of the target behavior. A wide variety of behavior
reduction procedures have been used that range from non-exclusionary time-out to
electric shock. Behavior reduction procedures include (a) extinction, the elimination
of reinforcing consequences of maladaptive behavior; (b) time-out from positive reinforcement; (c) response cost, the loss of a previously earned reward; (d) overcorrection,
restoring order after disrupting the environment or the repeated practice of an adaptive
behavior (e.g., dressing); (e) physical or mechanical restraint; and (f) visual screening.
Direct punishment procedures might include verbal reprimand, mild electric shock,
ammonia capsules, and mist spray. Punishment procedures show short-term efficacy
in suppressing maladaptive behaviors, at least under certain circumstances. However,
the stability and generalization of these effects are questionable because punishment
procedures primarily suppress behavior rather than teach adaptive solutions. The most
intrusive procedures typically have been reserved for the most dangerous behaviors
(e.g., serious aggression and self-injury).

Punishment procedures have been sharply criticized and are the source of considerable controversy. Many states have enacted regulations that either ban or seriously restrict the implementation of these procedures. These actions stem from ethical concerns
but also because behavior suppression or punishment alone does not teach self-
regulation or problem-solving skills that enhance future adaptive responses to stress.
In 1989, NIH (1990) sponsored a Consensus Development Conference on Treatment of
Destructive Behaviors in Persons with Developmental Disabilities. A panel of nationally recognized experts in the field of developmental disabilities reviewed the available
research and heard testimony from investigators and clinicians working with behavior
disorders in persons with intellectual disability disorder. The recommendations of
the panel for the treatment of severely disruptive behavior included the following
(NIH, 1990):

- Most successful approaches to treatment are likely to involve multiple elements
  of therapy (behavioral and psychopharmacologic), environmental change, and
  education.
- Treatment methods may require techniques for enhancing desired behaviors; for
  producing changes in social, physical, and educational environments; and for reducing or eliminating destructive behaviors.
- Treatments should be based on an analysis of medical and psychiatric conditions,
  environmental situations, consequences, and skill deficits. In the application of any

of these treatments, an essential step involves a functional analysis of existing behavioral patterns.

- Behavior reduction procedures should be selected for their rapid effectiveness *only* if the exigencies of the clinical situation require such restrictive interventions and *only* after appropriate review. These interventions should *only* be used in the context of a comprehensive treatment package.

Systematic research is ongoing to identify the specific behavioral interventions that are most efficacious for particular maladaptive behaviors. Most studies involve single-case designs with small sample sizes and rarely include clinical factors that might affect treatment outcome (e.g., clinical psychiatric syndromes and disorders, family history, and psychosocial circumstances). Overall, positive behavioral interventions are useful for social skills deficits; mild punishment procedures (e.g., extinction, disapproval, and overcorrection) for psychophysiologic symptoms (e.g., enuresis and encopresis); and more intrusive punishment procedures (e.g., restraint and time-out) for initial management of destructive behaviors (e.g., aggression and self-injurious behavior). Self-stimulatory behaviors, psychophysiologic symptoms, and noncompliance are the most responsive to behavioral treatment (65–75% success rate); destructive behaviors are next (45–65% success rate), and inappropriate social interactions are the least responsive (35–40% success rate). Although more than 50% of published studies focus on behavioral interventions, there are other approaches that are personalized to the individual and use cognitive therapy. These include skill training, mediation, technology-assisted interventions, and parent training (Woodcock & Blackwell, 2020).

## Psychotherapy

Individuals with mild cognitive impairments have been shown to benefit from individual, family, and group psychotherapy. Psychotherapeutic interventions are most effective in the treatment of emotional and behavioral disturbances in individuals who have experienced traumatic psychosocial experiences that lead to internalized conflict and maladaptive personality functioning. Repeated failure, social rejection, frequent losses, and dependency on others often result in feelings of inferiority, ambivalence, anxiety, and anger, and each of these symptoms may be targeted. Family conflicts involving feelings of jealousy toward normally developing siblings and tension with parents regarding issues of emancipation and independence are other targets. Psychotherapeutic interventions tend to be underutilized, primarily because of misconceptions about their effectiveness for persons with an IDD despite the fact that they are often good candidates for psychotherapy. They can be highly motivated to establish interpersonal relationships and often demonstrate a strong desire for enhancing their personal competence and independence.

The goals of psychotherapeutic treatment are like those for the general population and include the resolution of internalized conflict, improvement in self-esteem, and enhancement of personal competence and independence. Modifications of the usual treatment approaches may be necessary that take into account the developmental level of the patient. A supportive atmosphere, focused approaches by the therapist, and shorter and more frequent sessions may be needed.

## Psychopharmacology

Psychopharmacological management is an important treatment strategy and an adjunct to other forms of therapy for children and adults with an IDD (Ji & Findling, 2016). Psychotropic medications are effective in reducing the symptoms associated with a variety of psychiatric disorders and have been used quite extensively, especially in treating co-occurring aggression, self-injury, attentional problems, depression, anxiety, and mood disorders in people with IDD. Surveys indicate that between one-fifth and one-half of individuals with IDD residing in institutions and one-fourth to one-third residing in community settings receive some type of psychotropic medication. There are significant inter-institutional and inter-agency differences in prescribing patterns, ranging from less than 10% in some settings to more than 50% in others for patients with similar demographic and clinical characteristics. Overall, neuroleptics are prescribed most often and antidepressants and stimulants least often.

Despite the frequent use of psychopharmacologic interventions for individuals with IDD, relatively few studies include appropriate control groups. Single case reports and non-blind, open clinical trials make up the majority of these reports. Clinical reports often show evidence of methodological problems, such as reporting bias (underreporting of negative findings), retrospective or anecdotal data, lack of interrater reliability, and the concurrent use of other psychotropic medications that may be changed during the course of the drug trial. Antipsychotics, especially risperidone, are reported to be effective in reducing problem behavior in children with IDD, and methylphenidate and other dopamine receptor agonists are useful in ADHD. The following section discusses individual studies.

## Drug Treatment for Specific Disorders

### Attention-Deficit/Hyperactivity Disorder

As many as 40% of children and adolescents with IDD exhibit high activity levels, impulsive behavior, and inattentiveness. Epidemiologic studies show that for 8–39%, of cases (Baker et al., 2010), these symptoms are severe enough to warrant the diagnosis of ADHD (Ahuja et al., 2013; Strømme & Diseth, 2000). ADHD may be underdiagnosed due to "diagnostic overshadowing" (the tendency to overlook other diagnoses once the diagnosis of IDD is made). Therefore, stimulants are among the most frequently prescribed psychotropic medications for children with IDD. There is concurrence that the stimulants are useful for children and adolescents with mild IDD who meet diagnostic criteria for ADHD. Approximately 40–60% (Simonoff et al., 2013) of this group of children demonstrate a significant decrease in hyperactivity, impulsivity, and inattention and an increase in on-task behavior with drug treatment. This is lower than the 70–80% reported for typically developing children. Some studies have documented significant improvements on laboratory measures of attention, memory, and learning (e.g., continuous performance tasks, matching-to-sample tasks, and paired-associate learning). In contrast, little evidence shows that the stimulants improve behavior, learning, or performance among children with IDD, who either do not meet diagnostic criteria for ADHD or whose behavioral symptoms are characteristic of other disorders (e.g., ASD and anxiety disorders). In addition, side effects, which occur at a greater frequency than that reported in the general population (especially among nonresponders), include sleep problems, poor appetite, irritability, lethargy, internal preoccupation, social withdrawal, increased motor stereotypy, and overinclusive attention. Methylphenidate has reduced ADHD symptoms in fetal alcohol spectrum disorder, velocardiofacial syndrome, and fragile X syndrome. Clonidine and guanfacine are also reported to improve hyperactivity and global functioning (Ji & Findling, 2016).

## Schizophrenia

Community epidemiologic studies indicate that non-affective psychosis occurs in up to 3% of the population with IDD. The available literature documents the usefulness of neuroleptic medication for psychotic symptoms manifested by affected patients. Treatment responsiveness is similar to that found in typically developing persons.

## Mood Disorders

Although major depression and dysthymic disorder commonly occur among individuals with IDD, the evidence for efficacy of antidepressant medication is limited. Some case reports support the efficacy of antidepressant. Mood-stabilizing agents (e.g., lithium carbonate and valproate) have been studied for treatment of bipolar disorder and for the control of aggressive behavior. Several open trials and two controlled studies reported lithium to be effective in treating acute manic episodes and in reducing the frequency and duration of affective cycles. Controlled trials document the benefits of lithium to manage problem behaviors, especially aggression. Nausea, diarrhea, headache, and tremors are common side effects (Ji & Findling, 2016).

## Aggressive and Self-Injurious Behavior

Most medication trials have focused on the treatment of destructive behaviors, such as aggression and self-injury. Neuroleptics have been the most frequently subjected to clinical trials. Results are equivocal, particularly for the control of aggressive behavior. Although some studies have documented significant reductions in aggressive behavior with lithium, findings for self-injurious behavior are more consistent. The potential involvement of dopaminergic mechanisms in self-injurious behavior is supported by studies of the adenosine system. Caffeine, theophylline, and clonidine are adenosine antagonists that act indirectly to increase dopamine activity; they are also known to exacerbate self-injurious behavior. These data collectively indicate that self-injurious behavior might be successfully treated by medications that reduce dopamine transmission.

Findings regarding the efficacy of neuroleptics in the treatment of destructive behavior are equivocal; therefore, the use of these medications should be weighed against their potential adverse effects. However, neuroleptics are the most commonly prescribed psychotropic medication for people with IDD, targeting aggression, self-injury, sever stereotypies, and hyperactivity. There is good evidence for the efficacy of these medications, especially risperidone (M. Aman et al., 2002). Somnolence, headache,

436 HARRIS' DEVELOPMENTAL NEUROPSYCHIATRY

appetite increase, weigh gain, and extrapyramidal symptoms including parkinsonian symptoms and dystonic reactions are common side effects. Long-term side effects such as tardive dyskinesia have been reported (Turgay et al., 2002). The severity of cognitive impairment and the presence of other neurological conditions may increase the risk of tardive dyskinesia according to some, but not all, studies.

Serotonergic dysfunction also has been hypothesized to underlie some forms of destructive behavior. Reduced cerebrospinal fluid concentrations of the serotonin metabolite, 5-hydroxyindoleacetic acid, the principle metabolite of serotonin, are associated with aggressive behaviors (G. Brown & Linnoila, 1990). A number of case reports and several controlled studies have reported that lithium can reduce both aggressive and self-injurious behavior. These findings are supported by open clinical trials involving other medications that reportedly increase serotonergic activity, including buspirone, trazadone, and fluoxetine.

It has been suggested that the GABAergic system may play a role in self-injurious behavior. However, medications that affect GABA functioning (e.g., benzodiazepines) do not have consistent effects on aggression and self-injury. Some studies have reported that benzodiazepines reduce destructive behavior; others have reported an exacerbation of aggression and self-injurious behavior. Paradoxical excitement has also been reported.

Several lines of evidence implicate the endogenous opioid system in the pathogenesis of destructive behavior, especially self-injurious behavior (Gibson et al., 1995; Sandman et al., 1993). Two major hypotheses have been offered to explain the potential role of the endogenous opioid system. Preliminary studies suggest that some patients have elevated peripheral (and perhaps central nervous system) levels of endogenous opioids, leading to a high pain threshold and a tendency to persist in self-injurious behavior. According to another line of reasoning, self-injurious injury itself causes endogenous opioid levels to rise, resulting in stress-induced analgesia. Opioid antagonists have been recommended as a treatment either to increase the perception of pain (thereby serving as a natural deterrent to self-injurious behavior) or to extinguish the theoretically pleasurable effects of self-injurious behavior-induced elevations in endogenous opioid levels. Several studies (including several methodologically sound, controlled investigations) have assessed the efficacy of opioid antagonists (e.g., naloxone and naltrexone) in the treatment of individuals with an IDD diagnosis with self-injurious behavior. Although some of these studies have reported impressive beneficial effects, others have not (Rana et al., 2013; Symons et al., 2004). Additional investigations, employing larger samples of subjects, are necessary to identify the types of patients likely to benefit from such treatment.

Increased noradrenergic activity may lead to aggressive behavior, perhaps secondary to anxiety or a state of heightened arousal. Several case reports and open clinical trials suggest that both centrally and peripherally acting β-adrenergic blockers (e.g., propranolol and nadolol) may be helpful in reducing the frequency and intensity of explosive episodes of aggression (Kuperman & Stewart, 1987; Ratey et al., 1986).

The etiology and treatment of stereotypic behavior in children and adults with IDD have long been of interest. Both preclinical and clinical studies suggest involvement of the dopaminergic system (perhaps via postsynaptic dopamine supersensitivity) in the etiology of some forms of stereotypy. Dopamine agonists are known to induce stereotypic behavior, a response that can be blocked by treatment with dopamine D2 receptor antagonists. In addition, a relatively large number of studies indicate that neuroleptics may reduce stereotypic behavior among persons with an IDD diagnosis.

The initiation of psychotropic medication treatment requires a thorough psychiatric evaluation to identify a medication-responsive psychiatric disorder or a specific target behavior that may be responsive to medication. A drug-free baseline period during which the symptoms or behaviors identified for treatment are carefully defined and characterized (e.g., frequency, duration, intensity, etc.) is strongly recommended. Valid and reliable behavior rating scales should be selected and used at appropriate intervals during the medication trial to assess drug efficacy. Direct observational data and/or standardized rating scales should be used to monitor effects and potential side effects. The trial should include therapeutic doses of medication and be conducted for an adequate length of time.

## Conclusion

This chapter traces the history of IDD and summarizes recent developments in the field of IDD. Epidemiologic studies have demonstrated the increased prevalence of mental and behavior disorders in this population. When considering the complexity of psychiatric diagnosis and treatment, old questions persist and new ones arise. Among them are the following: (a) With the establishment of a phenomenological approach to the diagnosis of mental disorder, should clinical findings be clustered into diagnoses of neuropsychiatric disorders or simply considered dimensionally as aspects of cognitive and adaptive impairment or both, depending on the presentation? (b) How should diagnostic criteria be modified to take developmental symptoms into account? (c) Is there an association with certain genetic syndromes and specific psychiatric disorders? and (d) How should treatment be modified, based on the multiple etiologies of IDD?

Advances have been made in the treatment of both abnormal patterns of behavior and co-occurring neuropsychiatric disorders in individuals with IDD. Yet, treatment programs are often fragmented and need to be pulled together in a comprehensive fashion, involving an interdisciplinary team. In the future, better methods of assessment are needed that highlight the interface between environmental and neurobiological mechanisms involved in both affective and behavioral disturbances. This additional information may lead to more focused and effective treatment programs. Currently, full validation of specific treatment approaches for particular symptoms, or clusters of symptoms, is limited. To determine the efficacy of a treatment approach, larger clinical trials are needed with more subjects, greater homogeneity regarding symptoms, and the inclusion of neuropsychiatric diagnoses. In research, controlled procedures are necessary, which include randomization, double-blind designs, and standardized methods of assessment. With a better understanding of the efficacy of treatment for established homogeneous clinical groups, the long-term outcome can be established more predictably. Clinical testing and research focus on the recognition of the co-occurrence of mental disorders in persons with IDD, an area in which considerable progress has been made.

# References

Ahuja, A., Martin, J., Langley, K., & Thapar, A. (2013). Intellectual disability in children with attention deficit hyperactivity disorder. *Journal of Pediatrics, 163*(3), 890–895.

Akrami, L., & Davudi, M. (2014). Comparison of behavioral and sexual problems between intellectually disabled and normal adolescent boys during puberty in Yazd, Iran. *Iranian Journal of Psychiatry and Behavioral Sciences, 8*(2), 68–74.

Aman, H., Naeem, F., Farooq, S., & Ayub, M. (2016). Prevalence of nonaffective psychosis in intellectually disabled clients: Systematic review and meta-analysis. *Psychiatric Genetics, 26*(4), 145–155.

Aman, M. G., Burrow, W. H., & Wolford, P. L. (1995). The Aberrant Behavior Checklist–Community: Factor validity and effect of subject variables for adults in group homes. *American Journal on Mental Retardation, 100*(3), 283–292.

Aman, M. G., De Smedt, G., Derivan, A., Lyons, B., Findling, R. L., & Risperidone Disruptive Behavior Study Group. (2002). Double-blind, placebo-controlled study of risperidone for the treatment of disruptive behaviors in children with subaverage intelligence. *American Journal of Psychiatry, 159*(8), 1337–1346.

American Psychiatric Association. (2013). *Diagnostic and statistical manual of mental disorders* (5th ed.). American Psychiatric Publishing.

Baker, B. L., Neece, C. L., Fenning, R. M., Crnic, K. A., & Blacher, J. (2010). Mental disorders in five-year-old children with or without developmental delay: Focus on ADHD. *Journal of Clinical Child & Adolescent Psychology, 39*(4), 492–505.

Balboni, G., Battagliese, G., & Pedrabissi, L. (2000). The Psychopathology Inventory for Mentally Retarded Adults: Factor structure and comparisons between subjects with or without dual diagnosis. *Research in Developmental Disabilities, 21*(4), 311–321.

Barbey, A. K. (2018). Network neuroscience theory of human intelligence. *Trends in Cognitive Sciences, 22*(1), 8–20.

Barbey, A. K., Colom, R., & Grafman, J. (2013). Architecture of cognitive flexibility revealed by lesion mapping. *NeuroImage, 82*, 547–554.

Barbey, A. K., Colom, R., Paul, E. J., Chau, A., Solomon, J., & Grafman, J. H. (2014). Lesion mapping of social problem solving. *Brain, 137*(10), 2823–2833.

Barbey, A. K., Colom, R., Paul, E. J., & Grafman, J. (2014). Architecture of fluid intelligence and working memory revealed by lesion mapping. *Brain Structure and Function, 219*(2), 485–494.

Barbey, A. K., Colom, R., Solomon, J., Krueger, F., Forbes, C., & Grafman, J. (2012). An integrative architecture for general intelligence and executive function revealed by lesion mapping. *Brain, 135*(4), 1154–1164.

Belva, B. C., & Matson, J. L. (2015). Examining the psychometrics of the Psychopathology Inventory for Mentally Retarded Adults–II for individuals with mild and moderate intellectual disabilities. *Research in Developmental Disabilities, 36*, 291–302.

Bertelli, M. O., Cooper, S. A., & Salvador-Carulla, L. (2018). Intelligence and specific cognitive functions in intellectual disability: Implications for assessment and classification. *Current Opinion in Psychiatry, 31*(2), 88–95.

Bertelli, M. O., Salvador-Carulla, L., Scuticchio, D., Varrucciu, N., Martinez-Leal, R., Cooper, S. A., Simeonsson, R. J., Deb, S., Weber, G., Jung, R., Munir, K., Adnams, C., Akoury-Dirani, L., Girimaji, S. C., Katz, G., Kwok, H., & Walsh, C. (2014). Moving beyond intelligence in the revision of ICD-10: Specific cognitive functions in intellectual developmental disorders. *World Psychiatry, 13*(1), 93–94.

Binet, A., & Simon, T. (1904). Méthodes nouvelles pour le diagnostic du niveau intellectuel des anormaux. *L'année Psychologique, 11*(1), 191–244.

Bourneville, D.M. (1880). Sclérose tubereuse des convulsions c-vibrales: Idiotie et epilepsie bemiplgique. *Archives of Neurology, 1*, 81–91.

Brown, E. C., Aman, M. G., & Havercamp, S. M. (2002). Factor analysis and norms for parent ratings on the Aberrant Behavior Checklist–Community for young people in special education. *Research in Developmental Disabilities, 23*(1), 45–60.

Brown, G. L., & Linnoila, M. I. (1990). CSF serotonin metabolite (5-HIAA) studies in depression, impulsivity, and violence. *Journal of Clinical Psychiatry*, *51*(Suppl.), 31–43.

Bryan, C. (1930). *The papyrus Ebers*. Appleton.

Christoforou, A., Espeseth, T., Davies, G., Fernandes, C. P., Giddaluru, S., Mattheisen, M., Teneas, A., Harris, S., Liewald, D., Payton, A., Ollier, W., Horan, M., Pendleton, N., Haggarty, P., Djurovic, S., Herms, S., Hoffman, P., Cichon, S., Starr, J., . . . Le Hellard, S. (2014). GWAS-based pathway analysis differentiates between fluid and crystallized intelligence. *Genes, Brain and Behavior*, *13*(7), 663–674.

Colom, R., Karama, S., Jung, R. E., & Haier, R. J. (2010). Human intelligence and brain networks. *Dialogues in Clinical Neuroscience*, *12*(4), 489–501.

Conrad, E., & Knowlden, A. P. (2020). A systematic review of obesity interventions targeting anthropometric changes in youth with intellectual disabilities. *Journal of Intellectual Disabilities*, *24*(3), 398–417.

Davies, G., Tenesa, A., Payton, A., Yang, J., Harris, S. E., Liewald, D., Ke, X., Le Hellard, S., Christoforou, A., Luciano, M., McGhee, K., Lopez, L., Gow, A., Corley, J., Redmond, P., Fox, H., Haggarty, P., Whalley, L., McNeill, G., . . . Deary, I. J. (2011). Genome-wide association studies establish that human intelligence is highly heritable and polygenic. *Molecular Psychiatry*, *16*(10), 996–1005.

Deary, I. J., Penke, L., & Johnson, W. (2010). The neuroscience of human intelligence differences. *Nature Reviews Neuroscience*, *11*(3), 201–211.

Demetriou, A., Christou, C., Spanoudis, G., & Platsidou, M. (2002). The development of mental processing: Efficiency, working memory, and thinking. *Monographs of the Society for Research in Child Development*, *67*(1), 1–156.

Didden, R., VanDerNagel, J., Delforterie, M., & Van Duijvenbode, N. (2020). Substance use disorders in people with intellectual disability. *Current Opinion in Psychiatry*, *33*(2), 124–129.

Dodd, P., Doherty, A., & Guerin, S. (2016). A systematic review of suicidality in people with intellectual disabilities. *Harvard Review of Psychiatry*, *24*(3), 202–213.

Down, J. L. H. (1866). Observations on an ethnic classification of idiots. *London Hospital Reports*, *3*(1866), 259–262.

Dykens, E. M., Hodapp, R. M., Ort, S., Finucane, B., Shapiro, L. R., & Leckman, J. F. (1989). The trajectory of cognitive development in males with fragile X syndrome. *Journal of the American Academy of Child & Adolescent Psychiatry*, *28*(3), 422–426.

Einfeld, S., & Emerson, E. (2008). Intellectual disability. In M. Rutter (Ed.), *Rutter's child and adolescent psychiatry* (5th ed., pp. 820–840). Blackwell.

Einfeld, S. L., & Tonge, B. J. (1995). The Developmental Behavior Checklist: The development and validation of an instrument to assess behavioral and emotional disturbance in children and adolescents with mental retardation. *Journal of Autism and Developmental Disorders*, *25*(2), 81–104.

Emerson, E., Hatton, C., Baines, S., & Robertson, J. (2016). The physical health of British adults with intellectual disability: Cross sectional study. *International Journal for Equity in Health*, *15*(1), 1–9.

Emerson, E., Robertson, J., Baines, S., & Hatton, C. (2016). Obesity in British children with and without intellectual disability: Cohort study. *BMC Public Health*, *16*(1), 1–10.

Esquirol, E. (1845). *Mental maladies: A treatise on insanity* (E. K. Hunt, Trans.). Lea & Blanchard.

Evans, J. S. B. (2008). Dual-processing accounts of reasoning, judgment, and social cognition. *Annual Review of Psychology*, *59*, 255–278.

Finlayson, J., Morrison, J., Jackson, A., Mantry, D., & Cooper, S. A. (2010). Injuries, falls and accidents among adults with intellectual disabilities: Prospective cohort study. *Journal of Intellectual Disability Research*, *54*(11), 966–980.

Flanagan, D. P., & McGrew, K. S. (1997). A cross-battery approach to assessing and interpreting cognitive abilities: Narrowing the gap between practice and cognitive science. In D. P. Flanagan, J. L. Genshaft, & P. L. Harrison (Eds.), *Contemporary intellectual assessment: Theories, tests, and issues* (pp. 314–325). Guilford.

Gibson, A. K., Hetrick, W. P., Taylor, D. V., Sandman, C. A., & Touchette, P. (1995). Relating the efficacy of naltrexone in treating self-injurious behavior to the Motivation Assessment Scale. *Journal of Developmental and Physical Disabilities, 7*(3), 215–220.

Goddard, H. (1912). *The Kallikak family: A study in the heredity of feeble-mindedness*. Macmillan.

Gottfredson, L. S. (1997). Mainstream science on intelligence: An editorial with 52 signatories, history, and bibliography. *Intelligence, 24*(1), 13–23.

Greenspan, S. (2009). Assessment and diagnosis of mental retardation in death penalty cases: Introduction and overview of the special "Atkins" issue. *Applied Neuropsychology, 16*(2), 89–90.

Greenspan, S. (2016). Capturing the cognitive essence of IDD: Explaining the "relatedness" clause in DSM-5. *Psychology in Intellectual Disability and Autism, 42*(3), 23–26.

Greenspan, S. (2017). Borderline intellectual functioning: An update. *Current Opinion in Psychiatry, 30*(2), 113–122.

Greenspan, S., Brown, N. N., & Edwards, W. (2015). FASD and the concept of "intellectual disability equivalence." In M. Nelson & M. Trussler (Eds.), *Law and ethics in fetal alcohol spectrum disorder* (pp. 241–266). Springer.

Greenspan, S., Harris, J. C., & Woods, G. W. (2015). Intellectual disability is "a condition, not a number": Ethics of IQ cut-offs in psychiatry, human services and law. *Ethics, Medicine and Public Health, 1*(3), 312–324.

Greenspan, S., Loughlin, G., & Black, R. S. (2001). Credulity and gullibility in people with developmental disorders: A framework for future research. International *Review* of *Research* in *Mental Retardation, 24*, 101–135.

Greenspan, S., Switzky, H. N., & Woods, G. W. (2011). Intelligence involves risk-awareness and intellectual disability involves risk-unawareness: Implications of a theory of common sense. *Journal of Intellectual and Developmental Disability, 36*(4), 246–257.

Greenspan, S., & Woods, G. W. (2014). Intellectual disability as a disorder of reasoning and judgement: The gradual move away from intelligence quotient-ceilings. *Current Opinion in Psychiatry, 27*(2), 110–116.

Griesinger, W. (1876). *Die Pathologie und Therapie der psychischen Krankheiten für Ärzte und Studirende. 4. Aufl.* Wreden.

Griffin, J. C., Ricketts, R. W., Williams, D. E., Locke, B. J., Altmeyer, B. K., & Stark, M. T. (1987). A community survey of self-injurious behavior among developmentally disabled children and adolescents. *Psychiatric Services, 38*(9), 959–963.

Grossman, H. J. (1983). *Manual on terminology and classification in intellectual disability (intellectual developmental disorder)* (rev. ed.). American Association on Mental Deficiency.

Harris, J. C. (2006). *Intellectual disability: Understanding its development, causes, classification, evaluation, and treatment*. Oxford University Press.

Harris, J. C. (2010). Advances in understanding behavioral phenotypes in neurogenetic syndromes. American Journal of Medical Genetics Part C: Seminars in Medical Genetics, 154(4), 389–399.

Harris, J. C. (2014). Intellectual disability (intellectual developmental disorder). In G. O. Gabbard (Ed.), *Gabbard's treatment of psychiatric disorders* (5th ed., pp. 3–19). American Psychiatric Publishing.

Harris, J. C., & Greenspan, S. (2016). Nature and definition of intellectual and developmental disabilities. In N. N. Singh (Ed.), *Clinical handbook of evidence-based practices for individuals with IDD* (pp. 11–39). Springer.

Hastings, R. P., Brown, T., Mount, R. H., & Cormack, K. M. (2001). Exploration of psychometric properties of the Developmental Behavior Checklist. *Journal of Autism and Developmental Disorders, 31*(4), 423–431.

Haydt, N., Greenspan, S., & Agharkar, B. S. (2013). Advantages of DSM-5 in the diagnosis of intellectual disability: Reduced reliance on IQ ceilings in Atkins (death penalty) cases. *University of Missouri–Kansas City Law Review, 82*(2).

Hill, W. D., Marioni, R. E., Maghzian, O., Ritchie, S. J., Hagenaars, S. P., McIntosh, A. M., Gale, C. R., Davies, G., & Deary, I. J. (2019). A combined analysis of genetically correlated traits identifies 187 loci and a role for neurogenesis and myelination in intelligence. *Molecular Psychiatry, 24*(2), 169–181.

Inhelder, B. (1968). *The diagnosis of reasoning in the mentally retarded.* Day. (Original work published 1943)

Ireland, W. W. (1877). *On idiocy and imbecility.* Churchill.

Isler, A., Tas, F., Beytut, D., & Conk, Z. (2009). Sexuality in adolescents with intellectual disabilities. *Sexuality and Disability, 27*(1), 27–34.

Ji, N. Y., & Findling, R. L. (2016). Pharmacotherapy for mental health problems in people with intellectual disability. *Current Opinion in Psychiatry, 29*(2), 103–125.

Jung, R. E., & Haier, R. J. (2007). The Parieto-Frontal Integration Theory (P-FIT) of intelligence: Converging neuroimaging evidence. *Behavioral and Brain Sciences, 30*(2), 135–154.

Kaat, A. J., Lecavalier, L., & Aman, M. G. (2014). Validity of the Aberrant Behavior Checklist in children with autism spectrum disorder. *Journal of Autism and Developmental Disorders, 44*(5), 1103–1116.

Kanner, L. (1960). Itard, Seguin, Howe: Three pioneers in the education of retarded children. *American Journal of Mental Deficiency, 65*, 2–10.

Kanner, L. (1964). *A history of the care and study of the mentally retarded.* Charles C Thomas.

Kanner, L. (1967). Medicine in the history of mental retardation: 1800–1965. *American Journal of Mental Deficiency, 72*(2), 165–170.

Kaufmann, W. E., Capone, G. T., Carter, J. C., & Lieberman, D. N. (2008). Genetic intellectual disability: Neurobiological and clinical aspects. *Capute & Accardo's Neurodevelopmental Disabilities in Infancy and Childhood, 1*, 155–173.

King, P., & Kitchner, K. S. (2002). The reflective judgment model: 20 years of research about cognition, knowledge and knowing. In B. F. Hofer & P. R. Pintrich (Eds.), *Personal epistemology: The psychology of beliefs* (pp. 37–61). Erlbaum.

Kuperman, S., & Stewart, M. A. (1987). Use of propranolol to decrease aggressive outbursts in younger patients. *Psychosomatics, 28*(6), 315–319.

Lane, H. (1976). *The wild boy of Aveyron* (Vol. 149). Harvard University Press.

Lory, C., Mason, R. A., Davis, J. L., Wang, D., Kim, S. Y., Gregori, E., & David, M. (2020). A meta-analysis of challenging behavior interventions for students with developmental disabilities in inclusive school settings. *Journal of Autism and Developmental Disorders, 50*(4), 1221–1237.

Ludi, E., Ballard, E. D., Greenbaum, R., Bridge, J., Reynolds, W., & Horowitz, L. (2012). Suicide risk in youth with intellectual disability: The challenges of screening. *Journal of Developmental and Behavioral Pediatrics, 33*(5), 431–440.

Luteijn, I., Didden, R., & Van der Nagel, J. (2017). Individuals with mild intellectual disability or borderline intellectual functioning in a forensic addiction treatment center: Prevalence and clinical characteristics. *Advances in Neurodevelopmental Disorders, 1*(4), 240–251.

Margolis, H. (1987). *Patterns, thinking, and cognition: A theory of judgment.* University of Chicago Press.

Marshburn, E. C., & Aman, M. G. (1992). Factor validity and norms for the Aberrant Behavior Checklist in a community sample of children with mental retardation. *Journal of Autism and Developmental Disorders, 22*(3), 357–373.

Martinello, E. (2014). Reviewing strategies for risk reduction of sexual abuse of children with intellectual disabilities: A focus on early intervention. *Sexuality and Disability, 32*(2), 167–174.

McGrew, K. S. (2005). The Cattell–Horn–Carroll theory of cognitive abilities: Past, present, and future. In D. P. Flanagan, J. L. Genshaft, & P. L. Harrison (Eds.), *Contemporary intellectual assessment: Theories, tests, and issues* (pp. 314–325). Guilford.

Medina-Rico, M., López-Ramos, H., & Quiñonez, A. (2018). Sexuality in people with intellectual disability: Review of literature. *Sexuality and Disability, 36*(3), 231–248.

Mefford, H. C., Batshaw, M. L., & Hoffman, E. P. (2012). Genomics, intellectual disability, and autism. *New England Journal of Medicine, 366*(8), 733–743.

Menolascino, F. J. (1988). Mental illness in the mentally retarded: Diagnostic and treatment issues. In A. Stark, F. J. Menolascino, M. H. Albarelli, & V. C. Gray (Eds.), *Intellectual disability (intellectual developmental disorder) and mental health: Classification, diagnosis, treatment, services* (pp. 109–123). Springer.

Michelson, D. J., Shevell, M. I., Sherr, E. H., Moeschler, J. B., Gropman, A. L., & Ashwal, S. (2011). Evidence report: Genetic and metabolic testing on children with global developmental delay: Report of the Quality Standards Subcommittee of the American Academy of Neurology and the Practice Committee of the Child Neurology Society. *Neurology, 77*(17), 1629–1635.

Moss, J., & Howlin, P. (2009). Autism spectrum disorders in genetic syndromes: Implications for diagnosis, intervention and understanding the wider autism spectrum disorder population. *Journal of Intellectual Disability Research, 53*(10), 852–873.

Munir, K. M. (2016). The co-occurrence of mental disorders in children and adolescents with intellectual disability/intellectual developmental disorder. *Current Opinion in Psychiatry, 29*(2), 95–102.

National Institutes of Health. (1990). *Consensus conference on treatment of destructive behaviors in persons with developmental disabilities.* U.S. Government Printing Office.

Patja, K., Iivanainen, M., Vesala, H., Oksanen, H., & Ruoppila, I. (2000). Life expectancy of people with intellectual disability: A 35-year follow-up study. *Journal of Intellectual Disability Research, 44*(5), 591–599.

Rana, F., Gormez, A., & Varghese, S. (2013). Pharmacological interventions for self-injurious behaviour in adults with intellectual disabilities. *Cochrane Database of Systematic Reviews,* (4), CD009084.

Ratey, J. J., Mikkelsen, E. J., Smith, G. B., Upadhyaya, A., Zuckerman, H. S., Martell, D., Sorgi, P., Polakoff, S., & Bemporad, J. (1986). Beta-blockers in the severely and profoundly mentally retarded. *Journal of Clinical Psychopharmacology, 6*(2), 103–107.

Reed, G. M., First, M. B., Kogan, C. S., Hyman, S. E., Gureje, O., Gaebel, W., Maj, M., Stein, D., Maercker, A., Tyrer, P., Claudino, A., Garrarlda, E., Salvador-Carulla, L., Ray, R., Saunders, J., Dua, T., Poznyak, V., Medina-Mora, M., Pike, K., . . . Saxena, S. (2019). Innovations and changes in the ICD-11 classification of mental, behavioural and neurodevelopmental disorders. *World Psychiatry, 18*(1), 3–19.

Reiss, S. (1988). *Reiss Screen for Maladaptive Behavior: Test manual.* IDS.

Reiss, S., & Valenti-Hein, D. (1990). *Reiss scales for children's dual diagnosis.* IDS.

Reschly, D. J. (2009). Documenting the developmental origins of mild mental retardation. *Applied Neuropsychology, 16*(2), 124–134.

Roeleveld, N., & Zielhuis, G. A., & Gabreels, F. (1997). The prevalence of mental retardation: A critical review of recent literature. *Developmental Medicine & Child Neurology, 39*(2), 125–132.

Rutter, M., Tizard, J., & Whitmore, K. (Eds.). (1970). *Education, health and behaviour.* Longman.

Salvador-Carulla, L., & Bertelli, M. (2008). "Mental retardation" or "intellectual disability": Time for a conceptual change. *Psychopathology, 41*(1),10–16.

Salvador-Carulla, L., Bertelli, M., & Martinez-Leal, R. (2018). The road to 11th edition of the International Classification of Diseases: Trajectories of scientific consensus and contested science in the classification of intellectual disability/intellectual developmental disorders. *Current Opinion in Psychiatry, 31*(2),79–87.

Salvador-Carulla, L. S., Reed, G. M., Vaez-Aziz, L. M., Cooper, S. A., Martinez-Leal, M., Bertelli, M., Adnams, C., Cooray, S., Deb, S., Akoury-Dirani, L., Girimaji, S. C., Katz, G., Kwok, H., Luckasson, R., Simeonsson, R., Walsh, C., Munir, K., & Saxena, S., (2011). Intellectual developmental disorders: Towards a new name, definition and framework for "mental retardation/intellectual disability" in ICD-11. *World Psychiatry, 10*(3), 175–180.

Sandman, C. A., Hetrick, W. P., Taylor, D. V., Barron, J. L., Touchette, P., Lott, I., Crinella, F., & Martinazzi, V. (1993). Naltrexone reduces self-injury and improves learning. *Experimental and Clinical Psychopharmacology, 1*(1–4), 242–258.

Schalock, R. L. (2011). The evolving understanding of the construct of intellectual disability. *Journal of Intellectual and Developmental Disability, 36*(4), 227–237.

Schalock, R. L., Luckasson, R., & Tassé, M. J. (2021). *Intellectual disability: Definition, diagnosis, classification, and planning supports* (12th ed.). American Association on Intellectual and Developmental Disabilities.

Séguin, É. (1846). *Traitement moral, hygiène et éducation des idiots et des autres enfants arriérés ou rétardés dans leur développement, etc.* Baillière.

Séguin, É. (1866). *Idiocy and its treatment by the physiological method.* Wood.

Simonoff, E., Taylor, E., Baird, G., Bernard, S., Chadwick, O., Liang, H., Whitwell, S., Riemer, K., Sharma, K., Sharma, S., Wood, N., Kelly, J., Golaszewski, A., Kennedy, J., Rodney, L., West, N., Walwyn, R., & Jichi, F. (2013). Randomized controlled double-blind trial of optimal dose methylphenidate in children and adolescents with severe attention deficit hyperactivity disorder and intellectual disability. *Journal of Child Psychology and Psychiatry, 54*(5), 527–535.

Spearman, C. (1904). "General intelligence," objectively determined and measured. *American Journal of Psychology, 15,* 201–293.

Strømme, P., & Diseth, T. H. (2000). Prevalence of psychiatric diagnoses in children with mental retardation: Data from a population-based study. *Developmental Medicine & Child Neurology, 42*(4), 266–270.

Symons, F. J., Thompson, A., & Rodriguez, M. C. (2004). Self-injurious behavior and the efficacy of naltrexone treatment: A quantitative synthesis. *Mental Retardation and Developmental Disabilities Research Reviews, 10*(3), 193–200.

Tassé, M. J. (2009). Adaptive behavior assessment and the diagnosis of mental retardation in capital cases. *Applied Neuropsychology, 16*(2), 114–123.

Tassé, M. J., Luckasson, R., & Schalock, R. L. (2016). The relation between intellectual functioning and adaptive behavior in the diagnosis of intellectual disability. *Intellectual and Developmental Disabilities, 54*(6), 381–390.

Tassé, M. J., Schalock, R. L., Balboni, G., Bersani, H., Jr., Borthwick-Duffy, S. A., Spreat, S., Thissen, D., Widaman, K., & Zhang, D. (2012). The construct of adaptive behavior: Its conceptualization, measurement, and use in the field of intellectual disability. *American Journal on Intellectual and Developmental Disabilities, 117*(4), 291–303.

Thomas, S., & Wolfensberger, W. (1999). An overview of social role valorization. In R. J. Flynn & R. A. LeMay (Eds.), *A quarter century of normalization and social role valorization* (pp. 125–159). University of Ottawa Press.

Thomson, G. H. (1919). The hierarchy of abilities. *British Journal of Psychology, 9*(3), 337–344.

Torr, J. (2003). Personality disorder in intellectual disability. *Current Opinion in Psychiatry, 16*(5), 517–521.

Turgay, A., Binder, C., Snyder, R., & Fisman, S. (2002). Long-term safety and efficacy of risperidone for the treatment of disruptive behavior disorders in children with subaverage IQs. *Pediatrics, 110*(3), e34.

U.S. Public Health Service. (2001). *Closing the gap: A national blueprint for improving the health of individuals with mental retardation. Report of the Surgeon General's Conference on Health Disparities and Mental Retardation.* U.S. Department of Health and Human Services.

Watson, J. E., Aman, M. G., & Singh, N. N. (1988). The Psychopathology Instrument for Mentally Retarded Adults: Psychometric characteristics, factor structure, and relationship to subject characteristics. *Research in Developmental Disabilities, 9*(3), 277–290.

Wester Oxelgren, U., Myrelid, Å., Annerén, G., Westerlund, J., Gustafsson, J., & Fernell, E. (2019). More severe intellectual disability found in teenagers compared to younger children with Down syndrome. *Acta Paediatrica, 108*(5), 961–966.

Wing, L., & Gould, J. (1979). Severe impairments of social interaction and associated abnormalities in children: Epidemiology and classification. *Journal of Autism and Developmental Disorders, 9*(1), 11–30.

Wolfensberger, W. (1972). *The principle of normalization in human services.* National Institute on Intellectual Disability (Intellectual Developmental Disorder).

Wolfensberger, W. (1983). Social role valorization: A proposed new term for the principle of normalization. *Mental Retardation, 21*(6), 234–239.

Woodcock, K. A., & Blackwell, S. (2020). Psychological treatment strategies for challenging behaviours in neurodevelopmental disorders: What lies beyond a purely behavioural approach? *Current Opinion in Psychiatry, 33*(2), 92–109.

Woodward, M. (1959). The behaviour of idiots interpreted by Piaget's theory of sensori-motor development. *British Journal of Educational Psychology, 29*(1), 60–71.

Woodward, M. (1961). Concepts of number of the mentally subnormal studied by Piaget's method. *Journal of Child Psychology and Psychiatry, 2*(4), 249–259.

World Health Organization. (2011, April 2). *ICD-11 content model draft, Version 10.*

World Health Organization. (2018). *International statistical classification of diseases and related health problems* (11th rev.).

Yalon-Chamovitz, S., & Greenspan, S. (2005). Ability to identify, explain and solve problems in everyday tasks: Preliminary validation of a direct video measure of practical intelligence. *Research in Developmental Disabilities, 26*(3), 219–230.

Zigler, E. (1967). Familial intellectual disability (intellectual developmental disorder): A continuing dilemma. *Science, 155*, 292–298.

# 15

# Autism Spectrum Disorder

Leo Kanner published the first systematic description of autism in 1943 in his classic paper "Autistic Disturbances of Affective Contact." The following year, Kanner (1944) introduced the diagnostic term early infantile autism (Harris, 2018). However, early infantile autism was not included in the psychiatry diagnostic classification as a separate category until 1980 with the publication of the third edition of the *Diagnostic and Statistical Manual of Mental Disorders* (DSM-III; American Psychiatric Association [APA], 1980). The diagnosis has stood the test of time, and in the DSM-5 (APA, 2013) clinical features are essentially those described by Kanner in his original paper. Kanner generally excluded cases with known brain dysfunction and severe intellectual developmental disorder (IDD). The eponym "Kanner's syndrome" was used for many years but was abandoned with the publication of DSM-III. In DSM-5, the diagnostic term autism spectrum disorder (ASD) was introduced. When diagnosing, it is helpful to review Kanner's original description of 11 cases that were drawn from his observations and those of the children's parents. In his 1943 classic paper, Kanner wrote that we must "assume these children have come into the world with the innate inability to form the usual, biologically provided contact with people, just as other children come into the world with innate physical or intellectual handicaps."

From its beginnings, "autism" has been a term that focused on a neurodevelopmental disorder with deficits in social communication and restricted and repetitive patterns of behavior, interests, and activities. Recent developmental research has focused on deficits in social understanding, repetitive behaviors, affective development, social cognition, and interpersonal reciprocity. ASD may provide cues to a better understanding of how social cognition emerges in typical development and its relationship to a social cognitive network in the brain.

This chapter reviews the history, definition and classification, epidemiology, clinical features, etiologies (genetic and environmental), natural history, neurobiology, and treatment of ASD. It focuses on the spectrum of social communicative and social interaction deficits in ASD and examines the underlying neurobiology. The major emphasis is on social understanding and the development of social awareness and repetitive behavior from a neurobiological and a social interactional perspective.

## History

In his initial description, Kanner (1943) began,

> Since 1938, there have come to our attention a number of children whose condition differs so markedly and uniquely from anything reported so far, that each case

merits—and, I hope, will eventually receive—a detailed consideration of its fascinating peculiarities.

In this first paragraph of "Autistic Disturbances of Affective Contact," Kanner called for research into understanding ASD. His first patient, Donald T., had been first seen by Kanner on October 14, 1938, and was admitted to the Maryland Nursery and Child Study Home in Baltimore for evaluation of his unusual behavior. Kanner was on its board of directors. Donald T. was evaluated over a 2-week period alone, with staff, and in interaction with his mother. He was observed to be oblivious of people around him and indifferent to his parents' comings and goings. He spent his time spinning objects and tracing numbers and letters in the air. At age 5 years, he could count and was able to recite the alphabet forward and backward. His language lacked prosody; he avoided using the first-person pronoun "I," calling on the examiner to "give you blocks." Beyond repetitious acts, he had no desire to do anything. In observing him, Dr. Cameron (as cited in Vicedo & Ilerbaig, 2021), wrote, "In actual life performance, he is at the level of an idiot, in fund of information, he is a prodigy" p. 3). The examining physicians and Kanner initially thought Donald T.'s mother must have encouraged his memorizing and repetitive behavior. However, one of the examiners, psychiatrist Wendell Muncie, surprisingly said that his own daughter showed similar behavior. Muncie's daughter subsequently was included in Kanner's first publication as a female with early infant autism. Donald T.'s interest in numbers and letters had emerged unprompted and was not encouraged by his parents.

Adolf Meyer, the chairman of the Department of Psychiatry at Johns Hopkins Hospital, wondered if such continuous concentration of mental abilities in one area (numbers, letters) might be an obstruction of normal mental development (Vicedo & Ilerbaig, 2021). Kanner noted a lack of affective contact with people and emphasized the preservation of sameness in Donald T.'s stereotypies. By April 23, 1941, Kanner had seen five children who showed similar behavior; he presented his findings in a paper titled "Autistic Disturbances of Affective Contact" at a staff conference. The paper emphasized the lack of affective contact with other persons that included gestural, visual, and other kinds of sensory engagement. Kanner published his findings in 1943 after accumulating a total of 11 cases.

The following year, in the *Journal of Pediatrics*, Kanner (1944) described additional cases, proposing the diagnostic term early infantile autism. How affective contact develops in children with ASD remains a major theme in autism research more than three-fourths of a century later. Kanner's designation "autism" was chosen to highlight the sense of aloneness that seemed apparent to those who observed children with this neurodevelopmental disorder. However, autism does not refer to a retreat into fantasy but, rather, an absence of social awareness of themselves in relationship to others. Yet, autistic aloneness does not mean lonely; feeling lonely is a developmental acquisition that follows the emergence of a sense of self lacking in these children. Kanner believed this syndrome was congenital, an innate inability, present from the beginning of life, to develop social relationships with others. He noted that these children failed to initiate socially meaningful anticipatory gestures; children with ASD did not reach out to be picked up, did not respond to animated persons in the environment around them, and seemed to be "in a world of their own." Because social communicative interactions are among our most basic species-typical human characteristics, the lack of affective contact remains an intriguing topic for research. It is both perplexing and demoralizing to family members who attempt in vain to make meaningful contact with these children. Resistance to social contact and other characteristics that now define the syndrome were described in the first case report.

At one time, it was debated whether ASD was innate or a consequence of psychosocial deprivation. Based on psychoanalytic theory, the cause of autism was thought to result from having emotionally cold, distant mothers ("refrigerator mother"), leading to feelings of guilt and anger among mothers of autistic children. Early family studies did not find familial risk sibs of an autistic proband consistent with Mendelian genetics, supporting the notion that autism was caused by a toxic environment (Eisenberg, 2001). With the recognition that ASD is a neurobiologically based developmental disorder, child development research began to examine its genetics and developmental trajectory (Rutter, 1968). Because it is a neurodevelopmental disorder, the role of the family is crucial in facilitating child development. Teaching family members to understand the deficits allows them to respond more effectively to children with ASD. Parental motivation is important in helping these children emerge from the autistic withdrawn phase of the disorder. Parents have established parent support organizations throughout the world. In the United States, there are parent organizations such as Autism Speaks that facilitate parents coming together to help one another understand this perplexing condition, participate in treatment programs, and raise funds in support of treatment programs and research.

## Definition and Classification

Before DSM-III was published in 1980, there was no specific category of "autism spectrum disorder." Instead, the existing diagnosis terms "childhood schizophrenia" and "childhood psychosis" were broadly applied to children with severe psychiatric disturbances beginning in early life. In 1978, Michael Rutter highlighted the distinctions of autism in his paper, "Childhood Schizophrenia Reconsidered." Gradually, ASD was more clearly differentiated from schizophrenia with childhood onset, based on the age of onset, symptom presentation, and clinical course. ASD criteria are based on distortions in the development of multiple basic psychological functions involved in the acquisition of social skills and language, along with attention, perception, reality testing, and motor movement.

In 1980, more than 35 years after the original description, the basic criteria proposed by Kanner were incorporated in the DSM-III under the designation "early infantile autism," the term Kanner had proposed in 1944. The DSM-III definition for infantile autism specified onset before 30 months of age, pervasive lack of responsiveness to others, deviant language development, unusual responses to the environment, and the absence of hallucinations and delusions found in schizophrenia. However, because these original criteria were found to be too restrictive, they were most applicable for younger and more severely impaired individuals. Moreover, a residual category had been included in DSM-III; however, it was not commonly used because even the highest functioning adults with ASD continued to have difficulties with social adaptation and communication. Although individuals may emerge from the severe, socially autistic phase, they continue to remain sufficiently symptomatic as they grow older. The category "residual state" was not believed to describe them satisfactorily and was abandoned.

DSM-III-R, the first DSM revision (APA, 1987), recognized the importance of changes in syndrome expression during development and introduced more developmentally focused criteria, leading to a change in the name of the category from "early infantile autism" to "autistic disorder." Accordingly, the diagnostic criteria were broadened to include the entire age range and full spectrum of functioning. Three broad categories were included in DSM-III-R: abnormal reciprocal social relations, disturbances in communication and imaginative play, and restricted range of activities and interests. To receive a diagnosis of autistic disorder in DSM-III-R, a child or adult needed to demonstrate at least 8 of 16 criteria, with a specified distribution over the three categories. An age of onset before age 30 months was no longer required as a criterion, but the time of onset or time of recognition of symptoms needed to be recorded. Furthermore, differentiation from schizophrenia was further clarified in DSM-III-R so that an individual with an autistic disorder might be given both diagnoses if the diagnostic criteria for schizophrenia, such as the presence of hallucinations and delusions, were present. Essentially, the diagnosis of a schizophreniform disorder or of schizophrenia was recognized as potentially co-occurring in a vulnerable autistic person. Moreover, the diagnosis of autistic disorder could be made in DSM-III-R based on a current examination of the child without knowledge of the child's early history. The major changes in DSM-III-R, developmentally focused criteria, broadened the concept of autistic disorder substantially so that a greater number of false-positive cases were reported. Because DSM-III-R identified more atypical cases, its use for both clinical and research purposes was complicated. For that reason, additional modifications were proposed for a new DSM-IV classification (APA, 1994).

In addition, changes were made in DSM-IV to bring the diagnosis closer to criteria used in the *International Classification of Diseases* (ICD-10; World Health Organization, 1992). DSM-IV improved the diagnostic algorithm to address criteria problems DSM-III-R criticized as difficult to apply. However, operationalization of the criteria and the developmental orientation introduced in DSM-III-R were maintained. The changes in DSM-IV sought to provide greater simplicity in their application while maintaining compatibility with ICD-10. DSM-IV criteria sought to balance the too narrow DSM-III definition and the too broad DSM-III-R definition, maintaining the importance of considering symptoms that occurred at various ages during development.

In DSM-IV, influenced by research used in developing the ICD-10 classification, the overall term pervasive development disorder was used. Pervasive development disorder was subgrouped into four groups: autism disorder, Rett disorder, childhood disintegrative disorder, and Asperger syndrome. Criteria such as pervasive unrelatedness were not reintroduced because they apply primarily to the most severely autistic child and generally to the younger child. The age of onset or recognition criterion was reintroduced, whereas typical examples of autistic behavior that were previously included in DSM-III-R were removed. Finally, efforts were made to better operationalize criteria. Regarding the diagnostic algorithm, rather than 8 of 16 items, a total of 6 of 12 items were required for the DSM-IV diagnosis. A requirement for qualitative impairments in social interaction and in communication and restricted interests and activities was maintained. The word "stereotyped" was added. Delays or abnormal functioning were required prior to age 3 years in at least one of the following areas: social interaction, social communicative language, and symbolic or imaginative play. Moreover, with the inclusion of additional categories under the pervasive developmental disorder terminology, exclusionary criteria included Rett's disorder and childhood disintegrative disorder. In DSM-IV, diagnosis requires at least 2 items related to qualitative impairment in social interaction—one from the category of qualitative impairment in communication and one from the category of restricted repetitive and stereotyped patterns of behavior. The term Asperger syndrome was introduced in ICD-10 and DSM-IV to describe people with social communication deficits who were higher functioning. Asperger (1991) had clearly distinguished his subjects from Kanner's early infantile autism, viewing his syndrome as a personality spectrum disorder.

In 2013, DSM-5 was introduced. In DSM-5, all four of the DSM-IV-TR subgroups were eliminated. A new term, autism spectrum disorder, was introduced. Rett syndrome was removed because those with Rett syndrome have severe intellectual development disorder and show social behavior deficits unlike those in ASD. Moreover, in Rett syndrome, eye contact is maintained. Intense eye communication is a supportive diagnostic criterion for Rett syndrome (Neul et al., 2010). Revised diagnostic criteria for Rett syndrome do not list social deficits. Childhood disintegrative disorder was removed because unlike ASD, it involves severe continued cognitive decline. It is tempting to speculate that childhood disintegrative disorder was a form of pediatric-onset NMDA receptor encephalitis (Adang et al., 2014). Finally, Asperger's syndrome was eliminated. Asperger's syndrome was found not to be sufficiently distinguishable from high-functioning autism.

DSM-5 reduced DSM-IV's three diagnostic criteria into two criteria. These are social communication deficits and repetitive patterns of behaviors and restricted activities or interests (Szatmari et al., 2006). When the two revised DSM-5 criteria are compared to Kanner's original two key diagnostic features, autistic aloneness and preservation of sameness, the DSM-5 criteria appear to be closer to Kanner's original criteria than were the DSM-IV criteria. Previously, Kanner described sensory sensitivity and sensory integration problems. Such disordered sensory modulation, hypo- or hyper-reactivity to sensory input, is added as a new criterion in DSM-5. Ben-Sasson et al. (2009) provide a meta-analysis of sensory modulation symptoms in individuals with ASD justifying the addition. For the clinician who seeks to focus on ASD from the child's perspective, remembering Kanner's emphasis on autistic aloneness and preservation of sameness may allow the clinician to consider the autistic child's predicament, their inability to interpret social signals, and their difficulty in maintaining sensory stability, leaving them socially isolated. Preservative behaviors may be a means to cope. Considering the disorder from the child's perspective allows us to envision an isolated, socially perplexed child who does not socially engage and struggles to modulate sensory input from an ever-changing world. These advances in classification have led to broad-spectrum disorder diagnoses that set the stage for future subtyping (Harris, 2019).

## Differential Diagnosis

### Rett Syndrome

Children with Rett syndrome caused by mutations in *Mecp2* on the X-chromosome develop normally in the first months of life, but by the end of their first year, they fail to progress in their brain development. The diagnosis may not be made until somewhat later when it is often marked by seizure disorders. It occurs almost entirely in girls who are heterozygous for the mutation, whereas the hemizygous bearing the mutation die in utero. Social interaction deficits may emerge during the regressive phase (ages 1–4 years). Following the regressive phase, their social communication skills typically improve and autistic-like social deficits are no longer apparent. In Rett syndrome, microcephaly results from slowing in brain growth. In ASD, there may be a period of accelerated brain growth with macrocephaly. In Rett syndrome, there are simple hand clasping stereotypies, whereas in ASD these are peripheral and complex stereotypic movements. Girls with Rett syndrome fall into the severe/profound range of IDD.

### Selective Mutism

In selective mutism, early development typically is not disturbed. Communication skills are appropriate in some settings. Social reciprocity and gestures are not impaired. There are no restrictive or repetitive behaviors.

### Language Disorders and Social (Pragmatic) Communication Disorder

Specific language disorder (receptive and expressive) typically is not associated with abnormal nonverbal communication and not associated with restricted, repetitive patterns of behavior, interests, or activities. However, when there is impairment in pragmatic social communication and social interest without restricted repetitive behavior or interests, criterion for social (pragmatic) communication disorder, rather than ASD, may be met.

### Intellectual Developmental Disorder Without Autism Spectrum Disorder

Severe IDD without ASD may be difficult to establish in very young children. Kanner did not make the diagnosis of autism in those with severe IDD. In particular, children who have not developed language or symbolic skills are problematic because severe IDD is frequently associated with repetitive behaviors. A co-occurring diagnosis is only appropriate when social communitive deficits and interactions are unequivocally impaired with respect to the developmental level of that individual's nonverbal skills—for example, nonverbal problem-solving or motor skills. When intellectual development is not discrepant with level of social communitive skills, ASD is not diagnosed.

### Stereotypical Movement Disorder

Stereotypic movement disorders are repetitive, apparently purposeless, motor behaviors such as body rubbing, head banging, self-biting, and hand shaking movements that are more often found with severe IDD. The diagnosis is not made if the repetitive behaviors are better explained by ASD. Some repetitive behaviors—for example, lining up objects and hand flapping—are more often found in ASD. When stereotypies lead to self-injury and self-injury is a focus of treatment, both diagnoses can be given.

### Attention-Deficit/Hyperactivity Disorder

People diagnosed with ASD commonly have attentional abnormalities such as being easily distracted, overly focused, or hyperactive. A second diagnosis of attention-deficit/hyperactivity disorder (ADHD) can be made when attention deficits, impulsiveness, or hyperactivity exceeds that typically observed in children of comparable mental age.

### Social (Pragmatic) Communication Disorder

An individual with social (pragmatic) communication disorder has deficits in the social use of language, impaired social reciprocity in conversation, and impairment in using verbal language and nonverbal gestures to regulate social conversation or making inferences about other's social behavior. Individuals with this diagnosis are distinct from those with ASD because they do not demonstrate restricted and repetitive behaviors or interests.

### Schizophrenia

Unlike ASD, childhood-onset schizophrenia develops later in childhood after normal or near-normal development, although there may be a prodromal period with social impairment and atypical interests and beliefs. The diagnosis follows the DSM-5 criteria. The deficits in schizophrenia follow a different developmental trajectory than ASD. Hallucinations and delusions are characteristic of schizophrenia but not of ASD. Children with ASD are concrete in their thinking and may answer questions with word associations; however, this behavior is not a schizophrenia thought disorder. For example, a child with an ASD diagnosis was asked by a psychologist, "What do you do with a nail clipper?" The child's response concretely focused on the word "clipper." He said, "San Diego Clipper," which is a sports team. He went on to describe the members of the team. Hallucinations and delusion, characteristic of schizophrenia, are not a characteristic feature of ASD.

## Epidemiology

From the time of Leo Kanner through the 1990s, ASD was considered to be relatively rare. For example, in a epidemiologic study carried out by Lotter (1966) in Great Britain, the prevalence of ASD was reported as 0.45%. More recently, the Centers for Disease Control and Prevention provides regular updates of the prevalence of ASD among 8-year-olds through the Autism and Developmental Disabilities Monitoring Network, which was established in 2010. Estimates are drawn for 11 network sites located throughout the United States. The DSM-5 definition of ASD is used. For 2016, across all 11 sites, the prevalence of ASD for this group was 18.5/1,000 (1 in 54) among the 8-year-olds surveyed. A subset of 6 of the 11 sites monitored ASD among children aged 4 years. In 2016, the ASD prevalence was 15.6 per 1,000 (1 in 64). Prevalence between White and Black children did not differ by site. Epidemiologic investigations show that the rate is 4.3 times higher in boys than girls. More than half of those identified fall within the IDD severity. Although ASD was initially associated with higher social class, it is now evident that it is observed in families at all levels of education. The most common age of recognition is in the first 30 months of life. The diagnosis has also been made after a few months to a few years of apparently typical development. Although family factors and higher cognitive functioning may delay case recognition, when careful histories are taken, the early symptoms are often recognized. Autistic symptoms in toddlers at high genetic risk may be detected by age 18 months using the Checklist for Autism in Toddlers and other rating scales. Increased awareness of the diagnosis, inclusion of less severe cases along the spectrum, and changes in detection methods using standardized instruments are important in understanding the increasing rates. A link of increased prevalence to measles–mumps–rubella vaccine or the preservative thimerosal has been refuted. Approximately 10% of cases are associated neurogenetic disorders such as tuberous sclerosis and fragile X syndrome (Harris, 2016).

## Clinical Features

### Social Deficits

Autism spectrum disorder is characterized by persistent impairment in social communication and interaction and repetitive behaviors. The most essential feature of ASD is a qualitative abnormality in social interaction. The severity and nature of the social deficit vary with the child's age and developmental level, but the deficit is present from very early childhood and sustained through life.

In infancy, children with ASD may resist cuddling, not mold to the parent, and not utilize anticipatory gestures when approached or when approaching others. When engaged with others, they may lack joint attention, which is demonstrated through an absence of pointing and utilizing eye contact to engage others' interest (or in the failure to show pride of accomplishment in bringing items to show to others). As toddlers and preschoolers, they may ignore others or bump into them as if they were unaware of their existence. They may not turn when called and may not look at a person who is trying to engage them in conversation. This gaze avoidance may continue into school age and even into adulthood in a less striking form. Gaze avoidance can be attenuated by appropriate training.

When higher functioning children emerge from the autistic withdrawn phase, they may become socially intrusive rather than socially distant. The child may seem unaware of others' feelings and lack understanding of the negative impact of their behavior on others. There may be limited ability to interpret the tone of voice or facial expression of others, so the usual exchanges between child and parent that are used to convey wishes or show pleasure or displeasure may have little long-term effect on the child's behavior. The higher functioning child will have difficulty making friends and engaging other children in play, although at a younger age, the child seemingly is not distressed by social isolation and may seek solitude. But for those who do seek to find friends, ostracism may be the result of their awkward attempts to socialize. Moreover, children with ASD are rigid in their social responses and must be taught simple social forms, such as greeting another person. The verbal ASD child may learn the social rules often by rote but may not apply the rules appropriately in a social context.

## Deficits in Communication and Imaginative Activity

The failure to acquire language at an expected age is the most frequent presenting concern for parents of preschool autistic children. All preschool children with this disorder have some form of developmental language difficulty. The difficulties are not simply in expressive language but, rather, involve impaired comprehension of language. Some may be mute, and others may understand very little of conversation directed toward them. Some develop language later but may speak unintelligibly and not use appropriate sentence structure. Those who acquire speech later may have unintelligible jargon, which does not show communicative intent. This jargon may include bits and pieces of memorized information from cartoons, television commercials, or phrases they have heard. Their speech fluency may be misleading because they have comprehension problems, especially for questions that are addressed to them about their personal experiences. Others may speak more appropriately but become preoccupied with a narrow range of favorite topics and show little regard for the interest of the person with whom they are speaking. They may perseverate and ask the same question over and over, even though they know the answer. In other instances, they may recite phrases they have heard, imitating exactly the tone of voice and rhythm of the speaker from whom a phrase was learned. Early in life, verbal children with ASD may be echolalic and repeat a question rather than respond to it (immediate echolalic). This echolalia may be associated with a reversal of pronouns as the child refers to themself as "you" or by name, rather than using the word "I" appropriately.

Pragmatic language use, a form of nonverbal communication, is also deficient. This is seen most clearly when a child with ASD does not use gestures or pantomime in conversation. Although children normally begin to point with one finger to things that they like by approximately age 10 months and begin shaking their head "no" by age 1 year, many autistic children are limited in developing these nonverbal behaviors. Instead of pointing, they may get things themselves or take the hand of a parent and move it toward the preferred object. Being unable to gesture their communicative intent, they may become distressed and cry or have a tantrum until an adult has guessed, by trial and error, what the child needs.

Verbal children with ASD may speak in a monotone or sometimes in a singsong manner, either loudly or softly. They usually have a deficiency in using rhythm and intonation (prosody) to clarify the meaning of another's speech. They must be taught how to participate in conversation; maintain the topic; take turns; look at the conversational partner; and interpret tone of voice, facial expression, and body language. Imaginative activities are limited and often consist of the repetition of parts of commercials or cartoons the child has observed. The abnormality in inner language development is also a characteristic feature and is most often demonstrated in observations of play routines.

## Restricted and Repetitive Activities

Children with ASD routinely show repetitive patterns of movement (stereotypies and mannerisms) that include hand flapping (especially when excited), twirling, rocking, head banging, finger posturing, and sensory preoccupations. Commonly, they may resist changes in routines in the environment and become quite distressed when a small object is moved to another location. Stereotypies with objects are common, such as flicking a string, turning light switches on and off, tearing paper into shreds, or turning a toy car over and spinning the wheels rather than rolling it appropriately. Children who are higher functioning may become preoccupied with letters or numbers—for example, the yellow pages in the telephone book. Other children use verbal stereotypies and may repeat the same statements over and over again. When efforts are made to change their routines, the child may resist and have a tantrum. A lack of the use of imagination in creative play is apparent from the preschool years. Preference is for manipulating or stimulating with objects, lining them up, and utilizing the same play figures in repetitive ways. Recognition that figurines used in play represent people is delayed. When higher functioning ASD children do show some form of pretend play, such as feeding a stuffed animal or figurine and putting it to sleep, the pretending is repetitious and lacks flexibility.

The higher functioning verbal ASD child may become preoccupied with and become an expert on very limited topics, such as mapmaking or timetables. Once a topic is mastered, they may perseverate on a theme ideationally and want to speak about it continually. They become particularly preoccupied with classification and become collectors of small items such as stones.

## Intelligence

Initially, children with ASD were thought to show a broad range of intelligence. Others were considered untestable but potentially of normal intelligence. With better testing procedures, it became apparent that those with ASD are limited cognitively, and rather than normally intelligent, ASD children have discrepant cognitive profiles with striking differences between verbal and performance scores on IQ tests, with more than half diagnosed with IDD. Still, it is generally agreed that children with ASD do show the full range of intellectual competencies from profound IDD to superior intelligence. The modal IQ is in the moderately impaired range, and approximately 50% have an IQ of 70 or above when taking people with higher functioning into account.

Intelligence testing is complicated because the full-scale IQ measures the activities of multiple brain systems. The subtests that are utilized test different cognitive skills, and the profile for a person with ASD is uneven. Therefore, a full-scale IQ provides information that is of limited use and may be misleading in ASD. Most often, children with ASD have higher nonverbal or visual–spatial skills than auditory–verbal skills, which is most apparent for younger children. As the child advances in age, the abilities may show less discrepancy. Commonly, splinter skills for a narrow range of abilities, such as calculation, rote verbal memory, and puzzle completion, may be observed despite overall limited cognitive ability. Although it may be difficult to test children with ASD because of their distractibility, negativism, and difficulty comprehending, it should not be assumed they are untestable. If tasks are provided at the child's general cognitive level, they ordinarily can cooperate with an experienced tester.

## Mood and Affect

Because of their lack of responsiveness, children with ASD are often described as having a flat affect. Yet, preschool children in particular are generally described by parents as happy as long as environmental demands are not excessive. When demands are placed, they may become irritable, have tantrums, and be difficult to console. Older children with ASD may show labile affect, particularly when they are emerging from the socially withdrawn phase. Others may become aggressive and may pinch or hit without apparent provocation. Fearfulness can occur and phobias can develop if the child has been startled in a situation in which they do not understand the social context. Their fearfulness and anxiety may be situation-specific. Tantrums are common, particularly when their routines are disrupted. Tantrums may be so severe that the family becomes organized around the child's routines to try to reduce the frequency of tantrums.

## Attention and Arousal

Most children with ASD have attention deficits and may be highly distractible; some are hyperactive. It is difficult both to get their attention and to maintain it. The child may be observed to wander from one activity to the next and not become engaged in any activity. Yet, other children with ASD may show extremely long attention spans for activities that preoccupy them and perseverate on them. In these instances, they may stay with a single activity for long periods of time without apparent boredom.

## Sleep

Sleep disturbances are common in infants with ASD and may persist into school age. Approximately one-third of infants had sleep difficulties, with half reporting a worsening of sleep between ages 2 and 3 years. Waking once or twice at night is not uncommon. Alternations in sleep pattern may also be observed, with excessive sleepiness alternating with reduced sleep. Sleep disturbances typically show a poor response to medication, but melatonin may benefit sleep.

## Sensorimotor Abilities

Some children with ASD may show excellent coordination, whereas others are clumsy. The child who is well coordinated may be able to balance in remarkable ways—for example, standing on the edge of a chair and rocking back and forth. Both toe walking and hypotonia are frequently seen without evidence of specific neurological deficits. The child with ASD may be late in walking, have difficulty imitating movements, and have difficulty learning to use specific tools.

Abnormal response to sensory input is a common problem. It may be particularly evident when children with ASD place their hands over their ears to avoid auditory stimulation. A child with ASD may be intolerant of loud sounds but at other times may be unresponsive to sound and thought to be deaf. Difficulties in auditory processing may influence discrimination of speech sounds and affect language learning. Children with ASD may be fascinated with visual stimuli, such as watching a record turn or the rotation of a fan. They may spin wheels in order to watch the rotation and become fixated on moving lights. The visual modality may be better developed than the auditory one, as demonstrated through excellent visual–spatial skills.

There may also be other somatosensory abnormalities, such as insensitivity to pain. Children may bang their heads until there is a hematoma or bite their hands, leading to severe injury. In other instances, self-stimulation may involve excessive rubbing or masturbating. With the emergence from the autistic withdrawn phase, excessive sensitivity to pain may be noted in some instances. For example, an apparently minor toothache may lead to major changes in behavior until it is recognized. Some children may be tactually defensive and arch their backs and withdraw when touched or stroked. Other sensory modalities may also be involved; children may lick or smell objects they pick up and, in other instances, show strong taste aversions, leading to eating a very narrow range of foods.

## Seizure Disorder

The prevalence of seizures in children with ASD is greater than in the population at large. A systematic review and meta-analysis review of 19 studies found a prevalence of 6.3% compared to a general population prevalence of 0.4–0.8%. The U.S. National Survey of Children's Health study for the years 2011 and 2012 reported an 8.6% prevalence of epilepsy in ASD; the presence of epilepsy was associated with increasing age, female gender, intellectual disability, speech problems, and lower socioeconomic status (Thomas et al., 2017). By type, there is an increased risk for general epilepsy (4.7%), infantile spasms (19.9%), facial seizures (41.9%), and Dravet syndrome (47.4%). For those younger than age 18 years, there was a 13.2 times greater seizure risk in ASD (Strasser et al., 2018). The likelihood of seizures, however, is related to severity of IDD (4.9 times greater risk) and motor dysfunction (e.g., those who have more extensive brain damage). The onset of seizures increases gradually from childhood and reaches a peak during adolescence; the greatest risk for onset is before age 2 years. Approximately one-fourth of adults with ASD have been reported to have seizures. Seizures are least common in those with high-functioning ASD. When seizures do occur, there is no specific seizure type that is characteristic. Generalized, partial complex, atypical absence, and other types have been reported, either singularly or in combination. Syndromic ASD has the highest prevalence of epilepsy (55%), compared to 7% in idiopathic autism.

Autistic-like behavior has been associated with infantile spasms and the Lennox–Gastaut syndrome (El Achkar & Spence, 2015; Pavone et al., 2004). These disorders are associated with diffuse slow spike-wave complexes on electroencephalogram (EEG). Both are correlated with severity of IDD. Of interest is the fact that infantile spasms are related to abnormalities in the rapid eye movement sleep mechanism, a finding that seems unique to this form of seizure disorder. In addition, acquired epileptic aphasia (Landau–Kleffner syndrome), which is associated with unilateral or bilateral temporoparietal spike-wave discharges that may be activated during slow-wave sleep, also has been associated with autistic symptoms in a significant proportion of children. Finally, a family with a history of ASD or epilepsy has been linked to greater risk for the other disorder (Amiet et al., 2013). Multiplex families (12.8%), which are much more likely to have heritable causes of ASD, are reported to have greater risk for seizures than simplex families (2.4%).

## Etiologies

### Genetic Etiology

Although the autistic spectrum of behavioral and developmental features may be associated with a variety of genetic disorders (secondary or symptomatic autism) (Richards et al., 2015), it is the idiopathic classic presentation that Kanner described. Kanner was reluctant to diagnose children with severe IDD and those with known brain disorders as autistic. The most common genetic syndromes associated with autistic features are shown in Table 15.1. These symptomatic forms of ASD contribute less than 10% of those diagnosed with ASD.

ASD represents a striking example of the limitations of psychiatric categorical diagnoses. Children with several different genetic etiologies satisfy the diagnostic criteria for ASD, including autosomal recessive, autosomal dominant, X-linked trinucleotide repeat, and copy number variants (CNVs). The so-called Kanner form of autism without an obvious genetic cause comprises more than 90% of the ASD cases. However, recent appropriately powered genome-wide associations studies (GWAS) that require thousands of subjects have revealed that ASD is a disorder of complex genetics, with multiple risk genes of small effect interacting to produce the phenotype. The majority of the risk sites do not lie in the coding regions of the gene (exome) but presumably affect gene expression mRNA processing. Significant gene associations implicate

**Table 15.1** Genetic Syndromes Associated with Autism Spectrum Disorder Symptoms and Genetic Mechanisms

| Syndrome | Autism Spectrum Disorder Prevalence (%) | Mechanism |
| --- | --- | --- |
| Cohen's syndrome | 54 | Autosomal recessive |
| Cornelia de Lange syndrome | 43 | Autosomal dominant (spontaneous mutation) |
| Tuberous sclerosis complex | 36 | Autosomal dominant |
| Fragile X syndrome | Male only; 30 | X-linked-dominant trinucleotide repeat |
| Neurofibromatosis | 18 | Autosomal dominant |
| Noonan's syndrome | 12 | Autosomal dominant |
| 22q11.2 syndrome | 30 | Dominant: Spontaneous deletion |

neuronal function and corticogenesis (Grove et al., 2019). This complex genetics with risk genes coming from both parents now explain the clinical observations that a high percentage of the parents exhibit elements of the ASD phenotype (Eisenberg, 2001; Piven et al., 1994; Rutter, 1968; see below).

Importantly, the majority of individuals with these syndromes do not meet criteria for ASD. The natural history of symptom development (developmental trajectory) and outcome in these known genetic disorders differs from that of idiopathic autism. These disorders should be followed carefully to establish the course and developmental trajectory of autistic symptoms in each of them using non-affected individuals with those syndromes for comparison.

## Genetic Etiology

Kanner's recognition of autism as an innate neurodevelopmental disorder in 1943 stimulated subsequent study of genetics of autism. In 1977, genetic studies in identical twins confirmed a genetic basis of autism (Folstein & Rutter, 1977). A later review of more than 13 twin studies (Huguet et al., 2016) concluded that "the concordance for autism spectrum disorder is roughly 45% for monozygotic twins and 15% for dizygotic twins" (p. 103). Kanner's early recognition of autistic traits in parents, finding overfocus on details and limited interest in social interactions, is consistent with the identification of the "broader autism phenotype" in families. These family members may have mild ASD findings that do not meet full diagnostic criteria. The broader autism phenotype in family members has been studied using behavioral questionnaires and semistructured and blind interviews, neuropsychological tests, language testing, and brain imaging (Harris & Piven, 2016; Landa et al., 1992; Losh et al., 2009; Sasson et al., 2013; Yucel et al., 2015). Piven et al. (1990) studied 67 adult siblings of 37 autistic individuals. They found that 3% of the siblings were autistic, 4.4% had severe social dysfunction, 15% had cognitive disorders, and 15% had been treated for an autistic disorder.

Landa et al. (1992) studied social language use (pragmatics) in the parents of autistic individuals. Although mild in degree, disinhibited social communication, awkward/inadequate expression, and odd verbal interaction were reported. Landa et al. (1991) compared spontaneous discourse narratives of parents of autistic persons and controls. Although similar in length, the narratives of the autistic parents were less complex and coherent and, in some instances, rambling and difficult to comprehend. These narrative-discourse deficits may also be associated with genetic liability. Similarly, in the 1950s, Kanner and Eisenberg (1956) reported that 3% of the affected child's siblings met diagnostic criteria for autism. Current studies find the rate in siblings is nearer to 20% (Piven, et al., 1997, 2013). There are extensive clinical heterogeneity developmental trajectories in idiopathic autism.

Importantly, there is heterogeneity in symptom severity and adaptive functioning. One study examined developmental trajectories of both symptom severity and adaptive functioning longitudinally (Szatmari et al., 2015). The authors enrolled 421 newly diagnosed, 2- to 4-year-old children with ASD (355 male; mean age at study entry, 39.87 months). Prospective evaluations conducted at four time points from diagnosis to age 6 years were used to ascertain developmental trajectories using the Autism

Diagnostic Observation Schedule and for adaptive functioning using the Vineland Adaptive Behavior Scales, Second Edition. Two specific trajectory groups were identified. Group 1 (11.4%) had less severe symptoms and improving trajectories ($p <$ .05). Group 2 (88.6%) had severe symptoms and a stable trajectory. Regarding adapting functioning, there were three distinct trajectory groups. Group 1 (29.2%) showed lower functioning and a worsening trajectory, Group 2 (49.9%) had moderate functioning and a stable trajectory, and Group 3 (20.9%) had higher functioning and an improving trajectory ($p <$ .05). Sex was a predictor of symptom severity. Males were more likely to have several symptoms and a stable trajectory than females with less severity and improving trajectories. Age at diagnosis, language, and cognitive scores predicted adaptive functioning in the three groups. The authors demonstrated heterogeneity in developmental trajectories, noting improvement in 20%. Earlier age at diagnosis was associated with higher functioning and improvement. Higher baseline IQ or higher baseline language scores were associated with moderate functioning, stable trajectory, higher functioning, and improvement.

The cause of differences in symptom severity and adaptive functioning must be individualized. Another study of developmental trajectories found different trajectories for symptom severity in subjects with ASD when followed up from age 2 to 15 years, which supports heterogeneity in developmental trajectories (Gotham et al., 2012). Concordance rates based on monozygotic twins and siblings indicate an overall heritability of 0.70–0.80 (Colvert et al., 2015). However, a population-based study in Scandinavia shows a somewhat lower heritability estimate of 0.50–0.60 (Sandin et al., 2014). Although overall genetic liability is high, the genetic architecture is diverse and made up of alleles of various frequencies (common, rare, and very rare alleles), various patterns of inheritance (dominant, recessive, X-linked, and de novo), and variant type (large chromosomal rearrangements, CNVs, small insertions/deletions, and single nucleotide variants) (de la Torre-Ubieta et al., 2016; Ramaswami & Geschwind, 2018). To unravel this substantial genetic heterogeneity, advances in DNA sequencing technology are being applied to very large patient cohorts.

Genetic studies include the study of chromosomal rearrangements in children with ASD, recognition of CNVs, studies of common and rare variants, and whole exome/genome studies (Huguet et al., 2016). Still, at least 90% of cases are idiopathic—that is, nonsyndromal. Genetic linkage studies were initially carried out in multiplex families (those with more than one child with ASD), seeking to find chromosomal regions that are co-inherited by individuals diagnosed with ASD (Geschwind & State, 2015). Despite the identification of several potential loci for ASD, only two have been successfully replicated. One maps to chromosome 7q35 (Ramaswami & Geschwind, 2018), where language delay and social responsiveness have been linked to *CNTNAP2* on chromosome 7q35 (Alarcón et al., 2002; Geschwind, 2008). Approximately 10%, primarily in people with IDD, show inherited de novo CNVs or single nucleotide variants. Moreover, 100 rare Mendelian syndromes have been associated with ASD (Betancur, 2011). No variability is linked to finding both low-risk alleles (common variants that make up the genetic background) and low-risk in combination with rare deleterious variant mutations.

It is proposed that the major genetic contribution is from common variants. Common variants are genetic polymorphisms that are present in at least 5% of the population. The contribution of common variants has been examined using GWAS. It is estimated that common variants make up approximately 40–60% overall risk for ASD (Gaugler et al., 2014). Because the effect size of each individual variant is small, large sample sizes are required. Potentially, 50% of the risk is derived from common variants yet to be identified. For example, sample sizes in schizophrenia GWAS studies included more than 70,000 subjects with schizophrenia (Trubetskoy et al., 2022) and identified more than 100 risk sites. The most recent GWAS for ASD, which included slightly more than 75,000 subjects with ASD, identified five genome-wide significant loci (Grove et al., 2019). Thus, identifying common variants in ASD is only the beginning.

Rare variants make a smaller contribution to ASD risk (Huguet et al., 2016). Rare recessive mutations have been identified using linkage analyses and/or homozygosity mapping in consanguineous families—for example, the *CNTNAP2* mutation in Amish families. Other rare inherited variants have been identified in Phelen–McDermid syndrome, which involves a family of scaffolding proteins (Shank 1, Shank 2, and Shank 3) and also two members of the neurexin family (NRXN1 and NRXN3) (Ramaswami & Geschwind, 2018). Genetic background may compensate for a rare variant effect and reduce risk. Overall, the interaction of rare variants and genetic background leads to diversity in the phenotype with rare de novo mutations (Huguet et al., 2016).

Examining large cohorts with ASD, such as the Simons Simplex collection that includes single and multiple families, it is estimated that there are 400–1,000 ASD risk genes (Geschwind & State, 2015). Studies of families with several affected members reveal that a pertinent mutation may differ among siblings in a single family. Despite there being many ASD risk genes, these may converge and impact a limited number of biological pathways. On these pathways, genes linked to autism are involved in neuronal development, synaptic plasticity, and chromatin remodeling (Grove et al., 2019; Zoghbi & Bear, 2012).

In summary, advances in understanding genetic mechanisms are providing promising leads to discover the underlying neurobiology of ASD and how it relates to subtypes.

## Environmental Risk and Gene–Environment Interaction

Although genetic risk factors are well established for ASD, a specific genetic disorder diagnosis is not established for idiopathic autism. Environmental risk factors, gene–environment interaction, and intrauterine environmental factors all contribute (Deng et al., 2015). This approach is consistent with the neurodevelopmental continuum model that there is an early disturbance in intrauterine brain development, and the severity and timing of the disturbance determine abnormality in brain development. Thus, genetic and environmental "lesions" impact the developing brain. Subsequently, as the brain assumes new and more complex functioning during development, the impact of such neurodevelopmental pathology becomes apparent, resulting in ASD, schizophrenia, ADHD, or IDD based on the neurodevelopmental continuum. The severity of the disorder is indicated by the age of onset. In support of the neurodevelopmental continuum model is the finding that the same rare CNVs are in IDD, ASD, ADHD, and schizophrenia. Thus, these diagnoses share specific genetic risk genes with one another.

The model proposes that each of these neurodevelopmental disorders shows a range of outcomes that result from deviant or disrupted brain development (Owen & O'Donovan, 2017). However, the extent of impairment may be modified by other genetic and environmental factors. This model might lead to new approaches to classification in psychiatry drawn from evidence of shared genetic and environmental risk factors for these neurodevelopmental conditions consistent with a developmental neuropsychiatry (Owen, 2014). For example, IDD, depending on severity, may be recognized at birth or soon after, ASD is recognized as early as the second year of life extending into the preschool years, Tourette disorder is recognized in school-age children, and schizophrenia is recognized with onset of adolescence. ASD, schizophrenia, and bipolar disorder share etiological risk factors. For example, in studies involving Swedish, Israeli, and Danish patient cohorts, schizophrenia in parents was associated with increased risk of ASD in offspring. This finding supports shared common genetic risk factors (Sullivan et al., 2012). Further support for etiological overlap is reported in a comparative analysis of CNVs in ASD and schizophrenia. Kushima et al. (2018) identified multiple disease-relevant genes in eight well-recognized ASD-/schizophrenia-associated CNV loci in a Japanese cohort (). Thus, the co-occurrence of ASD with other psychiatric diagnoses such as schizophrenia is not surprising and vice versa.

## Environmental Risk Factors for Autism Spectrum Disorder

Thirty percent of the variance in ASD liability is determined by environmental factors, resulting in epigenetic interactions. Environmental factors typically are indicators of risk for disorder rather than causal, although drug exposure in early pregnancy at critical times in brain development may be potentially causal. For example, in a population-based Scandinavian study, exposure to thalidomide in early pregnancy resulted in 5% of 100 mothers exposed to the drug having a child diagnosed with ASD, a threefold increase in prevalence over the general population (Strömland et al., 1994). Yet, compared to genetic studies, environmental risk factors for ASD are less well studied. The environmental risk factors with the most evidence in ASD are advanced age in parents, both mothers and fathers; assisted reproductive technologies; metabolic risks such as preeclampsia; and complications of pregnancy such as anoxia, medication use in pregnancy, environmental chemicals and toxins, and nutritional factors (Gialloreti et al., 2019; Katz et al., 2021; Modabbernia et al., 2017). These risk factors have been examined at three time points deemed biologically relevant to brain development: the periconception, prenatal, and early postnatal periods. Potential protective factors that might modify or prevent the trajectory for ASD also have been examined. The role of epigenetic changes with regard to these risk and protective factors must be considered. In people who are genetically susceptible, environmental risks may combine to establish a threshold that results in dysfunction and identification as a risk for ASD.

First, at conception, older parental age is recognized as a risk factor. Advanced maternal and paternal age at birth ($\geq$35 years) is associated with increased risk, as is a combined parental age effect when both parents are older. For older fathers, there is increased risk for de novo mutations that increase risk. For mothers, the risk is not only genetic but also based on obstetrical complications that increase the risk for poor outcomes. A meta-analysis found that for each 10-year increase in maternal and paternal age, the ASD risk for offspring increases by 18–21% (Wu et al., 2017). Moreover, a meta-analysis of studies of assisted reproductive technology found an increase in risk for ASD (Liu et al., 2016). Exposure to chemical pollutants at critical times in utero may affects neural and behavioral development. Pollutant etiology may involve neurotoxicity but also may be linked to immune dysfunction, altered lipid metabolism, and mitochondrial dysfunction. Traffic-related pollution and pesticides are of particular concern (Gialloreti et al., 2019; Rossignol et al., 2014).

Studies of toxic exposure are, for the most part, limited by indirect and cross-sectional measures of exposure. Systematic reviews have been conducted on air pollution, thimerosal (methylmercury), and heavy metals. Multiple studies, including meta-analyses, find no evidence of an association between childhood thimerosal exposure in vaccines and ASD (Yoshimasu et al., 2014). In addition, meta-analyses of an association between childhood vaccines and ASD find no evidence of an association in children who have been vaccinated (Taylor et al., 2014). Meta-analyses of studies that compared a high concentration ratio of heavy metals in children with ASD and controls found no conclusive association.

Maternal obesity can lead to activation of the maternal immune system and chronic inflammation of the uterine environment. Undernutrition may activate a physiologic stress response and the expression of pro-inflammatory factors. Epidemiologic studies are needed to examine these effects. Folic acid has been systematically reviewed for risk for ASD (Castro et al., 2016). Although some evidence has been reported between foliate deficiency and ASD-like traits, the findings are inconclusive. Other studies have examined whether dietary supplements with foliate increase risk; results are inconsistent (Gialloreti et al., 2019).

Second, in the prenatal period, there are similar issues related to environmental chemicals and toxicants. Residential proximity to organophosphates during pregnancy has been reported to increase risk (Shelton et al., 2014). However, the overall air pollution and exposure to pesticides is not confirmed as a risk factor for ASD (Braun et al., 2014). Prenatal exposure to antiepileptic drugs is a risk factor, with valproate showing the most substantial association with neurodevelopmental outcomes and ASD (Roullet et al., 2013). Consequently, valproate is contraindicated as an antiepileptic or use as a mood stabilizer in pregnant women or in those who plan to become pregnant.

A potential relationship of ASD to prenatal exposure to selective serotonin reuptake inhibitors (SSRIs) has been proposed and extensively examined. A Danish longitudinal study with follow-up of more than 5 million person-years did not find a significant association between maternal use of SSRIs during pregnancy and ASD in offspring (Hviid et al., 2013). Similar findings are reported in other studies. Importantly, the diagnoses of depression and anxiety themselves could be risk factors for offspring rather than medication prescribed for treatment of these disorders (Rai et al., 2013). Antidepressant use in pregnancy must be balanced with the substantial adverse effects of untreated maternal depression. A major risk factor for pregnancy is gestational substance abuse. Alcohol abuse may lead to fetal alcohol spectrum disorder, in which ASD can co-occur (Eliasen et al., 2010).

Third, perinatal and early postnatal obstetric incidents are risk factors for ASD. Multiple studies have examined the association of maternal metabolic syndrome and risk for ASD in offspring. The most consistent evidence for an association is between maternal preeclampsia and ASD risk when examined in sufficiently powered population-based epidemiologic studies (Kate et al., 2021). Birth-related anoxia is a risk factor reported in numerous evidence-based reviews of links to ASD (Hisle-Gorman et al., 2018). Fetal anoxia and respiratory distress are reported to increase the risk for ASD in subgroups of twins (Froehlich-Santino et al., 2014). For example, out of 17 pairs discordant for autism, 12 with ASD had an associated biological hazard at birth that affected the autistic child's presentation but not the co-twin (Folstein & Rutter, 1977). These risk factors can be prevented by attention to maternal care during pregnancy and delivery. Other protective factors in the prenatal period include vitamin D supplements, omega-6 supplements, a diet rich in fatty acids, appropriate folic acid supplements, breast-feeding, and optimal support at delivery.

In summary, risk factors at conception for ASD are late parental age, possibly hormonal induction in assisted reproduction, environmental chemical exposure, and nutritional factors. Prenatal risk factors also include environmental toxin exposure and nutrition, as well as parental exposure to medications, infections, maternal immune activation, maternal metabolic factors, and preeclampsia. Perinatal risks relate to complications of delivery. Studies of environmental risk will benefit by clarifying the nature of the risks. Is the risk related to social deficits, repetitive behaviors, or both? It is important to consider environmental risk as part of a complex network of factors that can have epigenetic effects rather than as an independent element. Critically, increasing focus is on shifting from association studies to examining and establishing cause–effect relationships linking environmental factors to ASD (Modabbernia et al., 2017). With regard to mechanism, some environmental factors, including toxins and vitamin D deficiency, may increase the risk of a gene mutation that could lead to ASD. For example, a polychlorinated biphenyl conger, PCB-95, might genetically modify the number of CNVs, such as duplications of 15q11–q13, which is associated with symptomatic autism (Mitchell et al., 2012).

Epigenetic mechanisms are modifications of DNA methylation and histones that affect gene expression but do not change the base sequence of DNA. Overall, normal epigenetic markers are modifiable by environmental exposures, which alter the regulation of gene expression and impact pathways that are essential in brain development. Epigenetics is an essential genome-wide regulatory layer that modulates gene transcription initiation, mRNA splicing, and the binding of transcription factors. With regard to ASD risk, valproate inhibits histone deacetylase and interferes with folate metabolism; this is an epigenetic modification. Folate deficiency also affects methylation, an epigenetic mechanism. Epigenetic dysregulation of the oxytocinergic system plays a role in social behavior disruption in ASD. General communication and social communication scores have been associated with DNA methylation of the oxytocin receptor (OXTR) (Siu & Weksberg, 2017). The complexity of potential epigenetic mechanisms and their intermediary role in bridging the range of multifaceted risk factors through gene–environment interactions are ongoing challenges in the study of the etiology of ASD. In summary, the broad heterogeneity of ASD is an obstacle for identifying genetic and environmental risk factors (Harris, 2019).

## Neurobiology

Multiple brain regions are relevant to core features of ASD. These brain regions are linked to social behavior, social communication, and repetitive behaviors in animal studies, in neuroimaging studies in humans, and in lesion studies in humans. As shown in Figure 15.1, these regions include the frontal lobe, the superior temporal sulcus, the parietal cortex, and the amygdala.

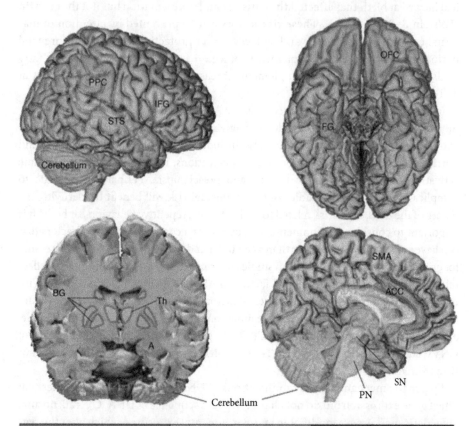

| Social impairment | Communication deficits | Repetitive behaviors |
|---|---|---|
| OFC – Orbitofrontal cortex<br>ACC – Anterior cingulate cortex<br>FG – Fusiform gyrus<br>STS – Superior temporal sulcus<br>A – Amygdala mirror neuron regions<br>IFG – Interior frontal gyrus<br>PPC – Posterior parietal cortex | IFG – Inferior frontal gyrus<br>(Broca's area)<br>STS – Superior temporal sulcus<br>SMA – Supplementary motor area<br>BG – Basal ganglia<br>SN – Substantia nigra<br>Th – Thalamus<br>PN – Pontine nuclei cerebellum | OFC – Orbitofrontal cortex<br>ACC – Anterior cingulate cortex<br>BG – Basal ganglia<br>Th – Thalamus |

**Figure 15.1** Major brain regions relevant to the core features of autism. The frontal lobe, superior temporal cortex, parietal cortex, and amygdala are regions linked to core autism features. Expressive language functioning is typically linked to Broca's area in the inferior frontal gyrus and parts of the supplementary motor cortex, whereas Wernicke's area is key for receptive language function. The superior temporal sulcus plays a role in both language and social attention. Repetitive or stereotyped behaviors of autism may be linked to the orbitofrontal cortex and caudate nucleus.

From Amaral et al. (2008).

## Neuroimaging

Neuroimaging studies have established important neurobiological underpinnings of ASD in the developing brain of affected children. Neuroimaging studies facilitate our understanding of atypical trajectories of brain maturation across early stages of neurodevelopment from infancy to adulthood. Although there are similarities in neurodevelopmental abnormalities, ASD is a heterogeneous disorder with variability in neuroanatomical phenotypes among affected individuals. Such heterogeneity might be reduced by future stratification into biologically homogeneous subtypes (Ecker, 2017; Harris, 2019). Neuroimaging studies benefit from careful identification of cases using Autism Diagnostic Interview–Revised (ADI-R) research criteria. These studies have been carried out cross-sectionally and longitudinally in both children and adults. Adult neuroimaging studies have examined regional brain changes that persist into adult life in people with ASD. Our understanding of the relationship between ASD and the anatomy of specific brain regions is complicated by failure to replicate findings among some studies and the small sample sizes of many studies.

A large-scale multicenter magnetic resonance imaging (MRI) study was conducted in the United Kingdom to clarify neuroimaging findings in ASD. Comparisons were made between 89 men with ASD and 89 age-matched male controls. All were high functioning, with full-scale IQ means of 110 in those with ASD and 113 in controls. Males with ASD were not significantly different from the control group in measures of global brain volume. However, there were regionally specific differences in gray and white matter volume. Increased gray matter volume was demonstrated in the anterior temporal and dorsolateral prefrontal regions; decreased gray matter density was found in the occipital and medial parietal regions in the ASD subjects. When the gray matter was further examined, adults with ASD showed changes in the cingulate gyrus, supplementary motor area, basal ganglia, amygdala, inferior parietal lobule, and cerebellum. Additional regional differences were found in the dorsolateral prefrontal, lateral orbitofrontal, and dorsal and ventral medial prefrontal cortices. These were accompanied by spatially distributed reductions in regional white matter volume (Ecker et al., 2012). In this study, regional differences in neuroanatomy correlated with the severity of specific autistic symptoms based on the ADI-R criteria. Thus, ASD is a syndrome that involves atypical neural connectivity (Ecker et al., 2013).

Structural brain mapping is being used to study morphological connectivity in ASD. Because ASD manifests differently in males and females, differences between genders must be considered as one source of heterogeneity. Males with ASD have been disproportionately represented in research, consistent with the threefold greater prevalence in males. Indeed, neuroanatomical differences have been demonstrated between high-functioning males and females with ASD (when intelligence is in the average to the above average range). Lai et al. (2013) studied the brains of 30 right-handed males and 30 right-handed females and matched controls. Differences between males and females were found in gray matter and white matter regions of interest. Nevertheless, brain structures in the females that showed evidence of sexual dimorphism overlapped. Although gender-dependent neuroanatomy in ASD requires replication, these findings highlight the importance of stratifying by sex in neuroimaging studies. Clarification with regard to whether differences between males and females are related to cognition and whether such differences generalize to males and females whose intelligence is in the mild to severe ranges of intellectual developmental disorder is needed.

Understanding brain connectivity in ASD is necessary because brain structures are tightly coupled in development. Correlations between frontal lobe gray matter volume and temporal lobe, parietal lobe, and subcortical gray matter are shown to be disrupted in ASD. However, the nature of the altered brain connectivity deficit is poorly understood. Functional brain phenotypes are characterized by both hypoconnectivity and hyperconnectivity involving large-scale brain systems. Studies of connectivity focus on task-based functional connectivity—for example, synchronization of activation of a brain region when the subject is presented with a cognitive challenge. In addition, examination of resting-state functional connectivity in the absence of a task has been carried out.

A developmental perspective is important in examining hyperconnectivity and hypoconnectivity during brain development. A review of functional MRI (fMRI) studies of functional connectivity in children, adolescents, and adults from a developmental perspective finds dynamic changes with aging. In younger children, functional connectivity seems to be increased, whereas in adolescents and adults with ASD, connectivity seems to be reduced compared with age-matched controls. Future studies of a developmental framework in prepubertal, adolescent, and adult subjects are needed to resolve conflicting findings on hypoconnectivity and hyperconnectivity to a better understand the neurobiology of ASD (Uddin et al., 2013).

Abnormal integration of information in distributed brain networks could result in core clinical features of ASD. Before the stage of higher order integration, neural dysfunction in primary sensory and motor cortical areas and in the thalamus also may underlie these clinical features (Uddin et al., 2013). Younger children with ASD have reduced long-range connectivity between default mode network nodes and increased local connectivity within default mode network nodes. This includes the visual and motor resting-state networks and the salience network. As long-distance connections are studied during adolescence, such findings will provide further support for the developmental disconnection model of ASD (Washington et al., 2014). In addition, resting-state connectivity studies can be used to distinguish ASD from schizophrenia (Mastrovito et al., 2018).

## Longitudinal Trajectory of Brain Growth

Despite heterogeneity and multiple behavioral and biological phenotypes, accelerated brain growth during early childhood is a well-established feature in idiopathic ASD. Macrocephaly is found in approximately 20% of affected individuals and is considered to be megalencephaly (abnormal enlargement of the brain). The increased head circumference was recognized in Kanner's original 1943 publication. Although, at birth, head circumference is in the typical range, overgrowth becomes apparent in the first 18 months of life with acceleration of head growth. In affected cases, by age 3 or 4 years, there is an average increase in brain size of approximately 10%. Accelerated brain growth is apparent before the recognition of most of the clinical features. MRI and other imaging methods demonstrate an overall increase in the mean volume of the brain resulting from increased white matter and gray matter in the cerebral cortex. This is not linked to intellectual disability, psychotropic medication use, or other co-occurring psychopathology (Lainhart & Lange, 2011).

Cortical thickness, like brain volume, also shows early overgrowth followed by arrested growth. When head circumference measurements collected longitudinally between birth and age 18 months in 35 male children with ASD and a comparison group of 22 typically developing control subjects were examined, there was significantly thinner cortex in the ASD group, predominantly located in the left temporal and parietal lobes. In another ASD study, participants had thinner cortex in the left fusiform/inferior temporal cortex compared to typically developing individuals. This suggests a second period of abnormal cortical growth with greater thinning (Wallace et al., 2010).

Neurogenesis is completed by the end of pregnancy throughout the entire cerebral cortex, including the prefrontal cortex. Developmentally, programmed cell death (apoptosis), one possible mechanism for these findings of volume differences, affects the number of neurons in the brain in childhood. An increase in neurons would be consistent with prenatal origin (Courchesne et al., 2011). Postmortem cortical gray matter in the prefrontal cortex in an autopsy study of seven boys with ASD found 79% more neurons in the dorsolateral prefrontal cortex and 29% more in the mesial prefrontal cortex compared with matched controls (Courchesne et al., 2011). Courchesne et al. suggested that increased neuron number in the prefrontal cortex correlated with accelerated postnatal brain growth and macrocephaly in ASD in early childhood. With regard to specificity, comparison studies are required for those with ASD, who do not have brain overgrowth, and non-autistic children with benign megalencephaly. Such studies are needed to clarify whether increased prefrontal neuron count in ASD is associated only with ASD. However, because cortical neurons are generated in prenatal life, a pathological overabundance of neurons indicates early developmental disturbances in critical brain regions in ASD.

The relationship between total brain volume and onset of ASD symptoms has been examined. Failure of developmental progression with loss of acquired skills is documented in 25–35% of affected children in epidemiological studies. Typically, in the second year of life in affected children, attention become less focused, acquired word use is lost, and motor stereotypes appear. Comparisons were made between 61 children with ASD who regressed and 53 cases who did not regress, along with a comparison group (Nordahl et al., 2011). Early onset ASD is typically diagnosed by approximately age 18 months. Head circumference measurements from birth to age 18 months revealed that abnormal brain enlargement occurred most often in boys with behavioral and language regression. Moreover, brain enlargement was associated with ASD in preschool-age boys but not in girls. In boys without regression, the brain did not differ from that of typical controls. Nordahl et al. concluded that rapid head growth may be a risk factor in boys with the onset of regression in the second year of life, potentially identifying a regression subgroup.

The defining symptoms of ASD are not present in the first year of life. Because little information is available on brain development at ages 6 and 12 months before the appearance of ASD symptoms, a prospective study of high-risk infants, who have an older sibling with ASD, was initiated: the Baby Sibs study. In the Baby Sibs study, brain changes were observed at age 6 months before the appearance of ASD symptoms. At that age, there is also increased volume of cerebrospinal fluid in these children (Shen et al., 2018; Wolff et al., 2012). This was shown in infant sibling studies with longitudinal MRI scans carried out at three time points along with comprehensive behavioral assessments. Fifty-five "high-risk" (with an affected sibling) and 22 "low-risk" infants were imaged at ages 6–9 months. A total of 43 of these (27 high-risk and 16 low-risk) were imaged at ages 6–9, 12–15, and 18–24 months. Among these, 10 infants, who developed ASD, had significantly greater extra-axial cerebrospinal fluid at ages 6–9 months, which remained elevated at ages 12–15 and 18–24 months. There was excessive cerebrospinal fluid in the subarachnoid space, particularly over the frontal lobes. Extra-axial cerebrospinal fluid, detected as early as age 6 months, was predictive of more severe ASD symptoms at the time of outcome. Infants who developed ASD also had significantly large total cerebral volumes at both 12–15 and 18–24 months of age (Shen et al., 2017).

There are altered functional networks and white matter track diffusion as assessed by diffusion tensor imaging. Between ages 6 and 12 months, there is a hyper-expansion of cortical surface area that is regionally specific. Between ages 12 and 24 months, there is increased total brain volume growth. Therefore, structural MRI changes from ages 6 to 12 months can predict individual outcomes with high accuracy (Hazlett et al., 2017). Important neuronal connections correlate with later ASD-related behavior (Emerson et al., 2017). These correlations include social communication, cognitive ability, and re-petitive behavior (Elison et al., 2013). Correlates of functional connectivity MRI can be recognized with initiation of joint attention in infants (Eggebrecht et al., 2017). Specific networks are involved in specific forms of restricted and repetitive behaviors at each age as well as within restricted and repetitive categories across age (McKinnon et al., 2019).

The next aim in the Baby Sibs study was to predict measures of social responsiveness, joint attention, language, and repetitive behaviors with the goal of establishing efficient pre-symptomatic intervention trials. The next step was to build on longitudinal neu-roimaging of high-risk siblings of ASD cases that have demonstrated a specific pattern of brain development in infant siblings subsequently diagnosed with ASD. The pattern of brain development identified so far shows cortical surface area hyper-expansion in the first year of life. This is followed by overgrowth brain volume in the second year of life that is associated with the emergence of social deficits characteristic of ASD. These findings, combined with earlier genetic ones and those from animal models, support a hypothesis for abnormal early postnatal development in ASD resulting from an increase in proliferation of neural progenitor cells and the hyper-expansion of cortical surface area during the pre-symptomatic first year when a disruption in sensorimotor and at-tentional processes becomes apparent. This finding suggests an alteration in experience-dependent neuronal development with reduced elimination of neuronal processes. The recognition of the timing of developmental brain and behavior mechanisms during in-fancy before the emergence of clinical features is important in planning interventions for the first year of life (Piven et al., 2017).

## Neuropathology of Autism Spectrum Disorder

The investigation of neuropathology of ASD is necessary for the identification by brain ASD brain pathology not apparent with neuroimaging (Palmen et al., 2004).

Neuropathologic studies have demonstrated abnormalities in cortical and noncortical brain areas, including the archicortex, brain stem, cerebellum, and other subcortical structures. Twenty-one of 29 brains studied showed a decreased number of Purkinje cells in the cerebellum. More than half of the brains showed features of cortical dysgenesis (Palmen et al., 2004). In contrast, most of the cases evaluated in earlier post-mortem studies involved brains from individuals with a diagnosis of severe intellectual disability or who had comorbid seizure disorders. Epilepsy is usually associated with pathology of the cerebral cortex, amygdala, cerebellum, and hippocampal formation—regions also implicated in ASD. Therefore, co-occurring conditions may confound the interpretation of the neuroanatomy of ASD. Thus, it is important to include younger subjects free of co-occurring conditions such as severe IDD and epilepsy in examining neuropathology of ADD.

A hypothesis-based approach to neuropathology is being pursued in many studies by examining cell differentiation and migration, neuronal morphology, and alterations in cytoarchitecture. The considerable etiologic and phenotypic heterogeneity of ASD requires large sample sizes to achieve statistical power for subclassification. The findings from small studies need to be replicated before uncritical acceptance.

Despite the diversity of findings, there are many consistent results that can help address the heterogeneity of ASD and can contribute to identifying subgroups derived from structural, neurochemical, and genetic studies. There are clues to the timing of ASD/developmental features. In cortical areas, abnormalities are found in neuronal differentiation and migration, cytoarchitecture, and neuronal number. As reviewed above, the increase in brain size and head circumference occurs in a subset of cases. There are global developmental anomalies in archicortex, cerebellum, brain stem, and other subcortical areas. There is disorganization of gray and white matter with subependymal thickening. People with ASD have smaller and a greater number of minicolumns in Brodmann areas. Young children have reduced neuronal cytoplasmic volume, particularly in idiopathic ASD. There is an increase in the frontal polar region and anterior cingulate but not in visual, motor, somatosensory, and dorsolateral prefrontal cortex. Slower pruning of spines in the temporal lobe leads to differences in higher spine densities compared to controls (Tang et al., 2014). Although dendritic spine density in ASD and control brains was similar in early life (ages 2–9 years), the density declined in controls (ages 13–20 years) but not in the ASD brains. There is loss of cortical lamination in the fusiform gyrus and abnormal morphology in the temporal cortex, amygdala, and hippocampus involving dystrophic serotonin neurons in ASD (Azmitia et al., 2011).

The prefrontal cortex—the brain region that coordinates memory, planning, and executive functions—consistently has been shown to exhibit abnormal overgrowth in ASD in children aged 2–5 years (Sparks et al., 2002, p. 334). In the inferior frontal cortex—the brain region involved in language production, empathy, and social processing—people with ASD have been shown to have significantly smaller pyramidal neurons without a decrease in number (Jacot-Descombes et al., 2012). The reduction in size correlates with reductions in long-range communication with the inferior frontal cortex. The fusiform gyrus is the brain region primarily involved in our ability to process faces important in social interactions. Functional MRI studies have found hypoactivation of the fusiform gyrus in ASD, which may be an indicator of reduced energy metabolism and reflect a reduction in neuron number or neuronal density. People with ASD have been reported to have significantly lower neuronal density in layer III of the fusiform gyrus and reduced total neurons in layers III, V, and VI, along with reduced perikaryal volume (Varghese et al., 2017). These findings are consistent with reduced connectivity to cortical regions involved in analyzing facial expression and rewarding valid facial contact. Moreover, the fusiform gyrus projects to the amygdala, which is important in understanding emotional significance. Findings vary depending on the age of subjects, emphasizing the importance of a developmental approach.

The fronto-insular cortex is a brain region involved in self-awareness and emotion regulation. Von Economo neurons (VENs), found almost exclusively in the fronto-insular cortex and anterior cingulate cortex, are affected in ASD. VENs largely emerge after birth and increase in numbers to age 4 years. These neurons are involved in the integration of bodily feelings, emotion regulation, and goal-directed behaviors, as well as the intuitive grasp and evaluation of complex situations and the "embodied" dimension of social cognition. VENs project from the fronto-insular and anterior cingulate cortex to the frontal and temporal cortex, regions implicated in theory of mind. These brain regions are also involved in finding the intuitive gist judgments, which are potentially modulated cognitively by more deliberative judgments.

In a neuropathological stereological (three-dimensional) study of young patients with ASD involving four postmortem brains and three control brains, a higher ratio of VEN pyramidal neurons ($p = .02$) was found in postmortem patients than in control subjects, which suggests neuronal overgrowth that might be linked to neuronal migration, cortical lamination in layers (neocortex is characterized by lamination of neuron cell bodies in six layers), and apoptosis. Changes in VENs correlate with heightened introspection and disrupted information processing in ASD (Santos et al., 2011). The anterior cingulate cortex (ACC) is involved in motion processing and integration of information for decision-making. Alterations in ACC activation patterns have been shown in neuroimaging studies in ASD, including reduced thickness, functional connectivity, and levels of creatinine/phosphocreatine/GABA metabolites (Ito et al., 2017). A qualitative assessment of neuronal size and density carried out in anterior cingulate cortex in nine ASD cases using stereotypical techniques revealed significantly decreased cell size and cell packing density in ASD. However, three of the nine brains showed increased VEN density and six of the nine brains showed reduced VEN density compared to controls, indicating heterogeneity in neuropathological findings in a disorder that clinically shows heterogeneity. The presence of excess cells in the white matter adjacent to layer VI in the cingulate cortex along with changes in cytoarchitectural of limbic and neocortical areas suggest involvement in late prenatal and early postnatal periods.

The hippocampus is primarily involved in long-term memory storage and in spatial processing and navigation. In ASD, there is a difficulty remembering social information, a lack of flexibility in making decisions based on past experiences, but a possible enhancement of memory for factual details. Pathological studies in ASD have revealed decreases in neuronal size, increased cell packing density, and less complex dendrite arborization. These findings are consistent with a disruption of neuronal maturation. In some individuals with ASD, there are neuronal abnormalities in the entorhimal cortex and disruption of layers of the dentate gyrus of the hippocampus (Varghese et al., 2017).

Neuropathological studies in ASD also reveal abnormalities in extracortical brain regions, especially the amygdala, cerebellum, and brain stem. Changes in the amygdala are pertinent because of its role in social behavior and establishment of emotional salience. Early pathological studies of individuals diagnosed with ASD revealed decreased size and increased packing density of neurons in medial cortex and cortical nuclei (Bauman & Kemper, 1994). Subsequent quantification studies have revealed a significant reduction in neuronal numbers in the amygdala overall and in the lateral nucleus (Schumann & Amaral, 2006). Reduction in neuronal number may result from fewer neurons being produced or subsequent cell loss. Differences from earlier to later studies may be accounted for by epileptic comorbidity in earlier studies. Consistent findings of neuropathology in the amygdala and connected brain regions abnormal pathways in ASD.

The cerebellum plays a role in cognition and the regulation of emotion as well as in motor coordination. The cerebellum is one of the most completely examined brain region with regard to ASD neuropathology. The focus of these investigations is on the number, size, and density of Purkinje cells, which were found to be smaller than those in control subjects (Whitney et al., 2009). Studies in ASD also indicate overall cerebellar hypoplasia and flocculonodular dysphasia.

Finally, disruption in cell morphology occurs in the brain stem in ASD. The medial superior olivary nucleus, an auditory brain stem structure, shows disrupted cell morphology, especially in cell body orientation and shape. The misalignment of inferior olivary neurons along the border of the primary olivary ribbon of neurons indicates a prenatal insult, possibly in the first trimester in a subset of cases (Blatt, 2012).

In summary, ASD brains have neocortical differences in structure, including cortical mini-columns (Casanova & Trippe, 2009; Opris & Casanova, 2014) and overgrowth, face processing areas in the fusiform gyrus of the temporal lobe, anterior and posterior cingulate cortex, limbic hippocampus, entorhinal cortex, amygdala in the forebrain and hindbrain cerebellum, and inferior olivary complex (Blatt, 2012). Increasing the number of specimens in brain banks with precise medical histories for each case with accompanying genetic background will likely lead to finding additional pathology. Study of genetic and environmental influences is expected to lead to better understanding of why genes are dysregulated, where they are expressed, and how this information can be correlated with neuropathological findings.

## Neurochemistry

Neurotransmitters and neuropeptides play a critical role in normal brain development. They influence neuronal cell migration, differentiation, synaptogenesis, and synaptic pruning, in addition to their role in neurotransmission in the mature brain. Therefore, dysfunction of neurotransmitters must be considered in brain development in ASD (Marotta et al., 2020). Neurotransmitters and neuropeptides examined in ASD include γ-aminobutyric acid (GABA), glutamate, serotonin (5-HT), dopamine, acetylcholine, N-acetyl asparate, oxytocin, and arginine vasopressin. GABA is an excitatory neurotransmitter in immature neurons, in contrast to its role as the main inhibitory neurotransmitter in the mature brain. GABA is involved in neuronal proliferation, migration, synapse maturation, differentiation, and cell death. Glutamate is the main excitatory neurotransmitter in the central nervous system (CNS). Serotonin is involved in cell division, cortical proliferation, migration, differentiation, cortical plasticity, and synaptogenesis. It is involved in brain functions that include memory and learning, mood regulation, and sleep.

The most consistent finding in ASD is increased 5-HT levels in blood platelets, which occurs in 30–50% of ASD individuals and results in elevated whole blood 5-HT levels (Gabriele et al., 2014; Piven et al., 1991; Ritvo et al., 1970). Increases in blood 5-HT have also been noted in the broader ASD phenotype but not in IDD. Dietary tryptophan depletion and positron emission tomography (PET) studies support central 5-HT deficits in ASD. Acute depletion of dietary tryptophan reduces 5-HT in the brain and leads to a worsening of symptoms of ASD. PET studies using a radiolabeled 5-HT precursor showed reduced synthesis, consistent with developmental dysregulation of 5-HT synthesis. Moreover, there is a significant reduction in 5-HT$_{1A}$ receptor binding density in superficial and deep layers of the posterior cingulate cortex and fusiform gyrus and also in the density of 5-HT$_{2A}$ receptors in these layers. Polymorphisms in the *SL6A4* gene that encodes for platelet and neuronal transport of 5-HT are associated with ASD (Jaiswal et al., 2015).

In addition to 5-HT, dopamine and norepinephrine have also been studied. Levels of homovanillic acid, the primary dopamine metabolite in blood, urine, and cerebrospinal fluid, have been reported to be abnormal in subjects with ASD compared to controls. Persons with ASD have reductions in the mesocorticolimbic dopaminergic signaling pathway, as demonstrated in a PET study. Dopamine modulates motor activity, attention, and reward and social behaviors. A PET scan study measured the accumulation of fluorine-8-labeled DOPA (FDOPA) in the caudate, putamen, midbrain, prefrontal cortex, and occipital cortex in 14 medication-free children with ASD aged 13 years (8 male, 6 female) and 10 control subjects. Regional FDOPA accumulation was reduced by 39% in the anterior medial prefrontal cortex in the ASD group compared to controls. No other differences were observed between the two groups.

It is abundantly apparent from genetic and imaging studies that ASD is a heterogeneous disorder, and PET studies help identify subtypes. Findings in the dopamine mesocorticolimbic striatal circuit point to its link to stereotypical behavior. For example, a single nucleotide polymorphism (SNP) of the gene *(rs16771)* encoding the DRD3 receptor, which is highly expressed in the striatum, has been associated with stereotypical behavior in ASD. In this study involving 86 participants diagnosed with ASD with a mean age of 15.3 years, the DRD3 rs16771 SNP correlated with the volumes of the caudate and putamen, which correlated with stereotypical behavior. This association may be a biological marker for a subtype of ASD (Staal et al., 2015). These findings require replication.

Magnetic resonance spectroscopy (MRS) is a noninvasive way to study brain neurochemistry. It allows in vivo quantification of biochemical and metabolite concentrations in the brain, including glutamate and GABA. MRS has been carried out in the striatum and medial prefrontal cortex in humans, mice, and rats for cross-species comparisons of glutamate and GABA signaling. In humans diagnosed with ASD, the concentration of glutamate was found to be reduced in the striatum, which correlated with severity of social deficits. GABA levels were not reduced within this brain region.

Mice prenatally exposed to valproate, an ASD animal model with face validity, showed reduction in striatal glutamate, as did mice carrying the *NRXN1* risk gene microdeletion for ASD, a genetic animal model.

Glutamate/GAA codon abnormalities in corticostriate circuitry may be important pathological mechanisms in ASD (Horder et al., 2018). Elevations in blood glutamate levels in people with ASD provide further support for the role of glutamate in ASD. A systematic review and meta-analysis of 12 studies involving 880 participants and 446 incident cases found higher blood glutamate levels in ASD with considerably heterogeneity across studies (Zheng et al., 2016). A subgroup analysis revealed higher plasma glutamate levels in ASD compared to control subjects. Assays using highly sensitive high-performance liquid chromatography and mass spectrometry have also demonstrated higher levels.

In other MRS studies, reductions in GABA have been found in ASD. Reductions in GABA levels have been reported in an age-dependent manner in motor, visual, auditory, somatosensory area, and perisylvian brain regions of the left hemisphere (Puts et al., 2017; Rojas et al., 2014). An imbalance between GABAergic and glutamatergic levels (excitatory:inhibitory ratio [E:I]) was also examined in 40 male children with ASD and 38 age- and gender-matched neurotypical controls using standardized rating scales for social responsiveness and ASD behaviors. In this study, children with ASD had a significant elevation of plasma GABA and the glutamate-to-glutamine ratio. Although no significant relationship was found between glutamate levels and severity of ASD, glutamate did appear to be the best prognostic marker for ASD. Overall, the results suggest an increased GABA:glutamate ratio (reduced E:I ratio) in ASD (Al-Otaish et al., 2018). Nevertheless, there have been only a few clinical trials of GABA-modulating drugs such as arbaclofen or acamprosate in ASD, which have led to inconclusive or mixed results. A randomized trial of arbaclofen yielded negative results; results with acamprosate were mixed. However, study sample sizes were small. Currently, there is insufficient evidence to recommend GABA modulation for children with ASD (Brondino et al., 2016).

ASD is associated with widespread reductions in *N*-acetylaspartate (NAA), creatine and phosphocreatine, choline-containing compounds, and *myo*-inositol. These reductions suggest impaired neuronal function and/or metabolism. However, findings vary depending on the study and region of interest. Studies should control for variability in subjects' age and level of functioning to address neurodevelopmental levels and findings specifically associated with ASD. A meta-analysis identified 22 articles on ASD satisfying the criteria with measures of NAA, creatine, choline-containing compounds, *myo*-inositol, glutamate, and glutamine in the frontal, temporal, and parietal regions; amygdala–hippocampus complex; thalamus; and cerebellum (Aoki et al., 2012) . Random effect analyses showed significantly lower NAA levels in all the brain regions examined except the cerebellum in childhood; yet, there was no significant difference in metabolite levels in adulthood. These findings are consistent with early transient brain expansion in ASD that may be caused by an increase in nonneuronal tissues, such as glial cell proliferation.

Other investigators have correlated MRS changes with social and cognitive functioning in ASD. In one study involving 77 young children with ASD (23 boys and 8 girls), reductions in NAA were found in the left amygdala and in the orbitofrontal cortex bilaterally compared to those in a control group (Mori et al., 2015). NAA levels correlated with ratings of the social quotient in the children with ASD, suggesting that neuronal dysfunction in these brain regions contributes to these symptoms. Another study of 54 children diagnosed with ASD (aged 8–13 years) and 56 controls showed correlation of NAA and glutamate with striatal volume in ASD subjects, indicting reduced neuronal integrity or impaired neuronal functioning in the striatum (Naaijen et al., 2018).

## Oxytocin

Oxytocin, vasopressin, and related peptides are pertinent to both social and repetitive behavior symptoms in ASD. Oxytocin is involved with social cognition, interpersonal bonding, trust, and stress management from infancy to old age. Its release is sensitive to the emotional and social context. Oxytocin plays an important role in emotional regulation through facilitating parent–child attachment. Polymorphisms of the oxytocin receptor have been implicated in sensitivity to social cues. Oxytocin modulates emotions and social judgments through actions on the hypothalamic–pituitary–adrenal axis and autonomic nervous system responsiveness. It may alter perceptions of the social environment as safe or threatening. Accordingly, oxytocin is being studied as an adjunctive treatment to behavioral interventions to facilitate social cognition and emotion regulation in ASD.

Any theory regarding the risk for ASD must consider the nearly fourfold male bias in risk. The gender differences in the central regulation and expression of oxytocin and vasopressin may contribute to the sex difference in ASD risk. Estrogen modulates the oxytocin system, with levels of the peptide and its receptor being higher in females. Oxytocin enhances the corticostriatal functional connectivity in women (Bethlehem et al., 2017). Levels of vasopressin in the extended amygdala–lateral septal axis of the nervous system are sexually dimorphic, being higher in males. Nevertheless, males are more sensitive than females to the actions of vasopressin, especially during early development. In females, insensitivity to vasopressin or a lack of dependence on this peptide could be protective against ASD, whereas oxytocin may be protective either directly or indirectly. Its anti-anxiety effects reduce fear and increase a sense of safety or trust. Vasopressin is associated with both parenting behavior and social bonding, where higher levels are associated with anxiety and aggression (Iovino et al., 2018). In addition, vasopressin may play a role in the integration of sensory input during complex social behavior (Bester-Meredith et al., 2015). Moreover, vasopressin amplifies reaction to stressors by increasing arousal. Both intranasal oxytocin and vasopressin antagonists are being studied in clinical trials to improve social communication in ASD (Umbright et al., 2017).

## Animal Studies

Animal models are utilized to advance our understanding of disease mechanisms that underlie ASD and are important for the development of potential treatments. Mice with mutations of risk genes for ASD are commonly used to study genetic or environmental risk factors for ASD (Ergaz et al., 2016). These models can express features of the disorder but not the full human condition. Mutant mouse models of neurogenetic syndromes including ASD have demonstrated that some symptoms of the disorder can be reversed. Thus, studying rare syndromic disorders may be pertinent to some features of idiopathic ASD (Harris, 2016; Sztainberg & Zoghbi, 2016). Despite reversal of symptoms in adult mutant mouse models of human neurogenetic syndromes such as Rett syndrome, human treatment trials based on genetic manipulation in these purported animal models have not always been successful. A striking example is fragile X syndrome. Studies of the mGluR5 antagonist mavoglurant (AFQ056) in mice bearing the fragile X mutation demonstrated substantial reduction in symptoms (Bear et al., 2004). However, two large international clinical trials found that mavoglurant was ineffective in reducing symptoms in fragile X patients. One trial involved adults with fragile X syndrome, and the other involved adolescent subjects with the syndrome (Berry-Kravis et al., 2016). Questions have been raised whether clinical trials may need to begin in infancy because fragile X syndrome involves the development and maturation of dendritic branching. Another approach has been to study single nucleotide variants of *SHANK3* responsible for Phelan–McDermid syndrome, which exhibits ASD symptoms. Mice with *SHANK3* mutations exhibit ASD-like behaviors and have deficits in synaptic development (Mei et al., 2016; Monteiro & Feng, 2017).

The mouse brain differs substantially from the human brain. There are more than 83 million years in evolutionary distance between humans and mice. Over the millennia, cognitive and emotional capacity has advanced, and complex behavior has evolved to establish two functional domains in the human brain. The first domain is conserved in all mammals and involves reward, emotion, and memory. The second functional domain is unique to primates. It evolved with the growth in size of the cerebral cortex, which established new cognitive capacities, language, tool use, and self-awareness. The frontoparietal attention network, the capacity for imitation, tactile use of the hands to grasp, social systems, and social hierarchies are products of brain evolution. Primates and mice also differ in that mice do not have a retinal fovea, which pinpoints visual attention. The primate fovea facilitates eye movement that allows the eyes to align binocular vision and attend to a specific visual target. The fovea not only enhances visual acuity but also fundamentally establishes how the world can be seen in three dimension (Belmonte et al., 2015).

The evolved CNS in nonhuman primates (NHPs) makes them a better choice than mice to model human brain diseases. In recent years, genetic manipulation of NHPs has become feasible to study human genetic diseases (Jennings et al., 2016; Sasaki et al., 2009). For example, in the marmoset, neuroimaging studies are mapping marmoset brain regions for comparison with human brains (Okano et al., 2016; Seki et al., 2017). The development of the orbitofrontal cortex, cingulate cortex, amygdala, and hippocampus has also been characterized in the common marmoset (*Callithrix jacchus*) (Sawiak el al., 2018; Uematsu et al., 2017). This information lays the foundation for studies of genetic models of developmental disorders in the marmoset. Genetic silencing of *MECP2*, the gene responsible Rett syndrome, in the marmoset re-created the physiological, behavioral, and structural abnormalities of the disorder (Y. Chen et al., 2017). Eye tracking studies also revealed decreased social attention (Zhang et al., 2019). A *SHANK3* mutation was established in cynomolgus monkeys using the

CRISPR/Cas9 genome editing method. The *SHANK3*-deficient monkey fetus showed a significant loss of neuronal cells, differentiating it from Shank3-knockout mice. This nonhuman primate model is consistent with a clinical role for the *SHANK3* gene in early brain development, which may be pertinent for understanding aspects of ASD (Tu et al., 2019; Zhao et al., 2017).

In summary, there is considerable interest in animal models of ASD. Mutant mouse models and transgenic NHPs are being studied with the aim to identify biochemical pathways and/or brain circuit changes pertinent to ASD behaviors and targets for drug development.

## Developmental Hypotheses

Kanner proposed that early infantile autism is an inborn neurodevelopmental disorder. Several theoretical models have been proposed to account for the primary social deficits in ASD. Recognized models include the emotional, intersubjective, and meta-representational models (cognitive); executive function; and the weak coherence models (Rogers & Pennington, 1991). The emotional model addresses affective attunement with others. The intersubjectivity model focuses on impaired formation/coordination of self–other representations in social interactions. The meta-representational or cognitive models address the theory of mind or mentalizing deficits in ASD. Theory of mind refers to the ability to attribute mental states to oneself and others. In doing so, we anticipate what others are thinking. Individuals diagnosed with ASD often do not understand that other people may have distinct plans, intentions, thoughts, feelings, and points of view that differ from their own. Essentially, they cannot put themselves in the place of others. Central coherence is defined as a limited ability to understand psychological context or to see the big picture. Executive functioning involves thinking used in cognitive control of emotions and behavior. Executive functions focus attention, utilizing working memory, and emphasize planning and flexibility in thinking (Happé, 1999; Happé & Frith, 2006). Kanner's hypothesis of autistic disturbance of affective contact places emphasis on developmental milestones linked to early social engagement and social reciprocity rather than meta-cognitive processes. Social milestones include social attachment, use of gestures in social engagement, and the emergence of social pragmatic interpersonal communication.

Pragmatic communication includes turn-taking conversations, shaking the head no, and nodding yes. Moreover, the emergence of self-conscious emotions (embarrassment, shaking, guilt, and probably blushing) represents important social developmental milestones. Imaginative play serves as a means to integrate interpersonal experiences through role-playing to consolidate personal identity (Davidson et al., 2017; Heerey et al., 2003). Self-conscious emotions such as embarrassment and shame are associated with aspects of theory of mind. These are the ability to understand that behavior has consequences and understanding social norm violations. Hobson's emotional theory (Hobson, 1991b, 1993; Hobson & Lee, 1999), the polyvagal model of social engagement (Porges, 2001), and findings of neuroendocrine hormones (oxytocin and vasopressin) (Carter et al., 2008) further our understanding of emotional development pertinent to ASD. Hobson's emotional model highlights the importance of the developing self in social engagement (Hobson & Meyer, 2005). Individuals with ASD fail to recognize the meaning of emotional expressions in others. Observations of people with ASD found that they express emotions inappropriately by not using them to regulate social interactions with others (Gaigg, 2012). Hobson suggested that typically developing people do not simply interact with one another. Instead, they engage interpersonally with others. They identify with the other person and recognize others' attitudes and psychological orientations as distinct from their own (Hobson et al., 2007; Hobson & Lee, 1999).

Affective attunement emerges soon after birth when the infant synchronizes their movements to the rhythms of the mother's speech as she slows her speech in synchrony with the infant's movements. Synchronized and emotionally patterned early social interaction and biobehavioral synchrony provide the basis for interpersonal engagement. Gradually, the infant discovers a connection between their behavior and that of others and links behavior to subjective experiences (Trevarthen, 1979; Trevarthen & Aitken, 2001). Interactional synchrony facilitates the emergence of the infant's understanding that other people are "like me." It is the beginning of a sense of "we-ness" in relationships—that is, that we are doing this together. This capacity to identify and to synchronize with others is impaired in individuals with ASD (Hobson et al., 2007). As children with ASD grow older, such innate affective deficits in biobehavioral synching are important impediments in the development of symbolic play and language (J. Hobson et al., 2009).

Social, emotional, and behavioral difficulties in ASD interfere with the establishment of biobehavioral synchrony. Educational interventions to facilitate physiological interactional attunement in children with ASD can promote emotional development. For example, often children with ASD like to spin themselves around. Picking the child up and deliberately spinning around with them until the child makes eye contact with the therapist is a way to make use of a preferred spinning behavior to facilitate interactional attunement. Now socially engaged when put down, the child can be encouraged to raise their arms to be picked up to continue this game of social engagement and shape a social-appropriate behavior.

Physiological synchrony involves enteroception. The role of enteroception in the physiology of social communication and engagement can be better understood based on Porges' polyvagal model (Porges et al., 2013, 2014; Porges & Lewis, 2009). Porges et al. studied deficits in interoceptive integration in people with ASD (Garfinkel et al., 2016), who have difficulty identifying others' emotions and regulating their own emotions. Such affective deficits may result from abnormalities in interoceptive processing. Individuals with ASD have an impaired ability to identify and objectively detect their own bodily signals, suggesting that emotional deficits and affective symptoms involve the interoceptive interface between body and mind (Garfinkel et al., 2016; Quattrocki & Friston, 2014).

The social bond between mother and child is modulated by the hormones oxytocin and vasopressin. These hormones facilitate social engagements and mother–infant attachment (Carter et al., 2008; Feldman, 2012b; Feldman et al., 2011; Quattrocki & Friston, 2014). Intranasal oxytocin has been shown to have short-term effects in children with ASD (Huang et al., 2021). It has also been found to enhance intrinsic corticostriatal functional connectivity in women (Bethlehem et al., 2017). However, long-term oxytocin use is less effective (Tachibana et al., 2013), and its use in clinical settings is complex because its effects are context-dependent (Harris & Carter, 2013; Huang et al., 2021). Moreover, vasopressin is associated with parenting behavior and social bonding. Although high levels of vasopressin cause anxiety and aggression, intranasal administration in low doses increases social behavior (Carson et al., 2015; Iovino et al., 2018). Vasopressin can play a role in enhancing social behavior integration of sensory input during complex social behavior (Bester-Meredith et al., 2015).

Vasopressin amplifies reactivity to stressors by increasing arousal to enhance attention, verbal learning, and memory (Iovino et al., 2018). Vasopressin 1A receptor antagonists have improved social communication in ASD in clinical trials (Umbricht et al., 2017). The understanding of interactional synchrony, affective engagement, and intersubjectivity is being incorporated to developmentally oriented ASD treatment programs. For example, the Early Start Denver Model (ESDM) is a comprehensive early intervention approach that provides a developmentally based curriculum intervention for children with ASD aged 12–48 months based on our understanding of social deficits (Dawson et al., 2010; Rogers & Dawson, 2009; Rogers, Dawson, et al., 2012). The educational skills taught are carefully defined. Teaching procedures have been standardized to apply them in clinical settings (Rogers, Estes, et al., 2012).

ESDM combines a developmentally focused intervention with carefully planned and applied behavior analysis procedures. The goal is to facilitate shared interpersonal engagement in the context of joint attention to develop an interpersonal sense of "we-ness"; attunement is facilitated with parent or teacher. This approach seeks to enhance social communication and language development.

In summary, interventions are increasingly based on developmental neurophysiological concepts and are tailored to the needs of individual children. Notably, a recent meta-analysis of 12 studies on the efficacy of ESDM found a modest significant effect on cognition and language but regrettably no effects on autistic symptoms, adaptive behavior, social communication, or restrictive and repetitive behaviors (Fuller et al., 2020).

## Assessment

The confirmation of the diagnosis of ASD is generally based on the clinical history, neuropsychiatric interview, and observational assessment. A variety of psychometric instruments are available for the assessment of ASD in children. Among these are the Childhood Autism Rating Scale–Second Edition (CARS-2), which is composed of 15 elements that include different symptoms of ASD (Schopler et al., 2010). The CARS-2 distinguishes mildly to moderately and severely symptomatic ASD children. It is based on direct observation of the child. The CARS-2 is useful for research and administrative classification and also for deriving a descriptive summary of the ASD behaviors. It should be used in conjunction with diagnostic information from the child's history and information from home, school, and community. For research purposes, the most comprehensive interview and observation scales are the ADI-R (de Bildt et al., 2015; Kim & Lord, 2012) and the Autism Diagnostic Observation Schedule (Lord et al., 2012). Frequently, parents will ask about electrophysiologic studies, neuroimaging, and blood and urine tests to establish a diagnosis. Only a minority of ASD children require extensive testing. The tests are done to reassure the family that the condition is not a known metabolic disorder or neurological condition.

The history focuses on behaviors typically found in children. The themes mentioned include the development of sociability, language, play, the presence of stereotypies, and abnormal responses to sensory stimuli. Although autistic symptoms ordinarily are not related to perinatal difficulties, birth history and history of infections and accidents that may involve the brain must be included in the history. Because of the potential genetic disorder, questions are asked about other family members with autism and other developmental disorders as well as specific psychiatric disorders, such as mood disorders, which have, in some instances, been related to autistic disorder in family studies (Piven et al., 2013).

The purpose of the physical examination is to identify potential disorders that have been associated with autistic-like behavior, such as tuberous sclerosis, congenital rubella, and fragile X syndrome. The mental status examination is primarily observational for younger children. It begins with engaging the child in meaningful interactions and, for verbal children, in conversation. Assessment for imaginative play with representational toys is important. Although the diagnosis may be apparent in those who are severely affected, for those who are less severely affected, attention must focus on more subtle difficulties in the child's relatedness and play. Attention must also be paid to gaze avoidance, difficulty in initiating social communication, problems with joint attention, and stereotypies.

Testing should be carried out by an interdisciplinary team to establish the needed interventions. This includes psychological tests and speech and language tests that are done to establish baseline information about the child and to clarify the nature of the deficits. In some instances, a hearing test is necessary because of the complaint of language and speech delays. If the child cannot cooperate in standard behavioral audiometry, then brain stem auditory evoked response measures are carried out.

## Assessment for Co-Occurring Psychiatric Disorders

The assessment of individuals with ASD includes careful consideration for co-occurring psychiatric disorders that more commonly occur in ASD than in the general population. A comprehensive systematic review and meta-analysis of prevalence of co-occurring psychiatric disorders included 96 studies. Lai et al. (2019) found that subjects with ASD had a pooled prevalence of 28% with ADHD; 20% with anxiety disorders; 13% with sleep–wake disorder; 12% with disruptive, impulse control, and conduct disorders; 11% with depressive disorders; 9% with obsessive–compulsive disorders; 5% with bipolar disorder; and 4% with schizophrenia spectrum disorder. In this study, heterogeneity was an issue with regard to age, gender, and intellectual level of functioning. Up to 70% of those studied were diagnosed with at least one co-occurring diagnosis, and approximately 50% were given multiple diagnoses. In the studies examined, prevalence of co-occurring conditions was higher in those ascertained in referred clinics than in population-based and registry-based studies. Thus, particular attention is needed to carefully examine clinic-referred cases for co-occurring diagnoses. Although heterogeneity may be related to age, gender, and intelligence level, there is a substantial heterogeneity that is unexplained. ADHD diagnoses are more prevalent in younger age groups. Those with IDD had a higher probability of co-occurring schizophrenia spectrum disorder. With neurodevelopmental disorders, there can be diagnostic ambiguity. Therefore, revised diagnostic procedures are recommended. The co-occurrence of ADHD with ASD might be related to a shared genetic contribution (Ghirardi et al., 2019). This may also be the case with ASD and anxiety (Shephard et al., 2019).

Suicidality and self-injurious behavior are of particular concern in people with ASD because the prevalence of self-injurious behavior is substantially increased in people with ASD and severe IDD (Minshawi et al., 2014). During the past four decades, the prevalence of ASD has increased substantially in the general population with current diagnostic criteria, with greater numbers diagnosed whose intelligence is in the normal range. With increased prevalence, it is apparent that both self-injurious behavior and suicidality are public health problems in ASD. A retrospective population study (1995–2016) conducted in Denmark included 6.5 million individuals aged 10 years or older and identified 35,020 individuals (73% male) with a diagnosis of ASD. Individuals with ASD had greater than threefold higher rates of both suicide attempts and completed suicides than those not diagnosed with ASD. Suicide attempts were more common in females than males, but increased rates were found across all age groups (Kõlves et al., 2021). Rates were substantially higher in the 72% with co-occurring psychiatric disorders than those with ASD alone. Ninety percent of those who attempted suicide had at least one other co-occurring disorder, thus identifying an important risk factor for suicide in ASD. However, despite higher rates of co-occurring conditions, no difference was found if there was co-occurring IDD using adjusted incidence rate ratios (aIRRs). Highest rates were also found for post-traumatic stress disorder (33 aIRR), substance abuse disorder (25 aIRR), and borderline personality disorder (21 aIRR). Rates were increased for affective disorders (13 aIRR) and co-occurring depression (13 aIRR) that, when combined, had the highest rate. If the parent had a psychiatric disorder, rates were doubled for those who did not have an ASD diagnosis and somewhat increased (1.3-fold) if they were diagnosed with ASD.

Overall, the most common co-occurring psychiatric diagnosis was affective disorders (50.9%). This was followed by anxiety disorders, dissociative disorders, stress-related disorders, and somatoform disorders. The overall incidence risk for suicide was found to be highest for co-occurring depression and substance abuse. Several studies find that suicide attempts are increased in adolescence (ages 12–17 years) and young adulthood (ages 18–29 years) and among those with higher cognitive functioning (M. Chen et al., 2017; Hannon & Taylor, 2013). Although problems in mood regulation and co-occurring mood and anxiety disorders are most commonly associated with suicide and suicide attempts, the clinical features of ASD increase the risk. These include impaired social communication, impulsivity, perseveration on a specific train of thought or behavior, and problems with imagining alternatives to suicide (Arwert & Sizoo, 2020). With regard to the assessment of suicidal thoughts and behavior, so far there is no validated suicide susceptibility assessment tool for ASD (Howe et al., 2020).

Protective factors against suicide in the general population, such as older age and higher education level, were not found to be protective for those with ASD. Similarly, marriage, cohabitating, and employment were also found to be less protective against suicide in ASD. Importantly, early intervention to enhance social skills in children with

ASD may lower risk for suicidal behavior. In addition, it is essential that support services be expanded for people with ASD, especially in adult life after leaving protective school settings. Screening for and treatment of co-occurring conditions, especially anxiety disorder and depression, are important for suicide prevention. Finally, personalized interventions are key, with an emphasis on teaching safety planning and help-seeking behavior when distressed (Jager-Hyman et al., 2020).

## Neuropsychological Testing

Kanner (1943) suggested that autistic disorder is "inborn," and this judgment is confirmed by genetic research. In his original description, Kanner highlighted both deficits and talents. Kanner found precocious decoding of words in reading, excellent memory, well-developed visual–spatial skills, a failure to use language to convey meaning, inability to relate to others, and an obsessive desire for sameness. Subsequently, the neuropsychological phenotype has focused on attention/arousal, long-term episodic memory, executive function, and social cognitive deficits (Oliveras-Rentas et al., 2012). Specific patterns of cognitive and affective developmental profiles are recognizable in persons with ASD. They have uneven profiles on subtests of versions of the Wisconsin Card Sorting Test (WISC) and Wechsler Adult Intelligence Scale, in contrast to IQ-matched controls. The major differences are on subtests dealing with verbal abstraction, sequencing, visual–spatial skills, and rote memory. These deficits are thought to impair normal language acquisition and social functioning.

The fourth edition of the WISC (WISC-IV) has four indices: the Verbal Comprehension Index, the Perceptual Reasoning Index, the Working Memory Index, and the Processing Speed Index. There are 10 core subsets: Similarities, Vocabulary, Comprehension, Block Design, Picture Concepts, Matrix Reasoning, Digit Span, Letter–Number Sequencing, Coding, and Symbol Search. There are five complimentary subsets: Information, Word Reasoning, Picture Completion, Arithmetic, and Cancellation (Wechsler, 2003). To determine the cognitive profile of ASD with the WISC-IV, 51 autistic cases, 15 Asperger syndrome cases, and 42 typically developing children were enrolled in a study by Nader et al. (2015). Although there was no significant difference in IQ among the groups, children diagnosed with ASD scored higher on the Perceptual Reasoning Index than the Verbal Comprehension Index. Those diagnosed with Asperger syndrome scored higher on the Verbal Comprehension Index than the other indices; their lowest score was on the Processing Speed Index. For the autistic group, Block Design, Matrix Reasoning, and Picture Concepts were the strongest subsets. The weakest subsets were Comprehension, Digit Span, Letter–Number Sequence, and Coding. In the Asperger syndrome group, Vocabulary and Similarities had the best performance score, whereas Digit Span and Coding were weakest. This is consistent with other studies comparing Asperger syndrome, a diagnosis eliminated in DSM-5, with high-functioning autism. Their neurocognitive profiles are similar; however, those diagnosed with Asperger syndrome were found to have stronger verbal and abstract reasoning skills and better performance on theory of mind tests (Koyama et al., 2007). Still, both groups had greater deficits in meta-cognition, abstract reasoning, and nonverbal communication compared to typically developing children (Meyer &

Minshew, 2002). Overall, in DSM-5, despite better performance in some areas, Asperger syndrome is included as an ASD. For the typically developing comparison group, the indices showed no significant differences. Overall, for the typical group, Picture Concepts and Vocabulary were the strongest subsets. This is consistent with an even profile in typically developing children, in contrast to the subset scatter in ASD subjects.

Social cognitive functioning has been studied in ASD persons with the theory of mind paradigm (Baron-Cohen et al., 1985), in which meta-representational deficits are thought to impair the ASD person's comprehension of the mental states of others. Theory of mind refers to the ability to attribute mental states—that is, beliefs, desires, and intentions—to one's self and to other people as a way of predicting and understanding the behavior of others. ASD individuals show significantly poorer performance on tests of their understanding of others' beliefs and knowledge. Disruption in brain circuitry underlying theory of mind has been shown at multiple levels with fMRI and includes decreased activation and decreased functional connectivity between frontal and posterior brain regions (Kana et al., 2015). Yet these deficits are not specific to social cognition; autistic persons also perform poorly on executive function tasks, such as the WCST and the Tower of Hanoi test (Ozonoff et al., 1991). These tests are designed to identify an impaired ability to anticipate others' intentions, systematically plan actions, or respond spontaneously to novel events.

Frontally mediated executive function abilities are the basis for performance on cognitive tasks, such as joint attention and theory of mind tasks, which is impaired in ASD. In nonverbal joint attention, the child uses gestures and eye contact to coordinate attention with another person to share their interest with them—for example, making eye contact and then pointing to a picture in a book. Deficient joint attention is the most pronounced deficit in nonverbal communication in ASD and is consistently present across developmental levels. Although necessary for performance, executive dysfunction is not a core neuropsychological deficit in ASD disorder, which primarily affects affective and social cognitive domains.

Kanner's emphasis on disturbances in affective contact has been challenged by this focus on cognitive deficits. In keeping with Kanner, Hobson and Meyer (2005) maintain that many problems of ASD children are related to a lack of capacity to form affective contact with others and a lack of the ability to develop intimate friendships as they grow older despite their motivation to do so. Individuals with ASD have difficulty recognizing and understanding emotional expressions in others and rarely use them to regulate social interaction with others (Gaigg, 2012). In addition, they lack creative symbolic play and "flexible, context-sensitive" thinking and language. An ASD person's social problems are not fully accounted for by conceptual impairment in interpersonal understanding, although this may be an essential aspect of ASD. Their lack of understanding of others' beliefs and desires based in the theory of mind is not an adequate explanation for the quality of their nonverbal communication disorder and relationship difficulties.

Hobson's emotional conceptualization for ASD emphasizes the importance of the developing self in understanding autistic social engagement (Hobson & Meyer, 2005). Rather than simply interact developmentally, infants and children engage interpersonally with others. In doing so, they identity with and share attitudes with others. In early life, perception and action are linked in affective attunement and engaging in biobehavioral synchrony as the infant synchronizes their movements with the prosody of the mother's speech (Kato et al., 1983; Leclère et al., 2014; Trevarthen & Aitken, 2001). These experiences facilitate the infant's sense that other people are "like me" and are the beginning of a sense of "we-ness" in relationships (Harris, 2018). Children with severe IDD with mental ages of less than 3 years can be socially responsive despite the absence of meta-representational ability that becomes established by the mental age of 3 or 4 years.

The underlying neurobiological abnormality involves both higher level cognitive processes and responses to affective stimuli. The lack of social relatedness in ASD is the result of an innate incapacity to recognize and respond to emotional state expression in others. This is a difficult hypothesis to evaluate using neuropsychological tests because standard emotional recognition tasks are quite sensitive to cognitive influences. An alternative approach is to assess affective responsivity because individuals who do not understand a social or emotional event may show a decreased affective response.

Most children with ASD are impaired in attending to and recognizing simple emotions and their expression, and they show abnormal emotional expression themselves. This leads to a disturbance of affective contact—that is, a severe disruption in the experience of "interpersonal relations as interpersonal" (Hobson & Meyer, 2005). Here, *affective* refers to the domain in which body and mental inner coordination are linked, and intra-individual forms of expressed bodily feelings are understood between persons as a social experience. Stern (1985) uses the term "attunement" to describe these experiences of contact, and Trevarthen and Aitken (2001) refer to them as "intersubjectivity."

## Developmental Issues

The establishment of interactional synchrony between parent and child is a critical component of early development. From age 2 months onward, nonverbal interchanges between parent and child are stimulated by temporal patterns of spoken conversation. This early affective attunement is thought to be essential to facilitate language development. Interactional synchrony is beginning to be studied systematically in ASD children, based on concepts of attunement and intersubjectivity. Biobehavioral synchrony has been assessed in ASD by examining covariation in psychophysiological arousal levels between interacting parents and children (Baker et al., 2015).

## Natural History

The autistic child can have a period of apparently normal early development. However, all elements of the behavioral syndrome have been recognized in the early months of life. Problems with feeding, lack of responsiveness to others, absent anticipatory gestures, and excessive quietness and cooperativeness during infancy have been reported, as have excessive irritability and screaming.

The impairments in ASD involve all aspects of language and not only speech. In most ASD children, language development is deviant, with difficulties in both the comprehension of speech and the expression of ideas in speech. ASD persons may be markedly impaired in their vocal and nonvocal symbolic processes. Yet they may be good at nonsymbolic matching and assembly tasks.

The prognosis of ASD children is based on intelligence scores and the level of functional language development. Language development at age 5 years is a useful marker. Verbal and full-scale IQ scores are generally taken as an index of severity of the disorder; however, nonverbal IQ is essential to monitor because there may be discrepancies of 60 or more points between nonverbal and verbal scores in the preschool years. During the school years, academic achievement for the higher functioning group may be benefited by their memory skills. However, the presence of hyperlexia may lead to an overestimate of ability (Whitehouse & Harris, 1984).

Academic achievement and social adaptability have improved with advances in comprehensive treatment. Early intensive intervention, behavioral interventions, and evidence-based practice guidelines are parts of that comprehensive treatment model (Hyman et al., 2020). Children on the autistic spectrum may be obsessed with letters and endlessly arranging them. Hyperlexia refers to the ability to decode and sound out words without understanding their meaning. Venter et al. (1992) studied 58 high-functioning ASD children over an 8-year period. Verbal skills were the best predictor of social adaptive functioning, whereas academic achievement was related to intellectual functioning. However, academic achievement declined when task demands for abstract reasoning exceeded rote memory skills.

Despite their academic achievement, high-functioning ASD children may be placed in special education classes for social and emotional disturbances because of their deficits in interpersonal skills. In some instances, high-functioning ASD children who have been mainstreamed in grade school will return to special education during the high school years. Persons with mild and moderate IDD benefit from special education with teachers who have training to understand the ASD-associated behaviors.

Approximately 20% of children who show some autistic behavior in their early years gradually emerge from the autistic phase. Some make a relatively good social adjustment, although they may continue to have unusual and eccentric behaviors as adults. However, for the majority, symptoms of ASD persist into adult life. Adult adjustment is judged based on independent living and employability. Moderately impaired individuals may work successfully when their careful attention to detail and preoccupations can be channeled into jobs requiring completion of repetitive tasks. In job settings that require the least interaction with others, they may be most successful. Other employees who are aware of an obvious disability may help and support them. Achievement by those who are most successful academically may be limited by their social deficits, particularly by difficulty in language comprehension and poor judgment in social situations. Employers often do not appreciate the extent of their limitations in problem-solving and social adjustment. Social adjustment requires self-awareness of difference from others by the ASD person, and special education programs specifically focus on social, language, and cognitive impairment.

In recent years, the prevalence of ASD has substantially increased, with higher rates in all age groups. Data from the UK Adult Psychiatric Morbidity Study found a prevalence of 11/1,000 (Brugha et al., 2016). In adulthood, people with ASD face many challenges because social and health services are inadequate (Murphy et al., 2016).

There is a wide heterogeneity in adult outcomes, making it difficult to determine what proportion find adequate social integration and what proportion experience a good psychological and physical life and show resilience to stress (Howlin & Magiati, 2017). With aging, individuals with ASD exhibit a decline in cognitive skills, processing speed, attention, verbal memory, cognitive flexibility, planning, and theory of mind; however, they are less prone to decline in visual and working memory than the typical elderly population (Lever & Geurts, 2016).

## Affective Responses in Autistic Individuals

It is essential to monitor affective development in ASD children. Aggression toward others, sadness in the context of frustration, and apparent joy are frequently reported. Although fear of specific objects, such as animals, may be expressed, a more general awareness of danger and understanding of dangerous situations are lacking. In general, an enhanced expression of affect precedes the emergence of social awareness of others. On emergence from the autistic phase, social perplexity and social intrusiveness are common. The transition from lack of social awareness and inattention to others is often heralded by exaggerated emotions and behavioral difficulty.

ASD persons generally do not attend to faces or utilize information from faces in the same way as others do, and they often simply respond to faces as perceptual patterns (Fein et al., 1992). They perform better than matched control subjects when faces are shown to them upside down. This suggests the lower portion of the face is used to recognize peers, in contrast to normal children, who use the upper portion (Langdell, 1978). Moreover, the ASD person's performance declines on these tasks when the mouth and forehead are covered, suggesting they may focus more on the mouth than on the eyes to identify facial expressions (Yeung, 2022). They have more difficulty than IQ-matched persons with IDD in matching videotaped segments or pictures of gestures, vocalizations, and understanding the situational context of photographed or drawn pictures of facial expressions.

Older subjects who are neurotypically developing and have emerged from the autistic phase can show little difficulty comprehending emotional content in pictures of faces. Moreover, if given a choice on which cue to use to identify others, ASD children use items of dress, such as hats, rather than facial expression. ASD children are less able to imitate an affect when asked or to imitate an affect demonstrated by another person. Although ASD persons do not process affective and facial stimuli in the same way as neurotypical comparators, this could be a comprehension problem. If, for example, an ASD person does not view another person as having feelings or thoughts, then facial expressions are not be meaningful indicators for them.

ASD children's affective responses must be observed in a variety of situations to clarify whether these children show a full range of emotions. ASD children show all affective states except surprise. However, their affective responses are generally reported to be flat and not contingent on the particular situation. In addition, parents have reported that their ASD children's vocalizations are idiosyncratic and can only be understood by those who know the child. When ASD children's own spontaneous facial expressions are observed—for example, how they respond to seeing their image in a mirror—they exhibit less positive affect and less self-consciousness than neurotypically developing children. ASD children in the preschool years (ages 2–4 years) showed fewer observed intervals of affective response, positive or negative, when interacting with familiar adults than with IDD comparators. Observing how ASD children respond to affective signals when interacting with others in an ambiguous situation is an essential aspect of their assessment. Learning to respond to another's affect is a major developmental milestone.

## Theoretical Approaches

Despite apparent neurotypical development for the first few months of life, there are differences that can be documented in the latter part of the first year confirmed in the Baby Sibs study in infants later diagnosed with ASD. There are advantages to evaluating the deficits in ASD within the framework of typical development, including deficits in imitation, emotional perception, meta-representation, intersubjectivity, pragmatics, and symbolic play. The following three general models have been proposed: cognitive models (Baron-Cohen et al., 1985), the emotion theory (Hobson, 1989, 1991a), and the intersubjectivity model (Rogers & Pennington, 1991; Trevarthen, 1979).

## Cognitive Models

Cognitive models include the meta-representation model (theory of mind or mentalizing), weak control coherence, and executive function model. The meta-representational model is a cognitive conceptualization of ASD based on a variety of measures of theory of mind. These include false belief tasks, appearance reality tests, and storage sequencing tasks. The theory of mind (mentalizing) refers to the ability to anticipate and predict the behavior of others in terms of the other's mental state, being aware of another's intentions, desires, and beliefs. From the child's point of view, knowing another person, having wishes with regard to another person, and pretending are aspects of theory of mind.

The ability to understand others' intentions is not manifest at birth and apparently cannot be taught. At age 1 year, infants attend to behavior and internally represent physical states of the world. For example, infants can remember what they perceive in the external environment, which is referred to as "first-order representation." In the second year of life, a second-order representational ability develops that allows children to represent mental states as well as physical states of mind. This advance is known as the establishment of representational thought. Children not only attend to the behavior of others but also have the capacity to make sense of others' behavior by anticipating and deducing the other person's underlying mental states. By age 4 years, children normally acquire a concept of belief as they come to understand that people have different beliefs, including false beliefs. Most ASD individuals fail these tasks, whereas a majority of age-matched IDD comparators and neurotypically developing controls succeed. Consequently, the ASD child may be unable to represent another's mental state in their own mind.

The meta-representational theory predicts that ASD children will be able to recognize themselves and recognize others but are impaired in understanding and making assumptions about another person's internal mental state. One example of the establishment of meta-representation during development is in the capacity to substitute symbolically one object for another in play (Baron-Cohen et al., 1985). Play emerges in the second year of life. The meta-representation hypothesis helps explain deficits in symbolic play, communication pragmatics, joint attention, and theory of mind in autistic subjects.

Rogers and Pennington (1991) raise several questions in a critique of the meta-representational theory of ASD. First, the meta-representational theory does not provide an adequate account for deficits in imitation, a capacity that develops earlier than joint attention and symbolic play in infants. Second, they argue that a specific link between meta-representational ability and symbolic ability has not been proven. Third, meta-representational theory implies a specific discontinuity in the establishment of a theory of others' minds, whereas other developmental theories propose that development of intersubjectivity is a continuous process (Stern, 1985). Finally, although meta-representation has been linked to joint attention by some authors, joint attention is not necessarily related to the establishment of meta-representation. Therefore, the meta-representational approach also does not fully account for the presence of sensorimotor imitation, affective deficits, or the possible continuous development of intersubjectivity during development.

Although meta-representation does not account for all the developmental features of ASD, a theory of mind deficit may account for certain symptoms of ASD because the majority of young autistic children exhibit this deficit. That awareness of others' minds is a special human interpersonal ability is a position that has been taken by ethologists, attachment theorists, philosophers, and object relations theorists.

## Central Coherence Model

The "weak central coherence" hypothesis refers to the limitation in the ability to understand context in ASD. In other words, it is the failure to see the "big picture." Weak central coherence is basically evidenced by the overly detailed processing characteristic of ASD and the inability to extract meaning from experience. A review of empirical studies of coherence found that there is a local bias in processing in ASD. It is not considered to be a side effect of executive dysfunction and may be independent of theory of mind (Happé & Frith, 2006). Attentional and perceptual abnormalities have been recognized since its first description with an intense focus in detail. For example, in completing a jigsaw puzzle, a child with ASD tends to focus on the shape of the pieces rather than the printed picture and could complete the puzzle with the picture upside down rather than right side up. Similarly, people with ASD score well on the embedded figured task and block design subset on the WISC, with performance superior to that of neurotypically developing children and those matched for mental age (Jolliffe & Baron-Cohen, 1997). Thus, this is an acute ability to process fine detail. An alternative to weak central coherence is that people with ASD have a reduced ability to process similarity at the perceptual and attentional level that may lead to abnormalities at the conceptual level of central coherence (Plaisted et al.,1998). This is consistent with perceptual mechanisms underlying the proposed weak central coherence model.

## Executive Dysfunction Model

Executive-focused cognitive hypotheses have been proposed to explain symptom clusters in ASD as a potential cognitive endophenotype. There is a broad impairment in executive functioning in ASD; however, the heterogeneity of executive function performance is not consistent with there being an executive dysfunction as cognitive endophenotype (Geurts et al., 2014). The variability in executive function performance may be persistent for subtyping within ASD. Atypical executive functioning in ASD may include difficulties in shifting set (capacity to shift mindset to new concepts), response inhibition (ability to inhibit a response that becomes dominant), and working memory (retaining and updating information in short-term memory) (Demetriou et al., 2019).

## Emotion (Affective Deficit) Theory

Like Kanner, Hobson and many others suggest that an impairment in affectively patterned, intersubjective personal relations is basic to ASD. Hobson (1989) suggested that the ASD child's deficits in symbolic play, cognition, and language result primarily from a problem in affective development that involves constitutionally based emotional reactivity. This includes deficits in emotional expression and perception and an inability to develop reciprocal affectively based relationships with others. Because of these deficits, the ASD child does not develop intersubjective awareness of self and others, which results in the child's failure to recognize other people as distinct people with their own feelings, thoughts, wishes, and intentions. In addition, it leads to a severe impairment in the capacity to think abstractly and symbolically.

There are demonstrable deficits in an ASD person's perception and understanding of affect. Specific deficits in expression of affect in ASD children, compared to control groups, include difficulty in recognizing and understanding emotional expression in others; reduced affective response toward a social partner; less use of gaze to communicate affect; and less mirroring of social signals from others, such as smiles (Gaigg, 2012). Although emotional perception deficits have been found in subjects with IDD, they are not primary as in ASD.

Hobson emphasized that instead of simply interacting, people engage interpersonally by sharing psychological orientation and attitudes with others (Hobson & Lee, 1999). This capacity to identify with others is lacking in ASD and leads to core ASD deficits (Hobson & Lee, 2007). Neurotypical development proceeds with ongoing intersubjectivity in attuned parent–child interactions to make sense of the relationship. In developmental naturalistic interventions, such as ESDM, a goal is to establish intersubjectivity to the extent possible.

## Intersubjectivity Model

Intersubjectivity refers to reciprocal sharing of one's internal subjective experiences, whether they are affective or cognitive, with another person through imitative, affective, and communicative modes. In ASD, an intersubjective deficit may be combined with other developmental deficits, such as IDD. The intersubjective hypothesis posits that the ASD child does not choose to withdraw from the social world or to avoid it but, rather, has difficulty in accessing the social world through "physically mirroring affective mutuality," shared meanings and understanding of the interior life of others. This hypothesis further posits that the basis for ASD is in the deficient capacity to form or to manipulate particular internal representations of the self and others. These representations are basic to the infant's body imitation, affective mirroring, and sharing with others, as well as awareness of others' subjective states.

When ASD children are considered in the context of the interpersonal hypothesis proposed by Stern (1985), they have an impairment in the development of the verbal self and disorders of language area consequence. Sigman (1989) proposed that the young ASD child does not develop an intersubjective self and has only a partial realization that inner subjective experiences may be shared with others. It is possible that intersubjective experiences are not shared with others because ASD children do not recognize others have separate minds. This may be related to the ASD child being unable to experience affective attunement—that is, biobehavioral synchrony.

In Stern's (1985) proposal, in the earliest phase of life, an infant has only subjective experiences of the various internal organizations that are forming. Gradually, through internal and external perceptions, the infant distills and begins to organize the general qualities of experience. This emergent organization is active as the various domains of the self are formed. From 2 to 7 months of age, the infant develops a sense of a core self and a core other. Basic experiences that lead to the integration of the core self include (a) an impression of coherence among the infant's own experiences and behaviors, (b) a sense of affect as belonging to the infant, (c) memory of the self over a brief period, and (d) an initial view of the self as an agent of action. These experiences take place as a consequence of intense social interactions between the infant and others. A sense of a core other develops concurrently through experiences of being with another person, who helps regulate the infant's affect, attention, somatic state, or degree of cognitive engagement. The adult's role as a self-regulating other may allow the infant to construct the sense of an "evoked companion" or to internalize a working model of interpersonal relationships.

The sense of a subjective self begins to emerge between ages 7 and 9 months; the autistic child may show distortions in the sense of self during this developmental period. Stern (1985) states,

> The next . . . leap in the sense of self occurs when the infant discovers that he or she has a mind and other people have minds as well . . . infants gradually come upon the momentous realization that inner subjective experiences, subject matter of mind, are potentially sharable with someone else.

Therefore, intersubjective relatedness involves not only the sharing of intentions and motives but also an activation of experiences, which includes changes in internal states of arousal and affect. The sharing of interpersonal activation experiences, which has been called affective attunement by Stern and biobehavioral synchrony by others, results in the infant's sensing forms of feelings based on the subjective state of another person (Feldman, 2012a). The behaviors of others can then be recognized as signifying an interior state. The next stage in self-development takes place at approximately age 15–18 months. Now the child's ability to coordinate sensorimotor schemas with external actions or words allows the child's self to be an object of reflection, to engage in symbolic actions, and to acquire language. The infant now can establish shared meaning with another about personal knowledge (Sigman, 1989).

For the ASD child, the emergent self appears to have developed, but it is uncertain whether the ASD child forms a core self and a core other in early life. ASD individuals are able to differentiate between themselves and others and show some coherence in their sense of themselves. They are able to use themselves and others as agents of action as well as to demonstrate that they have memories of themselves in action; consequently, limited working models of internalized relationships may develop in people with ASD. In neurotypical people, development of the core self and core other may continue normally in infancy until a major developmental distortion occurs related to the intersubjective self.

Failure to form an intersubjective self may be based on cognitive and/or affective deficits. This might involve a modal perception that Stern (1985) describes as an innate capacity to take information from one sensory modality and translate it into another. What may be translated is an encoded representation that might be recognized by the various sensory modalities. In Stern's theory, this "amodal" information processing is needed to establish the self. It is possible that ASD individuals are limited in their ability for amodal information processing, or their lack of affective attunement could be central to an inherent affective unresponsiveness. Although the mechanisms of early self-development remain hypothetical, a critical developmental task for the 7- to 9-month-old child apparently is not fully mastered by the ASD child.

The intersubjectivity hypothesis acknowledges the importance of sharing of emotions during development and the incorporation of early and later self–other experiences. It incorporates areas not accounted for by the affective and meta-representational models. For example, the affective deficit model does not fully account for the role of the imitation impairment and the development of social processes, such as attachment, and the meta-representational hypothesis does not account for deficits in imitation and in the sharing of emotions. Intersubjectivity theory also differs from the meta-representational model because these meta-representational deficits are considered to be primary and discontinuous. Still, intersubjectivity theory recognizes, as does the meta-representational approach, the importance of having a theory of others' minds as a landmark in social development.

Overall, the intersubjectivity model integrates the major impairments in ASD into a developmental framework. It includes both intact and deficient social skills and integrates other competing theories of ASD, thereby accounting for similarities and differences between ASD children and comparison groups throughout development. In addition, it offers an alternative interpretation of the pragmatic and symbolic play deficits in ASD. Each of the theoretical approaches recognizes that social deficits in ASD are primary, long-lasting, and reflect dysfunction in the neurobiological mechanisms that underlie human sociability. It is hypothesized that these deficits are linked to proposed dysfunction in the limbic and orbitofrontal brain regions.

## Treatment

A comprehensive approach to treatment recognizes that each child diagnosed with ASD is unique. An understanding of the development trajectory of a child with ASD and the functioning of the ASD nervous system must be considered in establishing treatments. Programs that are developmentally based, affectively and interpersonally oriented, and tailored to specific known deficits in individual children with ASD can lead to positive changes in development with compensation made for areas of deficit and the reduction of autistic behavior.

The goals of treatment are based on the extent of disabilities found in each child (Howlin et al., 1987). Treatment programs must be sensitive to the needs and perceptions of each child (Simons & Oishi, 1987) and must provide guidance to parents. The primary treatment goal is to foster neurotypical development to the extent possible. In doing so, what is known about neurotypical developmental processes is considered when addressing behaviors that interfere with neurotypical development. Because the neurobiological basis of ASD is better understood, interventions focus on helping children compensate for their developmental deficits.

Four general aims to be pursued in treatment are to promote cognitive development, language development, social development, and overall learning. In addition to these, reduction of aberrant behavior and behavioral enhancement strategies are needed, as is appropriate use of pharmacological medications to address behavioral problems that interfere with these aims (Hyman et al., 2020).

Cognitive development is promoted through the facilitation of meaningful experiences to reduce isolation. Neurotypical development may be facilitated through planned periods of interaction and correction and addressing impaired understanding through simplified communication and individualized treatment approaches. The child's lack of initiative for social interaction requires structured direct learning experiences. Specific cognitive deficits can be targeted by choosing appropriate learning tasks. Reduced cognitive capacity requires interventions that focus on direct teaching at the appropriate developmental level.

Language interventions target social/conversational exchanges to reduce social isolation by social engagement. Planned periods of interaction should be scheduled to promote social development. The problem of social reciprocity is addressed by encouraging interactions that involve joint attention and structure the exchange of reciprocal language. Deficits in social communication and pragmatic language refer to failure to use language socially. Direct intervention is necessary to teach the social use of language. Behavioral approaches include differential reinforcement of reciprocal communication rather than simply focusing on reinforcing speech. Pragmatic language enhancement includes teaching turn-taking and other aspects of social communication. Because language development is limited, direct teaching must appreciate the child's level of language comprehension. Augmented communication, such as the use of sign language and communication boards, is beneficial.

Promotion of social development requires intense positive personal interaction with the child that is comforting and enjoyable. Addressing the lack of social approach and social reciprocity in social interactions in children with ASD requires structured settings. The therapist may intrude to help the child remain focused on the social exchange. Joint attentional exercises are needed; the adult attracts the child's attention and then requires the child to gesture or point to items of interest. They are encouraged to show things to the examiner. Personal caretaking may be required, particularly if the child has not been instructed in personal hygiene and other aspects of personal care. Overall, a lack of social awareness that is characteristic of ASD is addressed through direct teaching of skills that can lead to social competence.

A general approach to learning is necessary. First, focusing attention on environmental cues is essential. Because children with ASD lack self-direction, structured learning is necessary with an effort to break down learning tasks into small steps. There may be difficulty in remaining focused on the task because of deviant behaviors that require concomitant behavior reduction strategies. Moreover, children with ASD often are overselective in their choice of activities, and considerable effort may be necessary to keep them on task. It is important to be aware of their specific interests. Facilitating generalization of learning to new situations is particularly important and requires that context specificity be considered. The goal is learning in natural environments at home and at school, limited use of residential treatment, and structure and routine to facilitate generalization from one situation to another. A central problem in promoting learning is the child's difficulty in understanding the meaningfulness of events. This comprehension deficit requires that the teaching staff monitor learning carefully and focus on meaningfulness of events by putting them in context. Finally, lack of persistence to cope with challenges and the aversive responses to failure require, as much as possible, the provision of error-free learning.

The basic principles of behavior modification are utilized in the treatment of ASD. Behavioral techniques must be developed based on a clear understanding of the child's deficits and the types of abnormal behavior associated with ASD because these will determine what can be targeted for change and the best approach to the individual patient. Attempts to use behavior management techniques without considering the specific characteristics of the neurologic deficits in ASD, especially problems with sensory integration, may lead to difficulty and potentially might result in failure or worsening of the affected child's behavior. Moreover, the environment must often be adapted to the person with ASD rather than expecting the autistic individual to adapt to it. The nature of the autistic deficit makes adaptability and generalization of targeted behaviors across settings difficult. A stable environment is necessary for treatment, and once this environment is established, it should not be changed without careful consideration of the contingencies that led to improvement.

When behavioral difficulties develop, the first step is to determine whether they are the result of environmental factors, which might include excessive social contacts, excessive demand for change, or staff who do not appreciate the individual characteristics of the person with ASD. Stereotypies, which are characteristic feature of ASD, may themselves be used as reinforcers as part of the behavioral program. It is often helpful to find a context for these behavioral patterns. For example, a child's repetitive hand movements may be redirected to a meaningful use.

Behavior management strategies are utilized to target the development of new skills and eliminate nonspecific maladaptive behaviors. The behavioral approach is based on an evidence-based applied behavioral analysis through application of learning theory (Roane et al., 2016). A careful functional analysis considers the possible concurrent use of medication, impact of intercurrent illnesses, and seizure disorders. It requires a careful evaluation of preceding circumstances (antecedents, behavior, and consequences) that increase or decrease the likelihood of the occurrence of a maladaptive behavior together with an analysis of succeeding circumstances that seem to be associated with either diminution or prolongation of the behavior. To employ a behavioral technique, it is essential to determine which environmental features influence a behavior, not in children in general but for the particular child.

For the most severely impaired individuals with ASD, behavioral approaches are based on operant conditioning procedures rather than on cognitive understanding of rewards. A comprehensive applied behavioral analysis approach to younger children, referred to as early intensive applied behavioral analysis, has been studied in controlled trials and single-subject trial literature (Smith & Eikeseth, 2011). There is limited evidence for efficacy in children younger than age 12 years, for whom more time must be invested to meet treatment goals (Linstead et al., 2017).

For individuals who are less impaired, consequences are better understood cognitively and token economies for behavior management may be established. Still, generalization of treatment to new settings may be limited. Therefore, it is extremely important to address the individual's understanding regardless of level of intelligence. The types of challenging behaviors most frequently addressed in behavior management programs are aggression and self-injurious behavior. For these and other disruptive behaviors, avoidance of precipitants, provision of help to establish coping skills, and differential reinforcement strategies are used as interventions. Differential reinforcement involves feedback to the child, rewards for positive behaviors, and behavior reduction procedures for negative behaviors. Fears may be addressed through controlled exposure, with desensitization, modeling, and the teaching of coping skills to deal with them.

## Parent-Mediated Treatment/Parent Management Training

The role of the parent is crucial in interventions for the child with ASD. The parent may function as co-therapist and has an integral role in treatment. Parent counseling begins with clarification of the diagnosis and an explanation of the characteristic symptoms of ASD. A detailed history is essential. It is reassuring to the parent to know that perplexing behaviors that they have observed in their child are part of a known disorder. An important part of a therapeutic program is focused interventions provided by trained parents and caregivers. Parent-mediated therapies are described in detail by Oono et al. (2013). Parent-mediated therapies have been shown to be effective in toddlers (Beaudoin et al., 2014) and older children (Bearss et al., 2015). Parent management training typically is described as either parent support or parent-mediated interventions. Parent support is focused on providing knowledge to the parent that is of indirect benefit to the child. Parent support includes psychoeducation and care coordination, whereas parent-mediated interventions are technique-focused and provide direct benefit to the child. These interventions target core symptoms of ASD. These parent-mediated approaches may be coordinated with applied behavior analysis in the home and other natural settings (Bearss et al., 2015).

Parent sessions are delivered in the home, clinic, school, or community settings (Oono et al., 2013). Parent-mediated training, including training for challenging behaviors, can be carried out remotely through telehealth (Lindgren et al., 2016). Benefits of parent-mediated intervention for toddlers with ASD have been demonstrated in a randomized controlled trial involving 86 toddlers and their primary caregivers. A 10-week course of hands-on parent training in joint attention, symbolic play, engagement, and regulation was compared to a parent-only psychoeducation intervention for increasing joint child–parent engagement (Kasari et al., 2015). Including parents in intervention and treatment was shown to be essential to facilitate compliance with instruction, to enhance social communication, and for redirection of maladaptive and other behaviors (Hyman et al., 2020).

## Educational Approaches and Interventions

By federal law, education of children with ASD is carried out in classrooms that provide support in the least restrictive environment and an Individualized Education Program (IEP). The IEP goals are set by the school team in collaboration with the ASD student and family. If the child does not meet criteria for an IEP, classroom-level accommodations are provided through a Section 504 plan. Children with ASD may be placed in inclusive classrooms with neurotypical students but with classroom supports. Others benefit from ASD-focused classrooms. These include Learning Experiences and Alternative Program (LEAP) for preschoolers and their parents and Treatment and Education of Autistic and Related Communication Handicapped Children (TEACCH) programs. LEAP combines applied behavior analysis with special education teaching methods in elementary school in inclusive classrooms. In one randomized study of LEAP, 294 preschool children were evaluated. Compared to treatment as usual, LEAP resulted in greater improvement in socialization, language, cognition, and challenging behaviors (Strain & Bovey, 2011).

TEACCH was developed at the University of North Carolina as an evidence-based program for individuals with ASD at all ages and skill levels to promote meaningful engagement in activities, independence, and efficacy. A 2011 review of more than 150 ASD intervention studies found that the TEACCH program had the strongest education benefits among recognized education programs (Warren et al., 2011). TEACCH classes are organized in a manner so as to focus young children with ASD to socially engage as they learn (Boyd et al., 2014). TEACCH is an assessment-based curriculum placing emphasis on structure, visual use of schedules, and an optimized environment to minimize distractions by minimizing auditory and other sensory stimuli that trigger sensory dysregulation. There is a routine that is organized to be predictable. Tasks are oriented to facilitate independence from adult prompts and directions (Boyd et al., 2014; Virues-Ortega et al., 2013). TEACCH has been shown to provide measurable benefit for perceptual, motor, verbal, and cognitive skills but less so for adaptive functioning and challenging behaviors. Compared to standard special education classes taught by teachers trained in ASD, studies of TEACCH have found better improvement in ASD severity for children with greater cognitive delay. This benefit is attributed to the environmental and behavioral supports utilized in TEACCH. Studies of LEAP and TEACCH interventions address elements needed to provide the best evidence-based practices for ASD school education (Hyman et al., 2020).

## Interpersonal Approaches to Treatment: Interpersonal Developmental Behavioral Intervention

A treatment program for ASD based on the intersubjectivity model considers the child's age and developmental level. The treatment program for preschool children with ASD addresses the development of interpersonal relationships, pragmatic language, and the establishment of symbolic thought with the use of play techniques. These interventions include naturalistic developmental behavioral interventions, which incorporate elements of applied behavioral analysis informed by developmental principles. The emphasis is on developmentally guided learning targets focused on social learning skills. Interventions are carried out during naturally occurring social activities in everyday settings. Importantly, child-initiated teaching is included. Turn-taking interactions are facilitated within play using behavioral analysis to set measurable goals (Schreibman et al., 2015). The best study of these naturalistic approaches is the ESDM, which was organized to prepare children to learn in real-life settings (Estes et al., 2015). In a multisite trial of ESDM, children with early age of entry to treatment showed the greatest improvement (Rogers, Estes, et al., 2012). Forty-eight children in the original trial were randomly assigned to ESDM or community treatment and were studied using event-related potentials and spectral power on EEG while viewing faces versus inanimate objects and were compared to neurotypical community controls on each of these tasks. The children enrolled in ESDM showed improvement in the neurophysiologic measures along with improvement in social behavior (Dawson et al., 2012; Hyman et al., 2020).

ESDM is a day treatment program for children with ASD aged 12–48 months that is grounded in the intersubjectivity model. The emphasis is placed on providing positive affective experiences to aid in the development of interpersonal relationships and on using pragmatic language therapy offered in a structured and predictable school setting while providing these services through the medium of play. Play is emphasized as a means to facilitate assimilation and generalization of social–emotional, cognitive, and communicative skills just as it does for non-impaired children. Adult–child social relationships are promoted through a specific adult working with an individual child on activities. The one-to-one adult–child contact, involving social games and reciprocal interactions, is essential to maintain the child's attention and engagement. Other social relationships that must be encouraged focus on peer awareness and close proximity during play among children. The adult's role is to direct the ASD child's attention to their peers' activities. If conflicts between children emerge, the adult provides verbal and behavioral "scripts" to facilitate negotiation and problem-solving. Moreover, the effect of one child's behavior on another is explicitly described to highlight what had occurred. In adult–child interactions, positive affect is essential to enhance the child's attention to specific experiences and particularly to motivate them to continue activities. Close physical proximity facilitates imitation, is more likely to provide meaning to learning experiences, and should result in relationships that are pleasing to both adult and child. ESDM also uses a developmentally based behavior management program that incorporates applied behavior analysis with play and joint attention to enhance language, cognitive, and social skills (Estes et al., 2015).

Because communication difficulties are a component of ASD, adults working with children with ASD must utilize specific language strategies. With this approach, the adult interprets the child's potential verbal communicative and nonverbal gestural behaviors at the child's developmental level. This includes clarification and explanation about the child's feelings, actions, apparent desires, and responses, which are then reflected back to them at the child's developmental language level. Children lacking in speech are taught simple signs from the American Sign Language system, and preverbal gestures are used or prompted. Consistency is essential and repetition critical in teaching communication. The transition from sensorimotor intelligence to representational or symbolic intelligence is essential for language development and is particularly impaired in these children. Educationally oriented activities that demand mental representation are incorporated into the program. This includes activities organized around the establishment of symbolic play and preoperational grouping activities.

Play, adult–child social relationships, stimulation of positive affective experiences, communicative training, and an emphasis on representational thinking are carried out in a structured classroom with a well-established daily routine. The social structure, the physical arrangements, and the rhythm of the day's activities are used to provide an external structure to facilitate self-regulation and to help the child mediate, select, focus, and organize sensory stimuli. Distractors are identified for each child by evaluating activities with respect to their primary goals. Sensory stimulation is reduced when it becomes apparent the child is overly sensitive to that sensory modality. The treatment programs involve child psychiatrists, speech and language therapists, occupational therapists, and clinical child psychologists, who work with teachers in the classroom and develop individualized treatment programs for each child.

This comprehensive approach is an alternative to a strict behavior management approach, which focuses on acquisition of specific skills. The behavioral approach is typically not developmentally oriented and may fail to recognize the specific deficits of an individual child with ASD or place those targeted skills in a clearly meaningful developmental framework. If development is not considered in the establishment of treatment goals, then isolated skills may be trained that do not generalize well to other situations or to other skills. The comprehensive preschool approach emphasizes the individual child's specific deficits and considers symbolic processes, social relationships, and communication and provides a structured environment to help remediate and compensate for them.

ESDM promotes change in cognitive, communicative, social–emotional, perceptual–motor, and motor domains by using early intervention incorporating preschool profiles, the Play Observation Scale, and CARS (Schopler et al., 2010). Ratings of symbolic play were significantly improved, although the effects were relatively modest. These changes are important because symbolic activities of children with ASD are related to their cognitive and communicative abilities as they grow older. In addition, the symbolic play occurs in the context of environmental exploration of both the physical and the social world. The enhancement of these skills over time can improve long-term outcome.

Social relatedness improved using this approach. The elements most essential were sensitivity by the adult to the child's verbal and nonverbal communications, structured social reciprocal interactions with the child, an emphasis on positive affective experiences, and the use of play in interaction with the child (Schopler et al., 2010). Long-term follow-up is needed to determine whether the effects of treatment endure.

For the older verbal child, who has emerged from the autistic phase and is socially perplexed, a social cognitive approach focused on the intersubjectivity and meta-representational deficits can be helpful. Intersubjectivity is conceptualized as an appreciation of self–other representations and the ability to put oneself in the place of another person and empathetically respond. Issues that relate to understanding others' minds may be interpreted for the higher functioning child in the context of affective awareness. It is not uncommon for older and higher functioning individuals with ASD to complain that they are not able to read other people's thoughts and have difficulty anticipating the response of others to their overtures. The person with ASD finds it difficult to gauge the depth of another's feeling about something, although they may recognize the feeling state itself in the other person.

When mental state concepts are successfully taught, specific instruction can be given to the person with ASD on how to cope socially—that is, social survival skills. Treatment based on the cognitive theory of mind approach can focus on compensating for and the remediation of possible insensitivity to others' feelings, the inability to take into account what other people know during a conversation, the inability to read others' intentions, the inability to appreciate the listener's level of interest in one's own conversation directed toward them, and the inability to anticipate what others might think of their actions.

Difficulties in reading others' intentions may make the person with ASD the butt of jokes by others. They may not appreciate when they are being teased or deceived after complying without question to an inappropriate request. Difficulty with reading the listener's level of interest in one's speech may lead to monologues boring to the listener about the limited special interests of the ASD person. Often, individuals with ASD are unaware that others do not share their enthusiasm for topics that interest them. An inability to anticipate others' responses to one's speech or actions is common in the social interactions of individuals with ASD.

Examples of some communicative errors by people with ASD include unwanted and inappropriate comments about the other's personal appearance; this may be interpreted by others as personal insensitivity rather than curiosity based on the child's simple observation. A lack of sense of the personal space with others, and persistent requests for information about them or their family, can be viewed as too intimate by others and as intrusive. The inability to consider what other people may already know in conversation is problematic and results from a lack of understanding by the person with ASD that another individual's experiences are different from their own. The person with ASD must be taught that when referring to events, the provision of background information to the other person is essential to establish a context for the conversation.

An approach to the teaching of social skills is to break down mental state understanding into simple principles that are taught through intensive training. For the neurotypically developing child, these principles do not need to be explicitly taught. The use of stories and discussion about their life experiences may also be used in teaching. The following fundamental basic principles are recommended to be taught to persons with ASD about mental states (Baron-Cohen & Howlin, 1993):

- *Perception causes knowledge.* An individual will know that something happened only if it was seen or heard. This approach can be applied by introducing stories in which the central character does not know that something has happened unless they have actually seen that it occurred.
- *Desires are satisfied by actions or objects.* If a person wants something, they will look to obtain it; but if they do not want it, they will refuse or avoid it. In children's stories, for example, if the child wants their parents, they will look at them. When unpleasant problems occur, such as when someone is chasing them, they will move away.
- *Pretense involves object substitution or outcome suspension.* If a person pretends something will happen, they may do so to solve a problem or for fun. An example is when someone pretends an object is another thing, such as when a child pretends a block is a car.
- *Deception involves making someone think something is false.* For example, if someone needs something, they may not try to obtain it directly but, rather, use indirect means.
- *Understanding emotion involves an awareness that someone carries out a particular behavior based on how they are feeling at the time.* For example, if someone is grieving, their crying means that they are sad.

Teaching of mental state concepts requires that the person with ASD has attained the mental age when these concepts are normally acquired—a mental age of at least 3½ to 4 years. Teaching how beliefs, desires, new knowledge, pretense, deception, and emotion are experienced by another person may involve a variety of techniques, including imaginative play with figurines, drama, explanation, pictures, the use of computer graphics, and the use of television.

## Pharmacotherapy

Currently, there are no specific pharmacological treatments for the core deficits of ASD. However, because the neuropeptides oxytocin and vasopressin play an important role in modulating social communicative and prosocial behavior, the effects of intranasal administration of these two neuropeptides on behavior have been studied in individuals with ASD. A meta-analysis of the effects of intranasal oxytocin composed of 28 studies with 726 subjects with ASD showed positive effects in social functioning but not in nonsocial domains (Huang, 2021). An important consideration in the use of intranasal oxytocin is that its effects are context-dependent and that it may best be used to extend periods of social engagement rather than initiate them. Notably, intranasal oxytocin was shown to significantly reduce anxiety and some repetitive behaviors with minimal side effects in subjects with ASD. Arginine vasopressin also promotes social behavior in ASD (Parker et al., 2019). A double-blind, randomized, placebo-controlled study examined the efficacy of intranasal vasopressin in 30 children with ASD aged 6–9.5 years with a dose of 24 IU and children aged 9.6–12.9 years with a dose of 32 IU. Compared to placebo, there were significant positive effects on the Social Responsiveness Scale ($p = .005$).

Psychiatric disorders and behavioral symptoms co-occurring with ASD are often amenable to pharmacologic management. These include attention deficits, hyper-activity, aggression, affective lability, anxiety, obsessive–compulsive behaviors, self-injurious behavior, psychotic symptoms, and depression (Hyman et al., 2020; Ji & Findling, 2015). Before instituting pharmacotherapy, it is essential that the underlying cause of the troubling behaviors be identified. Medication should be considered following accurate diagnosis of co-occurring psychiatric disorder and problem behaviors, a functional behavioral assessment, and careful history to rule out medical problems that may exacerbate challenging behaviors (pain, gastrointestinal reflux, otitis media, etc.). It is important to carefully review medication management with family members and the patient.

ADHD is frequently comorbid in children and teenagers with ASD. DSM-5 permits both diagnoses to be made (Sturman et al., 2017). Children with ASD respond to stimulant medication, although side effects (appetite suppression and insomnia) must be carefully monitored. Heterocyclic antidepressants may also be helpful for symptoms of ADHD. Clonidine has been successfully utilized for some features of ADHD in children with ASD (Goel et al., 2018; Ming et al., 2008).

Low doses of neuroleptics (risperidone, aripiprazole, and olanzapine) have been recommended for treating hyperactivity, aggression, and for brief reactive and schizophreniform psychosis (Fallah et al., 2019; Fung et al., 2016; Hollander et al., 2006; McCracken et al., 2002). The effectiveness of low-dose neuroleptics is well documented. Earlier studies found that reduction in symptoms during short-term haloperidol treatment was not related to whether children developed dyskinesias later in long-term haloperidol administration. Currently, based on a multisite randomized placebo-controlled clinical trial, risperidone and aripiprazole are more frequently used (McCracken et al., 2002). Caution is required in the use of neuroleptics because ASD is a lifelong condition. Thus, the risk of tardive dyskinesia must be considered, particularly when high doses of atypical neuroleptics such as risperidone are prescribed. The neuroleptics may be necessary to maintain a child with severe aggressive symptoms in their school program but should only be used on a short-term basis.

Two other medications that have been used in the treatment of ASD are buspirone (Ceranoglu et al., 2019) and propranolol (Sagar-Ouriaghli et al., 2018). Both medications have been recommended to reduce aggression and anxiety in children with ASD. Clomipramine was found to be superior to placebo and desipramine in reducing anger and compulsive and ritualistic behavior, whereas clomipramine was equal to desipramine and both drugs were superior to placebo in reducing hyperactivity (Gordon et al., 1993). However, these pharmacologic treatment recommendations are based on relatively small clinical trials. Attention deficit disorder can be diagnosed in children and teenagers with ASD, according to DSM-5 (Sturman et al., 2017).

Mood stabilizers, such as lithium, sodium valproate, and carbamazepine, have been used to treat mood disorders and aggressive behavior in ASD (Hirota et al., 2014). However, results are mixed because the primary indication for sodium valproate and carbamazepine is for seizure disorders. Naltrexone, an opiate antagonist, has been successfully used as an adjunctive treatment for children with ASD for aggression and self-injurious behavior, but the evidence is not compelling (Elchaar et al., 2006). In choosing the use of an opiate antagonist, it is important to consider sensory abnormalities in the child with ASD. Because the opiate receptors mediate the effects of sensory neurotransmitters, some children will have an enhancement of their sensitivity to sound as a side effect of the use of naltrexone.

Anxiety in ASD is typically treated with SSRIs, including citalopram and fluoxetine (Strawn et al., 2015; Vasa et al., 2016). Findings with the use of SSRIs for depression in ASD are mixed in children and less so in adults. The use of psychotropic medication typically is greater in older children, those with co-occurring disorders, those more cognitively impaired, and those with high rates of challenging behaviors such as aggression and self-injury. In addition to co-occurring psychiatric and behavioral disorders, medical management is essential for problems such as seizures, sleep disorders, gastrointestinal disorders, and dental problems. Notably, recent research has documented the high prevalence of gastrointestinal disorders that can exacerbate behavioral symptoms in ASD (Madra et al., 2021).

Children with ASD are at risk for accidents, including drowning (Guan & Li, 2017). They have limited awareness of community rules and social conventions. Impulsivity and preservative interests can lead them into dangerous situations. Wandering (elopement) is a particular risk, which, because of its prevalence, should be included in the child's problem list for monitoring. A survey of parents carried out online with 1,200 families revealed that almost half of the children between ages 4 and 10 years eloped (Anderson et al., 2012). Most of these children were missing for extended times, leading the parents to contact the police. Among them, two-thirds were at risk for traffic accidents and nearly one-third were reported to have a near drowning. Moreover, in a national survey inquiring about elopement attempts in the prior years, approximately one-third of parents of children with ASD, with or without IDD, reported their elopement (Rice et al., 2016). The most common reason that children eloped was their enjoyment of running, seeking to go to a favorite place (e.g., the park), pursuant of a favorite interest (playing in sand or water), and to avoid sensory overstimulation. Many became lost. Those at greatest risk were nonverbal or had limited language. Prevention is key in addressing wandering with regular observation, physical barriers, and constant supervision. Fencing, alarm systems, and personal identification bracelets providing phone number and address are advised. Monitoring sleep is needed for children who wander at night. Finally, teaching safety skills and appropriate behavior in the community is important for prevention.

## Impact of Etiologic Heterogeneity on Treatment

When initially described, ASD was considered a rare disorder with an "innate," probably genetic cause(s) (Eisenberg, 2001; Kanner & Eisinberg, 1956; Rutter, 1968). By the turn of the 21st century, several secondary or syndromic causes of the ASD phenotype were described in several genetic disorders, including fragile X syndrome, tuberous sclerosis, and neurofibromotosis, as well as fetal insults such as congenital rubella. With the completion of the human genome sequencing, which led to technical improvements that made more efficient searches for genetic causes of ASD, rare CNVs were found to be highly penetrant causes (Rees & Kirov, 2021). More recently, sufficiently powered GWAS are disclosing an increasing number of risk genes that likely account for the more common "idiopathic" forms of ASD (Grove et al., 2019). Thus, ASD comprises numerous etiologies, which belie the uniformity of the syndromic diagnosis implicated by the categorical diagnostic schema of DSM-5 (Lombardo & Mandelli, 2022). One implication of this reality is that ASD patients identified for early intervention may differ in their response to generally used cognitive–behavioral interventions. Lombardo et al., (2021) examined this possibility by carrying out assays of ASD-associated leukocyte gene expression to compare outcomes for ASD-diagnosed children enrolled in the Strategies for Teaching Based on Autism Research (STAR) curriculum (Arick et al., 2004) before or after age 24 months. They confirmed that starting the intervention before age 24 months was associated with better outcomes. They also found that the leukocyte ASD associated gene expression pattern could also explain 13% of the variance in treatment response slopes. Polygenic risk scores to further subtype ASD children to tailor interventions will likely play a greater role in the future (Morneau-Vaillancourt et al., 2021).

## Future Directions

Substantial progress has been made since autistic disorder was first described in 1943 by Leo Kanner. However, much remains to be done. Future research will emphasize genetic aspects, refinements in classification, identification of better diagnostic techniques, identifying biomarkers, and the development of more effective treatments. Better characterization of cases is essential to conduct genetic studies that will be benefited by a better understanding of underlying pathophysiological mechanisms involved in social cognition. Advances in classification neuroimaging, particularly in MRI, fMRI, and PET scanning, will also be helpful in the characterization of subtypes.

## References

Adang, L. A., Lynch, D. R., & Panzer, J. A. (2014). Pediatric anti-NMDA receptor encephalitis is seasonal. *Annals of Clinical and Translational Neurology, 1*(11), 921–925.

Alarcón, M., Cantor, R. M., Liu, J., Gilliam, T. C., Geschwind, D. H., & the Autism Genetic Resource Exchange Consortium. (2002). Evidence for a language quantitative trait locus on chromosome 7q in multiplex autism families. *American Journal of Human Genetics, 70*(1), 60–71.

Al-Otaish, H., Al-Ayadhi, L., Bjørklund, G., Chirumbolo, S., Urbina, M. A., & El-Ansary, A. (2018). Relationship between absolute and relative ratios of glutamate, glutamine and GABA and severity of autism spectrum disorder. *Metabolic Brain Disease, 33*(3), 843–854.

American Psychiatric Association. (1980). *Diagnostic and statistical manual of mental Disorders* (3rd ed.).

American Psychiatric Association, Committee on Nomenclature and Statistics. (1987). *Diagnostic and statistical manual of mental disorders* (3rd ed., rev.).

American Psychiatric Association. (1994). *Diagnostic and statistical manual of mental disorders* (4th ed.).

American Psychiatric Association. (2013). *Diagnostic and statistical manual of mental disorders* (5th ed.). American Psychiatric Publishing.

Amiet, C., Gourfinkel-An, I., Laurent, C., Bodeau, N., Génin, B., Leguern, E., Tordjman, S., & Cohen, D. (2013). Does epilepsy in multiplex autism pedigrees define a different subgroup in terms of clinical characteristics and genetic risk? *Molecular Autism, 4*(1), Article 47.

Anderson, C., Law, J. K., Daniels, A., Rice, C., Mandell, D. S., Hagopian, L., & Law, P. A. (2012). Occurrence and family impact of elopement in children with autism spectrum disorders. *Pediatrics, 130*(5), 870–877.

Aoki, Y., Kasai, K., & Yamasue, H. (2012). Age-related change in brain metabolite abnormalities in autism: A meta-analysis of proton magnetic resonance spectroscopy studies. *Translational Psychiatry, 2*(1), e69.

Arick, J., Loos, L., Falco, R., & Kung, D. (2004). *The STAR Program: Strategies for teaching based on autism research.* Pro-Ed.

Arwert, T. G., & Sizoo, B. B. (2020). Self-reported suicidality in male and female adults with autism spectrum disorders: Rumination and self-esteem. *Journal of Autism and Developmental Disorders, 50*(10), 3598–3605.

Asperger, H. (1991). "Autistic psychopathy" in childhoos. In U. Frith (Ed.), *Autism and Asperger syndrome* (pp. 37–92). Cambridge University Press.

Azmitia, E. C., Singh, J. S., & Whitaker-Azmitia, P. M. (2011). Increased serotonin axons (immunoreactive to 5-HT transporter) in postmortem brains from young autism donors. *Neuropharmacology, 60*(7–8), 1347–1354.

Baker, J. K., Fenning, R. M., Howland, M. A., Baucom, B. R., Moffitt, J., & Erath, S. A. (2015). Brief report: A pilot study of parent–child biobehavioral synchrony in autism spectrum disorder. *Journal of Autism and Developmental Disorders, 45*(12), 4140–4146.

Baron-Cohen, S., & Howlin, P. (1993). The theory of mind deficit in autism: Some questions for teaching and diagnosis. In S. Baron-Cohen, H. Tager-Flusberg & D. Cohen (Eds.), *Understanding other minds: Perspectives from autism* (pp. 466–480). Oxford University Press.

Baron-Cohen, S., Leslie, A. M., & Frith, U. (1985). Does the autistic child have a "theory of mind"? *Cognition, 21*(1), 37–46.

Bauman, M. L., & Kemper, T. L. (1994). Neuroanatomic observations of the brain in autism. In M. L. Bauman & T. L. Kemper (Eds.), *The neurobiology of autism* (pp. 119–145). Johns Hopkins University Press.

Bear, M. F., Huber, K. M., & Warren, S. T. (2004). The mGluR theory of fragile X mental retardation. *Trends in Neurosciences, 27*, 370–377

Bearss, K., Johnson, C., Smith, T., Lecavalier, L., Swiezy, N., Aman, M., McAdam, D., Butter, E., Stillitano, C., Minshawi, N., Sukhodolsky, D., Mruzek, D., Turner, K., Neal, T., Hallett, V., Mulick, J., Green, B., Handen, B., Deng, Y., . . . Scahill, L. (2015). Effect of parent training vs parent education on behavioral problems in children with autism spectrum disorder: A randomized clinical trial. *JAMA, 313*(15), 1524–1533.

Beaudoin, A. J., Sébire, G., & Couture, M. (2014). Parent training interventions for toddlers with autism spectrum disorder. *Autism Research and Treatment, 2014*, 839890.

Belmonte, J. C. I., Callaway, E. M., Caddick, S. J., Churchland, P., Feng, G., Homanics, G. E., Lee, K., Leopold, D., Miller, C., Mitchell, J., Mitalipov, S., Moutri, A., Movshon, J., Okano, H., Reynolds, J., Ringach D., Sejnowski, T., Silva, A., Strick, P., . . . Zhang, F. (2015). Brains, genes, and primates. *Neuron, 86*(3), 617–631.

Ben-Sasson, A., Hen, L., Fluss, R., Cermak, S. A., Engel-Yeger, B., & Gal, E. (2009). A meta-analysis of sensory modulation symptoms in individuals with autism spectrum disorders. *Journal of Autism and Developmental Disorders, 39*(1), 1–11.

Berry-Kravis, E., Des Portes, V., Hagerman, R., Jacquemont, S., Charles, P., Visootsak, J., Brinkman, M., Rerat, K., Koumaras, B., Zhu, L., Barth, G., Jaecklin, T., Apostol, G., & Von

Raison, F. (2016). Mavoglurant in fragile X syndrome: Results of two randomized, double-blind, placebo-controlled trials. *Science Translational Medicine, 8*(321), 321ra5.

Bester-Meredith, J. K., Fancher, A. P., & Mammarella, G. E. (2015). Vasopressin proves es-sensetial: Vasopressin and the modulation of sensory processing in mammals. *Frontiers in endocrinology, 6*, Article 5.

Betancur, C. (2011). Etiological heterogeneity in autism spectrum disorders: More than 100 genetic and genomic disorders and still counting. *Brain Research, 1380*, 42–77.

Bethlehem, R. A. I., Lombardo, M. V., Lai, M. C., Auyeung, B., Crockford, S. K., Deakin, J., Soubramanian, S., Sule, A., Kundu, P., Voon, V., & Baron-Cohen, S. (2017). Intranasal oxytocin enhances intrinsic corticostriatal functional connectivity in women. *Translational Psychiatry, 7*(4), e1099.

Blatt, G. J. (2012). The neuropathology of autism. *Scientifica, 2012*, 703675.

Boyd, B. A., Hume, K., McBee, M. T., Alessandri, M., Gutierrez, A., Johnson, L., Sperry, L., & Odom, S. L. (2014). Comparative efficacy of LEAP, TEACCH and non-model-specific special education programs for preschoolers with autism spectrum disorders. *Journal of Autism and Developmental Disorders, 44*(2), 366–380.

Braun, J. M., Kalkbrenner, A. E., Just, A. C., Yolton, K., Calafat, A. M., Sjödin, A., Hauser, R., Webster, G., Chen, A., & Lanphear, B. P. (2014). Gestational exposure to endocrine-disrupting chemicals and reciprocal social, repetitive, and stereotypic behaviors in 4- and 5-year-old children: The HOME study. *Environmental Health Perspectives, 122*(5), 513–520.

Brondino, N., Fusar-Poli, L., Panisi, C., Damiani, S., Barale, F., & Politi, P. (2016). Pharmacological modulation of GABA function in autism spectrum disorders: A systematic review of human studies. *Journal of Autism and Developmental Disorders, 46*(3), 825–839.

Brugha, T. S., Spiers, N., Bankart, J., Cooper, S. A., McManus, S., Scott, F. J., Smith, J., & Tyrer, F. (2016). Epidemiology of autism in adults across age groups and ability levels. *British Journal of Psychiatry, 209*(6), 498–503.

Carson, D. S., Garner, J. P., Hyde, S. A., Libove, R. A., Berquist, S. W., Hornbeak, K. B., Jackson, L., Sumiyoshi, R., Howerton, C., Hannah, S., Partap, S., Phillips, J., Hardan, A., & Parker, K. J. (2015). Arginine vasopressin is a blood-based biomarker of social functioning in children with autism. *PLoS One, 10*(7), e0132224.

Carter, C. S., Grippo, A. J., Pournajafi-Nazarloo, H., Ruscio, M. G., & Porges, S. W. (2008). Oxytocin, vasopressin and sociality. *Progress in Brain Research, 170*, 331–336.

Casanova, M., & Trippe, J. (2009). Radial cytoarchitecture and patterns of cortical connectivity in autism. *Philosophical Transactions of the Royal Society Series B: Biological Sciences, 364*(1522), 1433–1436.

Castro, K., Klein, L. D. S., Baronio, D., Gottfried, C., Riesgo, R., & Perry, I. S. (2016). Folic acid and autism: What do we know? *Nutritional Neuroscience, 19*(7), 310–317.

Ceranoglu, T. A., Wozniak, J., Fried, R., Galdo, M., Hoskova, B., DeLeon Fong, M., Biederman, J., & Joshi, G. (2019). A retrospective chart review of buspirone for the treatment of anxiety in psychiatrically referred youth with high-functioning autism spectrum disorder. *Journal of Child and Adolescent Psychopharmacology, 29*(1), 28–33.

Chen, M. H., Pan, T. L., Lan, W. H., Hsu, J. W., Huang, K. L., Su, T. P., Li, C., Lin, W., Wei, H., Chen, T. J., & Bai, Y. (2017). Risk of suicide attempts among adolescents and young adults with autism spectrum disorder: A nationwide longitudinal follow-up study. *Journal of Clinical Psychiatry, 78*(9), 1174–1179.

Chen, Y., Yu, J., Niu, Y., Qin, D., Liu, H., Li, G., Hu, Y., Wang, J., Lu, Y., Kang, Y., Jiang, Y., Wu, K., Li, S., Wei, J., He, J., Wang, J., Liu, X., Luo, Y., Si, C., . . . Sun, Y. E. (2017). Modeling Rett syndrome using TALEN-edited MECP2 mutant cynomolgus monkeys. *Cell, 169*(5), 945–955.

Colvert, E., Tick, B., McEwen, F., Stewart, C., Curran, S. R., Woodhouse, E., Gillan, N., Hallett, V., Lietz, S., Garnett, T., Ronald, A., Plomin, R., Rijsdijk, F., Happe, F., & Bolton, P. (2015). Heritability of autism spectrum disorder in a UK population-based twin sample. *JAMA Psychiatry, 72*(5), 415–423.

Courchesne, E., Mouton, P. R., Calhoun, M. E., Semendeferi, K., Ahrens-Barbeau, C., Hallet, M. J., Barnes, C. C., & Pierce, K. (2011). Neuron number and size in prefrontal cortex of children with autism. *JAMA, 306*(18), 2001–2010.

Davidson, D., Vanegas, S. B., & Hilvert, E. (2017). Proneness to self-conscious emotions in adults with and without autism traits. *Journal of Autism and Developmental Disorders, 47*(11), 3392–3404.

Dawson, G., Jones, E. J., Merkle, K., Venema, K., Lowy, R., Faja, S., Kamara, D., Murias, M., Greenson, J., Winter, J., Smith, M., Rogers, S., & Webb, S. J. (2012). Early behavioral intervention is associated with normalized brain activity in young children with autism. *Journal of the American Academy of Child & Adolescent Psychiatry, 51*(11), 1150–1159.

Dawson, G., Rogers, S., Munson, J., Smith, M., Winter, J., Greenson, J., Donaldson, A., & Varley, J. (2010). Randomized, controlled trial of an intervention for toddlers with autism: The Early Start Denver Model. *Pediatrics, 125*(1), e17–e23.

de Bildt, A., Sytema, S., Zander, E., Bölte, S., Sturm, H., Yirmiya, N., Yaari, M., Charman, T., Salomone, E., LeCouteur, A., Green, J., Bedia, R., Primo, P., van Daalen, E., de Jonge, M., Guomundsdottir, E., Johannsdottir, S., Raleva, M., Boskovska, M., . . . Oosterling, I. J. (2015). Autism Diagnostic Interview–Revised (ADI-R) algorithms for toddlers and young preschoolers: Application in a non-US sample of 1,104 children. *Journal of Autism and Developmental Disorders, 45*(7), 2076–2091.

de la Torre-Ubieta, L., Won, H., Stein, J. L., & Geschwind, D. H. (2016). Advancing the understanding of autism disease mechanisms through genetics. *Nature Medicine, 22*(4), 345–361.

Demetriou, E. A., DeMayo, M. M., & Guastella, A. J. (2019). Executive function in autism spectrum disorder: History, theoretical models, empirical findings, and potential as an endophenotype. *Frontiers in Psychiatry, 10*, Article 753.

Deng, W., Zou, X., Deng, H., Li, J., Tang, C., Wang, X., & Guo, X. (2015). The relationship among genetic heritability, environmental effects, and autism spectrum disorders: 37 pairs of ascertained twin study. *Journal of Child Neurology, 30*(13), 1794–1799.

Ecker, C. (2017). The neuroanatomy of autism spectrum disorder: An overview of structural neuroimaging findings and their translatability to the clinical setting. *Autism, 21*(1), 18–28.

Ecker, C., Ronan, L., Feng, Y., Daly, E., Murphy, C., Ginestet, C. E., Brammer, M., Fletcher, P., Bullmore, E., Suckling, J., Baron-Cohen, S., Williams, S., Loth, E., MRC AIMS Consortium, & Murphy, D. (2013). Intrinsic gray-matter connectivity of the brain in adults with autism spectrum disorder. *Proceedings of the National Academy of Sciences of the USA, 110*(32), 13222–13227.

Ecker, C., Suckling, J., Deoni, S. C., Lombardo, M. V., Bullmore, E. T., Baron-Cohen, S., Catani, M., Jezzard, P., Barnes, A., Bailey, A., Williams, S., Murphy, D., & MRC AIMS Consortium. (2012). Brain anatomy and its relationship to behavior in adults with autism spectrum disorder: A multicenter magnetic resonance imaging study. *Archives of General Psychiatry, 69*(2), 195–209.

Eggebrecht, A. T., Elison, J. T., Feczko, E., Todorov, A., Wolff, J. J., Kandala, S., Adams, C., Snyder, A., Lewis, J., Estes, A., Zwaigenbaum, L., Botteron, K., McKinstry, R., Constantino, J., Evans, A., Hazlett, H., Dager, S., Paterson, S., Schultz, R., . . . Pruett, J. R., Jr. (2017). Joint attention and brain functional connectivity in infants and toddlers. *Cerebral Cortex, 27*(3), 1709–1720.

Eisenberg, L. (2001). The past 50 years of child and adolescent psychiatry: A personal memoir. *Journal of the American Academy of Child and Adolescent Psychiatry, 40*(7), 743–748.

El Achkar, C. M., & Spence, S. J. (2015). Clinical characteristics of children and young adults with co-occurring autism spectrum disorder and epilepsy. *Epilepsy & Behavior, 47*, 183–190.

Elchaar, G. M., Maisch, N. M., Augusto, L. M., & Wehring, H. J. (2006). Efficacy and safety of naltrexone use in pediatric patients with autistic disorder. *Annals of Pharmacotherapy, 40*(6), 1086–1095.

Eliasen, M., Tolstrup, J. S., Nybo Andersen, A. M., Grønbæk, M., Olsen, J., & Strandberg-Larsen, K. (2010). Prenatal alcohol exposure and autistic spectrum disorders—A population-based prospective study of 80,552 children and their mothers. *International Journal of Epidemiology, 39*(4), 1074–1081.

Elison, J. T., Wolff, J. J., Heimer, D. C., Paterson, S. J., Gu, H., Hazlett, H. C., Styner, M., Gerig, G., Piven, J., & IBIS Network. (2013). Frontolimbic neural circuitry at 6 months predicts individual differences in joint attention at 9 months. *Developmental Science, 16*(2), 186–197.

Emerson, R. W., Adams, C., Nishino, T., Hazlett, H. C., Wolff, J. J., Zwaigenbaum, L., Constantino, J., Shen, M., Swanson, M., Elison, J., Kandala, S., Estes, A., Botteron, K., Collins, L., Dager, S., Evans, A., Gerig, G., Gu, H., McKinstry, R., . . . Piven, J. (2017). Functional neuroimaging of high-risk 6-month-old infants predicts a diagnosis of autism at 24 months of age. *Science Translational Medicine, 9*(393), eaag2882.

Ergaz, Z., Weinstein-Fudim, L., & Ornoy, A. (2016). Genetic and non-genetic animal models for autism spectrum disorders (ASD). *Reproductive Toxicology, 64,* 116–140.

Estes, A., Munson, J., Rogers, S. J., Greenson, J., Winter, J., & Dawson, G. (2015). Long-term outcomes of early intervention in 6-year-old children with autism spectrum disorder. *Journal of the American Academy of Child & Adolescent Psychiatry, 54*(7), 580–587.

Fallah, M. S., Shaikh, M. R., Neupane, B., Rusiecki, D., Bennett, T. A., & Beyene, J. (2019). Atypical antipsychotics for irritability in pediatric autism: A systematic review and network meta-analysis. *Journal of Child and Adolescent Psychopharmacology, 29*(3), 168–180.

Fein, D., Lueci, D., Braverman, M., & Waterhouse, L. (1992). Comprehension of affect in context in children with pervasive developmental disorders. *Journal of Child Psychology and Psychiatry, 33*(7), 1157–1162.

Feldman, R. (2012a). Bio-behavioral synchrony: A model for integrating biological and microsocial behavioral processes in the study of parenting. *Parenting, 12*(2–3), 154–164.

Feldman, R. (2012b). Oxytocin and social affiliation in humans. *Hormones and Behavior, 61*(3), 380–391.

Feldman, R., Magori-Cohen, R., Galili, G., Singer, M., & Louzoun, Y. (2011). Mother and infant coordinate heart rhythms through episodes of interaction synchrony. *Infant Behavior and Development, 34*(4), 569–577.

Folstein, S., & Rutter, M. (1977). Infantile autism: A genetic study of 21 twin pairs. *Journal of Child Psychology and Psychiatry, 18*(4), 297–321.

Froehlich-Santino, W., Tobon, A. L., Cleveland, S., Torres, A., Phillips, J., Cohen, B., Torigoe, T., Miller, J., Fedele, A., Collins, J., Smith, K., Lotspeich, L., Croen, L., Ozonoff, S., Lajonchere, C., Grether, J., O'Hara, R., & Hallmayer, J. (2014). Prenatal and perinatal risk factors in a twin study of autism spectrum disorders. *Journal of Psychiatric Research, 54,* 100–108.

Fuller, E. A., Oliver, K., Vejnoska, S. F., & Rogers, S. J. (2020). The effects of the Early Start Denver Model for children with autism spectrum disorder: A meta-analysis. *Brain Sciences, 10*(6), Article 368.

Fung, L. K., Mahajan, R., Nozzolillo, A., Bernal, P., Krasner, A., Jo, B., Coury, D., Whitaker, A., Veenstra-Vanderweele, J., & Hardan, A. Y. (2016). Pharmacologic treatment of severe irritability and problem behaviors in autism: A systematic review and meta-analysis. *Pediatrics, 137*(Suppl. 2), S124–S135.

Gabriele, S., Sacco, R., & Persico, A. M. (2014). Blood serotonin levels in autism spectrum disorder: A systematic review and meta-analysis. *European Neuropsychopharmacology, 24*(6), 919–929.

Gaigg, S. B. (2012). The interplay between emotion and cognition in autism spectrum disorder: Implications for developmental theory. *Frontiers in Integrative Neuroscience, 6,* Article 113.

Garfinkel, S. N., Tiley, C., O'Keeffe, S., Harrison, N. A., Seth, A. K., & Critchley, H. D. (2016). Discrepancies between dimensions of interoception in autism: Implications for emotion and anxiety. *Biological Psychology, 114,* 117–126.

Gaugler, T., Klei, L., Sanders, S. J., Bodea, C. A., Goldberg, A. P., Lee, A. B., Mahajan, M., Manaa, D., Pawitan, Y., Reichert, J., Ripke, S., Sandin, S., Sklar, P., Svantesson, O., Reichenberg, A., Hultman, C., Devlin, B., Roeder, K., & Buxbaum, J. (2014). Most genetic risk for autism resides with common variation. *Nature Genetics, 46*(8), 881–885.

Geschwind, D. H. (2008). Autism: Many genes, common pathways? *Cell, 135*(3), 391–395.

Geschwind, D. H., & State, M. W. (2015). Gene hunting in autism spectrum disorder: On the path to precision medicine. *Lancet Neurology, 14*(11), 1109–1120.

Geurts, H., Sinzig, J., Booth, R., & Happé, F. (2014). Neuropsychological heterogeneity in executive functioning in autism spectrum disorders. *International Journal of Developmental Disabilities, 60*(3), 155–162.

Ghirardi, L., Pettersson, E., Taylor, M. J., Freitag, C. M., Franke, B., Asherson, P., Larsson, H., & Kuja-Halkola, R. (2019). Genetic and environmental contribution to the overlap between ADHD and ASD trait dimensions in young adults: A twin study. *Psychological Medicine, 49*(10), 1713–1721.

Gialloreti, E. L., Mazzone, L., Benvenuto, A., Fasano, A., Garcia Alcon, A., Kraneveld, A., Moavero, R., Raz, R., Riccio, M., Siracusano, M., Zachor, D., Marini, M., & Curatolo, P. (2019). Risk and protective environmental factors associated with autism spectrum disorder: Evidence-based principles and recommendations. *Journal of Clinical Medicine, 8*(2), Article 217.

Goel, R., Hong, J. S., Findling, R. L., & Ji, N. Y. (2018). An update on pharmacotherapy of autism spectrum disorder in children and adolescents. *International Review of Psychiatry, 30*(1), 78–95.

Gordon, C. T., State, R. C., Nelson, J. E., Hamburger, S. D., & Rapoport, I. L. (1993). A double-blind comparison of clomipramine, desipramine, and placebo in the treatment of autistic disorder. *Archives of General Psychiatry, 50,* 441–447.

Gotham, K., Pickles, A., & Lord, C. (2012). Trajectories of autism severity in children using standardized ADOS scores. *Pediatrics, 130*(5), e1278–e1284.

Grove, J., Ripke, S., Als, T. D., Mattheisen, M., Walters, R. K., Won, H., Pallesen, J., Agerbo, E., Andreassen, O. A., Anney, R., Awashti, S., Belliveau, R., Bettella, F., Buxbaum, J. D., Bybjerg-Grauholm, J., Bækvad-Hansen, M., Cerrato, F., Chambert, K., Christensen, J. H., . . . Børglum, A. D. (2019). Identification of common genetic risk variants for autism spectrum disorder. *Nature Genetics, 51*(3), 431–444.

Guan, J., & Li, G. (2017). Injury mortality in individuals with autism. *American Journal of Public Health, 107*(5), 791–793.

Hannon, G., & Taylor, E. P. (2013). Suicidal behaviour in adolescents and young adults with ASD: Findings from a systematic review. *Clinical Psychology Review, 33*(8), 1197–1204.

Happé, F. (1999). Autism: Cognitive deficit or cognitive style? *Trends in Cognitive Sciences, 3*(6), 216–222.

Happé, F., & Frith, U. (2006). The weak coherence account: Detail-focused cognitive style in autism spectrum disorders. *Journal of Autism and Developmental Disorders, 36*(1), 5–25.

Harris, J. C. (2016). The origin and natural history of autism spectrum disorders. *Nature Neuroscience, 19*(11), 1390–1391.

Harris, J. C. (2018). Leo Kanner and autism: A 75-year perspective. *International Review of Psychiatry, 30*(1), 3–17.

Harris, J. C. (2019). The necessity to identify subtypes of autism spectrum disorder. *JAMA Psychiatry, 76*(11), 1116–1117.

Harris, J. C., & Carter, C. S. (2013). Therapeutic interventions with oxytocin: Current status and concerns. *Journal of the American Academy of Child and Adolescent Psychiatry, 52*(10), 998–1000.

Harris, J. C., & Piven, J. (2016, April 26). Correcting the record: Leo Kanner and the broad autism phenotype. *Spectrum News.* Retrieved January 29, 2021, from https://www.spectrumnews.org/opinion/viewpoint/correcting-the-record-leo-kanner-and-the-broad-autism-phenotype

Hazlett, H. C., Gu, H., Munsell, B. C., Kim, S. H., Styner, M., Wolff, J. J., Elison, J., Swanson, M., Zhu, H., Botteron, K., Collins, D., Constantino, J., Dager, S., Estes, A., Evans, A., Fonov, V., Gerig, G., Kostopoulos, P., McKinstry, R., . . . IBIS Network. (2017). Early brain development in infants at high risk for autism spectrum disorder. *Nature, 542*(7641), 348–351.

Heerey, E. A., Keltner, D., & Capps, L. M. (2003). Making sense of self-conscious emotion: Linking theory of mind and emotion in children with autism. *Emotion, 3*(4), 394–400.

Hirota, T., Veenstra-VanderWeele, J., Hollander, E., & Kishi, T. (2014). Antiepileptic medications in autism spectrum disorder: A systematic review and meta-analysis. *Journal of Autism and Developmental Disorders, 44*(4), 948–957.

Hisle-Gorman, E., Susi, A., Stokes, T., Gorman, G., Erdie-Lalena, C., & Nylund, C. M. (2018). Prenatal, perinatal, and neonatal risk factors of autism spectrum disorder. *Pediatric Research*, *84*(2), 190–198.

Hobson, J. A., Harris, R., García-Pérez, R., & Hobson, R. P. (2009). Anticipatory concern: A study in autism. *Developmental Science*, *12*(2), 249–263.

Hobson, R. P. (1989). Beyond cognition: A theory of autism. In G. Dawson (Ed.), *Autism: Nature, diagnosis and treatment* (pp. 22–48). Guilford.

Hobson, R. P. (1991a). What is autism? *Psychiatric Clinics of North America*, *14*, 1–18.

Hobson, R. P. (1991b). Against the theory of "theory of mind." *British Journal of Developmental Psychology*, *9*(1), 33–51.

Hobson, R. P. (1993). The emotional origins of social understanding. *Philosophical Psychology*, *6*(3), 227–249.

Hobson, R. P., & Lee, A. (1999). Imitation and identification in autism. *Journal of Child Psychology and Psychiatry*, *40*(4), 649–659.

Hobson, R. P., Lee, A., & Hobson, J. A. (2007). Only connect? Communication, identification, and autism. *Social Neuroscience*, *2*(3–4), 320–335.

Hobson, R. P., & Meyer, J. A. (2005). Foundations for self and other: A study in autism. *Developmental Science*, *8*(6), 481–491.

Hollander, E., Wasserman, S., Swanson, E. N., Chaplin, W., Schapiro, M. L., Zagursky, K., & Novotny, S. (2006). A double-blind placebo-controlled pilot study of olanzapine in childhood/adolescent pervasive developmental disorder. *Journal of Child and Adolescent Psychopharmacology*, *16*(5), 541–548.

Horder, J., Petrinovic, M. M., Mendez, M. A., Bruns, A., Takumi, T., Spooren, W., Barker, G., Kunnecke, B., & Murphy, D. G. (2018). Glutamate and GABA in autism spectrum disorder—A translational magnetic resonance spectroscopy study in man and rodent models. *Translational Psychiatry*, *8*, Article 106.

Howe, S. J., Hewitt, K., Baraskewich, J., Cassidy, S., & McMorris, C. A. (2020). Suicidality among children and youth with and without autism spectrum disorder: A systematic review of existing risk assessment tools. *Journal of Autism and Developmental Disorders*, *50*(10), 3462–3476.

Howlin, P., & Magiati, I. (2017). Autism spectrum disorder: Outcomes in adulthood. *Current Opinion in Psychiatry*, *30*(2), 69–76.

Howlin, P., Rutter, M., Berger, M., Hemsley, R., Hersov, L., & Yule, W. (1987). *Treatment of autistic children*. Wiley.

Huang, Y., Huang, X., Ebstein, R. P., & Yu, R. (2021). Intranasal oxytocin in the treatment of autism spectrum disorders: A multilevel meta-analysis. *Neuroscience and Biobehavioral Reviews*, *122*, 18–27.

Huguet, G., Benabou, M., & Bourgeron, T. (2016). The genetics of autism spectrum disorders. In P. Sassone-Corsi & Y. Christen (Eds.), *A time for metabolism and hormones* (pp. 101–129). Springer.

Hviid, A., Melbye, M., & Pasternak, B. (2013). Use of selective serotonin reuptake inhibitors during pregnancy and risk of autism. *New England Journal of Medicine*, *369*(25), 2406–2415.

Hyman, S. L., Levy, S. E., & Myers, S. M.; Council on Children with Disabilities, Section on Developmental and Behavioral Pediatrics. (2020). Identification, evaluation, and management of children with autism spectrum disorder. *Pediatrics*, *145*(1), e20193447.

Iovino, M., Messana, T., De Pergola, G., Iovino, E., Dicuonzo, F., Guastamacchia, E., Giagulli, V., & Triggiani, V. (2018). The role of neurohypophyseal hormones vasopressin and oxytocin in neuropsychiatric disorders. *Endocrine, Metabolic & Immune Disorders Drug Targets*, *18*(4), 341–347.

Ito, H., Mori, K., Harada, M., Hisaoka, S., Toda, Y., Mori, T., Goji, A., Abe, Y., Miyazaki, M., & Kagami, S. (2017). A proton magnetic resonance spectroscopic study in autism spectrum disorder using a 3-Tesla clinical magnetic resonance imaging (MRI) system: The anterior cingulate cortex and the left cerebellum. *Journal of Child Neurology*, *32*(8), 731–739.

Jacot-Descombes, S., Uppal, N., Wicinski, B., Santos, M., Schmeidler, J., Giannakopoulos, P., Heinsen, H., Schmitz, C., & Hof, P. R. (2012). Decreased pyramidal neuron size in Brodmann areas 44 and 45 in patients with autism. *Acta Neuropathologica*, *124*(1), 67–79.

Jager-Hyman, S., Maddox, B. B., Crabbe, S. R., & Mandell, D. S. (2020). Mental health clinicians' screening and intervention practices to reduce suicide risk in autistic adolescents and adults. *Journal of Autism and Developmental Disorders, 50*(10), 3450–3461.

Jaiswal, P., Guhathakurta, S., Singh, A. S., Verma, D., Pandey, M., Varghese, M., Sinha, S., Ghosh, S., Mohanakumar, K., & Rajamma, U. (2015). SLC6A4 markers modulate platelet 5-HT level and specific behaviors of autism: A study from an Indian population. *Progress in Neuro-Psychopharmacology and Biological Psychiatry, 56*, 196–206.

Jennings, C. G., Landman, R., Zhou, Y., Sharma, J., Hyman, J., Movshon, J. A., Qiu, Z., Roberts, A., Roe, A., Wang, X., Zhou, H., Wang, L., Zhang, F., Desimone, R., & Feng, G. (2016). Opportunities and challenges in modeling human brain disorders in transgenic primates. *Nature Neuroscience, 19*(9), 1123–1130.

Ji, N. Y., & Findling, R. L. (2015). An update on pharmacotherapy for autism spectrum disorder in children and adolescents. *Current Opinion in Psychiatry, 28*(2), 91–101.

Jolliffe, T., & Baron-Cohen, S. (1997). Are people with autism and Asperger syndrome faster than normal on the Embedded Figures Test? *Journal of Child Psychology and Psychiatry, 38*(5), 527–534.

Kana, R. K., Maximo, J. O., Williams, D. L., Keller, T. A., Schipul, S. E., Cherkassky, V. L., Minshew, N. J., & Just, M. A. (2015). Aberrant functioning of the theory-of-mind network in children and adolescents with autism. *Molecular Autism, 6*(1), Article 59.

Kanner, L. (1943). Autistic disturbances of affective contact. *Nervous Child, 2*(3), 217–250.

Kanner, L. (1944). Early infantile autism. *Journal of Pediatrics, 25*, 211–217.

Kanner, L., & Eisenberg, L. (1956). Childhood schizophrenia; symposium, 1955: VI. Early infantile autism, 1943–55. *American Journal of Orthopsychiatry, 26*, 556–566.

Kasari, C., Gulsrud, A., Paparella, T., Hellemann, G., & Berry, K. (2015). Randomized comparative efficacy study of parent-mediated interventions for toddlers with autism. *Journal of Consulting and Clinical Psychology, 83*(3), 554–563.

Kato, T., Takahashi, E., Sawada, K., Kobayashi, N., Watanabe, T., & Ishh, T. (1983). A computer analysis of infant movements synchronized with adult speech. *Pediatric Research, 17*(8), 625–628.

Katz, J., Reichenberg, A., & Kolevzon, A. (2021). Prenatal and perinatal metabolic risk factors for autism: A review and integration of findings from population-based studies. *Current Opinion in Psychiatry, 34*(2), 94–104.

Kim, S. H., & Lord, C. (2012). New Autism Diagnostic Interview–Revised algorithms for toddlers and young preschoolers from 12 to 47 months of age. *Journal of Autism and Developmental Disorders, 42*(1), 82–93.

Kõlves, K., Fitzgerald, C., Nordentoft, M., Wood, S. J., & Erlangsen, A. (2021). Assessment of suicidal behaviors among individuals with autism spectrum disorder in Denmark. *JAMA Network Open, 4*(1), e2033565.

Koyama, T., Tachimori, H., Osada, H., Takeda, T., & Kurita, H. (2007). Cognitive and symptom profiles in Asperger's syndrome and high-functioning autism. *Psychiatry and Clinical Neurosciences, 61*(1), 99–104.

Kushima, I., Aleksic, B., Nakatochi, M., Shimamura, T., Okada, T., Uno, Y., Morikawa, M., Ishizuka, K., Shiino, T., Kimura, H., Arioka, Y., Yoshimi, A., Takasaki, Y., Yu, Y., Nakamura, Y., Yamamoto, M., Iidaka, T., Iritani, S., Inada, T., . . . Ozaki, N. (2018). Comparative analyses of copy-number variation in autism spectrum disorder and schizophrenia reveal etiological overlap and biological insights. *Cell Reports, 24*(11), 2838–2856.

Lai, M. C., Kassee, C., Besney, R., Bonato, S., Hull, L., Mandy, W., Szatmari, P., & Ameis, S. H. (2019). Prevalence of co-occurring mental health diagnoses in the autism population: A systematic review and meta-analysis. *Lancet Psychiatry, 6*(10), 819–829.

Lai, M. C., Lombardo, M. V., Suckling, J., Ruigrok, A. N., Chakrabarti, B., Ecker, C., Deoni, S., Craig, M., Murphy, D., Bullmore, E., MRC AIMS Consortium, & Baron-Cohen, S. (2013). Biological sex affects the neurobiology of autism. *Brain, 136*(9), 2799–2815.

Lainhart, J. E., & Lange, N. (2011). Increased neuron number and head size in autism. *JAMA, 306*(18), 2031–2032.

Landa, R., Folstein, S. E., & Isaacs, C. (1991). Spontaneous narrative-discourse performance of parents of autistic individuals. *Journal of Speech, Language, and Hearing Research, 34*(6), 1339–1345.

Landa, R., Piven, J., Wzorek, M. M., Gayle, J. O., Chase, G. A., & Folstein, S. E. (1992). Social language use in parents of autistic individuals. *Psychological Medicine, 22*(1), 245–254.

Langdell, T. (1978). Recognition of faces: An approach to the study of autism. *Journal of Child Psychology and Psychiatry, 19*(3), 255–268.

Leclère, C., Viaux, S., Avril, M., Achard, C., Chetouani, M., Missonnier, S., & Cohen, D. (2014). Why synchrony matters during mother–child interactions: A systematic review. *PLoS One, 9*(12), e113571.

Lever, A. G., & Geurts, H. M. (2016). Age-related differences in cognition across the adult lifespan in autism spectrum disorder. *Autism Research, 9*(6), 666–676.

Lindgren, S., Wacker, D., Suess, A., Schieltz, K., Pelzel, K., Kopelman, T., Lee, J., Romani, R., & Waldron, D. (2016). Telehealth and autism: Treating challenging behavior at lower cost. *Pediatrics, 137*(Suppl. 2), S167–S175.

Linstead, E., Dixon, D. R., French, R., Granpeesheh, D., Adams, H., German, R., Powell, D. A., Stevens, E., Tarbox, J., & Kornack, J. (2017). Intensity and learning outcomes in the treatment of children with autism spectrum disorder. *Behavior modification, 41*(2), 229–252.

Liu, L., Zhang, D., Rodzinka-Pasko, J. K., & Li, Y. M. (2016). Environmental risk factors for autism spectrum disorders. *Der Nervenarzt, 87*(2), 55–61.

Lombardo, M. V., Busuoli, E. M., Schreibman, L., Stahmer, A. C., Pramparo, T., Landi, I., Mandelli, V., Bertelsen, N., Barnes, C. C., Gazestani, V., Lopez, L., Bacon, E. C., Courchesne, E., & Pierce, K. (2021). Pre-treatment clinical and gene expression patterns predict developmental change in early intervention in autism. *Molecular Psychiatry, 26*(12), 7641–7651.

Lombardo, M. V., & Mandelli, V. (2022). Rethinking our concepts and assumptions about autism. *Frontiers in Psychiatry, 13*, 903489.

Lord, C., Rutter, M., DiLavore, P. C., Risi, S., Gotham, K., & Bishop, S. (2012). *Autism Diagnostic Observation Schedule, 2nd Edition manual.* Western Psychological Services.

Losh, M., Adolphs, R., Poe, M. D., Couture, S., Penn, D., Baranek, G. T., & Piven, J. (2009). Neuropsychological profile of autism and the broad autism phenotype. *Archives of General Psychiatry, 66*(5), 518–526.

Lotter, V. (1966). Epidemiology of autistic conditions in young children: I. Prevalence. *Social Psychiatry, 1*, 124–137.

Madra, M., Ringel, R., & Margolis, K. G. (2021). Gastrointestinal issues and autism spectrum disorder. *Psychiatric Clinics of North America, 44*(1), 69–81.

Marotta, R., Risoleo, M. C., Messina, G., Parisi, L., Carotenuto, M., Vetri, L., & Roccella, M. (2020). The neurochemistry of autism. *Brain Sciences, 10*(3), Article 163.

Mastrovito, D., Hanson, C., & Hanson, S. J. (2018). Differences in atypical resting-state effective connectivity distinguish autism from schizophrenia. *NeuroImage: Clinical, 18*, 367–376.

McCracken, J. T., McGough, J., Shah, B., Cronin, P., Hong, D., Aman, M. G., Arnold, L., Lindsay, R., Nash, P., Hollway, J., McDougle, C., Posey, D., Swiezy, N., Kohn, A., Scahill, L., Martin, A., Koenig, K., Volkmar, F., Carroll, D., . . . McMahon, D.; Research Units on Pediatric Psychopharmacology Autism Network. (2002). Risperidone in children with autism and serious behavioral problems. *New England Journal of Medicine, 347*(5), 314–321.

McKinnon, C. J., Eggebrecht, A. T., Todorov, A., Wolff, J. J., Elison, J. T., Adams, C. M., Snyder, A., Estes, A., Zwaigenbaum, L., Botteron, K., McKinstry, R., Marrus, N., Evans, A., Hazlett, H., Dager, S., Paterson, S., Pandey, J., Schultz, R., Styner, M., . . . Pruett, J., Jr.; IBIS Network. (2019). Restricted and repetitive behavior and brain functional connectivity in infants at risk for developing autism spectrum disorder. *Biological Psychiatry: Cognitive Neuroscience and Neuroimaging, 4*(1), 50–61.

Mei, Y., Monteiro, P., Zhou, Y., Kim, J. A., Gao, X., Fu, Z., & Feng, G. (2016). Adult restoration of Shank3 expression rescues selective autistic-like phenotypes. *Nature, 530*(7591), 481–484.

Meyer, J. A., & Minshew, N. J. (2002). An update on neurocognitive profiles in Asperger syndrome and high-functioning autism. *Focus on Autism and Other Developmental Disabilities*, *17*(3), 152–160.

Ming, X., Gordon, E., Kang, N., & Wagner, G. C. (2008). Use of clonidine in children with autism spectrum disorders. *Brain and Development*, *30*(7), 454–460.

Minshawi, N. F., Hurwitz, S., Fodstad, J. C., Biebl, S., Morriss, D. H., & McDougle, C. J. (2014). The association between self-injurious behaviors and autism spectrum disorders. *Psychology Research and Behavior Management*, *7*, 125–136.

Mitchell, M. M., Woods, R., Chi, L. H., Schmidt, R. J., Pessah, I. N., Kostyniak, P. J., & LaSalle, J. M. (2012). Levels of select PCB and PBDE congeners in human postmortem brain reveal possible environmental involvement in 15q11–q13 duplication autism spectrum disorder. *Environmental and Molecular Mutagenesis*, *53*(8), 589–598.

Modabbernia, A., Velthorst, E., & Reichenberg, A. (2017). Environmental risk factors for autism: An evidence-based review of systematic reviews and meta-analyses. *Molecular Autism*, *8*(1), Article 13.

Monteiro, P., & Feng, G. (2017). SHANK proteins: Roles at the synapse and in autism spectrum disorder. *Nature Reviews Neuroscience*, *18*(3), 147–157.

Mori, K., Toda, Y., Ito, H., Mori, T., Mori, K., Goji, A., Hashimoto, H., Tani, H., Miyazaki, M., Harada, M., & Kagami, S. (2015). Neuroimaging in autism spectrum disorders: [1]H-MRS and NIRS study. *Journal of Medical Investigation*, *62*(1–2), 29–36.

Morneau-Vaillancourt, G., Andlauer, T. F. M., Ouellet-Morin, I., Paquin, S., Brendgen, M. R., Vitaro, F., Gouin, J. P., Séguin, J. R., Gagnon, É., Cheesman, R., Forget-Dubois, N., Rouleau, G. A., Turecki, G., Tremblay, R. E., Côté, S. M., Dionne, G., & Boivin, M. (2021). Polygenic scores differentially predict developmental trajectories of subtypes of social withdrawal in childhood. *Journal of Child Psychology and Psychiatry, and Allied Disciplines*, *62*(11), 1320–1329.

Murphy, C. M., Wilson, C. E., Robertson, D. M., Ecker, C., Daly, E. M., Hammond, N., Galanopoulos, A., Dud, I., Murphy, D. G., & McAlonan, G. M. (2016). Autism spectrum disorder in adults: Diagnosis, management, and health services development. *Neuropsychiatric Disease and Treatment*, *12*, 1669–1686.

Naaijen, J., Zwiers, M. P., Forde, N. J., Williams, S. C., Durston, S., Brandeis, D., Glennon, J. C., The Tactics Consortium, Franke, B., Lythgoe, D. J., & Buitelaar, J. K. (2018). Striatal structure and its association with N-acetylaspartate and glutamate in autism spectrum disorder and obsessive compulsive disorder. *European Neuropsychopharmacology*, *28*(1), 118–129.

Nader, A. M., Jelenic, P., & Soulières, I. (2015). Discrepancy between WISC-III and WISC-IV cognitive profile in autism spectrum: What does it reveal about autistic cognition? *PLoS One*, *10*(12), e0144645.

Neul, J. L., Kaufmann, W. E., Glaze, D. G., Christodoulou, J., Clarke, A. J., Bahi-Buisson, N., Leonard, H., Bailey, M., Schanen, N., Zappella, M., Renieri, A., Huppke, P., Percy, A., & RettSearch Consortium. (2010). Rett syndrome: Revised diagnostic criteria and nomenclature. *Annals of Neurology*, *68*(6), 944–950.

Nordahl, C. W., Lange, N., Li, D. D., Barnett, L. A., Lee, A., Buonocore, M. H., Simon, T., Rogers, S., Ozonoff, D., & Amaral, D. G. (2011). Brain enlargement is associated with regression in preschool-age boys with autism spectrum disorders. *Proceedings of the National Academy of Sciences of the USA*, *108*(50), 20195–20200.

Okano, H., Sasaki, E., Yamamori, T., Iriki, A., Shimogori, T., Yamaguchi, Y., Kasai, K., & Miyawaki, A. (2016). Brain/MINDS: A Japanese national brain project for marmoset neuroscience. *Neuron*, *92*(3), 582–590.

Oliveras-Rentas, R. E., Kenworthy, L., Roberson, R. B., Martin, A., & Wallace, G. L. (2012). WISC-IV profile in high-functioning autism spectrum disorders: Impaired processing speed is associated with increased autism communication symptoms and decreased adaptive communication abilities. *Journal of Autism and Developmental Disorders*, *42*(5), 655–664.

Oono, I. P., Honey, E. J., & McConachie, H. (2013). Parent-mediated early intervention for young children with autism spectrum disorders (ASD). *Evidence-Based Child Health*, *8*(6), 2380–2479.

Opris, I., & Casanova, M. F. (2014). Prefrontal cortical minicolumn: From executive control to disrupted cognitive processing. *Brain, 137*(7), 1863–1875.

Owen, M. J. (2014). New approaches to psychiatric diagnostic classification. *Neuron, 84*(3), 564–571.

Owen, M. J., & O'Donovan, M. C. (2017). Schizophrenia and the neurodevelopmental continuum: Evidence from genomics. *World Psychiatry, 16*(3), 227–235.

Ozonoff, S., Pennington, B. F., & Rogers, S. J. (1991). Executive function deficits in high-functioning autistic individuals: Relationship to theory of mind. *Journal of Child Psychology and Psychiatry, 32*(7), 1081–1105.

Palmen, S. J., van Engeland, H., Hof, P. R., & Schmitz, C. (2004). Neuropathological findings in autism. *Brain, 127*(12), 2572–2583.

Parker, K. J., Oztan, O., Libove, R. A., Mohsin, N., Karhson, D. S., Sumiyoshi, R. D., Summers, J., Hinman, K., Motonaga, K., Phillips, J., Carson, D., Fung, L., Garner, J., & Hardan, A. Y. (2019). A randomized placebo-controlled pilot trial shows that intranasal vasopressin improves social deficits in children with autism. *Science Translational Medicine, 11*(491), eaau7356.

Pavone, P., Incorpora, G., Fiumara, A., Parano, E., Trifiletti, R. R., & Ruggieri, M. (2004). Epilepsy is not a prominent feature of primary autism. *Neuropediatrics, 35*(04), 207–210.

Piven, J., Elison, J. T., & Zylka, M. J. (2017). Toward a conceptual framework for early brain and behavior development in autism. *Molecular Psychiatry, 22*(10), 1385–1394.

Piven, J., Gayle, J., Chase, G. A., Fink, B., Landa, R., Wzorek, M. M., & Folstein, S. E. (1990). A family history study of neuropsychiatric disorders in the adult siblings of autistic individuals. *Journal of the American Academy of Child & Adolescent Psychiatry, 29*(2), 177–183.

Piven, J., Palmer, P., Jacobi, D., Childress, D., & Arndt, S. (1997). Broader autism phenotype: Evidence from a family history study of multiple-incidence autism families. *American Journal of Psychiatry, 154*(2), 185–190.

Piven, J., Tsai, G. C., Nehme, E., Coyle, J. T., Chase, G. A., & Folstein, S. E. (1991). Platelet serotonin, a possible marker for familial autism. *Journal of Autism and Developmental Disorders, 21*(1), 51–59.

Piven, J., Vieland, V. J., Parlier, M., Thompson, A., O'Conner, I., Woodbury-Smith, M., Huang, Y., Walters, K., Fernandez, B., & Szatmari, P. (2013). A molecular genetic study of autism and related phenotypes in extended pedigrees. *Journal of Neurodevelopmental Disorders, 5*(1), Article 30.

Piven, J., Wzorek, M., Landa, R., Lainhart, J., Bolton, P., Chase, G. A., & Folstein, S. (1994). Personality characteristics of the parents of autistic individuals. *Psychological Medicine, 24*(3), 783–795.

Plaisted, K., O'Riordan, M., & Baron-Cohen, S. (1998). Enhanced discrimination of novel, highly similar stimuli by adults with autism during a perceptual learning task. *Journal of Child Psychology and Psychiatry, 39*(5), 765–775.

Porges, S. W. (2001). The polyvagal theory: Phylogenetic substrates of a social nervous system. *International Journal of Psychophysiology, 42*(2), 123–146.

Porges, S. W., Bazhenova, O. V., Bal, E., Carlson, N., Sorokin, Y., Heilman, K. J., Cook, E., & Lewis, G. F. (2014). Reducing auditory hypersensitivities in autistic spectrum disorder: Preliminary findings evaluating the listening project protocol. *Frontiers in Pediatrics, 2*, Article 80.

Porges, S. W., & Lewis, G. F. (2010). The polyvagal hypothesis: Common mechanisms mediating autonomic regulation, vocalizations and listening. Handbook of *Behavioral Neuroscience, 19*, 255–264.

Porges, S. W., Macellaio, M., Stanfill, S. D., McCue, K., Lewis, G. F., Harden, E. R., Handelman, M., Denver, J., Bazhenova, O., & Heilman, K. J. (2013). Respiratory sinus arrhythmia and auditory processing in autism: Modifiable deficits of an integrated social engagement system? *International Journal of Psychophysiology, 88*(3), 261–270.

Puts, N. A., Wodka, E. L., Harris, A. D., Crocetti, D., Tommerdahl, M., Mostofsky, S. H., & Edden, R. A. (2017). Reduced GABA and altered somatosensory function in children with autism spectrum disorder. *Autism Research, 10*(4), 608–619.

Quattrocki, E., & Friston, K. (2014). Autism, oxytocin and interoception. *Neuroscience & Biobehavioral Reviews, 47*, 410–430.

Rai, D., Lee, B. K., Dalman, C., Golding, J., Lewis, G., & Magnusson, C. (2013). Parental depression, maternal antidepressant use during pregnancy, and risk of autism spectrum disorders: Population based case–control study. *BMJ, 346*, f2059.

Ramaswami, G., & Geschwind, D. H. (2018). Genetics of autism spectrum disorder. Handbook of *Clinical Neurology, 147*, 321–329.

Rees, E., & Kirov, G. (2021). Copy number variation and neuropsychiatric illness. *Current Opinion in Genetics & Development, 68*, 57–63.

Rice, C. E., Zablotsky, B., Avila, R. M., Colpe, L. J., Schieve, L. A., Pringle, B., & Blumberg, S. J. (2016). Reported wandering behavior among children with autism spectrum disorder and/or intellectual disability. *Journal of Pediatrics, 174*, 232–239.

Richards, C., Jones, C., Groves, L., Moss, J., & Oliver, C. (2015). Prevalence of autism spectrum disorder phenomenology in genetic disorders: A systematic review and meta-analysis. *Lancet Psychiatry, 2*(10), 909–916.

Ritvo, E. R., Yuwiler, A., Geller, E., Ornitz, E. M., Saeger, K., & Plotkin, S. (1970). Increased blood serotonin and platelets in early infantile autism. *Archives of General Psychiatry, 23*(6), 566–572.

Roane, H. S., Fisher, W. W., & Carr, J. E. (2016). Applied behavior analysis as treatment for autism spectrum disorder. *Journal of Pediatrics, 175*, 27–32.

Rogers, S. J., & Dawson, G. (2009). *Play and engagement in early autism: The Early Start Denver model.* Guilford.

Rogers, S. J., Dawson, G., & Vismara, L. A. (2012). *An early start for your child with autism: Using everyday activities to help kids connect, communicate, and learn.* Guilford.

Rogers, S. J., Estes, A., Lord, C., Vismara, L., Winter, J., Fitzpatrick, A., Guo, M., & Dawson, G. (2012). Effects of a brief Early Start Denver Model (ESDM)–based parent intervention on toddlers at risk for autism spectrum disorders: A randomized controlled trial. *Journal of the American Academy of Child & Adolescent Psychiatry, 51*(10), 1052–1065.

Rogers, S. J., & Pennington, B. F. (1991). A theoretical approach to the deficits in infantile autism. *Development and Psychopathology, 3*(2), 137–162.

Rojas, D. C., Singel, D., Steinmetz, S., Hepburn, S., & Brown, M. S. (2014). Decreased left perisylvian GABA concentration in children with autism and unaffected siblings. *NeuroImage, 86*, 28–34.

Rossignol, D. A., Genuis, S. J., & Frye, R. E. (2014). Environmental toxicants and autism spectrum disorders: A systematic review. *Translational Psychiatry, 4*(2), e360.

Roullet, F. I., Lai, J. K., & Foster, J. A. (2013). In utero exposure to valproic acid and autism—A current review of clinical and animal studies. *Neurotoxicology and Teratology, 36*, 47–56.

Rutter, M. (1968). Concepts of autism: A review of research. *Journal of Child Psychology and Psychiatry, and Allied Disciplines, 9*(1), 1–25.

Rutter, M. (1978a). Diagnosis and definition of childhood autism. *Journal of Autism and Childhood Schizophrenia, 8*(2), 139–161.

Rutter, M. (1978b). Diagnosis and definition. In M. Rutter & E. Schopler (Eds.), *Autism* (pp. 1–25). Springer.

Sagar-Ouriaghli, I., Lievesley, K., & Santosh, P. J. (2018). Propranolol for treating emotional, behavioural, autonomic dysregulation in children and adolescents with autism spectrum disorders. *Journal of Psychopharmacology, 32*(6), 641–653.

Sandin, S., Lichtenstein, P., Kuja-Halkola, R., Larsson, H., Hultman, C. M., & Reichenberg, A. (2014). The familial risk of autism. *JAMA, 311*(17), 1770–1777.

Santos, M., Uppal, N., Butti, C., Wicinski, B., Schmeidler, J., Giannakopoulos, P., Heinsen, H., Schmitz, C., & Hof, P. R. (2011). Von Economo neurons in autism: A stereologic study of the frontoinsular cortex in children. *Brain Research, 1380*, 206–217.

Sasaki, E., Suemizu, H., Shimada, A., Hanazawa, K., Oiwa, R., Kamioka, M., Tomioka, I., Sotomaru, Y., Hirakawa, R., Eto, T., Shiozawa, S., Maeda, T., Ito, M., Ito, R., Kito, C., Yagihashi, C., Kawai, K., Miyoshi, H., Tanioka, Y., . . . Nomura, T. (2009). Generation of transgenic non-human primates with germline transmission. *Nature, 459*(7246), 523–527.

Sasson, N. J., Lam, K. S., Childress, D., Parlier, M., Daniels, J. L., & Piven, J. (2013). The Broad Autism Phenotype Questionnaire: Prevalence and diagnostic classification. *Autism Research*, *6*(2), 134–143.

Sawiak, S. J., Shiba, Y., Oikonomidis, L., Windle, C. P., Santangelo, A. M., Grydeland, H., Cockcroft, G., Bullmore, E., & Roberts, A. C. (2018). Trajectories and milestones of cortical and subcortical development of the marmoset brain from infancy to adulthood. *Cerebral Cortex*, *28*(12), 4440–4453.

Schopler, E., Van Bourgondien, M. E., Wellman, G. J., & Love, S. R. (2010). *CARS-2: Childhood Autism Rating Scale–Second Edition*. Western Psychological Services.

Schreibman, L., Dawson, G., Stahmer, A. C., Landa, R., Rogers, S. J., McGee, G. G., Kasari, C., Ingersoll, B., Kaiser, A., Bruinsma, Y., McNerney, E., Wetherby, A., & Halladay, A. (2015). Naturalistic developmental behavioral interventions: Empirically validated treatments for autism spectrum disorder. *Journal of Autism and Developmental Disorders*, *45*(8), 2411–2428.

Schumann, C. M., & Amaral, D. G. (2006). Stereological analysis of amygdala neuron number in autism. *Journal of Neuroscience*, *26*(29), 7674–7679.

Seki, F., Hikishima, K., Komaki, Y., Hata, J., Uematsu, A., Okahara, N., Yamamoto, M., Shinohara, H., Sasaki, E., & Okano, H. (2017). Developmental trajectories of macroanatomical structures in common marmoset brain. *Neuroscience*, *364*, 143–156.

Shelton, J. F., Geraghty, E. M., Tancredi, D. J., Delwiche, L. D., Schmidt, R. J., Ritz, B., Hansen, R., & Hertz-Picciotto, I. (2014). Neurodevelopmental disorders and prenatal residential proximity to agricultural pesticides: The CHARGE study. *Environmental Health Perspectives*, *122*(10), 1103–1109.

Shen, M. D. (2018). Cerebrospinal fluid and the early brain development of autism. *Journal of Neurodevelopmental Disorders*, *10*(1), Article 39.

Shephard, E., Bedford, R., Milosavljevic, B., Gliga, T., Jones, E. J., Pickles, A., Johnson, M., & Charman, T.; BASIS Team. (2019). Early developmental pathways to childhood symptoms of attention-deficit hyperactivity disorder, anxiety and autism spectrum disorder. *Journal of Child Psychology and Psychiatry*, *60*(9), 963–974.

Sigman, M. (1989). The application of developmental knowledge to a clinical problem: The study of childhood autism. In D. Cicchetti (Ed.), *The emergence of a discipline: Rochester Symposium on Developmental Psychopathology* (Vol. 1, pp. 165–187). Erlbaum.

Simons, J., & Oishi, S. (1987). *The hidden child: The Linwood method for reaching the autistic child*. Woodbine House.

Siu, M. T., & Weksberg, R. (2017). Epigenetics of autism spectrum disorder. *Advances in Experimental Medicine and Biology*, *978*, 63–90.

Smith, T., & Eikeseth, S. (2011). O. Ivar Lovaas: Pioneer of applied behavior analysis and intervention for children with autism. *Journal of Autism and Developmental Disorders*, *41*(3), 375–378.

Sparks, B. F., Friedman, S. D., Shaw, D. W., Aylward, E. H., Echelard, D., Artru, A. A., Maravilla, K., Giedd, J., Munson, J., Dawson, G., & Dager, S. R. (2002). Brain structural abnormalities in young children with autism spectrum disorder. *Neurology*, *59*(2), 184–192.

Staal, W. G., Langen, M., Van Dijk, S., Mensen, V. T., & Durston, S. (2015). DRD3 gene and striatum in autism spectrum disorder. *British Journal of Psychiatry*, *206*(5), 431–432.

Stern, D. N. (1985). *The interpersonal world of the infant: A view from psychoanalysis and developmental psychology*. Basic Books.

Strain, P. S., & Bovey, E. H. (2011). Randomized, controlled trial of the LEAP model of early intervention for young children with autism spectrum disorders. *Topics in Early Childhood Special Education*, *31*(3), 133–154.

Strasser, L., Downes, M., Kung, J., Cross, J. H., & De Haan, M. (2018). Prevalence and risk factors for autism spectrum disorder in epilepsy: A systematic review and meta-analysis. *Developmental Medicine & Child Neurology*, *60*(1), 19–29.

Strawn, J. R., Welge, J. A., Wehry, A. M., Keeshin, B., & Rynn, M. A. (2015). Efficacy and tolerability of antidepressants in pediatric anxiety disorders: A systematic review and meta-analysis. *Depression and Anxiety*, *32*(3), 149–157.

Strömland, K., Nordin, V., Miller, M., Akerström, B., & Gillberg, C. (1994). Autism in thalido-mide embryopathy: A population study. *Developmental Medicine & Child Neurology*, *36*(4), 351–356.

Sturman, N., Deckx, L., & van Driel, M. L. (2017). Methylphenidate for children and adolescents with autism spectrum disorder. *Cochrane Database of Systematic Reviews*, *11*(11), CD011144.

Sullivan, P. F., Magnusson, C., Reichenberg, A., Boman, M., Dalman, C., Davidson, M., Fruchter, E., Hultman, C., Lundberg, M., Langstrom, N., Weiser, M., Svensson, A., & Lichtenstein, P. (2012). Family history of schizophrenia and bipolar disorder as risk factors for autism. *Archives of General Psychiatry*, *69*(11), 1099–1103.

Szatmari, P., Georgiades, S., Bryson, S., Zwaigenbaum, L., Roberts, W., Mahoney, W., Goldberg, J., & Tuff, L. (2006). Investigating the structure of the restricted, repetitive behaviours and interests domain of autism. *Journal of Child Psychology and Psychiatry*, *47*(6), 582–590.

Szatmari, P., Georgiades, S., Duku, E., Bennett, T. A., Bryson, S., Fombonne, E., Mirenda, P., Roberts, W., Smith, I., Vaillancourt, T., Volden, J., & Waddell, C., Zwaigenbaum, L., Elsabbagh, M., Thompson, A., & Pathways in ASD Study Team. (2015). Developmental trajectories of symptom severity and adaptive functioning in an inception cohort of preschool children with autism spectrum disorder. *JAMA Psychiatry*, *72*(3), 276–283.

Sztainberg, Y., & Zoghbi, H. Y. (2016). Lessons learned from studying syndromic autism spec-trum disorders. *Nature Neuroscience*, *19*(11), 1408–1417.

Tachibana, M., Kagitani-Shimono, K., Mohri, I., Yamamoto, T., Sanefuji, W., Nakamura, A., Oishi, M., Kimura, T., Onaka, T., Ozono, K., & Taniike, M. (2013). Long-term administration of intranasal oxytocin is a safe and promising therapy for early adolescent boys with autism spectrum disorders. *Journal of Child and Adolescent Psychopharmacology*, *23*(2), 123–127.

Tang, G., Gudsnuk, K., Kuo, S. H., Cotrina, M. L., Rosoklija, G., Sosunov, A., Sonders, M., Kanter, E., Castagna, C., Yamamoto, A., Yue, Z., Arancio, O., Peterson, B., Champagne, F., Dwork, A., Goldman, J., & Sulzer, D. (2014). Loss of mTOR-dependent macroautophagy causes autistic-like synaptic pruning deficits. *Neuron*, *83*(5), 1131–1143.

Taylor, L. E., Swerdfeger, A. L., & Eslick, G. D. (2014). Vaccines are not associated with autism: An evidence-based meta-analysis of case–control and cohort studies. *Vaccine*, *32*(29), 3623–3629.

Thomas, S., Hovinga, M. E., Rai, D., & Lee, B. (2017). Brief report: Prevalence of co-occurring epi-lepsy and autism spectrum disorder: The U.S. National Survey of Children's Health 2011–2012. *Journal of Autism and Developmental Disorders*, *47*(1), 224–229.

Trevarthen, C. (1979). Communication and cooperation in early infancy. A description of pri-mary intersubjectivity. In M. Bullowa (Ed.), *Before speech: The beginnings of human communi-cation* (pp. 321–346). Cambridge University Press.

Trevarthen, C., & Aitken, K. J. (2001). Infant intersubjectivity: Research, theory, and clinical applications. *Journal of Child Psychology and Psychiatry*, *42*(1), 3–48.

Trubetskoy, V., Pardiñas, A. F., Qi, T., Panagiotaropoulou, G., Awasthi, S., Bigdeli, T. B., Bryois, J., Chen, C. Y., Dennison, C. A., Hall, L. S., Lam, M., Watanabe, K., Frei, O., Ge, T., Harwood, J. C., Koopmans, F., Magnusson, S., Richards, A. L., Sidorenko, J., & Wu, Y.; Schizophrenia Working Group of the Psychiatric Genomics Consortium. (2022). Mapping genomic loci implicates genes and synaptic biology in schizophrenia. *Nature*, *604*(7906), 502–508.

Tu, Z., Zhao, H., Li, B., Yan, S., Wang, L., Tang, Y., Li, Z., Bai, D., Li, C., Lin, Y., Li, Y., Liu, J., Xu, H., Guo, X., Jiang, Y., Zhang, Y., & Li, X. J. (2019). CRISPR/Cas9-mediated disruption of SHANK3 in monkey leads to drug-treatable autism-like symptoms. *Human Molecular Genetics*, *28*(4), 561–571.

Uddin, L. Q., Supekar, K., & Menon, V. (2013). Reconceptualizing functional brain connectivity in autism from a developmental perspective. *Frontiers in Human Neuroscience*, *7*, Article 458.

Uematsu, A., Hata, J., Komaki, Y., Seki, F., Yamada, C., Okahara, N., Kurotaki, Y., Sasaki, E., & Okano, H. (2017). Mapping orbitofrontal–limbic maturation in non-human primates: A longi-tudinal magnetic resonance imaging study. *NeuroImage*, *163*, 55–67.

Umbricht, D., del Valle Rubido, M., Hollander, E., McCracken, J. T., Shic, F., Scahill, L., Noeldeke, J., Boak, L., Khwaja, O., Squassante, L., Grundschober, C., Kletzl, H., & Fontoura, P. (2017). A single dose, randomized, controlled proof-of-mechanism study of a novel vasopressin 1a receptor antagonist (RG7713) in high-functioning adults with autism spectrum disorder. *Neuropsychopharmacology, 42*(9), 1914–1923.

Varghese, M., Keshav, N., Jacot-Descombes, S., Warda, T., Wicinski, B., Dickstein, D. L., Harony-Nicolas, H., De Rubeis, S., Drapeau, E., Buxbaum, J., & Hof, P. R. (2017). Autism spectrum disorder: Neuropathology and animal models. *Acta Neuropathologica, 134*(4), 537–566.

Vasa, R. A., Mazurek, M. O., Mahajan, R., Bennett, A. E., Bernal, M. P., Nozzolillo, A. A., Arnold, L., & Coury, D. L. (2016). Assessment and treatment of anxiety in youth with autism spectrum disorders. *Pediatrics, 137*(Suppl. 2), S115–S123.

Venter, A., Lord, C., & Schopler, E. (1992). A follow-up study of high-functioning autistic children. *Journal of Child Psychology and Psychiatry, 33*(3), 489–597.

Vicedo, M., & Ilerbaig, J. (2021). Autism in Baltimore, 1938–1943. *Journal of Autism and Developmental Disorders, 51*(4), 1157–1172.

Virues-Ortega, J., Julio, F. M., & Pastor-Barriuso, R. (2013). The TEACCH program for children and adults with autism: A meta-analysis of intervention studies. *Clinical Psychology Review, 33*(8), 940–953.

Wallace, G. L., Dankner, N., Kenworthy, L., Giedd, J. N., & Martin, A. (2010). Age-related temporal and parietal cortical thinning in autism spectrum disorders. *Brain, 133*(12), 3745–3754.

Warren, Z., McPheeters, M. L., Sathe, N., Foss-Feig, J. H., Glasser, A., & Veenstra-VanderWeele, J. (2011). A systematic review of early intensive intervention for autism spectrum disorders. *Pediatrics, 127*(5), e1303–e1311.

Washington, S. D., Gordon, E. M., Brar, J., Warburton, S., Sawyer, A. T., Wolfe, A., Mease-Ference, E., Girton, L., Hailu, A., Mbwana, J., Gaillard, W., Kalbfleisch, M., & VanMeter, J. W. (2014). Dysmaturation of the default mode network in autism. *Human brain mapping, 35*(4), 1284–1296.

Wechsler, D. (2003). *Wechsler Intelligence Scale for Children–Fourth Edition (WISC-IV).* Psychological Corporation.

Whitehouse, D., & Harris, J. C. (1984). Hyperlexia in infantile autism. *Journal of Autism and Developmental Disorders, 14*(3), 281–289.

Whitney, E. R., Kemper, T. L., Rosene, D. L., Bauman, M. L., & Blatt, G. J. (2009). Density of cerebellar basket and stellate cells in autism: Evidence for a late developmental loss of Purkinje cells. *Journal of Neuroscience Research, 87*(10), 2245–2254.

Wolff, J. J., Gu, H., Gerig, G., Elison, J. T., Styner, M., Gouttard, S., Botteron, K., Dagar, S., Dawson, G., Estes, A., Evans, A., Hazlett, H., Kostopoulos, P., McKinstry, R., Paterson, S., Schultz, R., Zwaigenbaum, L., Piven, J., & IBIS Network. (2012). Differences in white matter fiber tract development present from 6 to 24 months in infants with autism. *American Journal of Psychiatry, 169*(6), 589–600.

World Health Organization. (1992). *The lCD-10 classification of mental and behavioural disorders: Clinical descriptions and diagnostic guidelines.*

Wu, S., Wu, F., Ding, Y., Hou, J., Bi, J., & Zhang, Z. (2017). Advanced parental age and autism risk in children: A systematic review and meta-analysis. *Acta Psychiatrica Scandinavica, 135*(1), 29–41.

Yeung, M. K. (2022). A systematic review and meta-analysis of facial emotion recognition in autism spectrum disorder: The specificity of deficits and the role of task characteristics. *Neuroscience and Biobehavioral Reviews, 133*, 104518.

Yoshimasu, K., Kiyohara, C., Takemura, S., & Nakai, K. (2014). A meta-analysis of the evidence on the impact of prenatal and early infancy exposures to mercury on autism and attention deficit/hyperactivity disorder in the childhood. *Neurotoxicology, 44*, 121–131.

Yucel, G. H., Belger, A., Bizzell, J., Parlier, M., Adolphs, R., & Piven, J. (2015). Abnormal neural activation to faces in the parents of children with autism. *Cerebral Cortex, 25*(12), 4653–4666.

Zhang, B., Zhou, Z., Zhou, Y., Zhang, T., Ma, Y., Niu, Y., Ji, W., & Chen, Y. (2019). Social-valence-related increased attention in Rett syndrome cynomolgus monkeys: An eye-tracking study. *Autism Research, 12*(11), 1585–1597.

Zheng, Z., Zhu, T., Qu, Y., & Mu, D. (2016). Blood glutamate levels in autism spectrum disorder: A systematic review and meta-analysis. *PLoS One, 11*(7), e0158688.

Zhao, H., Tu, Z., Xu, H., Yan, S., Yan, H., Zheng, Y., Yang, W., Zheng, J., Li, Z., Tian, R., Lu, Y., Guo, X., Jiang, Y., Li, X., H., & Zhang, Y. Q. (2017). Altered neurogenesis and disrupted expression of synaptic proteins in prefrontal cortex of SHANK3-deficient non-human primate. *Cell Research*, 27(10), 1293–1297.

Zoghbi, H. Y., & Bear, M. F. (2012). Synaptic dysfunction in neurodevelopmental disorders associated with autism and intellectual disabilities. *Cold Spring Harbor Perspectives in Biology*, 4(3), a009886.

# 16

# Attention-Deficit/Hyperactivity Disorder

Attention-deficit/hyperactivity disorder (ADHD) is the most common neurodevelopmental disorder diagnosed in children who are seen in psychiatric clinics. It is estimated to affect children worldwide with an overall prevalence of 5% and is a factor in one-third of referrals to child psychiatric clinics. In addition to their attentional problems, difficulties with social perception and social awareness commonly occur, leading to psychosocial difficulties. Still, it is not simply attention deficits but, rather, impulsivity, overactivity, executive dysfunction, inappropriate social behavior, and problems in interpersonal relationships that lead to these clinic referrals. Oppositional defiant disorder, conduct problems, poor self-attitude, mood disorder, and anxiety symptoms are frequently comorbid.

This chapter reviews ADHD with an emphasis on the associated social cognitive and affect regulation problems that lead to dysfunctional relationships in the family and at school. It reviews the history, classification, epidemiology, etiology, environmental risk factors, neuroimaging, neurochemistry, social cognitive domain, interpersonal aspects, effect of the disorder on others, developmental course, diagnostic assessment, and treatment for this disorder. The fifth edition of the *Diagnostic and Statistical Manual of Mental Disorders* (DSM-5; American Psychiatric Association [APA], 2013) designation for this disorder is ADHD. This abbreviation is used throughout the chapter.

## History

Attentional difficulties and overactivity were recognized in disabled children during the second half of the 19th century. The first reports are in textbooks on intellectual developmental disorder (IDD; Ireland, 1877; Tredgold, 1908). The hyperactive child entered the folklore of the late 1800s with Reverend Dr. Heinrich Hoffmann's (1862) popular poem, "The Story of Fidgety Phillip." Yet the associated behavioral aspects in typically developing children were not well described until the beginning of the 20th century when George Still, assistant physician to the Hospital for Sick Children in London, gave three lectures under the title, "Some Abnormal Psychical Conditions in Children." In these Goulstonian Lectures, Still (1902) described as "abnormal incapacity for sustained attention, restlessness, fidgetiness, violent outbursts, destructiveness, noncompliance, choreiform movements, and minor congenital anomalies." His focus, however, was on a defect in moral self-control in children. He emphasized the psychosocial aspects of their attentional problems when he wrote, "Interesting as these disorders may be as an abstruse problem for the professed psychologist to puzzle over, they have a real practical—shall I say social—importance which I venture to think has been hardly sufficiently recognized." He went on to describe their problems in self-control in social situations. It is in this area that the child's difficulty impacts on family functioning.

Still's (1902) stated intention was to describe a morbid defect in volition. He used the term "moral self-control" to refer to "the control of action for the good of all" and noted that moral control can exist only when there is a sufficient cognitive understanding of one's relationship to others. However, Still maintained that intellectual understanding is not enough; volitional control is also necessary. He went on to describe developmental aspects of these conditions and referred to the slow and gradual development of inhibitory volition as the child grows older. He suggested it is a lack in the inhibitory nature of volition to "overpower" a stimulus that leads to excessive activity. He also noted that inhibitory volition becomes directed toward those forms of activity that are the most instinctive—for example, the expression of emotions.

Still (1902) viewed moral control as multidetermined and acknowledged that later outcome depended on the cognitive interrelationship with the environment, with moral consciousness, and with volition. In his subsequent lectures, he provided examples to demonstrate that IDD, a purely cognitive defect, was not the cause of a self-control deficit because neurotypically developing individuals may show far more severe behavioral defects than those with IDD. He offered a series of case examples of defects in moral control and categorized them as congenital cases: those acquired following brain injury, those with permanent symptoms, those with temporary symptoms, and those in which behavioral control was cyclical.

In subsequent years, different aspects of Still's original description have been emphasized (E. A. Taylor, 1986). Barkley (1990) describes several periods, noting an initial focus on the brain-damaged child (1900–1960), then a specific emphasis on hyperactivity (1960–1969), followed by the ascendance of attention deficits (1970–1979), and, finally, the establishment of diagnostic criteria and the waning of attention deficits (1980–1989). Barkley (1990) offers a renewed focus on volitional control and emphasizes the importance of rule-governed behavior along with problems associated with inhibitory control.

In the United States, attention deficits came to medical attention following the 1917–1918 influenza pandemic. Children who survived often had significant behavioral and cognitive difficulties (Bender, 1942; Bond & Appel, 1931; Ebaugh, 1923; Hohman, 1922; Kessler, 1980). The children who were affected during the influenza epidemic often developed overactivity, attention deficits, and impulse control problems, whereas affected adults were more likely to develop parkinsonian symptoms as a sequelae. Such different presentations, depending on the age of the insult, highlighted the importance of the onset of the disorder during the developmental period. The fact that the occurrence of an infectious disease in infancy or in childhood could lead to a different behavioral presentation than the onset in adulthood was an early basis for a developmental perspective on brain–behavior relationships.

These early studies concluded that not only the influenza infection during the Great Pandemic of 1918 but also other cerebral insults, such as measles infection, birth trauma, lead toxicity, head trauma, and seizures, can cause severe restlessness; less severe behavioral symptoms may result from interpersonal difficulties or stress. The term "organic driveness" was used by Kahn and Cohen (1934) to describe the behavioral abnormality thought to be a consequence of brain stem involvement that led to behavioral disorganization. Levin (1938) suggested that severe restlessness in children resulted from pathological changes in forebrain structures. With regard to treatment, Bradley (1937) and Bradley and Bowen (1940) reported that benzedine (amphetamine sulfate) reduced hyperactivity and improved attention in children with behavioral difficulties.

By the 1940s, the concept of hyperactivity and inattention had been broadened further so that hyperactivity alone was often considered adequate evidence for a diagnosis of brain damage (Strauss & Werner, 1943). Strauss and Lehtinen (1947) attributed brain injury to children who presented with these behavioral characteristics although brain pathology was not clearly documented by history or physical examination. Yet Strauss and Werner (1943) did see similarities between hyperactive children and adults who lost control after neurological injury or stroke. Strauss referred to this as the "brain-injured child syndrome," and Strauss and Lehtinen suggested approaches to education. In the 1950s, it came to be known as the "Strauss syndrome."

By the late 1950s (Laufer & Denhoff, 1957; Laufer et al., 1957), the diagnostic term "hyperkinetic impulsive disorder" was used for children with emotional and conduct problems. Hyperkinetic impulse disorder was identified as a condition involving the brain in children who had no overt evidence of brain damage; its designation as a disorder was considered to be a corrective to the prevailing psychodynamic view that focused primarily on the parents' contribution to causing children's problems. The identification of positive drug treatment effects on behavior and findings of abnormalities on physiologic testing in affected children were followed by a dramatic increase in both biological and pharmacological research on this condition.

Critical reviews began to appear in the 1960s that questioned whether there was an identifiable brain syndrome in children, suggesting instead multiple syndromes. These reviews (Birch, 1964; Rapin, 1964) acknowledged that behavioral symptoms may result from brain damage but questioned whether the term "brain damage" was appropriate for children with behavioral problems who had only equivocal evidence of dysfunction on neurological examination. The confusion about the appropriate label was highlighted by a task force that found 37 different labels were being used for the same type of clinical presentation (Clements, 1966). The task force found that neurological, psychiatric, and educational terms were all being applied to the same children and suggested the name of the disorder be changed. Recommendations included "minimal brain dysfunction" (MBD), "minimal cerebral dysfunction," and "central nervous system dysfunction." In each instance, the word "damage" was removed from the diagnostic label. Of these, MBD became the most commonly used term (Wender, 1971). Minimal was used to distinguish it from major cerebral dysfunction, such as that seen in cerebral palsy, some IDD syndromes, and other brain-related syndromes.

The prevailing view on hyperactivity was that it was part of a brain dysfunction syndrome but of milder degree than previously considered. Despite the lack of agreement regarding etiology, the term MBD gained widespread use. Moreover, it was recognized that although brain damage could cause behavioral symptoms, genetic factors are important. Because many children do not have evidence of prenatal, perinatal, or postnatal insults, a genetic and developmental etiology was considered. Moreover, parents were noted to have similar problems as those of their children during their own childhood and, in some instances, into adulthood. It was thought that the environment played a role in modifying its behavioral presentation. Current evidence indicates that ADHD has heritability approaching 90% (Geschwind & Flint, 2015).

Like the prior brain damage explanation, MBD gradually was also recognized as too vague, overly inclusive, and not supported by evidence of neurological dysfunction. With increasing scrutiny, MBD was gradually replaced by labels that focused on specific cognitive, learning, and behavior disorders, such as dyslexia, learning disability, and, finally, hyperactivity. In this period, the emphasis increasingly shifted to hyperactivity as the most important symptom of MBD. Still, affected children continued to be recognized as at the mercy of background stimulation, having difficulty in concentrating and inhibiting activity. Chess (1960), in discussing hyperactivity as the defining feature, stressed the need for objective evidence, separated hyperactivity from brain damage, and concurred that the behavior was not the result of dysfunctional parenting. These distinctions prepared the way for the inclusion of hyperkinetic behavior into the APA's 1968 diagnostic and classification system.

## Classification

With the introduction of the DSM-II (APA, 1968), a new section was added on child and adolescent disorders, and the syndrome of childhood hyperactivity formally entered the system of classification as "hyperkinetic reaction of childhood or adolescence." In DSM-I (APA, 1952), the term "reaction" accompanied many diagnostic categories— for example, affective reaction and schizophrenic reaction—because of concerns about prematurely creating a rigid nosological concept of disease. With the publication of DSM-II, the term reaction was, for the most part, eliminated so that affective disorder and schizophrenia were introduced as specific diagnostic categories. However, the term reaction continued to be applied to the newly created childhood category, hence the designation "hyperkinetic reaction" under the category of behavior disorders of childhood and adolescence. These disorders were considered to be more stable, internalized, and resistant to treatment than transient situational disturbances—that is, they were considered more pervasive. The hyperkinetic reaction was characterized by "overactivity, restlessness, distractibility, and short attention span, especially in young children; the behavior usually diminishes in adolescence" (p. 50).

In North America, with the introduction of DSM-II, the "hyperkinetic reaction of childhood or adolescence" was viewed as a behavioral syndrome with characteristic excessive activity. It was thought to be a common disturbance that was not necessarily associated with brain damage and, in fact, was possibly a normal variant of temperament in some instances. In Great Britain, however, hyperkinetic disorder continued to be viewed as extremely uncommon. In the Isle of Wight survey, Rutter et al. (1970) found that hyperkinetic behavior was infrequent in 9-year-olds. In Great Britain, the brain-damaged model seems to have persisted, and the syndrome was thought to be quite uncommon. When present, it was associated primarily with epilepsy, IDD, and hemiplegia (E. A. Taylor, 1988).

During the 1970s, features other than the hyperactivity emphasized in DSM-II were increasingly addressed, especially distractibility and short attention span. The existence of a pure syndrome of hyperactivity was questioned (August & Stewart, 1982).

The concept of MBD faded as critical reviews appeared, such as those of Rutter (1977, 1982) emphasizing that MBD symptoms were not well defined, the condition was heterogeneous, there was poor internal correlation among symptoms, and the symptoms lacked specific etiological significance and showed no common course or outcome. During the 1970s, additional research (Douglas, 1972) highlighted the importance of sustained attention and impulse control in the diagnosis. Using a continuous performance test, Douglas found that these children had difficulty on vigilance tasks and tasks of sustained attention. Variability in their task performance was the most significant feature. She emphasized deficits in investment, organization, and maintenance of attention; inability to inhibit impulsive responding; inability to modulate arousal levels to meet specific situational demands; and a strong inclination to seek immediate environmental reinforcement. This and subsequent research on attention led to the renaming of the disorder "attention deficit disorder" (ADD) in 1980, with the publication of the DSM-III (APA, 1980). Deficits in sustained attention and impulse control were recognized as having greater clinical significance than hyperactivity. This new focus provided some increased specificity because research on hyperactivity had shown no clear delineation between normal and abnormal levels of activity, although Porrino and colleagues (1983) subsequently did demonstrate that activity was quantitatively greater in a group of affected children.

The DSM-III criteria provided greater emphasis on inattention and impulsivity as defining features and included a specific symptom list with numerical cutoff points for symptoms, guidelines for age of onset and duration of symptoms, and exclusionary criteria. DSM-III also created subtypes of attention deficit disorder with hyperactivity (ADDH) and without hyperactivity. Children with attention deficit disorder without hyperactivity were characteristically less active than those with ADDH, lethargic, learning disabled, and tended to daydream (Carlson, 1986).

During the 1980s, research criteria also were developed (Barkley, 1982; Loney, 1983). Loney and others (Loney et al., 1978; Milich et al., 1982; Milich & Landau, 1989) focused on differentiating the symptoms of hyperactivity from those of aggression or conduct disorder. Loney demonstrated that a short list of symptoms for hyperactivity could be empirically separated from a short list of aggressive symptoms. The demonstration of a separate aggression cluster established that negative outcomes of hyperactivity during adolescence and young adulthood most likely may be due to the concurrent presence and extent of aggression because both symptoms co-occur. Purely aggressive children did not show substantial problems with attention; purely hyperactive children did. In addition, greater psychopathology in the families of hyperactive children was found to be related to the extent of aggressiveness in the children. Aggression was more likely to be associated with environmental circumstances and family dysfunction; hyperactivity was linked to developmental immaturity. Efforts to subtype ADDH increasingly focused on associated language-based learning disabilities; pervasive versus situational hyperactivity; and co-occurring symptoms of anxiety, depression, and compulsive behavior. Co-occurring symptoms began to be studied in reference to response to pharmacological interventions.

An international symposium on research diagnostic criteria for ADD was convened (Sergeant, 1988), and the following criteria were proposed for subjects enrolled in research study: (a) reports of problems with activity and attention from two independent sources (e.g., home, school, and psychiatric clinic), (b) endorsement of at least three or four difficulties with activity and three or four with attention, (c) age of onset before 7 years, (d) duration of 2 years, (e) significantly elevated scores on parent–teacher ratings of ADD symptoms, and (f) exclusion of autistic disorder and psychosis.

The diagnostic criteria in the DSM-III revision published in 1987 (DSM-III-R; APA, 1987) were changed. ADDH was now designated "attention deficit hyperactivity disorder" (ADHD). This change took place because ADDH was more common and better defined than the syndrome without hyperactivity. In the DSM-III-R classification, a single-item list of symptoms and a single cutoff score replaced the three DSM-III clusters (i.e., inattention, impulsivity, and hyperactivity) and the cutoff scores used individually for them in DSM-III. In DSM-III-R, the item list was based on empirically derived dimensions of child behavior drawn from behavior rating scales. The cutoff scores and the items were chosen following a large field trial conducted to evaluate their sensitivity, specificity, and distinguishing features. In DSM-III-R, it was emphasized that the symptoms were developmentally inappropriate to the child's mental age, and the coexistence of affective disorders with ADHD was no longer an exclusionary criterion for the diagnosis of ADHD. Finally, the category of ADD without hyperactivity was removed and a new category, "undifferentiated attention deficit disorder," was added to incorporated as a reminder that additional subtyping might be possible. ADHD was classified as part of a new grouping, the disruptive behavior disorders, along with oppositional defiant disorder and conduct disorder.

In DSM-IV (APA, 1994), the categorization was further revised and refined. Three general designations were introduced: attention deficit/hyperactivity disorder, predominantly inattentive type; attention deficit/hyperactivity disorder, predominantly hyperactive–impulsive type; and attention deficit/hyperactivity disorder, combined type. In addition, there was a residual category, attention deficit/hyperactivity disorder not otherwise specified.

In DSM-5 (APA, 2013), ADHD is defined as a persistent pattern of inattention and/or hyperactivity–impulsivity that interferes with functioning or development. For inattention, six or more symptoms of inattention for children up to age 16 years or five or more for adolescents aged 17 years and older and adults are required. The symptoms of inattention must be present for at least 6 months, and they are inappropriate for the developmental level. For hyperactivity and impulsivity, six or more symptoms of hyperactivity–impulsivity for children up to age 16 years or five or more for adolescents aged 17 years and older and adults are required. The symptoms of hyperactivity–impulsivity must have been present for at least 6 months to an extent that is disruptive and inappropriate for the person's development level.

There are three presentations. Combined presentation is used if enough symptoms of both criteria in attention and hyperactivity–impulsivity are present for the past 6 months. Predominately inattentive is used if enough symptoms of inattention but not hyperactivity–impulsivity were present for the past 6 months. Predominately hyperactive–impulsive presentation is used if enough symptoms of hyperactivity–impulsivity but not inattention were present for the past 6 months. Moreover, symptoms can change over time. Symptoms look different at older ages. For example, in adults, hyperactivity is extreme restlessness.

DSM-5 introduced several significant changes in relation to the DSM-IV Text Revision (DSM-IV-TR; APA, 2000). First, the threshold in the number of symptoms (Criterion A) necessary for the diagnosis in older adolescents and adults was reduced from six to five. Despite a reduction in the number of symptoms during development, adults with ADHD in childhood also contributed the majority of adults diagnosed with ADHD. The required age of onset was increased from prior to age 7 years in DSM-IV TR to prior to age 12 years. Another pivotal change in DSM-5 is the removal of the veto around the dual diagnosis of ADHD and autism spectrum disorders that was present in previous editions of the DSM. This change is supported by evidence (Visser et al., 2016).

These changes in DSM-5 reflect recent empirical evidence and/or practical needs in the diagnostic process. However, there are issues that still need to be addressed in future classifications. Importantly, current criteria continue to focus on the number of symptoms rather than on a more precise definition of functional impairment. Second, each of the symptoms listed in the DSM Criterion A carries the same weight; it has been argued that inattention should be more heavily weighted than hyperactivity–impulsivity.

## Extended Definition of Attention Deficit Disorder: Executive Dysfunction

Although not included in the DSM-5 classification, Barkley (Barkley, 1997, 2010; Barkley & Fischer, 2019) proposed a consensus definition of ADHD that highlights the developmental nature of behavioral inhibition, self-regulation of motivation, and working memory. His theoretical model links inhibition to four executive neuropsychological functions that depend on it for their effective execution: (a) working memory, (b) self-regulation of affect–motivation–arousal, (c) internalization of speech, and (d) reconstitution (behavioral analysis and synthesis). Extended to ADHD, the model predicts that ADHD is associated with secondary impairments in these four executive functions and the motor control that results. Barkley emphasized the issue of volition and extended the definition of ADD. In the extended definition, a functional aspect is added by highlighting deficient rule-governed behavior and difficulties in maintaining work performance. Barkley's (1997) extended definition is as follows:

> Attention-deficit/hyperactivity disorder is a developmental disorder characterized by developmentally inappropriate degrees of inattention, overactivity, and impulsivity. These difficulties are typically associated with deficits in executive rule governed behavior and in maintaining a consistent pattern of work performance over time. Rule-governed behavior refers to the capacity for language, i.e., commands, directions, instructions, descriptions to act as "discriminative stimulus for behavior." Rules specify contingencies for action. Understanding the ways in which deficits in executive function contribute to the symptoms of ADHD can help in differentiating ADHD from disorders that share similar characteristics.

## Motivational Deficit Disorder: Executive Dysfunction

Barkley's (1997, 2010) extended definition suggests that ADHD should be viewed as a disorder of motivation rather than only of attention and that deficits in rule-governed behavior may account for many of the behaviors. In this view, ADHD might stem from an insensitivity to environmental consequences, either reinforcement or punishment. A motivational model provides greater explanatory value to account for situational variability in attention and is consistent with recent neuroanatomic studies that suggest decreased activation of brain reward centers and associated corticolimbic regulating circuits (Lou et al., 1989). It is also consistent with neurotransmitter studies implicating dopamine pathways in regulating not only locomotor behavior but also learning based on incentives.

Another view consistent with deficits in rule-governed behavior, as described by Barkley, is that of Denckla (1989), who extends the definition further when she suggests that many children with ADHD have features of executive dysfunction. In keeping with this proposal, she has used neuropsychological tests to identify difficulty with planning and sequencing complex behaviors, difficulty paying attention to several features at once, reduced capacity to grasp the gist of a complex situation, resistance to distraction and interference, inhibition of inappropriate response tendencies, and reduced ability to maintain behavioral output over time. Particular problems were noted with organizing, planning, and managing time.

## Epidemiology

Attention-deficit/hyperactivity disorder is the most common neurodevelopmental disorder in children, with an estimated worldwide prevalence of approximately 5% (Polanczyk et al., 2007). Although it has long been considered a childhood disorder, it is now well established that impairing ADHD symptoms persist into adulthood in 65% of cases (Sibley et al., 2016). The disorder occurs more commonly in boys than in girls and more often in lower socioeconomic settings. ADD without hyperactivity is more common in adolescence than in childhood (Szatmari et al., 1989).

There is a high co-occurrence between ADHD and other disruptive behavior disorders, particularly conduct disorder. In the Ontario Child Health Survey (Szatmari et al., 1989), 42% of boys with ADDH, aged 4–11 years, and 36% of girls with ADDH, aged 4–11 years, had co-occurring conduct disorder, with higher rates reported for adolescents. Anderson et al. (1987) found that 47% of children with ADHD in a New Zealand study had co-occurring diagnoses of either oppositional disorder or conduct disorder, and in a study in Puerto Rico, Bird et al. (1989) found that 54% of children with ADHD had co-occurring disruptive behavior disorders. Moreover, comorbidity between ADHD and anxiety or emotional disorders ranges from 17% to 26%, depending on the study (Anderson et al., 1987; Bird et al., 1989; Szatmari et al., 1989). In the Ontario Child Health Survey, children with pure ADHD had more developmental problems than those with pure conduct disorder. Those with conduct disorder came from more disadvantaged backgrounds and had a greater family history of aggressive behavior. Those with co-occurring disorders had higher rates of both developmental disorders and psychosocial problems, and they had a worse prognosis (Szatmari, 1992).

Future epidemiologic studies need to consider the best way to combine data from several informants and to clarify whether behaviors can simply be pooled. Should each source (e.g., parent and teacher) contribute independently to the diagnosis, and should subthreshold diagnoses from one or two separate sources be considered together?

## Etiology

### Attention

Brain systems that may be involved in attention, inhibition, activity, and their control are the subject of ongoing investigation. The attention systems are extensive and, therefore, vulnerable to damage and dysfunction. Attention is based on arousal; attention involves vigilance, a span of apprehension, perseverance to maintain it, and the capacity to resist distractions (Denckla, 1989). There are various aspects of attention, including focusing, executing, sustaining, and shifting attention. The reticular activating system mediates the attentional state involved in the rapid modulation of information processing (brain stem and midbrain) as attention is channeled to higher levels of the brain. These attentional functions involve brain regions that are interconnected and organized into systems. Depending on the locus of the insult, various aspects of attention may be affected. The capacity to shift attention from one aspect of the environment to another is supported by the prefrontal cortex (PFC); focusing attention on environmental events is shared by the superior temporal and inferior parietal cortices as well as by the components of the corpus striatum (i.e., the caudate putamen and globus pallidus). In addition, the inferior parietal and corpus striatal regions are involved in motoric executive function. The hippocampus is involved in encoding stimuli that are related to memory, which may be required for some aspects of attention.

Denckla (1989) suggested that these various components of attention must be assessed to study the heterogeneity of ADHD. This might include study of the state/channel dimension (arousal), the dimension involving the right and left hemispheric contributions to attention (right hemispheric damage has greater effect than left hemispheric damage), the motivational aspects of attention (cingulate/limbic), the sensory-representational aspects (mainly posterior parietal cortex), and the motor-exploratory aspects that depend on the frontal lobe and its subcortical connections. The frontal lobe is central to attention, yet it is the last part of the brain to develop and has the longest period of vulnerability.

### Executive Dysfunction Syndrome

Children with executive dysfunction have difficulty organizing and managing time. These abilities depend on the integrity of the frontal lobes and their subcortical connections, including the basal ganglia and particularly the striatum. Barkley's view that ADHD is a disability involving rule-governed behavior is consistent with this view.

The conceptualization of ADHD as an executive function syndrome has the advantage of focusing specifically on brain regions that may be evaluated using neuropsychological testing. Dennis (1991) suggested that frontal lobe systems are involved in the general areas of attention/inhibition, self-monitoring, and the regulation of social discourse. Problems in all three of these areas are commonly present in children with ADHD. Self-monitoring and the maintenance of rule-governed behavior are involved in attentional processes and inhibition, and they are linked to Barkley's emphasis on a motivational deficit. Finally, problems in maintenance of social discourse have been highlighted when pragmatic language and narrative production have been assessed. Attention deficits and self-monitoring can be assessed with the Test of Variables of Attention (TOVA), and narrative abilities may be assessed in children using a story retelling task (Tannock et al., 1993). Although no specific battery of tests has been absolutely identified to demonstrate executive dysfunction, Denckla (1989) proposed a neuropsychological approach to evaluate the psychological or cognitive processes. The test utilizes systematic assessment of the executive function domain, including, but not limited to, continuous performance tasks. Using this approach, specific qualitative errors are detected that are pathognomonic if a deficiency in psychological processes involved in rule-governed performances is found. One proposal for accomplishing this is the use of constructs of initiating (planning), sustaining (concentrating), inhibiting (self-monitoring), and shifting (cognitive flexibility) on a battery of tests. For example, a continuous performance test, such as the TOVA, measures concentration, as do the Trail Making Test Parts A and B. The Stroop Color and Word Interference Test evaluates concentration, self-monitoring, and cognitive flexibility. Verbal fluency is useful in assessing all four of these constructs. From these tests, Denckla developed a neuropsychological equivalent of attention deficit disorder.

## Genetic Factors

Genetic factors are strongly implicated in the cause of ADHD, with heritability approaching 90% (Geschwind & Flint, 2015). Four lines of evidence support a role for genetic factors: family studies, twin studies, adoption studies, and genome-wide association studies (GWAS). Family studies are consistent with there being a robust genetic component for hyperactivity in that there is a higher rate of disorders in the families of children identified with ADHD (Biederman et al., 1986). Biederman et al. (1991) evaluated 73 males with ADHD and 264 of their first-degree relatives along with 26 male pediatric normal controls and their 92 relatives. This study used structured interviews, age-corrected analyses of risks, and blinded interviewers and found evidence for familial transmission of both ADHD and co-occurring mood disorders. The risk for ADHD in relatives of identified children with ADHD and identified children with both ADHD and mood disorder was 27% and 22%, respectively, whereas the rate in the control population was 5%. The co-occurrence of mood disorder was thought to be related to nonfamilial stressful environmental circumstances as the authors emphasize the importance of environmental factors as well as genetic ones.

Adoption studies provide a control for the similar rearing environments of monozygotic twins. Morrison and Stewart (1973) compared adoptive parents of children with ADHD with biological parents of other children with ADHD. These authors found that the adoptive parents and their biological relatives had lower levels of childhood hyperactivity; the adoptive parents showed low rates of pathological behavior (2.1%). Cadoret and Stewart (1991) collected data on the biological parents of adoptees from two adoption agencies with regard to both psychiatric and criminal histories. A total of 283 male adoptees and their adoptive parents were assessed with reference to their genetic background; environmental factors; and outcomes in relation to ADHD, aggression, and antisocial personality features. The authors concluded that there is a genetic component for ADHD, but they did not demonstrate a genetic component for aggression. This is consistent with other reports that aggression and hyperactivity are independent dimensions.

Twin studies indicate that ADHD represents the extreme tail of one or more heritable quantitative traits. Moreover, family and twin studies find genetic overlap between ADHD and other disorders, including antisocial personality disorder/behaviors, cognitive impairment, autism spectrum disorder, schizophrenia, bipolar disorder, and major depressive disorder. As with other mental disorders, the genetics of ADHD involves a complex interaction of many risk genes, each with a relatively small effect, with environmental factors.

GWAS involve the analysis of a large number of common single nucleotide polymorphisms that are present at greater than 5% frequency in the population and roughly equally distributed across the genome. Because of the high number of comparisons involved in scanning the entire genome for differences between the affected and the controls, a quite stringent threshold for significance has been set at $5 \times 10^{-8}$. Subsequently, 12 independent loci have been identified through GWAS (Demontis et al., 2019).

Associations were enriched in evolutionarily constrained genomic regions and loss-of-function intolerant genes and around brain-expressed regulatory marks. These findings are supported by analyses of three replication studies: a cohort of individuals diagnosed with ADHD, a self-reported ADHD sample, and a meta-analysis of quantitative measures of ADHD symptoms in the population. The strong concordance with GWAS of quantitative population measures of ADHD symptoms supports that clinical diagnosis of ADHD is an extreme expression of continuous heritable traits (Demontis et al., 2019).

An epigenome-wide prospective meta-analysis identified DNA methylation sites associated with ADHD symptoms. Neumann et al. (2020) found evidence that DNA methylation at birth predicted ADHD symptoms in childhood, whereas DNA methylation at school age did not. The association of DNA methylation at birth with ADHD symptoms in 2,477 children aged 4–15 years from five cohorts and the association of DNA methylation at school age with concurrent ADHD symptoms in 2,374 children aged 7–11 years from nine cohorts were examined, with three of these cohorts included in both assessments. Additional research is needed to confirm the utility of methylation variations as biomarkers and to clarify any role in causal mechanisms.

Genetic associations have been extensively studied in ADHD. In retrospect, the results remain tentative until confirmed by the agnostic, sufficiently powered GWAS. Several studies have found that intronic variants in the *ADGRL3* (*LPHN3*) gene are associated with ADHD with poor outcomes. Significant homogeneous genetic effects of *ADGRL3* variants predisposing to ADHD in children, adolescents, and adults and predicting the response to stimulant medication have been identified and independently replicated (Arcos-Burgos et al., 2010, 2012; Fallgatter et al., 2013; Ribases et al., 2011). This association was also found in the Multimodal Treatment Study of Children with ADHD (MTA), which was initiated as a 14-month randomized clinical trial of 579 children diagnosed with DSM-IV ADHD combined type(ADHD-C) (Acosta et al., 2016). The MTA study transitioned to a 16-year prospective observational follow-up. An additional 289 classmates were added at the 2-year assessment to serve as a local normative comparison group. Diagnostic evaluations at entry were based on the Diagnostic Interview Schedule for Children–Parent (DISC-P). This was repeated several times throughout the years. In an add-on genetic study, blood samples were collected from 232 subjects in the MTA group and 139 in the local normative comparison group. In the 205 MTA participants, 15% retained the DISC-P diagnosis of ADHD in adolescence. For 127 local normative comparison group participants, 88% remained undiagnosed by the DISC-P. The authors genotyped 15 polymorphic single nucleotide polymorphism markers harbored in the *ADGRL3* gene in this sample and compared allele frequencies for the 30 cases with continued diagnosis of ADHD-C in adolescence to the other participants. The authors found replication of the association of rs2345039 *ADGRL3* variant ($p = .004$) and concluded the detection of susceptibility conferred by *ADGRL3* variants in the extreme phenotype of continued diagnosis of ADHD-C from childhood to adolescence (Acosta et al., 2016), although this association has not been replicated in the the largest GWAS to date (Demontis et al., 2019).

## Environmental Risk Factors

With regard to environmental risk factors, prenatal and postnatal factors such as maternal smoking and alcohol use, low birth weight, premature birth, and exposure to environmental toxins (e.g., organophosphate pesticides, polychlorinated biphenyls, and zinc) have been associated with risk for ADHD (Cortese & Coghill, 2018). However, other than preterm birth, genetics studies have implicated unmeasured familial confounding factors, which are not in keeping with a causal role of environmental factors (Thapar et al., 2017). A better understanding of how genes interact with each other and of the interplay between environmental factors and genes is needed.

## Neuroimaging

Initial pathophysiological models of ADHD published more than 20 years ago were largely focused on a limited number of brain areas, primarily the frontal cortex and the basal ganglia (Cortese & Coghill, 2018). During the past two decades, there has been a major paradigm shift from focusing on alterations in individual brain regions to focusing on dysfunction in brain networks for understanding the pathophysiology of ADHD. Meta-analyses and mega-analyses of the structural MRI studies conducted during the past two decades consistently address replicated alterations in the basal ganglia (Nakao et al., 2011) and in several other subcortical areas (Hoogman et al., 2017).

A comprehensive meta-analysis found that the ADHD-related hypoactivated areas are related. Conversely, the majority of ADHD-related hyperactivated areas fall within the default mode network, and other hyperactivated areas are within the visual network and dorsal attention networks. This supports the view that the attentional lapses which characterize ADHD result from an inappropriate intrusion of the default network in the activity of task-positive networks frontoparietal, ventral, or dorsal attention networks of ADHD (Sonuga-Barke & Castellanos, 2007).

Despite this research, neuroimaging in ADHD is still far from informing clinical practice (Pereira-Sanchez & Castellanos, 2021). Neuroimaging research on ADHD has documented that children with ADHD have smaller global and regional brain structures than typically developing controls, involving both cortical and subcortical areas. However, effect sizes are small. Functional imaging results are far less clear, although some meta-analytic approaches do indicate an interplay of several key networks is associated with ADHD. However, this finding is not supported by the most comprehensive and unrestricted analyses. Thus, meta-analyses of functional neuroimaging research have failed to provide spatial convergence across studies, with the exception of a meta-analysis focused on a few areas of interest. Machine-learning approaches hold promise to identify multimodal markers related to the diagnosis and prognosis of ADHD, although methodological challenges need to be worked out. Multimodal approaches integrating imaging, genetic, and phenotypic data are in process; however, their replicability has not been confirmed (Pereira-Sanchez & Castellanos, 2021). Adoption of open science and best reporting practices is needed to make ADHD neuroimaging research more methodologically sound and relevant to improve patient care.

## Neurochemistry

The symptoms of ADHD involve impairments in prefrontal cortical top-down regulation of attention and behavior. All current pharmacological treatments for ADHD facilitate catecholaminergic neurotransmission, and basic research suggests that these drugs, such as methylphenidate, dextroamphetamine, and atomoxetine, have prominent actions in the PFC. Dopamine and norepinephrine, which play a major role in high-level executive functions, act as neuromodulators of fronto-striato-cerebellar circuits. The prefrontal cortical and subcortical mechanisms through which these medications exert their therapeutic effects are an ongoing area of study (Del Campo et al., 2011).

The dorsolateral PFC is especially sensitive to dopaminergic and noradrenergic neurotransmission so that either too little or too much impairs PFC function. Physiological studies show that norepinephrine strengthens PFC network connectivity and maintains persistent firing during a working memory task through stimulation of postsynaptic $\alpha_{2A}$ adrenoceptors on PFC neurons. Conversely, dopamine acts at D1 receptors to stabilize network inputs. The stimulant medications and atomoxetine enhance PFC function via indirectly increasing catecholamine actions through blockade of norepinephrine and/ or dopamine transporters. Guanfacine mimics the enhancing effects of norepinephrine at postsynaptic $\alpha_{2A}$ receptors in the PFC and strengthens network connectivity.

Such PFC regulation of attention, behavior, and emotion contributes to the therapeutic effects of these medications for the treatment of ADHD.

Evidence from positron emission tomography (PET) studies highlights the utility of quantifying dopaminergic markers at baseline and following drug administration in striatal subregions. This approach focuses on the neurobiological underpinnings of ADHD (and associated cognitive dysfunction) and its treatment by considering specific neural circuits. These PET imaging studies reveal that therapeutic doses of stimulants increase endogenous dopamine's stimulation of D2 receptors in the striatum (Volkow et al., 2002). They are effective under conditions when dopaminergic neurons would be activated—that is, in response to a salient stimulus (Volkow et al., 2005). However, PET imaging is unable to detect dopamine's interactions with receptors in the human PFC, but biochemical studies in rats indicate that methylphenidate is even more effective in increasing dopamine release in PFC than in striatal structures.

## Social Cognitive Domain

Social cognition is an important function to consider in children with ADHD because it is not only an off-task behavior vulnerable to distraction but also affects social perception (interpreting nonverbal cues such as facial expression), role-taking (taking another's point of view), social problem-solving (generating alternative solutions), and social communication (social pragmatics; e.g., maintaining a conversation) that may be problematic for these children. Thus, social cognition has an intimate tie to affective or emotional relations with others and has evolved in response to the demands of a complex social environment. The possibility of there being a social cognitive network in the brain has received new emphasis with the identification of feature recognition cells in the temporal lobe in primates. The linkage of these cells to the PFC suggests a selective response of single neurons or groups of neurons to social contact. Although the existence of a specific social cognitive network in the brain has not been demonstrated in humans, deficits in response inhibition have been suggested to be the result of dysfunction in the right frontostriatal system.

## Dysfunctional Affect Discrimination

Another aspect of the social deficit in ADHD relates to affect discrimination. A variety of affective responses are normally recognized, including joy, anger, fear, sadness, and disgust (Izard, 1991). Verbal labeling of the emotions is a task that follows a developmental sequence. Damasio and colleagues (1990) have argued that failure to activate somatic (bodily) states deprives an individual of an automatic device to signal the ultimately deleterious consequences of decisions. Longer term consequences can go unrecognized, even though impulsive decisions might bring immediate reward. Normally, activation of somatic or bodily states might focus an individual's attention on the negative consequences of their choices based on past experiences. With this awareness, one would choose to inhibit the behavior. The experience of the body in the mind is commonly referred to as "gut feelings" or Kahneman's (2011) "thinking fast."

Clinically, the automatic response to social stimuli appears to be deficient in ADHD. Some children with ADHD cannot adequately discriminate bodily feeling states and/ or can misperceive social situations. Alternatively, the child or adolescent might experience inappropriate negative or aversive bodily sensations and have difficulty linking the affective state to cognition. The child might say to themself (and then to others to justify the behavior) that another child "looked at him the wrong way" to justify his fighting.

## Narrative Production

Difficulties in self-organization are associated with executive dysfunction. Children with ADHD often have difficulty organizing their schoolwork and other activities. This lack of organization may extend to individuals with ADHD having difficulty in narrative production but not in narrative comprehension (Tannock et al., 1993; Zentall, 1988). Assessing narrative production in ADHD is necessary because narratives play a central role in social interactions and in academic activities. Narrative production involves storytelling and retelling, describing past experiences and giving directions; narratives require comprehension and extended language production. To meet the listener's needs, an oral monologue is maintained while the listener remains relatively passive. Information must be presented by the speaker that is accurate, organized, and complete. Such narrative accounts require metacognitive functions or executive control of processes of online monitoring, planning, and organization in addition to linguistic ability (Tannock et al., 1993).

Executive control allows the speaker to integrate and adapt to information from relevant sources that include the social context, the meaning of what is said, the content of what is said, and the characteristics of the speaker. Deficits in internal planning, organizing, and online monitoring have been reported in ADHD. These deficits can be identified through the use of a story retelling task to evaluate narrative abilities. Boys with ADHD have been found to provide less information overall and to produce poorly organized stories that are less cohesive and contain more inaccuracies. Consequently, their stories may be confusing and difficult to follow. Because organization and monitoring of information require executive functioning, these deficits reflect deficiencies in metacognitive processing.

In the analysis of a story, sequence errors, misinterpretations, substitutions, ambiguous references, and embellishment are evaluated. Tannock et al. (1993) evaluated the narrative abilities of 30 boys with ADHD and 30 neurotypically developing boys who were matched for age and IQ. The authors evaluated whether the idea unit was retold in a different order than the original story, which affected the story theme (sequence error); whether the meaning of an action was incorrectly interpreted (misinterpretation); whether a word used for an object, character, or event in the original story was replaced with an inappropriate word that was not a synonym; whether ambiguous references were present (a person is not linked to a specific character so its referent is ambiguous); and whether new events or characters were introduced that were not part of the original story event (embellishment). Tannock et al. confirmed previous research suggesting that children with ADHD did not differ in comprehension of narratives and had the ability to differentiate important and relevant information from nonessential detail. However, they also confirmed a narrative production deficit, as had been found in previous studies.

Studies that have presented test stories through the auditory route are more likely to demonstrate the deficit. However, studies of narration in which the provision of content support is offered by allowing a child to read along with the tester, using a copy of the test story, may not show differences between groups (O'Neill & Douglas, 1991). Overall, storytelling in children with ADHD showed a higher frequency of sequence errors and cohesion errors that reflect a breakdown in the ability to globally organize a story's theme. Affected children also produced more local errors of information processing across story production. Misinterpreted information and the use of inappropriate word substitutions were unlikely to reflect problems in comprehension because there was no difference from controls on comprehension measures. Rather, these abnormalities more likely reflected a failure to monitor information because of deficits in executive control.

The interpretation of results of these narrative story findings must consider whether the problems are attributable to deficits in executive processes or language impairment or both. Some children with ADHD could show production deficits that could be quantitatively linked to those produced by others with language impairment, whereas their linguistic competence appears superior to that of children with a language disorder. Word substitutions, delays, and problems in cohesion may be associated with both language disorders and deficits in executive processes. Most studies on narration have not assessed language abilities other than those involved in narratives. Although there is no specific evidence that children with ADHD exhibit deficits in verbal memory span or memory capacity (Weingartner et al., 1980), they may have co-occurring learning disorders. Still, Purvis and Tannock (1997) have suggested that the presence of learning disability leads to a different pattern of deficits than they found in children with the ADHD diagnosis using the narrative assessment method. Moreover, narrative deficits persist into adulthood (Coelho et al., 2018). Stimulant medication, through its ability to enhance executive processes (Douglas et al., 1988), may improve narrative production and coherence.

## Interpersonal Aspects: Social Behavior

Whalen and Henker (1992) identified five aspects related to the interpersonal behavior of children with ADHD: response patterns, style of approach, social information processing, peer appeal, and interpersonal impact of the disorder. These authors note that although a sample of children with ADHD is necessarily heterogeneous and the children evaluated commonly have associated behavioral difficulties, these interpersonal patterns described are generally applicable if the child meets the diagnostic criteria for ADHD.

First, the individual response pattern tends to be one of an increased rate of social contact that heightens awareness of the child's presence by others. Persistent excessive contact increases the likelihood of inappropriate interpersonal interactions that place the child at risk for being in conflict and being rejected. Most children with ADHD engage in socially objectionable acts, such as noncompliance, intrusiveness, rule-breaking, bossiness, and disruptive behavior. Although these behaviors seem intentional, they may not be. In the intentional group, co-occurring oppositional defiant disorder may be identified. For the non-intentional group, there may be a high level of social interest, impulsive rather than planned social approaches, and/or an emotionally labile temperament. These children are action oriented, and the effects of their behavior on others can be largely inadvertent. They tend to be less likely to evaluate the social context when they enter a new group, consider the social norms, or wait for an appropriate invitation to enter. Rather than wait, they may make demands and attempt to redirect or revise the rules of the group. Some children with ADHD seem socially awkward rather than deliberately intrusive, and their responses may relate to problems in social perception or immaturity. These characteristic responses, which are not interpersonally matched to ongoing events, may result in the individual appearing insensitive to others' needs and not responsive to feedback from peers or adults.

An assessment procedure that includes evaluation of interpersonal social transactions may be more clinically useful than a more classical behavioral approach that involves monitoring frequency counts of excessive and deficit behaviors. Children with ADHD seem less likely to watch peers, more likely to attempt contact and interrupt when peers are working independently, and more likely to respond to unauthorized questions when asked by teachers to work without talking. In addition, less joint activity and more aggression with peers, lower rates of verbal reciprocity, and more social withdrawal following aggression have been noted.

Prosocial behaviors may or may not be in the behavioral repertoire of children with ADHD. Although inappropriate behavior is commonly emphasized in research studies, there is no clear-cut evidence for deficiencies in prosocial behavior. An evaluation of prosocial behavior and the identification of the presence or absence of prosocial dysfunction are crucial in treatment planning. Prosocial behaviors involve helping others, empathy toward others in distress, and capacity to maintain friendships. Prosocial behaviors are particularly important to evaluate in cases of a co-occurring conduct disorder.

Problems in response pattern and dyadic communication may not be evident on first office visits but, rather, become apparent later as additional tasks are introduced. Normal responsiveness is also commonly seen on initial evaluation visits with professionals. There may be several reasons to account for the apparent worsening of behavior with repeated assessment. These include decreasing novelty and loss of interest, inability to sustain social attention, problems with goal orientation, or simply fatigue. During unstructured activities and free play, no differences in behavior are noted between affected and non-affected children. Differences become apparent in situations in which there are task demands and increasing constraints. This occurs particularly when certain rules must be followed or the task, such as a set of math problems, must be completed.

The style that the child with ADHD uses to approach others has been studied. This involves assessment of the intensity of response, behavioral modulation of responses, and modulation of affect. Although children with ADHD may know the appropriate social norms and may even have an adequate repertoire of interpersonal routines, the modulation of their responses and the timing of their interactions can be inappropriate. They show more intense interactions that are forceful, vigorous, and loud, with atypical levels of intensity not only in the classroom but also when playing alone. The child's intensity is decreased with stimulant medication. In addition, teachers may be more intense when interacting with children with ADHD, whereas the level of teachers' intensity is normalized when children with ADHD are on medication, which suggests reciprocal influences.

The modulation of behavior as situational demands change has been documented. In structured situations in which roles must be reversed, boys with ADHD have difficulty in shifting. Problems in role shifting were demonstrated in a simulated space flight communication task in which boys took turns as mission control and astronaut. The messages given by the boys with ADHD were more rigidly consistent across roles as they moved from one role to the other, suggesting a failure to modulate role requirements based on variations in task demands.

Dysregulation or modulation of affect is pertinent to style and intensity of interaction. Children with ADHD are commonly found to be emotionally labile and inappropriately responsive to both physical and social stimulation in social situations. Efforts are commonly made by teachers and parents to prevent affective arousal because arousal may build up rapidly and make it difficult to redirect the child. The emotionality of the child with ADHD may lead to excessive enthusiasm or explosive, intrusive behavior. Dysregulation of affect may decrease interpersonal contact and further remove the child from involvement with peers. Treatment with stimulant drugs can dampen the expression of affect, produce a decrease in affective communication between peers and lead to disengagement with others, and produce a mild dysphoria. This includes assessment of whether or not the child infers hostile intent to ambiguous actions by peers, understands the assignment of responsibility for behavior, appreciates the extent of their own aggressiveness, and assumes blame for inappropriate behavior. Problems in social information processing that relate to inaccurate appraisals of others' intentions and inappropriate attributions regarding others' behavior should be identified. These inaccurate appraisals influence ongoing interactions and color future expectations about others' behavior. Finally, children with ADHD may have difficulty with general social competencies that relate to social problem-solving skills. There is variability among children with ADHD regarding the extent of their noncompliance and aggression; in fact, a significant proportion of children with ADHD have few externalizing difficulties.

Unpopularity with peers is an ongoing problem for children with ADHD. Behavioral patterns of inattention and impulsivity apparently make independent contributions to peer rejection. Although both aggression and overactivity are related to rejection, hyperactivity has been found to be the more important determinant of low peer acceptance (Pope et al., 1989). Whalen and Henker (1992) suggest that there are two subtypes of children with ADHD who are unpopular: The first are actively rejected by peers, and the second are passively neglected. The actively rejected group rapidly re-establish their rejected status when they move into a new group setting. The passively neglected children, however, interact less frequently with peers and generally do not do things to offend others. Of the two groups, the rejected subgroup is least responsive to intervention and has the greatest risk at long-term follow-up. These authors suggest that children diagnosed with ADHD are more often actively rejected, and those with the diagnosis of ADD without hyperactivity are more often passively neglected. Although both groups have social impairment, the differences between them with regard to peer status and peer relationships are factors in prognosis.

The social impact of the behavior of children with ADHD on others is a major concern because children with ADHD markedly impact their social environment. Assessment must consider not only the child's level of distress and dysfunction but also the social response and disharmony that are produced by the child's behavior and change the overall atmosphere of a classroom (Whalen et al., 1980). Moreover, parents show increased levels of negative and controlling behaviors as they interact with untreated children with ADHD. In evaluating behavioral change, the assessment must take into account changes in others' behavior toward the child as well as changes in their own behavior. An adult's overreaction, lack of response, or constraint in relation to the child may increase or decrease the responsiveness of the child. Peer reactions may prevent or provoke behavioral escalation. Peer experiences over time may provide social learning opportunities or prevent them and, consequently, impair interpersonal competence.

## Effect of the Disorder on Others

The presence of prosocial behaviors, the capacity for psychological reflectivity, the ability to self-monitor, the ability to self-regulate, the capacity to identify and label affect, responsiveness to medication, and concurrent language and learning disabilities are all factors that influence the family relationship. As the result of problems in social cognition and affect discrimination, the child with ADHD is unaware of the effect of their behavior on others. Children with ADHD generally do not complain of a sense of psychological suffering or express conflict about their symptoms. This lack of awareness of the effect of one's behavior on others may lead to misunderstanding in the family and reduced self-esteem when others respond negatively toward them.

The family relationship is influenced not only by associated social–emotional deficits but also by co-occurring diagnoses of oppositional disorder and/or conduct disorder. The co-occurrence of other disruptive behavior disorders and/or difficult temperament generally have a greater negative effect on others and lead to a worse prognosis (Harris et al., 1984). The recognition and treatment of associated language and learning disabilities are of particular importance to prevent or reduce antisocial behavior (Harris, 1989).

Problems with executive dysfunction that includes rule-governed behavior may interact with temperament and personality features associated with ADHD. These include low self-esteem, mood lability, low frustration tolerance, anhedonia (e.g., lack of pleasure in accomplishment or gratitude for gifts), and temper outbursts. These personality and temperament features predispose affected children to developing oppositional defiant behavior and conduct problems. Through their interactions with peers, family members, and others, they may become demoralized or possibly clinically depressed based on the learned helplessness model of depression.

## Developmental Course

Attention-deficit/hyperactivity disorder begins in infancy but is not ordinarily diagnosed then because the symptoms are nonspecific and may reflect a variety of disorders that occur later in life. Infants vary greatly in their level of activity. Individual differences in temperament in infants show limited stability; however, early recognition of symptoms may occur if careful assessment of activity is an aspect of a temperament measurement. Retrospective histories do include symptoms that began infancy, such as irritability, feeding and sleep problems, irregular rhythms, tantrums, stereotypies, over-activity, and disorganization. In the preschool child, behavior continues to be poorly differentiated; it can be difficult to distinguish ADHD as a component of generally dis-ruptive behavior at this age. Campbell (1985, 1987) and Campbell et al. (1986) followed preschool children who were difficult to manage and found that in approximately one-third, symptoms resolved in grade school, but that the other two-thirds had a later diag-nosis of disruptive disorders (ADHD, oppositional defiant disorder, conduct disorder, and others). Those whose symptoms had resolved by age 6 years previously had similar symptoms of short attention span and overactivity as seen in the persistent group, al-though their symptoms were less severe, and interpersonal difficulty with peers as well as the severity of conduct problems were also less severe. Overall, maternal reports were more reliable predictors of later behavior problems; behavior observed by the investigators did not specifically predict subsequent ADHD.

McGee et al. (1991) reported less difficulty making the diagnosis in the preschool years and identified 2% of a preschool sample as pervasively hyperactive, with persistent problems at follow-up 12 years later. Ross and Ross (1982) found that few preschool children presented with clinical symptoms, but those who did often had difficulty with peers and in preschool. However, because of the lack of specificity in the behavioral presentation, there is a risk of overdiagnosing ADHD in the preschool years.

Most ADHD research has been conducted with school-age children aged 6–10 years, and it is in this group that the classical symptoms of attention deficit, impulsivity, distractibility, and overactivity have been most clearly identified. Although the diag-nosis of ADHD is most commonly recognized in the early school years, when the child's prior development is reviewed, the onset is generally found to be before age 5 years and may be as early as age 2 years or younger. Although more common in boys, the disorder does occur in girls, who have been referred to as a "silent minority" with this disorder.

In adolescence, the tendency has been to underdiagnose ADHD because it was in-itially believed the disorder is residual by this age. Yet longitudinal studies show that symptoms persist into adolescence, although they may have to be specifically sought out, and that approximately 70% of adolescents who had ADHD in childhood continue to have difficulty. In adolescence, attentional and impulsive problems are more ap-parent, and hyperactivity may be reduced. Associated problems, such as mood changes, poor motivation, and delinquent behavior, often become the focus of attention in ado-lescence, thus overshadowing the attention deficit and impulsive symptoms. The more severe problems with substance abuse and aggression may draw more attention from caregivers and teachers.

## Diagnostic Assessment

The social/family/school context is basic to the diagnostic and assessment process. ADHD is identified in a family or at school by family members or teachers recognizing the condition and initiating the referral. The DSM-5 criteria for the diagnosis of ADHD are based on others' observations of the child. Both behavior rating scales and structured interviews rely on teacher ratings and the parental interview to confirm the diagnosis. Rating scales are particularly useful for parents to complete at the time of referral, or as part of the screening procedure, to allow them to designate the child's referral problem. Epidemiologic studies use parental ratings, such as the Child Behavior Checklist (Achenbach & Edelbrock, 1981), or teacher and parent ratings (Conners et al., 1998) to identify the externalizing symptoms of ADHD and co-occurring behavioral disturbances. The teacher's report of behavior in the classroom (Conners et al., 1998) is often needed to confirm the diagnosis of ADHD because behavioral problems are most apparent in a structured group setting. This is essential because children often will not show enough symptoms in a one-to-one office setting to make the diagnosis. Teachers benefit from their experience, making age-related comparisons between children and their peers in the classroom. Teacher reports can document the effects of the child's behavior on others and responses to the child from peers.

## Assessment of Family Functioning

The family assessment involves an evaluation of the interpersonal relationship between parent and child. Aversive/coercive interpersonal exchanges with parents are common because of the social, cognitive, and emotional recognition difficulties. The parent–child interaction can be marred by poor child compliance, time off task, negative responses to parent requests, poorly regulated rule-governed behavior, and less sustained attention to task. The child's negative response to requests leads to a vicious cycle of negativity with aversive and coercive interactions with the parent.

Specific family issues that must be considered in addressing the parent–child relationship include parental factors such as psychosocial background, parental psychiatric and developmental diagnosis (antisocial behavior, depression, alcohol abuse, and learning disability), parenting stress and the extent of parental acknowledgment of the child's disability, and parental motivation to participate in a multimodal treatment program. A description of parent–child interaction, ascertainment of parental psychological state, and evaluation of marital functioning are all recorded. Parents and siblings in families with a child with ADHD experience a higher rate of psychological distress. Mothers report lower levels of parenting self-esteem and higher levels of depression, especially with a preschool child with ADHD. There is an increased prevalence of antisocial behavior, depression, alcohol abuse, and learning disability in family members.

## Treatment

Children with ADHD have multiple difficulties involving social, emotional, and academic areas. Because of the complexity of their presentation, multimodal treatment interventions have been recommended. For any family, multimodal treatment must be individualized. Parent education and training will assist in their acknowledgment of the disability and in improving their self-esteem. The conduct of treatment in a family context is essential. A systematic multimodal approach should also incorporate a family therapy component. In addition, parents may need individual therapy for themselves, including pharmacotherapy for adult-onset ADHD or mood disorder.

## Combined Treatments and Pharmacotherapy

During the past few decades, there has been a substantial increase in the number of randomized controlled trials aimed at testing the short-term efficacy and tolerability of pharmacological treatments for ADHD (both stimulant and nonstimulant medications). Parallel research on nonpharmacological interventions are ongoing. In some instances, combined drug treatment may be indicated. This involves augmentation of stimulant medication for co-occurring diagnoses, such as intermittent explosive behavior, aggressive displays, and depression.

The most extensive study to examine treatment of ADHD is the MTA. It was initiated as a 14-month randomized clinical trial of 579 children diagnosed with ADHD-C, and it transitioned to a 16-year prospective observational follow-up. A total of 289 classmates were added at the 2-year assessment to serve as a local normative comparison group. Diagnostic evaluations at entry were based on the DISC-P, which was repeated at several time points throughout the years. For an add-on genetic study, blood samples were collected from 232 in the MTA group and 139 in the local normative comparison group. For the 205 MTA participants, 14.6% retained the DISC-P diagnosis of ADHD-C into adolescence (Acosta et al., 2016).

The MTA study showed that neither the type nor the intensity of treatment received during the initial 15-month randomized phase of the study—community treatment as usual; medication treatment (MED) plus a combination of strategies of parent training and child-focused or school-based behavioral therapies; strict behavioral therapy (BEH); medication plus strict behavioral therapy (COMBINED)— or exposure to medication during the subsequent observational periods predicted the functional outcome when follow-up was extended to 16 years. In the MTA, the treatments received in the three experimental arms (MED, BEH, and COMBINED) during the initial 15-month randomized phase were carefully organized to achieve optimal outcomes. Medication alone and the combined treatments were the most effective. After the initial phase, all participants were free to choose the type of treatment they received from their regular caregiver. However, because treatments were not as carefully optimized and monitored as in the original three experimental groups during the randomized phase, the long-term findings of the MTA need to be replicated. Acosta et al. (2016) and others report there was no statistical difference between combined treatment and medication alone at the end of the treatment-by-protocol (primary analyses).

A network meta-analysis including 190 randomized clinical trials of ADHD treatments supports the conclusion that psychostimulants are the most efficacious treatment available for ADHD, including pharmacologic and nonpharmacologic options (Catalá-López et al., 2017). The authors concluded that methylphenidate and dexamethasone had the best overall rankings.

## Atomoxetine

Atomoxetine (ATX) is considered an alternative treatment for ADHD when psychostimulants are contraindicated or not well tolerated. It should also be considered in some special situations, such as when ADHD is comorbid with bipolar disorder with high risk of mood destabilization with stimulants, substance abuse/dependence, or Tourette syndrome. Randomized clinical trials and meta-analyses find that ATX does have acceptable efficacy and tolerability; however, the effect size is smaller than that for psychostimulants (Liu et al., 2017).

A consideration is that different alleles of the cytochrome p450 2D6 (*CYP2D6*) gene confer extensive metabolic effects on ATX and have been shown to significantly affect clinical response (Brown & Bishop, 2015). Thus, patients with an indication for ATX but apparently refractory to treatment benefit from dose adjustments based on their classification between slow and fast metabolizers through *CYP2D6* genotyping.

## $\alpha_2$ Agonists

Guanfacine is a selective $\alpha_2$ agonist with less sedating and cardiovascular effects than clonidine. An extended-release preparation of guanfacine has been approved by the U.S. Food and Drug Administration (FDA) for the treatment of ADHD. Seven randomized clinical trials in children and adolescents support its efficacy compared to placebo. Meta-analyses indicate that the effect size of guanfacine is lower than that of psychostimulants but is comparable to that of ATX (Hirota et al., 2014; Joseph et al., 2017). Guanfacine is useful as an adjunctive treatment to psychostimulants, being more effective than placebo and each drug when administered alone (Findling et al., 2014; Wilens et al., 2015).

## Modafinil

Evidence of efficacy of modafinil for ADHD symptom reduction is mixed. Five short-term randomized clinical trials in children and adolescents have been published in a meta-analysis (Wang et al., 2017). The meta-analysis showed a moderate effect in reducing ADHD symptoms, with a dropout rate due to side effects similar to that for placebo. Adverse effects were insomnia and decreased appetite. However, studies on adults show contradictory results (Buoli et al., 2016). Moreover, clinical trials and post-surveillance reports associate modafinil with serious skin reactions, leading the FDA to request more data for the approval of the drug for ADHD treatment.

## Behavioral and Psychosocial Treatments

Behavior parent training and social skills training are the primary recommended alternatives to medication management of ADHD (Pliszka et al., 2007; E. Taylor et al., 2009). They are, for the most part, regarded as first-line treatments for very young

**Table 16.1** Treatment Strategies for Attention-Deficit/Hyperactivity Disorder

| Issue | Recommendation | Reasoning |
|---|---|---|
| Patient's age | Start with behavioral treatment in preschool children. | Less evidence of safety and efficacy for medication in preschool children. |
| | Prefer pharmacological treatment in children. | Lower efficacy of nonpharmacological interventions. |
| ADHD severity | Monotherapy with nonpharmacological treatment for mild disorder. | Expected efficacy of treatment ranges: Nonpharmacological < nonstimulants < stimulants < combination therapy. |
| | Combination treatments for severe disorder. | |
| Comorbidities | Tic disorders: Nonstimulants might be an option in cases in which methylphenidate increases tics. | Psychostimulants might exacerbate symptoms of tic disorders in some cases. |
| | Disruptive disorders: Prefer stimulants. | Psychostimulants reduce ODD/CD symptoms with large effect sizes. |
| | Mood and psychotic disorders: Prioritize comorbidity treatment. | Comorbid conditions may cause or exacerbate ADHD symptoms; use adjunctive medicine. |

ADHD, attention-deficit/hyperactivity disorder; CD, conduct disorder; OCD, oppositional defiant disorder.

children or those with mild to moderate ADHD (Pliszka et al., 2007; E. Taylor et al., 2009). The guidelines are outlined in Table 16.1.

Behavioral and psychosocial treatments are also the standard add-ons to medication treatment for severe presentations regardless of age (Pliszka et al., 2007; E. Taylor et al., 2009). These are the most frequently used nonpharmacological treatments among children and adolescents with ADHD (Danielson et al., 2018). Although intensive behavioral treatment may not add to the efficacy in treatment of well-managed interventions with medication, behavioral therapies have been found to be effective in improving positive parenting and addressing co-occurring conduct problems in children with ADHD.

New nonpharmacological treatment options and strategies tested for ADHD include coaching programs developed to help individuals with ADHD cope with the environment by focusing on improving executive functions such as time management, prioritization in planning, and maintaining sustained effort over time. Findings from small naturalistic trials (Prevatt & Levin, 2015; Prevatt & Yelland, 2015) need to be confirmed by randomized clinical trials. For adolescents, the Supporting Teens' Autonomy Daily (STAND) program uses motivational interviewing in adolescents with ADHD to enhance treatment adherence. A randomized clinical trial of STAND found promising acute and long-term (6 months after treatment ceased) effects not only on ADHD symptoms but also on parental stress and executive functioning skills.

Mindfulness-based therapies teach how to focus self-regulating attention on the current moment to stay on task (Goldberg et al., 2018). Mindfulness therapies address the deficits associated with ADHD by providing intensive training of attention to facilitate emotional regulation. This systematic demonstrated approach has a moderate to large effect for children with ADHD (Evans et al., 2018). Additional studies are needed because the overall quality of the studies taken together is very low. With regard to the duration of medication treatment, it must be emphasized that ADHD is a chronic disorder. There are long-term clinical follow-up studies of 6 years or more. Approximately 50% of the child-onset cases have been found to have persistent ADHD symptoms that are impairing (Faraone et al., 2006; Karam et al., 2015).

## School-Based Intervention

Because failure in school is common, it is important that psychiatric liaison with schools and awareness of special education needs be highlighted in every ADHD intervention. Furthermore, because of the negative feedback that these children receive, they often think of themselves as stupid. This may require counseling to help them deal specifically with problems in self-esteem. Specific interventions in the classroom are critical for long-term success. One well-developed program is the University of Washington's PATHS (Promoting Alternative Thinking Strategies) program. It uses educators and counselors to facilitate self-control, emotional awareness, and interpersonal problem-solving skills. Its goal is to enhance social competence in the classroom. The children's language developmental level must be considered in implementing this curriculum.

Kam et al. (2004) carried out an extensive evaluation of the PATHS program to investigate individual differences in emotional understanding and in children's behavioral response. The following specific goals are incorporated in the PATHS curriculum to address deficits in social cognition and affect regulation:

1. Increase self-control; the ability to stop and think before acting, especially when upset or coping with a conflict situation. This lesson also includes the recognition of upset feelings.
2. Teach attributional processes that lead to an appropriate sense of self-responsibility.
3. Enhance understanding of the vocabulary of logical reasoning and problem-solving (e.g., "if . . . then" and "why . . . because").
4. Increase understanding and use of the vocabulary of emotions and emotional states (e.g., excited, disappointed, confused, guilty, etc.), and increase use of verbal mediation.
5. Increase the ability to recognize and interpret similarities and differences in the feelings, reactions, and viewpoints of self and others.
6. Increase recognition and understanding of how one's behavior affects others.
7. Increase skills in social problem-solving: stopping and thinking; identifying problems and feelings; setting goals; generating alternative solutions; anticipating and evaluating consequences; and planning, executing, and evaluating a course of action and trying again if the first solution fails.
8. Increase the ability to apply social problem-solving skills to prevent and then resolve conflicts in social interactions.

Kam et al. examined the long-term effectiveness of the PATHS curriculum on the adjustment of school-age children with special needs, including ADHD. Because the PATHS curriculum focuses on enhancing children's emotional development, self-regulation, and social problem-solving skills, it is an important intervention. In this study, 18 special education classrooms were randomly assigned to treatment and control conditions in a controlled trial. Teachers received training and were provided ongoing consultation. Teachers provided PATHS to students in grades 1–3. Baseline data were collected before the intervention, and intervention data were collected for 3 successive years. Growth curve analysis demonstrated that the intervention reduced the rate of growth of teacher-reported internalizing and externalizing behaviors diagnosed in the children 2 years after the intervention and also resulted in a sustained reduction in depressive symptoms reported by the children. The intervention children showed significant improvement in frustration tolerance, improved assertive social skills, better task orientation, enhanced peer social skills, and improved emotional labeling. These findings suggest PATHS is effective for promoting adaptive classroom behavior and improving emotional understanding in special needs children.

## Conclusion

The child with ADHD has a disorder that requires comprehensive, long-term intervention. The child's difficulty in self-regulation and affect discrimination adversely impacts family functioning. Parental difficulties may compound the child's problems and increase the risk for co-occurring disorders. Treatment must involve family members in a multimodal treatment paradigm that may include individual medication, behavioral, social cognitive, family, and school-based interventions. Practice parameters for the assessment and treatment of ADHD have been developed by the American Academy of Child and Adolescent Psychiatry (2007).

With regard to medication and psychosocial interventions, all ADHD medications, although differing in their synaptic mechanisms, act on broader neurocognitive networks in the short term. Psychostimulants are highly effective compared to other psychiatric medications. Although less effective options, nonstimulants should be considered in special circumstances. Psychosocial interventions are especially useful for very young children, for mild ADHD, or as an add-on treatment to improve efficacy or reduce required stimulant dosage.

Treatment selection should rely on a shared decision-making process among the clinician, patient, and family. The primary issues to be considered by the clinician are age of the patient, severity of the disorder, and co-occurring psychiatric conditions. All patients are to be routinely followed to assess response to treatment and adverse events. Attention is paid to chronicity, disorder persistence over time, and changes in presentation in the progression from childhood to adolescence and then adulthood (Caye et al., 2019).

## References

Achenbach, T. M., & Edelbrock, C. S. (1981). Behavioral problems and competencies reported by parents of normal and disturbed children aged four through sixteen. *Monographs of the Society for Research in Child Development, 41*(1), 1–82.

Acosta, M. T., Swanson, J., Stehli, A., Molina, B. S., MTA Team, Martinez, A. F., Arcos-Burgos, M., & Muenke, M. (2016). *ADGRL3 (LPHN3)* variants are associated with a refined phenotype of ADHD in the MTA study. *Molecular Genetics & Genomic Medicine, 4*(5), 540–547.

American Psychiatric Association. (1952). *Diagnostic and statistical manual of mental disorders.*

American Psychiatric Association. (1968). *Diagnostic and statistical manual of mental disorders* (2nd ed.).

American Psychiatric Association. (1980). *Diagnostic and statistical manual of mental disorders* (3rd ed.).

American Psychiatric Association. (1987). *Diagnostic and statistical manual of mental disorders* (3rd ed., rev.).

American Psychiatric Association. (1994). *Diagnostic and statistical manual of mental disorders* (4th ed.).

American Psychiatric Association. (2000). *Diagnostic and statistical manual of mental disorders* (4th ed., text rev.).

American Psychiatric Association. (2013). *Diagnostic and statistical manual of mental disorders* (5th ed.) American Psychiatric Publishing.

Anderson, J. C., Williams, S., McGee, R., & Silva, P. A. (1987). DSM-III disorders in preadolescent children: Prevalence in a large sample from the general population. *Archives of General Psychiatry, 44*(1), 69–76.

Arcos-Burgos, Á., Jain, M., Acosta, M. T., Shively, S., Stanescu, H., Wallis, D., Domene, S., Velez, J., Karkera, J., Balog, J., Berg, K., Kleta, R., Gahl, W., Roessler, E., Long, R., Lie, J., Pineda, D., Londono, A., Palacio, J., . . . Muenke, M. (2010). A common variant of the latrophilin 3 gene, *LPHN3*, confers susceptibility to ADHD and predicts effectiveness of stimulant medication. *Molecular Psychiatry, 15*(11), 1053–1066.

August, G. J., & Stewart, M. A. (1982). Is there a syndrome of pure hyperactivity? *British Journal of Psychiatry, 140*(3), 305–311.

Barkley, R. A. (1982). Guidelines for defining hyperactivity in children. Advances in *Clinical Child Psychology, 5*, 137–180.

Barkley, R. A. (1990). *Attention-deficit disorder: A handbook for diagnosis and treatment.* Guilford.

Barkley, R. A. (1997). Behavioral inhibition, sustained attention, and executive functions: Constructing a unifying theory of ADHD. *Psychological Bulletin, 121*(1), 65–94.

Barkley, R. A. (2010). Differential diagnosis of adults with ADHD: The role of executive function and self-regulation. *Journal of Clinical Psychiatry, 71*(7), e17.

Barkley, R. A., & Fischer, M. (2019). Hyperactive child syndrome and estimated life expectancy at young adult follow-up: The role of ADHD persistence and other potential predictors. *Journal of Attention Disorders, 23*(9), 907–923.

Bender, L. (1942). Postencephalitic behavior disorders in children. In J. N. Neal (Ed.), *Encephalitis: A clinical study* (pp. 361–385). Grune & Stratton.

Biederman, J., Munir, K., Knee, D., Habelow, W., Armentano, M., Autor, S., Hoge, S., & Waternaux, C. (1986). A family study of patients with attention deficit disorder and normal controls. *Journal of Psychiatric Research, 20*(4), 263–274.

Biederman, J., Newcorn, J., & Sprich, S. (1991). Comorbidity of attention deficit hyperactivity disorder with conduct, depressive, anxiety, and other disorders. *American Journal of Psychiatry, 148*, 564–577.

Birch, H. G. (1964). *Brain damage in children: The biological and social aspects.* Williams & Wilkins.

Bird, H. R., Gould, M. S., Yager, T., Staghezza, B., & Canino, G. (1989). Risk factors for maladjustment in Puerto Rican children. *Journal of the American Academy of Child & Adolescent Psychiatry, 28*(6), 847–850.

Bond, E. D., & Appel, K. E. (1931). *The treatment of behavior disorders following encephalitis.* Commonwealth Fund.

Bradley, C. (1937). The behavior of children receiving benzedrine. *American Journal of Psychiatry, 94*(3), 577–585.

Bradley, C., & Bowen, M. (1940). School performance of children receiving amphetamine (benzedrine) sulfate. *American Journal of Orthopsychiatry, 10*(4), 782–788.

Brown, J. T., & Bishop, J. R. (2015). Atomoxetine pharmacogenetics: Associations with pharma-cokinetics, treatment response and tolerability. *Pharmacogenomics, 16*(13), 1513–1520.

Buoli, M., Serati, M., & Cahn, W. (2016). Alternative pharmacological strategies for adult ADHD treatment: A systematic review. *Expert Review of Neurotherapeutics, 16*(2), 131–144.

Cadoret, R. J., & Stewart, M. A. (1991). An adoption study of attention deficit/hyperactivity / aggression and their relationship to adult antisocial personality. *Comprehensive Psychiatry, 32*(1), 73–82.

Campbell, S. B. (1985). Hyperactivity in preschoolers: Correlates and prognostic implications. *Clinical Psychology Review, 5*(5), 405–428.

Campbell, S. B. (1987). Parent-referred problem three-year-olds: Developmental changes in symptoms. *Journal of Child Psychology and Psychiatry, 28*(6), 835–845.

Campbell, S. B., Breaux, A. M., Ewing, L. J., & Szumowski, E. K. (1986). Correlates and predictors of hyperactivity and aggression: A longitudinal study of parent-referred problem preschoolers. *Journal of Abnormal Child Psychology, 14*(2), 217–234.

Carlson, C. L. (1986). Attention deficit disorder without hyperactivity: A review of preliminary experimental evidence. Advances in Clinical Child Psychology, 9, 153–175.

Catalá-López, F., Hutton, B., Núñez-Beltrán, A., Page, M. J., Ridao, M., Macías Saint-Gerons, D., Catalá, M., Tabares-Seisdedos, R., & Moher, D. (2017). The pharmacological and non-pharmacological treatment of attention deficit hyperactivity disorder in children and adolescents: A systematic review with network meta-analyses of randomised trials. *PLoS One, 12*(7), e0180355.

Caye, A., Swanson, J. M., Coghill, D., & Rohde, L. A. (2019). Treatment for ADHD: An evidence-based guide to select optimal treatment. *Molecular Psychiatry, 24*(3), 390–408.

Chess, S. (1960). Diagnosis and treatment of the hyperactive child. *New York State Journal of Medicine, 60*, 2379–2385.

Clements, S. D. (1966). *Minimal brain dysfunction in children: Terminology and identifica-tion: Phase one of a three phase project* (Vol. 55). U.S. Department of Health, Education and Welfare.

Coelho, R., Mattos, P., & Tannock, R. (2018). Attention-deficit hyperactivity disorder (ADHD) and narrative discourse in older adults. *Dementia & Neuropsychologia, 12*(4), 374–379.

Conners, C. K., Sitarenios, G., Parker, J. D., & Epstein, J. N. (1998). The revised Conners' Parent Rating Scale (CPRS-R): Factor structure, reliability, and criterion validity. *Journal of Abnormal Child Psychology, 26*(4), 257–268.

Cortese, S., & Coghill, D. (2018). Twenty years of research on attention-deficit/hyperactivity disorder (ADHD): Looking back, looking forward. *Evidence-Based Mental Health, 21*(4), 173–176.

Damasio, A. R., Tranel, D., & Damasio, H. (1990). Individuals with sociopathic behavior caused by frontal damage fail to respond autonomically to social stimuli. *Behavioural Brain Research, 41*(2), 81–94.

Danielson, M. L., Visser, S. N., Chronis-Tuscano, A., & DuPaul, G. J. (2018). A national descrip-tion of treatment among United States children and adolescents with attention-deficit/hyper-activity disorder. *Journal of Pediatrics, 192*, 240–246.

Del Campo, N., Chamberlain, S. R., Sahakian, B. J., & Robbins, T. W. (2011). The roles of dopa-mine and noradrenaline in the pathophysiology and treatment of attention-deficit/hyperac-tivity disorder. *Biological Psychiatry, 69*(12), e145–e157.

Demontis, D., Walters, R. K., Martin, J., Mattheisen, M., Als, T. D., Agerbo, E., Baldursson, G., Belliveau, R., Bybjerg-Grauholm, J., Baekvad_Hansen, M., Cerrato, F., Chambert, K., Churchhouse, C., Dumont, A., Eriksson, N., Gandal, M., Goldstein, J., Grasby, K., Grove, J., . . . Neale, B. M. (2019). Discovery of the first genome-wide significant risk loci for attention deficit/hyperactivity disorder. *Nature Genetics, 51*(1), 63–75.

Denckla, M. B. (1989). Executive function, the overlap zone between attention deficit hyperac-tivity disorder and learning disabilities. *International Pediatrics, 4*(2), 155–160.

Dennis, M. (1991). Frontal lobe function in childhood and adolescence: A heuristic for assessing attention regulation, executive control, and the intentional states important for social discourse. *Developmental Neuropsychology, 7*(3), 327–358.

Douglas, V. I. (1972). Stop, look and listen: The problem of sustained attention and impulse control in hyperactive and normal children. *Canadian Journal of Behavioural Science, 4*(4), 259–282.

Douglas, V. I., Barr, R. G., Amin, K., O'Neill, M. E., & Britton, B. G. (1988). Dosage effects and individual responsivity to methylphenidate in attention deficit disorder. *Journal of Child Psychology and Psychiatry, 29*(4), 453–475.

Ebaugh, F. G. (1923). Neuropsychiatric sequelae of acute epidemic encephalitis in children. *American Journal of Diseases of Children, 25*(2), 89–97.

Evans, S., Ling, M., Hill, B., Rinehart, N., Austin, D., & Sciberras, E. (2018). Systematic review of meditation-based interventions for children with ADHD. *European Child & Adolescent Psychiatry, 27*(1), 9–27.

Fallgatter, A. J., Ehlis, A. C., Dresler, T., Reif, A., Jacob, C. P., Arcos-Burgos, M., Muenke, M., & Lesch, K. P. (2013). Influence of a Latrophilin 3 (*LPHN3*) risk haplotype on event-related potential measures of cognitive response control in attention-deficit hyperactivity disorder (ADHD). *European Neuropsychopharmacology, 23*(6), 458–468.

Faraone, S. V., Biederman, J., & Mick, E. (2006). The age-dependent decline of attention deficit hyperactivity disorder: A meta-analysis of follow-up studies. *Psychological Medicine, 36*(2), 159–165.

Findling, R. L., McBurnett, K., White, C., & Youcha, S. (2014). Guanfacine extended release adjunctive to a psychostimulant in the treatment of comorbid oppositional symptoms in children and adolescents with attention-deficit/hyperactivity disorder. *Journal of Child and Adolescent Psychopharmacology, 24*(5), 245–252.

Geschwind, D. H., & Flint, J. (2015). Genetics and genomics of psychiatric disease. *Science, 349*(6255), 1489–1494.

Goldberg, S. B., Tucker, R. P., Greene, P. A., Davidson, R. J., Wampold, B. E., Kearney, D. J., & Simpson, T. L. (2018). Mindfulness-based interventions for psychiatric disorders: A systematic review and meta-analysis. *Clinical Psychology Review, 59*, 52–60.

Harris, J. C. (1989). Interrelationship of learning and emotional difficulty: Their genesis and treatment. In M. B. Denckla (Ed.), *Attention-deficit disorder, hyperactivity, and learning disabilities: Current theory and practical approaches* (pp. 69–77). Ciba-Geigy.

Harris, J. C., King, S. L., Reifler, J. P., & Rosenberg, L. A. (1984). Emotional and learning disorders in 6–12-year-old boys attending special schools. *Journal of the American Academy of Child Psychiatry, 23*(4), 431–437.

Hirota, T., Schwartz, S., & Correll, C. U. (2014). Alpha-2 agonists for attention-deficit/hyperactivity disorder in youth: A systematic review and meta-analysis of monotherapy and add-on trials to stimulant therapy. *Journal of the American Academy of Child & Adolescent Psychiatry, 53*(2), 153–173.

Hoffmann, H. (1862). *Struwwelpeter*. Routledge.

Hohman, L. B. (1922). Post-encephalitic behavior disorders in children. *Johns Hopkins Hospital Bulletin, 33*, 372–375.

Hoogman, M., Bralten, J., Hibar, D. P., Mennes, M., Zwiers, M. P., Schweren, L., van Hulzen, K., Medland, S., Shumskaya, E., Jahanshad, N., Zeeuw, P., Szekely, E., Sudre, G., Wolfers, T., Onnink, A., Dammers, J., Mostert, J., Vives-Gilabert, Y., Kohls, G., . . . Franke, B. (2017). Subcortical brain volume differences of participants with ADHD across the lifespan: An ENIGMA collaboration. *Lancet Psychiatry, 4*(4), 310–319.

Ireland, W. H. (1877). *On idiocy and imbecility*. Churchill.

Izard, C. (1991). *The psychology of emotions*. Plenum.

Joseph, A., Ayyagari, R., Xie, M., Cai, S., Xie, J., Huss, M., & Sikirica, V. (2017). Comparative efficacy and safety of attention-deficit/hyperactivity disorder pharmacotherapies, including guanfacine extended release: A mixed treatment comparison. *European Child & Adolescent Psychiatry, 26*(8), 875–897.

Kahn, E., & Cohen, L. H. (1934). Organic drivenness a brain-stem syndrome and an experience. *New England Journal of Medicine, 210*(14), 748–756.

Kahneman, D (2011). *Thinking, fast and slow.* Macmillan.

Kam, C. M., Greenberg, M. T., & Kusché, C. A. (2004). Sustained effects of the PATHS curriculum on the social and psychological adjustment of children in special education. *Journal of Emotional and Behavioral Disorders, 12*(2), 66–78.

Karam, R. G., Breda, V., Picon, F. A., Rovaris, D. L., Victor, M. M., Salgado, C. A. I., Vitola, E., Silva, K., Guimaraes de Silva, P., Mota, N., Caye, A., Belmonte de Abreau, P., Rohde, L., Grevet, E., & Bau, C. H. D. (2015). Persistence and remission of ADHD during adulthood: A 7-year clinical follow-up study. *Psychological Medicine, 45*(10), 2045–2056.

Kessler, J. W. (1980). History of minimal brain dysfunction. In H. Rie & E. Rie (Eds.), *Handbook of minimal brain dysfunctions: A critical view* (pp. 18–52). Wiley.

Laufer, M. W., & Denhoff, E. (1957). Hyperkinetic behavior syndrome in children. *Journal of Pediatrics, 50*(4), 463–474.

Laufer, M. W., Denhoff, E., & Solomons, G. (1957). Hyperkinetic impulse disorder in children's behavior problems. *Psychosomatic Medicine, 19*(1), 38–49.

Levin, P. M. (1938). Restlessness in children. *Archives of Neurology & Psychiatry, 39*(4), 764–770.

Liu, Q., Zhang, H., Fang, Q., & Qin, L. (2017). Comparative efficacy and safety of methylphenidate and atomoxetine for attention-deficit hyperactivity disorder in children and adolescents: Meta-analysis based on head-to-head trials. *Journal of Clinical and Experimental Neuropsychology, 39*(9), 854–865.

Loney, J. (1983). Research diagnostic criteria for childhood hyperactivity. In S. B. Guze, F. J. Earls, & J. E. Barrett (Eds.), *Childhood psychopathology and development* (pp. 109–137). Raven Press.

Loney, J., Langhorne, J. E., & Paternite, C. E. (1978). An empirical basis for subgrouping the hyperkinetic/minimal brain dysfunction syndrome. *Journal of Abnormal Psychology, 87*(4), 431–441.

Lou, H. C., Henriksen, L., Bruhn, P., Børner, H., & Nielsen, J. B. (1989). Striatal dysfunction in attention deficit and hyperkinetic disorder. *Archives of Neurology, 46*(1), 48–52.

McGee, R., Partridge, F., Williams, S., & Silva, P. A. (1991). A twelve-year follow-up of preschool hyperactive children. *Journal of the American Academy of Child & Adolescent Psychiatry, 30*(2), 224–232.

Milich, R., & Landau, S. (1989). The role of social status variables in differentiating subgroups of hyperactive children. In L. M. Bloomingdale, J. M. Swanson, & R. Kiorman (Eds.), *Attention deficit disorder: Current concepts and emerging trends in attentional and behavioral disorders of childhood* (pp. 1–23). Pergamon.

Milich, R., Loney, J., & Landau, S. (1982). Independent dimensions of hyperactivity and aggression: A validation with playroom observation data. *Journal of Abnormal Psychology, 91*(3), 183–198.

Morrison, J. R., & Stewart, M. A. (1973). The psychiatric status of the legal families of adopted hyperactive children. *Archives of General Psychiatry, 28*(6), 888–891.

Nakao, T., Radua, J., Rubia, K., & Mataix-Cols, D. (2011). Gray matter volume abnormalities in ADHD: Voxel-based meta-analysis exploring the effects of age and stimulant medication. *American Journal of Psychiatry, 168*(11), 1154–1163.

Neumann, A., Walton, E., Alemany, S., Cecil, C., González, J. R., Jima, D. D., Lahti, J., Tuominen, S., Barker, E., Binder, E., Caramaschi, D., Carracedo, A., Czamara, D., Evandt, J., Felix, J., Fuemmeler, B., Gutzkow, K., Hoyo, C., Julvez, J., . . . Tiemeier, H. (2020). Association between DNA methylation and ADHD symptoms from birth to school age: A prospective meta-analysis. *Translational Psychiatry, 10*(1), Article 398.

O'Neill, M. E., & Douglas, V. I. (1991). Study strategies and story recall in attention deficit disorder and reading disability. *Journal of Abnormal Child Psychology, 19*(6), 671–692.

Pereira-Sanchez, V., & Castellanos, F. X. (2021). Neuroimaging in attention-deficit/hyperactivity disorder. *Current Opinion in Psychiatry, 34*(2), 105–111.

Pliszka, S., & AACAP Work Group on Quality Issues. (2007). Practice parameter for the assessment and treatment of children and adolescents with attention-deficit/hyperactivity disorder. *Journal of the American Academy of Child & Adolescent Psychiatry, 46*(7), 894–921.

Polanczyk, G., De Lima, M. S., Horta, B. L., Biederman, J., & Rohde, L. A. (2007). The worldwide prevalence of ADHD: A systematic review and metaregression analysis. *American Journal of Psychiatry, 164*(6), 942–948.

Pope, A. W., Bierman, K. L., & Mumma, G. H. (1989). Relations between hyperactive and aggressive behavior and peer relations at three elementary grade levels. *Journal of Abnormal Child Psychology, 17*(3), 253–267.

Porrino, L. J., Rapoport, J. L., Behar, D., Sceery, W., Ismond, D. R., & Bunney, W. E. (1983). A naturalistic assessment of the motor activity of hyperactive boys: I. Comparison with normal controls. *Archives of General Psychiatry, 40*(6), 681–687.

Prevatt, F., & Levrini, A. (2015). *ADHD coaching: A guide for mental health professionals.* American Psychological Association.

Prevatt, F., & Yelland, S. (2015). An empirical evaluation of ADHD coaching in college students. *Journal of Attention Disorders, 19*(8), 666–677.

Purvis, K. L., & Tannock, R. (1997). Language abilities in children with attention deficit hyperactivity disorder, reading disabilities, and normal controls. *Journal of Abnormal Child Psychology, 25*(2), 133–144.

Rapin, I. (1964). Brain damage in children. *Practice of Pediatrics, 4*, 123–141.

Ribases, Á., Ramos-Quiroga, J. A., Sanchez-Mora, C., Bosch, R., Richarte, V., Palomar, G., Gastaminza, X., Bielsa, A., Arcos-Burgos, M., Muenke, M., Castellanos, F., Cormand, B., Bayse, M., & Casas, M. (2011). Contribution of LPHN3 to the genetic susceptibility to ADHD in adulthood: A replication study. *Genes, Brain and Behavior, 10*(2), 149–157.

Ross, D. M., & Ross, S. A. (1982). *Hyperactivity: Current issues, research and theory* (2nd ed.). Wiley.

Rutter, M. (1977). Brain damage syndromes in childhood: Concepts and findings. *Journal of Child Psychology and Psychiatry, 18*(1), 1–21.

Rutter, M. (1982). Syndromes attributed to "minimal brain dysfunction" in childhood. *American Journal of Psychiatry, 139*, 21–33.

Rutter, M., Graham, P., & Yule, W. (1970). *A neuropsychiatric study in childhood.* Heinemann.

Sergeant, J. (1988). From DSM-III attentional deficit disorder to functional defects. In L. Bloomingdale & L. Sergeant (Eds.), *Attention deficit disorder: Criteria, cognition, intervention* (pp. 183–198). Pergamon.

Sibley, M. H., Mitchell, J. T., & Becker, S. P. (2016). Method of adult diagnosis influences estimated persistence of childhood ADHD: A systematic review of longitudinal studies. *Lancet Psychiatry, 3*(12), 1157–1165.

Sonuga-Barke, E. J., & Castellanos, F. X. (2007). Spontaneous attentional fluctuations in impaired states and pathological conditions: A neurobiological hypothesis. *Neuroscience & Biobehavioral Reviews, 31*(7), 977–986.

Still, G. F. (1902). The Goulstonian Lectures on Some abnormal psychical conditions in children. *Lancet, 159*, 1008–1013.

Strauss, A. A., & Lehtinen, L. E. (1947). *Psychopathology and education of the brain-injured child.* Grune & Stratton.

Strauss, A. A., & Werner, H. (1943). Comparative psychopathology of the brain-injured child and the traumatic brain-injured adult. *American Journal of Psychiatry, 99*(6), 835–838.

Szatmari, P. (1992). The epidemiology of attention-deficit hyperactivity disorders. *Child and Adolescent Psychiatric Clinics, 1*(2), 361–371.

Szatmari, P., Offord, D. R., & Boyle, M. H. (1989). Ontario Child Health Study: Prevalence of attention deficit disorder with hyperactivity. *Journal of Child Psychology and Psychiatry, 30*(2), 219–223.

Tannock, R., Purvis, K. L., & Schachar, R. J. (1993). Narrative abilities in children with attention deficit hyperactivity disorder and normal peers. *Journal of Abnormal Child Psychology, 21*(1), 103–117.

Taylor, E., Kendall, T., Asherson, P., Bailey, S., Bretherton, K., Brown, A., & Mavranezouli, I. (2009). *Attention deficit hyperactivity disorder: The NICE guideline on diagnosis and management of ADHD in children, young people, and adults: National clinical practice guideline Number 72*. British Psychological Society and Royal College of Psychiatrists.

Taylor, E. A. (1986). Childhood hyperactivity. *British Journal of Psychiatry*, *149*(5), 562–573.

Taylor, E. A. (1988). Diagnosis of hyperactivity: A British perspective. In L. Bloomingdale & J. Sergeant (Eds.), *Attention deficit disorder: Criteria, cognition, intervention* (pp. 141–160). Pergamon.

Thapar, A., Cooper, M., & Rutter, M. (2017). Neurodevelopmental disorders. *Lancet Psychiatry*, *4*(4), 339–346.

Tredgold, A. F. (1908). *Mental deficiency (amentia)*. Wood.

Visser, J. C., Rommelse, N. N., Greven, C. U., & Buitelaar, J. K. (2016). Autism spectrum disorder and attention-deficit/hyperactivity disorder in early childhood: A review of unique and shared characteristics and developmental antecedents. *Neuroscience & Biobehavioral Reviews*, *65*, 229–263.

Volkow, N. D., Fowler, J. S., Wang, G. J., Ding, Y. S., & Gatley, S. J. (2002). Role of dopamine in the therapeutic and reinforcing effects of methylphenidate in humans: Results from imaging studies. *European Neuropsychopharmacology*, *12*(6), 557–566.

Volkow, N. D., Wang, G. J., Fowler, J. S., & Ding, Y. S. (2005). Imaging the effects of methylphenidate on brain dopamine: New model on its therapeutic actions for attention-deficit/hyperactivity disorder. *Biological Psychiatry*, *57*(11), 1410–1415.

Wang, S. M., Han, C., Lee, S. J., Jun, T. Y., Patkar, A. A., Masand, P. S., & Pae, C. U. (2017). Modafinil for the treatment of attention-deficit/hyperactivity disorder: A meta-analysis. *Journal of Psychiatric Research*, *84*, 292–300.

Weingartner, H., Ebert, M. H., Mikkelsen, E. J., Rapoport, J. L., Buchsbaum, M. S., Bunney, W. E., Jr., & Caine, E. D. (1980). Cognitive processes in normal and hyperactive children and their response to amphetamine treatment. *Journal of Abnormal Psychology*, *89*(1), 25–37.

Wender, P. H. (1971). *Minimal brain dysfunction in children*. Wiley.

Whalen, C. K., & Henker, B. (1992). The social profile of attention-deficit hyperactivity disorder: Five fundamental facets. *Child and Adolescent Psychiatric Clinics of North America*, *1*(2), 395–410.

Whalen, C. K., Henker, B., & Dotemoto, S. (1980). Methylphenidate and hyperactivity: Effects on teacher behaviors. *Science*, *208*(4449), 1280–1282.

Wilens, T. E., Robertson, B., Sikirica, V., Harper, L., Young, J. L., Bloomfield, R., Lyne, A., Rynkowski, G., & Cutler, A. J. (2015). A randomized, placebo-controlled trial of guanfacine extended release in adolescents with attention-deficit/hyperactivity disorder. *Journal of the American Academy of Child & Adolescent Psychiatry*, *54*(11), 916–925.

Zentall, S. S. (1988). Production deficiencies in elicited language but not in the spontaneous verbalizations of hyperactive children. *Journal of Abnormal Child Psychology*, *16*(6), 657–673.

# 17

# Specific Learning Disorders

## Introduction

Specific learning impairments in reading, writing, and mathematics are recognized neurodevelopmental disorders in fifth edition of the *Diagnostic and Statistical Manual of Mental Disorders* (DSM-5; APA, 2013). Neurodevelopmental disorders are disorders of brain development and lifelong with early age of onset. They are distinct from acquired brain disorders resulting from trauma. To make these diagnoses, problems applying key academic skills to learning have an onset during the developmental period and must have persisted for at least 6 months despite targeted interventions. Such learning impairments, if not treated, increase the later risk for emotional and behavior disorders. In epidemiologic surveys of the general population, up to 15% of children in the school-age population have academic difficulty in reading, writing, or mathematics during their school careers (Altarac & Saroha, 2007; Centers for Disease Control and Prevention [CDC], 2016). Learning deficits are recognized in children who are typically developing as well as in children who have a variety of neurodevelopmental syndromes and who may have poor decoding skills regardless of IQ level. In specific learning disorders, intelligence is within the normal range and not secondary to an intellectual developmental disorder (IDD). The general terms "learning disabilities" and "learning disorders" include impairments in academic skills. It is essential to clearly designate the particular skill that is impaired. Academic impairments may involve reading, spelling, mathematics, and written expression.

This chapter reviews the history, epidemiology, definition and classification, assessment, etiology (genetics and neuroimaging), comorbid psychiatric disorders, and treatment for impairments in reading, hyperlexia, spelling, mathematics, and written expression. Specific evaluation instruments for assessment of academic achievement are reviewed Chapter 2.

## Reading Impairment

### History

Reading impairment has been described since the end of the 19th century. A detailed case report by a British physician, William Pringle Morgan, described a 14-year-old boy with a pronounced inability to read, which Morgan viewed to be a congenital defect. Morgan (1896) referred to this reading impairment as "congenital word blindness." That same year, an ophthalmologist, Hinshelwood (1896), published a paper on the care of dyslexia that he, too, referred to as a peculiar form of word blindness. Hinshelwood later published on two more similar cases. Early cases of word blindness were ascribed to brain damage based on what was then understood as alexia or reading loss in adults (Kirby, 2020). Subsequently, in the 20th century, theoretical explanations for learning disabilities, particularly reading disability, were offered, such as that by Orton (1928), who used the term *specific reading disability*. He proposed incomplete or mixed cerebral dominance and suggested that delayed development of specialization in the left hemisphere might be involved. Despite these early reports, before the 1940s, children in the United States who had reading problems were frequently considered to have an IDD, to be emotionally disturbed, or to be socially disadvantaged.

During the 1940s, learning disorders were more clearly recognized in children with neurological dysfunction. Historically, one group of studies focused on whether children with learning difficulties invariably had demonstrable brain damage. It was concluded that brain damage was minimal, and the term *minimal brain damage* was introduced (Strauss & Lehtinen, 1947). Others raised the possibility that learning difficulties reflected a brain that functioned differently, rather than being damaged, and suggested the term *minimal brain dysfunction*, which became the accepted designation (Clements, 1966). However, the minimal brain dysfunction syndrome proposal was not limited to learning problems. It included learning deficits, dyslexic errors, failing to read, spelling error, perceptual motor problems, poor coordination, overactivity, impulsivity, and subtle neurological signs.

Subsequently, the term *specific learning disability* was introduced to describe the same group of children (Farnham-Diggory, 1978; Kirk & Bateman, 1962). Although all these formulations emphasized brain dysfunction, standardized sensorimotor-based neurological examinations did not demonstrate neurologic abnormalities. Higher cortical functions were apparently involved in the learning disabled rather than motor and/or sensory neurological abnormalities. Neuropsychological and linguistic tests were introduced to measure academic skills to supplement traditional psychological examinations to identify children with these specific learning disorders. Stimulant medication was prescribed for minimal brain dysfunction and was found to improve the hyperactivity and attentional problems frequently associated with learning disorders. However, the specific learning problems themselves were not improved with these medications (Gittelman, 1983).

In 1968, a subcommittee of the World Federation of Neurology defined the term *specific developmental dyslexia* (Critchley, 1970) as "a disorder manifested by difficulty in learning to read despite conventional instruction, adequate intelligence, and sociocultural opportunity." It was attributed to "fundamental cognitive disabilities which are frequently of constitutional origin." Currently, the term *dyslexia* is used in DSM-5 to refer to a pattern of learning difficulties that involves problems with accurate or fluent word recognition, poor decoding, and poor spelling but not problems in reading comprehension or math as a broader term including both. The overall term *reading impairment* is currently preferred in DSM-5. Despite having the diagnosis of dyslexia due to demonstrable phonological deficits, children in families with a familial risk for dyslexia do not all have reading deficits despite deficits in phonological awareness (Snowling & Melby-Lervåg, 2016). The assessment of reading impairment is complicated because the predominant cause, a phonological deficit, may not be the only deficit observed that leads to poor reading. In addition, phonological skills are dimensional and may not affect one or more aspects of reading when phonological deficits are a "downstream" effect stemming from more primary problems. Reading comprehension and word decoding may also be significantly involved (Snowling et al., 2020).

The passage of U.S. Public Law 94-142 in 1975 was a major step forward in developing services and programs for these learning-disabled children in the United States. In Public Law 94-142, children with learning disorders are defined as follows:

> Those children who have a disorder in one or more of the basic psychological processes involved in understanding or in using language, spoken or written, which disorder may manifest itself in an imperfect ability to listen, think, speak, read, write, spell, or do math calculations. The term includes such conditions as perceptual handicaps, brain injury, minimal brain dysfunction, dyslexia, and developmental aphasia. The term does not include children having learning problems which are primarily the result of visual, hearing, or motor handicaps, of [intellectual developmental disorder], of emotional disturbances, or of environmental, cultural, or economic disadvantage.

Public Law 94-142 has been continually reauthorized and updated in the ensuing years with passage as the Individuals with Disability Education Act (IDEA) and the Education for All Handicapped Children Act. Additional emphasis was placed on education in the No Child Left Behind Act in 2001. The 2004 reauthorization of IDEA again allows the school system to study new approaches to identify and treat children by focusing on response-to-intervention methods. An additional focus on support was established in 2015 with the authorization of the Elementary and Secondary Education Act, which requires educational services be provided in a multitiered system of supports with the goal of coordinating general education and special education programming. The goals are to improve educational opportunities for all children with disabilities (Daniel et al., 2006; Klassen et al., 2011; Nelson & Harwood, 2011; Sexton et al., 2012).

## Epidemiology

The exact prevalence of learning disorders in the academic skills areas is unknown because various studies have used different criteria to define cases. However, the CDC (2016) concluded that based on the available data, 5–15% was a reasonable estimate of persons with specific learning impairments. Epidemiologic studies find that reading impairment affects approximately 20% of school-aged children. Although males outnumber females in clinic referrals (Rutter et al., 2007), reading impairment is found to affect boys and girls equally (B. Shaywitz & Shaywitz, 2020).

Reading impairment affects all ethnic, racial, and socioeconomic groups. In 2017–2018, 7 million students aged 3–21 years were enrolled in services under IDEA. This made up 14% of all public school students. One-third of these students or 4.6% had specific learning disabilities (National Center for Educational Statistics, 2017, 2018). Male children are more likely to have been diagnosed with a developmental disability than females, as are more non-Hispanic White and non-Hispanic Black children than Hispanic children or non-Hispanic children of other races, children living in rural areas compared to children living in urban areas, and children with public health insurance compared to uninsured children and children with private insurance. Reading impairment was typically linked to genetic factors. However, environmental factors, when they become apparent, must be considered. These include home literacy, language environment, and school quality (Fletcher et al., 2019).

The Connecticut Longitudinal Study is the most extensive epidemiological survey of prevalence of reading impairment in the United States. This survey involved 445 children enrolled in kindergarten on entry and followed since 1983. These children were given an IQ test (the Wechsler Intelligence Scale for Children–Revised) and in alternate years reading and mathematics achievement tests through 12th grade using the Woodcock–Johnson Achievement test battery. At the end of each school year, teachers completed the Multi-grade Inventory for Teachers, which included mastery of reading, arithmetic, and written expression. With ongoing follow-up, 80% (375 participants) were enrolled into their fifth decade. This study found a prevalence of 20% with equal distribution in boys and girls (B. Shaywitz & Shaywitz, 2020). The achievement gap between reading impaired and typically developing was recognized as early as first grade in this study. This study recommends that treatment of children at risk be implemented as early as possible in grades 1–3, when the learning slope is steepest.

## Definition and Classification

In contrast to the current IDEA definition of learning disorders, the DSM-5 definition requires specifiers for impairment in reading, mathematics, and written expression. The term dyslexia is more specific and characterized by problems in phonological processing. The 21st-century federal definition of dyslexia (reading impairment) is codified in Public Law 115-391 (2018):

> An unexpected difficulty in reading for an individual who has the intelligence to be a much better reader, most commonly caused by a difficulty in phonological processing (the appreciation of individual sounds of spoken language) which affects the ability of an individual to speak, read, and spell.

DSM-5 notes that when the term dyslexia is used, it is necessary to be specific if there also are difficulties with reading comprehension or math reasoning. Evidence suggests that problems in reading comprehension are distinct from dyslexia (Nation & Snowling, 1998).

In DSM-5, specific learning disorders are distinct from diagnoses of IDD, visual or hearing problems, other neurological or mental disorders, psychosocial adversity, or lack of educational instruction. Reading, expressive writing, and mathematics disorders involve different processing deficits, including visuospatial or linguistic processes that involve various brain regions. A synopsis of DSM-5 criteria is shown in Box 17.1. DSM-5, unlike DSM-IV, incorporates an important distinction between basic and complex academic skills.

---

**Box 17.1  Synopsis of DSM-5 Criteria for Specific Learning Disorder**

---

A. Persistent difficulties in one or more of these six academic skills:
  1. *Basic:* Single-word-reading accuracy and fluency (defining symptom of dyslexia)
  2. *Complex:* Reading comprehension ("poor comprehenders" have this defining symptom)
  3. *Basic:* Spelling (nearly always found in dyslexia; does not define a separate disorder)
  4. *Complex:* Written expression
  5. *Basic:* Number sense, math facts, and calculation skills (defining symptom of dyscalculia)
  6. *Complex:* Mathematical reasoning
B. The score on a test of the academic skill is substantially below the mean score for the patient's chronological age and causes functional impairment.
C. Problems begin in early school years, but complex learning disorders only become clinically significant in later academic years.
D. Not due to intellectual disability, peripheral sensory disorders, other mental or neurological disorders, psychosocial adversity, lack of proficiency in the second language used for instruction (e.g., child is a native Spanish speaker in the United States and is not yet proficient in English), or inadequate educational instruction.

---

## Assessment

An assessment of reading impairment examines each aspect of language. These are the pragmatic, semantic, syntactical/grammatical, and phonological (speech sounds) components. Pragmatics refers to social communication. To communicate, we engage socially, we speak and we listen. Denckla (2019) proposed a language pyramid with pragmatics, our capacity to adjust language to the needs of the listener, at the base of it. The next level of language is semantic, understanding the meaning of words. Children with poor language skills show weakness in learning to read words. Higher up on the pyramid still is syntax and grammar. the capacity to connect words together in a meaningful way. Finally, nouns, verbs, and adverbs are at the apex of the pyramid. This is where speech sounds are analyzed. Thus, impaired reading resides at the top of the language pyramid.

Children and adults with impairment in reading have deficits in the phonological component of language; they are impaired in processing speech sounds. Their difficulty lies in understanding how spoken words can be broken down, segmented into phenomes, the elemental units of sound. Essentially, they have "trouble with words" in the speech sound aspect of language (Denckla, 2019). Children and adults with phonological deficits may also have problems in spoken language. Here, the difficulty lies in miscommunication of words and in speech fluency. Affected children may have word fluency problems, with multiple hesitations or pauses when they speak. These

problems are based on an impairment of speech sound comprehension, not on semantic limitations. These problems in decoding words and in word recognition vary
by age and developmental level. Despite these difficulties, listening comprehension is
typically intact. Although with intervention, reading accuracy may improve; reading
fluency problems may persist. Those affected continue to be slow readers. Problems in
spelling may also reflect phonological problems, and written expression can also be
affected.

The psychological aspect to reading impairment that is best understood is weakness
in phonological awareness for spoken language. Phonology involves becoming aware
of the structure of words to map units of sound into corresponding letters in print.
Another phonological weakness is in rapid automatized naming. Such slowness in
naming may be linked to cognitive and linguistic processes that underlie fluent reading.
Children may have phonological problems or naming problems; those most severely
affected may have both. Finally, a third issue involved in severity concerns perceptual
processing, which may underlie the first two. Perceptual processes include visuospatial
attention and perceptual learning deficits. Developmentally, children in preschool and
kindergarten, who are at risk for later impairment, may have problems learning letters
and numbers and rhyming with words. Children may enjoy being read to but may avoid
reading aloud themselves. These findings of phonological deficits are consistent across
different languages.

## Etiology

There is an increased risk for reading impairment in families of affected children
(Snowling & Melby-Lervåg, 2016). A meta-analysis of 95 publications found a mean
prevalence of reading impairment (dyslexia) of 45%, with risk ranging from 29% to
66%. Typically, there is delayed language development in infancy and the toddler years.
By preschool, problems in phonological processing and more broadly limited phonological awareness, letter knowledge, and rapid automatized naming of words are
recognized. Children identified as having familial risk subsequently fulfill diagnosis
criteria for reading impairment in the school years, showing poor literary skills. Their
parents tend to have low educational levels and read less often themselves and to their
children. For those with severe reading difficulty, educational intervention can atten-
uate severity.

## Genetics

Twin studies of children diagnosed with reading impairment find that genetic factors
are significant (Pennigton & Olson, 2005; Scerri & Schulte-Körne, 2010). Genetic language studies have identified regions of nine chromosomes involved: 1p36–34p, 2p16–
15p, 3p12–13q, 6p22, 6q13–16.2, 11p15.5, 15q21.3, 18p11.2, and xq27.3 (Mascheretti
et al., 2017; Scerri & Schulte-Körne, 2010). Independent studies have replicated linkage
to candidate genes on several of these chromosomes (Paracchini, 2011). Genetic studies
implicate the *DYKZ* locus on chromosome 6p22, specifically the genes *DCDC2* and

*KIAA0319*, in reading impairment (Eicher et al., 2014). These genes may also influence language impairment, verbal language, and cognition. In addition, these genes may play a role in other neurodevelopmental disorders associated with reading impairment. The *DYX1C1*, *DCDC2*, and *KIAA0319* genes have been linked to variations in temporal white matter along with reading skill deficits (Darki et al., 2012). The associated genes affect neuronal migration, neurite outgrowth, and cortical morphogenesis. The *KIAA0319* gene, also associated with reading disability, is involved with axonal growth and neuronal migration (Deng et al., 2019). All of these risk genes have small effect size and must be verified with genome-wide association studies (GWAS).

With the identification of genes associated with reading impairment, there is considerable interest in studying pathways from genes to behavior using brain neuroimaging and in studying cognitive and sensory mechanisms (Mascheretti et al., 2017). The left hemisphere occipital region is found to act as an interactive node for reading, bringing together how the word looks, sounds, and what the word means. Investigators ask, What are the effects of risk genes on brain structure, brain circuits, and brain function? How might testing for cognitive and sensory deficits associated with reading impairment be best examined?

## Neuropathology and Neuroimaging Studies

Autopsy studies in the 1970s and 1980s (Galaburda et al., 1985; Galaburda & Kemper, 1979) found brain anomalies with reading disabilities. These studies led to the use of neuroimaging methods—magnetic resonance imaging (MRI), diffusion tensor imaging (DTI), and functional MRI (fMRI)—to study children with reading impairment to better understand their brain basis. Gray matter and white matter volumes have been quantified, and indirectly, fiber pathways have been studied. fMRI investigations have identified brain regions activated when at rest and during participation in cognitive and sensory tasks. However, most children with reading impairment do not show structural brain abnormalities. Functional brain imaging does show reduced brain activity in the left hemisphere temporoparietal cortex when reading in children with reading impairment compared to typically developing control subjects (Richlan, 2012; B. Shaywitz et al., 2004). These studies point to inefficient functioning of left hemispheric posterior brain systems in both children and adults with reading impairment.

The three brain systems involved in reading are (a) Broca's area (inferior frontal gyrus), involved in articulation and word analysis; (b) the occipitotemporal region, involved in word analysis; and (c) regions of the occipitotemporal word-form area that is involved in rapid, automatic, fluent identification of words. These hemispheric occipitotemporal regions serve as an interactive node for reading. B. Shaywitz and Shaywitz (2020) refer to the reduced functioning with underactivation of the two posterior occipitotemporal regions as a "neural signature" of dyslexia. Moreover, fMRI studies in children with a family history of dyslexia show reduced activation of the posterior reading area that predates poor reading (Figure 17.1). These functional brain changes are documented in languages using alphabetic (Indo-European) and logographic script (Chinese).

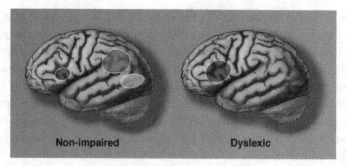

**Figure 17.1** The neural signature for dyslexia: Non-impaired readers (left) compared with dyslexic readers (right). Non-impaired readers activate each of the three important language areas on the left side of the brain. Broca's area is circled in the left inferior frontal gyrus anteriorly. Posterior circles designate the parietotemporal region above the occipitotemporal region below. These two posterior regions show significantly reduced brain activation in dyslexic readers.
From B. Shaywitz and Shaywitz (2020).

White matter networks that connect to components of the reading network can be visualized by DTI. The left arcuate superior longitudinal fasciculus connects the frontal and temporal language regions. The inferior longitudinal fasciculus connects the occipitotemporal lobes as well as the corona radiata that connects cortex to subcortical structures (Vendermosten et al., 2012).

DTI of brain connectivity has been used to clarify whether phonological representations are intact (Ramus & Szenkuvits, 2008). Ramus and Szenkuvits found that when phonemic representations were measured by activations in bilateral cortices (measured by DTI), connectivity between auditory cortices and left inferior frontal gyrus was reduced (Boets et al., 2013). This study found intact, but less accessible, phonetic representations in adults with reading impairment. With regard to brain connectivity, distant connections to frontal and parietal language regions were disrupted in dyslexic but not typical readers (Van der Mark et al., 2011). Brain imaging has also been used to examine the basis of rapid automatized naming. In one study in children, functional brain activation to a phonological awareness task found differences with phonological and rapid naming deficits (Norton et al., 2014). Activation in the left inferior parietal lobe was found to show a gradient that was associated with phonological awareness ability, whereas activation in the right cerebellar lobule VI showed a gradient with rapid naming ability.

These neuroimaging studies are important for identifying potential biomarkers that can be translated into interventions. Reading remediation is most effective in beginning readers. Early intervention is important before children experience phonological failure in reading. Neuroimaging studies are making progress in examining three major components of reading impairment: phonological awareness, rapid automatized naming, and reading fluency. Progress in this approach could facilitate early intervention (Maurer et al., 2009) and possibly the identification of poor readers as early as kindergarten (Bach et al., 2013). Neuroimaging could also predict children's reading acquisition by examining changes in white matter morphology (Myers et al., 2014) and facilitate identification of neural systems that predict long-term outcome (Norton et al., 2015).

## Associated Psychiatric Disorders

Approximately 60% children with reading impairment have a co-occurring disorder. The most frequently associated diagnosis with reading impairment is attention-deficit/ hyperactivity disorder (ADHD; Wadsworth et al., 2015), which is estimated to occur in between 20% and 40% of affected children, with the 40% prevalence of comorbid ADHD found in clinical referrals. A twin study examined genetic association of reading impairment and co-occurring ADHD symptoms of both inattention and hyperactivity (Greven et al., 2012). Twin pairs were examined in a study in which one twin in each pair met criteria for reading impairment, and the twins were followed up 5 years later. Reading analysis found that more than 60% of those initially diagnosed had familial risk, and essentially the same familial risk factors were reconfirmed at 5-year follow-up. Analysis of common genetic influences with co-occurrence of ADHD inattention and hyperactivity accounted for 20% of the variance at the initial assessment and 10% at 5-year follow-up. The authors concluded that familial influences on reading impairment are highly stable, with inattention largely related to familial influence but less robust for hyperactivity. Children with ADHD having a deficit in working memory are likely to exhibit impaired reading (Greven et al., 2012).

Another approach to examine the relationship between reading impairment and ADHD is a multidefect model of co-occurrence (McGrath et al., 2011). One study that examined phonological awareness, rapid automatized naming, and processing speed predicted untimed single-word reading. Processing speed predicted both reading impairment and inattention (Pennington et al., 2019). Processing speed accounted for 75% of variance in reading impairment (McGrath et al., 2011), a conclusion supported by other studies (Peterson et al., 2017). In another genetic follow-up study with twins, Willcutt et al. (2010) found that all of the shared genetic influence comparing reading and inattention involved processing speed. This is consistent with the generalist gene hypothesis that genes found for one learning disorder are associated with others (Pennington et al., 2019).

### Attention-Deficit/Hyperactivity Disorder and Reading Impairment

The relationship between reading impairment and ADHD symptoms primarily relates to the inattention disorder type (Plourde et al., 2017; Schuchardt et al., 2015). In neuropsychological testing, the co-occurrence of reading impairment and ADHD involves deficits in processing speed, verbal working memory, phonological short-term memory, naming speed, and central executive functions (primarily in working memory) (Moura et al., 2017). These findings are consistent with shared genetics, neural, and cognitive factors. However, neuroimaging studies show differences in both structural and functioning imaging when ADHD and reading impairment are examined separately, suggesting two pathways leading to impaired learning (Eden & Vaidya, 2008).

Stimulant medication improves attention in children and adolescents with ADHD and reading impairment (Tannock et al., 2018; Wietecha et al., 2013) and leads to improvement in reading. Mindfulness training and meditation are also beneficial (Tarrasch et al., 2016), although long-term effects need to be determined.

## Disruptive Impulsive Control and Conduct Disorder

Children with reading impairment may have co-occurring disruptive behavior, problems with impulse control, and oppositional defiant behaviors (Hendren et al., 2018). Most of the association is with problem behaviors rather than conduct disorder. It is not clear whether disruptive behavior is a primary diagnosis or secondary to emotional reaction to coping with the reading impairment. Conduct and behavioral problems are seen independent of reading impairment (Kempe et al., 2011; Russell et al., 2015). The co-occurrence may be a consequence of the increased rates of attention deficits in both disorders.

## Anxiety Disorder

Children with reading impairment have increased rates of general anxiety disorders compared to unaffected children (Mammarell et al., 2016). Moreover, the higher rates of anxiety persist despite a co-occurring ADHD diagnosis. Anxiety may be a result of coping with reading impairment and may compound the problem by increasing distraction. In a UK study, parents' and teachers' ratings on development and well-being of 9- to 15-year-olds documented that literacy difficulties were significantly associated with anxiety disorder (Carroll et al., 2005). In another epidemiological study in the United States, anxiety disorders were found to be significantly more common in 15-year-olds with reading impairment than in controls (Goldston et al., 2007). A systemic review and meta-analysis of 22 studies involving 1,700 poor readers and nearly 10,000 controls found elevated anxiety in poor readers independent of inattention (Francis et al., 2019). There may be a familial component because siblings with reading impairment are reported to have increased anxiety. Cognitive–behavioral therapy may reduce anxiety symptoms. Mindfulness training has also been shown to be effective in anxiety reduction (Beauchemin et al., 2008).

## Depressive Disorder

Children and adolescents exhibit increased rates of depression and mood disorders with reading impairment (Mammarella et al., 2016; Maughan et al., 2003). The depressive symptoms are not dependent on co-occurring ADHD. Low self-esteem is related to depression risk (Alexander-Passe, 2006), as are peer victimization and bullying. Moreover, difficulty in initiating and sustaining sleep has been reported in reading impairment (Carotenuto et al., 2016). Protective factors for co-occurring conditions include personal resilience to stress, social connections with peers, and self-advocacy (Haft et al., 2016).

In addition to ADHD and internalizing disorders, reading impairment co-occurs with disorders of language development, both language impairment and speech sound disorder (Nittrouer & Pennington, 2010). Language disorder involves structural language (syntax and grammar) and semantics (vocabulary). Speech sound disorder refers to the ability to accurately produce sounds of one's language. These co-occurring conditions, especially ADHD, language impairment, and speech sound disorder, may be recognized in preschool earlier than reading impairment, which is not diagnosed until school entrance. These risk factors may be assessed in preschool with early intervention. Moreover, children with reading impairment are at risk for reading comprehension disorder, math impairment, and writing impairment. This overlap is recognized in

DSM-5 criteria in that all three disorders are included under the overall term specific learning disorder. ADHD, anxiety, depression, disruptive impulse control, and conduct disorders may co-occur and require intervention (Hendren et al., 2018). Children and adolescents with reading disorder may also have other secondary emotional, social, and family problems. Finally, other neurodevelopmental disorders with associated specific academic skills include Tourette's disorder, neurofibromatosis, and seizure disorders.

## Treatment

Historically, intersensory integration models of reading dysfunction and intersensory perceptual training methods—such as the Fernald (1943) method, which utilizes auditory, visual, and tactile kinesthetic modalities, and the Frostig (1969) method on primary perceptual deficits—have been employed. These approaches focus on the neurophysiologic mechanisms that are involved in perceptual and motor development. This framework led to sensorimotor treatments, including the controversial Delacato (1966) approach, which involves creeping and crawling exercises to presumably retrain the brain by influencing hemispheric specialization. This approach has been demonstrated to be completely ineffective. The evidence from controlled studies does not support positive claims for these sensory integration approaches to remediate reading disability or their utility in teaching normal or disadvantaged readers (Robinson, 1972).

### Remediation of Impaired Reading

A variety of approaches have been advocated for treating reading impairment. Difficulty with phoneme awareness, identifying and mastering individual speech sounds in words, letter–sound correspondence, and letter–sound knowledge are the most important factors in enhancing word-level reading skills (Hulme et al., 2012). Interventions that target phoneme awareness and letter–sound knowledge are coupled with direct word recognition practice. Remediation of reading problems should begin early in development with an emphasis on language skills, including vocabulary and phonological skills, and continue throughout the life span. Early intervention is helpful in establishing reading accuracy for typically developing children and in those at risk for reading impairment. Intervention programs emphasize teaching alphabetics (phonemic awareness and phonics), reading fluency, vocabulary, and reading comprehension. The most effective interventions are specialized schools dedicated to teaching students with reading impairment (B. Shaywitz & Shaywitz, 2020), which include independent schools and public charter schools for dyslexia.

### Interventions
*Phonology*
The effectiveness of focused phonological interventions has been the subject of substantial research. A meta-analysis examined 83 controlled intervention studies. Phonological awareness, alphabet knowledge, and early decoding skills were assessed in preschool and kindergarten children with impaired decoding skills and those without difficulty in decoding. The interventions in these studies included phonological

awareness training offered individually or in small groups in which children were taught to identify phonemes in words by matching words with the same initial sound or to manipulate phonemes in words. These exercises were typically combined with reading instruction in phonics (training letter knowledge) and to relate this knowledge to printed words. These interventions supplemented regular school teaching for children with reading impairment. Overall, these interventions produced a major improvement of nearly 1 standard deviation (0.8 standard deviation) compared to typical phonological awareness approaches in control children, with improvement in both word reading and spelling (Lonigan & Shanahan, 2009). Another study examined older children and adults with impaired reading. Here, reading instructions in phonics, with or without phonological awareness training, led to enhanced word reading accuracy and greater word reading fluency (McArthur et al., 2012, 2018). Therefore, interventions addressing phonology along with letter–sound training and phonic reading instruction have positive benefits on reading, spelling, and phonological skills in children. The most effective phonological training targets phonemes, such as sounding out the word "cat": /k/ae/t/ . Starting children with reading connected text early in life is important (Melby-Lervåg et al., 2012).

*Fluency*

Reading fluency is the second critical element in reading instruction. With early intervention, older children with impairments in reading may master decoding at the word level yet reading still is not fluent but, rather, slow and labored. Fluency problems are more difficult to treat. Interventions that are most effective teach vocabulary and strategies to engage the reader with the text. One meta-analysis that examined how to remediate problems in fluency found that the most effective interventions involved guided repeat oral reading in which the student reads and rereads the same text repeatedly to a designated level of proficiency (Rasinski et al., 2011). The meta-analysis included children in grades 2–9, ages 6–14 years, and compared typical readers and those with reading impairment. There were moderate effects from repeated reading on decoding fluency, word recognition, and reading comprehension. These findings were supported by another study that examined repeated reading practices, finding substantial improvement in reading fluency and comprehension (Therrien, 2004). Better designed studies are needed with regard to the effectiveness of repeated practice on fluency and other interventions. However, all of these randomized control studies provide strong evidence that structured phoneme awareness and letter–sound knowledge interventions are highly effective.

For adolescent and college students, despite earlier intervention, educational accommodation continues to be needed as supported by neuroimaging studies. These students should be granted extra time for reading and writing assignments and for examinations. With continuing accommodations, reading accuracy may improve; however, slow reading often persist.

Another approach is systematic listening to spoken text. Text-to-speech programs include Voice Dream Reader, Immersive Reader, Reading out Loud, and Natural Reader. These word-to-text programs are available for smartphones and computers, including DragonDictate. Finally, an important accommodation is oral examination focused on content knowledge. With targeted early treatment and accommodations, accuracy improves, although fluency may continue to be problematic. With proper supports, children with impaired reading can be successful in the vocation of their choice.

In summary, treatment of reading impairment is based on helping the child compensate for both reading disorder and the frequently accompanying language disorder. The first step is to develop an individualized tutoring program that utilizes a phonics-based approach to reading. For younger children, training in segmental language skills may also be needed. If a phonics program is not successful, then tutoring in basic phoneme awareness skills may help.

The school setting may allow the child to compensate by providing extra time on written tests; spelling errors should be noted but not lead to reduced grades, foreign languages should not be required, and oral examinations are preferred over written exams. It is particularly important that all of the child's teachers be aware of the child's problem areas to avoid the child being labeled as lazy or incompetent. Parents must function as advocates for their child's treatment and help facilitate appropriate interventions as well as provide emotional support. The major adjustment difficulties related to reading disorder are reduced self-esteem, self-blame, anxiety, and mood disorder. Both parents and teachers need to provide for successes in the child's areas of strength and monitor the child for associated psychological symptoms (Silver, 1989). However, parents should not become their child's primary tutor, not only because of their lack of training in reading but also because of inherent conflicts between the role of parent and the role of teacher, which may lead to disagreements (Pennington, 1991).

### Pharmacological Treatment

Pharmacological approaches have been explored for treating reading disorders. Because attention is important for the development of fluent reading, associated ADHD has been treated pharmacologically. Psychostimulant medication, which is used to treat co-occurring ADHD, has been considered to be potentially effective for use in children with reading disorders. Gittelman et al. (1983) combined remedial reading instruction with either placebo or methylphenidate drug treatment. Their results suggested some benefit in academic task performance, such as in math computation. However, children with pure reading disorder did not show any clear benefit in reading performance. In this study, two measures of reading showed nonsignificant differences, and the one test that showed some advances did not lead to significant improvement in performance. Some studies have shown short-term improvement on laboratory tests of learning, but long-lasting improvement in academic achievement has not been demonstrated. The conclusion is that there is no justification for the use of stimulant medication alone, without academic treatment, and that the combined use of academic remediation with drug treatment may produce some improvement, although over a period of months, this advantage is neither "broad nor dramatic" (Gittelman et al., 1983). However, children with ADHD should be appropriately treated with stimulants, although expectations must be tempered in terms of educational improvement because the drug treatment is not targeted to the basic mechanism of the reading disorder.

More recently, pharmacological treatment of reading disorder has involved the use of piracetam, a drug structurally similar to the neurotransmitter γ-aminobutyric acid. It had been suggested that this medication may enhance performance on left hemispheric–dependent tasks (Tallal et al., 1986). Piracetam has been studied for the treatment of reading disorder because of suspected deficits involving left hemispheric function in some cases. A multisite, double-blind evaluation study with piracetam was conducted that involved 257 reading-disabled boys, who were assessed during a 12-week placebo-controlled study. Improved reading speed was observed in the peracitam-treated reading-disabled subjects, although no significant improvement was observed with reading accuracy or reading comprehension. A longer, 36-week multisite evaluation with 225 reading-disabled children showed small, but apparently reliable, improvement in oral passage reading (Wilsher et al., 1987). However, this study did not replicate the improvement in reading speed found in the original study. Additional measures of information processing, language, and memory did not show improvement with piracetam. Because learning-disabled children may show increased anxiety, anxiolytic medications have been prescribed. None of these studies have shown improvements in academic achievement related to drug use (Aman & Schroeder, 1990). Piracetam medication, in isolation, cannot be recommended as a treatment for developmental reading disorder. The evidence seems to indicate that pharmacotherapy is not indicated to treat specific learning disorders but may be useful for coexisting behavioral problems.

## Hyperlexia

Hyperlexia is a reading disorder in which there are advanced phonetic decoding skills relative to comprehension skills or general intelligence. Word reading skills are acquired early without specific teaching of these skills. There is a strong orientation by a child with hyperlexia toward written words. In hyperlexia, single-word reading precocity occurs in the absence of intensive instruction in children who have general cognitive and language deficiencies (Metsala & Siegel, 1992). Examination of hyperlexia, a disorder that is not infrequent in high-functioning children with autistic disorder (Whitehouse & Harris, 1984) and other children with developmental disorders, may further our understanding of neural processes involved in reading.

In early stages in reading acquisition, the semantic system is apparently more developed than decoding skills; however, in hyperlexia the opposite seems to be the case. In hyperlexia, knowledge of orthographic representations and sound–letter correspondences appear before semantic and syntactic processing. Reading appears to be mechanical and based on bottom-up processing without comprehension.

### Definition

The earliest description of what is now defined as hyperlexia was by Hollingworth and Winfold in 1918. The authors described a cognitively limited child who was innately gifted with special ability to master reading. Another similar case was described in 1930 (Phillips, 1930). Subsequently, definitions were proposed for hyperlexia. Silberberg and Silberberg (1967, 1968) used the term to refer to children who recognized written words that would not be expected to be known at their intellectual level. In hyperlexia, advanced word reading skills are observed in children who have language and cognitive delays. Speech development is generally severely delayed, and there may be no conversational speech. Precocious word recognition skills are observed as early in development as the first 2 or 3 years of life, prior to formal reading instruction. Abnormalities in expressive language, such as dysarthria, echolalia, and perseveration, are common. Rote memory skills may be well-developed (Ostrolenk et al., 2017).

Hyperlexia is generally viewed as a decoding skill with no or limited comprehension of the words that are sounded out. Thus, there can be a total absence of comprehension of single words and sometimes simple sentences. Typically, children score in the moderate to severe range of IDD on standardized tests. Yet, some studies have report hyperlexic children who tested in the typical range of intelligence (Goldberg & Rothermel, 1984; Richman & Kitchell, 1981; Welsh et al., 1987).

Richman and Kitchell (1981) identified children as hyperlexic whose word recognition on the Wide Range Achievement Test was 2 years above that expected for their full-scale cognitive ability. The most interest in hyperlexia has focused on children who test in the moderate to severe range of IDD. A more appropriate definition may be to focus on single-word reading precocity, in the absence of instruction, in children with cognitive and language deficiencies because this focus is on an ability that is not learned. Because of its occurrence in autism, hyperlexia has been described as a savant skill. Yet its neurocognitive basis and relation to autistic cognition and more typical reading acquisition are not established.

## Hyperlexia in Autism

Although there are no published data on the prevalence of hyperlexia in the general population, there is information available on autism spectrum disorder (ASD) and other neurodevelopmental disorders. These estimates vary considerably, with a prevalence of approximate 6% (Wei et al., 2015). Using less stringent criteria, a prevalence of 14–20% has been reported (Grigorenko et al., 2003). Criteria used for the higher rates were standardized reading decoding score at least 2 standard deviations above the level of intelligence and age-equivalent reading/decoding score at least 2 years above level of intelligence. In these studies, approximately 75% of the cases were male, consistent with the typical sex ratio in ASD. Nonverbal intelligence was typically within the normal range. In a systematic review of reported cases, Ostrolenk et al. (2017) found that 84% of the cases of hyperlexia were associated with ASD.

An MRI study sought to establish the neural basis of hyperlexia in a 9-year-old whose word reading was 6 years ahead of expectation for his age. The patient met criteria for ASD and was compared to two age-matched neurotypically developing children—one for chronological age and the other for reading age. Compared to the reading age-matched control, the patient scored greater activity in the right posterior inferior temporal sulcus, a brain region linked to visual word form recognition. This brain region typically is activated in the early phases of reading at a time when words are recognized by visual patterns. This region would typically no longer be engaged when reading becomes automatic. It is a letter-to-sound correspondence brain region (Turkeltaub et al., 2004). In addition, in this subject, phonological brain regions were hyperactivated along with phonemic awareness regions. Thus, the recognition systems are overactivated in hyperlexia. In a magnetoencephalographic study of 26 children with ASD aged 5–8 years, Kikuchi et al. (2013) reported that whereas the left hemispheric language areas were activated in cognitively neurotypical children, those with ASD showed mainly lateralized neurophysiological connectivity with visual cognition and phonological aspects of words. Overall, children with hyperlexia have orthographic representations mapped on phonological ones and essentially bypass the lexical–semantic route.

## Hyperlexia and Reading Disorder

Hyperlexia has led to considerable interest in understanding the mechanisms of word recognition skills in children with pervasive deficits in cognition. Central nervous system involvement is suggested by reports of dysarthria, perseveration, echolalia, poor motor functioning, and attention deficits.

There are two opposing views regarding the relationship between hyperlexic word decoding skills and the comprehension deficits. One view suggests that the same linguistic mechanism underlies both advanced word reading and deficient reading comprehension. The other proposes that the two processes are independent. In the unitary view, advanced word recognition is the result of bias in information processing, leading to an acute awareness of the physical features of stimuli and intense processing of physical attributes due to an inability to allocate processing capacity to higher level analysis. In this model, language consists of mechanical associations rather than semantic and syntactic processing. Children, then, would decode words but bypass the semantic analysis system. Comprehension is minimal because of the lack of interaction between top-down semantic information processing and bottom-up decoding.

The second view suggests that deficient comprehension skills occur independently of special word recognition abilities (Pennington et al., 1987; Welsh et al., 1987). In this model, word recognition skills are intact and do interact with semantic knowledge, if present. Poor comprehension, then, is the result of poor language and cognitive ability separate from intact word recognition abilities. Using this model, the underlying mechanism of isolated word reading may not be atypical. However, the processes that govern word recognition may function independently of general cognitive deficits in children with hyperlexia.

These two viewpoints have been considered with regard to the dual-route theory of reading, in which children may show exceptional decoding by one route but impaired semantic performance in the other. If hyperlexia is compared to surface (visual, orthographic, and dyseidetic) dyslexia, comprehension in surface dyslexics may not be as impaired as in hyperlexics. In surface dyslexia, there is difficulty with irregular words and semantic confusion of homophones. However, when hyperlexia is compared to direct (dyseidetic) dyslexia, in which fewer errors are reported on exceptional words than regular words, the words that are read are not understood. The direct (dysphonetic and auditory) dyslexics would read words through the lexical, whole-word route but not have access to lexical semantic knowledge. The ability of hyperlexic children to recognize exceptional words, in addition to making some visual errors, suggests that one or more levels of units higher than the grapheme–phoneme correspondence are functional. In hyperlexics, regular consistent words were recognized more accurately than inconsistent regular words. From these comparisons, it does not appear that hyperlexics represent an extreme form of reading impairment—that is, reading only by grapheme–phoneme correspondence or reading only by whole-word recognition—because they are able to recognize exceptional words that are not derived by grapheme–phoneme correspondences (Cobrinik, 1974). They are also able to read nonwords that are unfamiliar and not stored as whole-word units. It is suggested that hyperlexic children's isolated word recognition is deviant from normal only insofar as typical readers use other forms of word knowledge, such as semantic knowledge and spoken word knowledge. Cognitive and language deficits may impede the development of other sources of lexical knowledge.

Overall, there is not a unitary underlying style or mechanism, such as excessive attention to detail, that causes both lowered comprehension and advanced word recognition. Instead, hyperlexics may be differentiated from other developmentally disordered children by their unimpaired ability to acquire orthographic-to-phonological correspondences. Their oral language comprehension seems to be comparable to that of children with similar cognitive abilities. Essentially, these children appear to read as skilled word decoders. Decoding skills appear to develop independently of other types of lexical knowledge.

Compared to children with reading impairment, hyperlexic children are able to read nonwords but are not able to perform on some phonemic awareness tasks while children with reading impairments have difficulty reading nonwords and perform poorly on these tasks. These differences may relate to the child's accessibility to cognitive consciousness, which perhaps could be measured by phonemic awareness tasks that are thought to be an important aspect of normal reading acquisition and a predictor of reading success but may not be necessary for hyperlexic children.

For the normal reader, both the conceptual ability to understand a task and the stability of phonological representations allow intact sound-to-symbol structures to develop. Hyperlexic children may have difficulty understanding the task even though the phonological representations are well-developed. Although both groups perform poorly on tasks of phonemic awareness, it appears that children with reading impairment have an impairment in the development of specific phonological processes or a phonological processing that has been spared in children with hyperlexic disorder.

## Impairment in Spelling

Proficiency in reading is often considered the key to success in other academic areas. Reading achievement is highly correlated with mastery in spelling and mathematics. Lack of mastery in reading may prevent mastery in other basic skills areas. The greatest amount of research in learning disorders is on reading disorders; however, research on the other academic skills disorders is not far behind. Poor readers are almost invariably poor spellers, but the converse is not necessarily true.

There is no research base to support an isolated learning disorder in spelling (Pennington et al., 2019). Skills in phonological and/or graphic (conventional spelling of a language) processes are involved in spelling. Letter patterns in words that occur more frequently are learned first. Phonological information that occurs more frequently is recognized and mapped more quickly. Thus, both phonological and orthography are important in spelling. Essentially, orthography is the practice of correct spelling, recognizing the placement of letters one after another to make a word. Morphology is important to spelling as well. Morphology refers to studying words and parts of words. A morpheme is defined as the smallest unit of meaning in spelling and reading.

There is considerable overlap between reading and spelling difficulties; however, the processes involved in reading and spelling may be different. Frith (1978) suggested that there is no simple one-to-one sound–symbol correlation because sounds do not have natural segments and pronunciations frequently changes. Mastery of spelling requires a considerable degree of linguistic competence, and an understanding of "meaning in context" is important just as is knowledge of sound–symbol correspondences. Children may read aloud with accuracy and fluency yet have problems understanding what has been read. Spelling problems tend to last longer than reading problems. Phonological rather than visual skills are more important in the development of spelling, although visual memory for spelling patterns may play a major role in spelling proficiency. Thus, poor phonological awareness and poor phonological decoding are clearly correlated with the ability to spell (S. Shaywitz & Shaywitz, 2005). A longitudinal study of the development of spelling documented that proficiency in spelling is dependent on phoneme awareness and letter–sound knowledge (Caravolas et al., 2001).

Phonics, understanding that letters correspond to sounds, is applied to both reading and spelling. With this understanding of how letters map onto sounds, the next step is blending sounds together to read whole words. Spelling, however, requires that children segment words into pertinent sounds; for example, "dog" has three sounds, "d-o-g." To write words on a page, they use their understanding of how discrete sounds can appear on a page in written words.

The English language is more unpredictable for spelling than it is for reading (Caravolas et al., 2001). In English, learning to spell is more difficult because of the lack of one-to-one correspondence between letters and sounds. Some letters and words can be pronounced in more than one way, and sounds that can be written in more than one way. There is greater ambiguity in spelling and reading. Moreover, in spelling, a string of letters is produced from memory, but in reading, one deciphers print on a page (Ehri, 1997). Older adults with dyslexia whose word reading is improved generally will continue to have problems with spelling. In DSM-5, impairment in spelling is not a specific learning disorder. However, spelling accuracy is a feature of impairment in written expression and writing. Spelling accuracy is described as an element in an impairment of written expression.

## Interface Between Spelling and Reading

It is generally thought that if a child has learned to read, then spelling will naturally follow; however, this is not necessarily true. Children may read words that they cannot spell and may spell other words without being able to read them. These disassociations suggest reading and spelling skills have some independence from one another. Children who make spelling errors most commonly are poor readers rather than normal readers because reference to phonological cues is more common in spelling than in reading.

The examination of spelling errors identifies dysphonetic and/or phonetic misspelling. Children may be able to spell phonetically regular words that they are not able to read. Although a phonological analysis is essential in learning to spell, visual analysis is also required. To spell irregular words, word-specific knowledge is also required. In spelling as in reading, there is more than one approach. One code is based on the sound elements of the word and the other on the meaning and structure of the whole word (Temple, 1993).

Children with both reading and spelling difficulties tend to have a more generalized language disorder, whereas those with specific problems in spelling but few problems in reading more often have phonetically accurate spelling errors. Frith (1985) referred to children who had both reading and spelling difficulties as dyslexic and those who only had spelling errors as dysgraphic. In the dysgraphic group, phonetic spelling errors occurred twice as often as non-phonetic errors. In the reading-disordered group, the two types of errors were equally frequent. Consequently, in dysgraphics, the phono-logical route seemed intact because they were able to analyze speech sounds into phonemes. Although they did not show problems in reading, an increased difficulty in rhyming was noted. Phonological problems in spelling are associated with reading problems.

## Definition

The core neurodevelopmental issue in spelling difficulties includes deficits in phono-logical processing and decoding; orthographic problems (coding letters and words into memory and deficits in morphology); and use of suffixes, prefixes, and root words. The importance of phonological awareness in spelling is demonstrated by children's early attempts to invent the correct spelling of words and later when phonological skills are more developed for spelling progress. Training in sound categorization may have a greater effect on spelling than on reading, indicating that phonological awareness may be particularly important for spelling progress (Goswami & Bryant, 2016).

Several models have been introduced supporting the view that spelling is initially phonological. The integration of different strategies used in reading and spelling is needed for successful spelling. Frith (1985) suggests three stages in spelling: (a) logo-graphic, in which spelling is symbolic and not connected to phonology; (b) alphabetic, in which children spell words out by working out all the phonemes in the words and representing them with letters; and (c) orthographic, in which children work on larger segments, using analogies in spelling. Although this sequence is reasonable, the first stage may be brief and the methods used in the last two stages may overlap. As chil-dren approach these stages, the irregularities in the English writing system with its use of "th" and "sh" sounds, in addition to consonant clusters, make reading difficult; the irregularities are difficult to teach.

Children may utilize a phonological strategy in spelling in different ways. The con-stituent sounds, or phonemes, may be worked out alphabetically so each is represented by one letter, or the child may make analogies to similar-sounding words and see the similarity in spelling between the two words. The analogies are based on segments rather than phonemes. Rhymes are the most frequent phonological segments used for analogies in spelling. Beginning spellers may make use of rhymes but then attempt to represent the segment by a single letter, which leads to errors, such as "cr" for "car." When children learn to spell, they may categorize words at the phonemic or the rhyme level.

But when does visual memory for the appearance of words, gained through reading, become linked to spelling? There seems to be a normal developmental integration so that although younger children may be able to spell words, they cannot read; by age 10 years, this difference has essentially disappeared. For younger children, spelling is a more important contributor to this process of integration than reading. This may be because reflection on phonemic content that is necessary for spelling affects reading development by improving phonological awareness. As children grow older, they begin to use knowledge gained through reading as they approach spelling. Reading knowledge does result in the visual representation of particular letters and words. Consequently, these two skills influence each other at different times, and early spelling may help early reading. When reading is well-developed, children use their stored memories for spelling patterns; and this knowledge improves spelling.

## Spelling Disorders

Studies of children with phonological problems reveal difficulties in spelling. Children who become poor spellers may fail to integrate strategies that they already use in visual reading and spelling. Problems in phonology, coding words or letters into memory, and the use of suffixes, prefixes, and root words may present as dysphonetic spelling. This term refers to visually comparable approximations of words (e.g., "faght" for "fight"), phonetically correct but incorrectly spelled (e.g., "flite" for "flight"), or spelling that is not accurate (e.g., "played" spelled "plade"). Moreover, a child with memory problems may spell poorly due to weakness in coding. Other causes of misspelling occur if there is poor auditory working memory that interferes with processing letters properly. Difficulty with sequencing can lead to transposition spelling errors (Kelly & Natale, 2020).

Good readers who were poor spellers at age 14 years were worse at manipulating sounds than good readers who were good spellers. Poor spellers who are also poor readers have the most difficulty in remediation. These children tend to have difficulty working out the relationship between letters and sounds in both reading and spelling. A follow-up study of typical and poor readers first tested at age 14 or 15 years from the Isle of Wight epidemiological study and tested again in adulthood at age 44 or 45 years revealed persistent spelling errors at the 30-year follow-up for poor readers. By adolescence, individual differences in spelling were stable in these individuals (Maughan et al., 2009).

## Etiology and Genetics

Family studies have found that spelling abilities aggregate in families. In one study, spelling was found to aggregate in families, whereas handwriting did not aggregate (Raskind et al., 2000). The clearest evidence of heritability in spelling is found in twin studies, in which there is greater heritability than for reading (Stevenson et al., 1987). In one study of twins raised apart in separate families, heritability for word reading was 0.75, and it was 0.51 for reading comprehension and 0.76 for spelling (Johnson et al., 2005).

In genetic linkage studies, spelling has been linked to chromosome 15 (Nöthem et al., 1999; Schulte-Körne, 2001). Because impaired reading is also connected to chromosome 15, the genetic findings may represent a common factor to both. When spelling was examined as phenotype of impairment in reading (dyslexia) (Rubenstein et al., 2011), four genetic loci were identified that showed variation in both spelling and reading. These findings have yet to be confirmed by sufficiently powered GWAS. Spelling may make greater demand of the correct sequencing of letters and precision in letter recognition than the use of phonics applied to reading (Denckla, 2019).

## Treatment

### Spelling Remediation

The direct approach to remediate spelling difficulties is to train for phonological awareness. Specific training in phonological awareness does improve spelling. However, multisensory approaches are the most successful. In one method, the simultaneous oral spelling method, the child is shown the word to be learned on a small card. The word is read aloud by the teacher, and the child repeats the word and then copies it letter by letter, saying the name of each letter as it is written. Once the word has been written, the child repeats it once more and checks to see if the spelling is correct. This process is repeated twice. In this approach, a visual component (seeing the word), an auditory component (spelling out the letters), and a motor component (writing them) are all utilized. Poor spellers do best when taught using all components simultaneously. For example, using the complete approach, the children remembered 58% of words taught versus 30–35% taught when only one of the three components was included. Simultaneous oral spelling is important in learning because it connects reading and spelling. Although visual inspection alone may help typically developing children learn to spell, children with spelling disorder require integration of each of these components.

Children with impairment in spelling need support from the time of diagnosis. Interventions should target reading, spelling, and writing, as well as co-occurring disorders such as ADHD and anxiety disorder. A subgroup of children with both reading impairment and language impairment have more severe difficulty with phonetic spelling and poorer phonological skills than predicated from their receptive vocabulary (Larkin & Snowling, 2008).

## Impairment in Mathematics

Mathematics is essential in everyday life in calculating time and distance; using money; financial planning; and in science, technology, and engineering. It is a core subject in education. Numeracy refers to the knowledge and skills needed in all types of work in later life (Soares et al., 2018). Literacy in mathematics is essential for children and adolescents during the school years in preparation for entry into the workforce. Limited math skills affect self-esteem in the school years and are predictive of employment problems (Rivera-Batiz, 1992). In developmental psychology of typical and atypical math development, it is important to distinguish between approximate number sense and symbolic number sense (Pennington et al., 2019). The approximate number system is important to estimate, for example, the size of a group without any reliance on language or symbols. Conversely, the symbolic number system is essential in allowing a child to precisely represent quantities. The symbolic number sense is important as a predicator of later math skills.

Studies of preverbal infants and even nonhuman animals find that approximate number sense exists in the absence of language. Thus, mathematic approximate number sense is very different from reading and writing. Vertebrates such as fish and frogs have behavior consistent with a sense of numbers in that their decisions indicate a capacity to count or respond to "more or less." A frog can match type, length, and the number of mating calls of a rival by counting (Rose, 2018). Chimpanzees learn to associate Arabic numbers up to the number 9 and use visually based working memory (Denckla, 2019).

Infants seem to respond to the numerical properties of their visual world, without benefit of language, abstract reasoning, or real opportunity to manipulate their world (Butterworth, 2005). In the first months of life, infants can discriminate visual arrays on the basis of numerosity. Apparent numerosity in infants has led to a debate regarding whether there is a core deficit in numerosity (Geary et al., 2004). Most research is consistent with a general deficit rather than a core deficit in numerosity. A meta-analysis showed an association between symbolic number comparison tasks and later math achievement that is more consistent and stronger than the association with the approximate number system measured in dot matrix visual arrays in infants (Smedt et al., 2013). Others found that the symbolic number system is uniquely associated with subsequent skill in arithmetic when other variables are accounted for (Göbel et al., 2014). These studies are consistent with the multiple prediction model of development in math skill over time (Pennington et al., 2019).

Counting in early preschool years is learned to carry out more advanced math abilities such as arithmetic facts and math concepts. Counting speed improves with age. Children enter school understanding informal concepts of number and arithmetic from their experiences of counting and calculation. Development proceeds with an increasingly sophisticated understanding of numerosity and its implications for learning. In school, focused educational practice advances knowledge by drills teaching basic arithmetical facts. Children learn arithmetic in the following order: addition (single-digit to multidigit numbers), subtraction, multiplication, and division. Fractions and percentages are added after whole numbers are mastered. Children with math impairment have problems with counting and, once school instruction begins, difficulty mastering addition and subtracting. Thus, mathematics is a core subject taught in primary and higher education that builds on a foundation of mathematical skills for real-life situations (Butterworth, 2005).

Specific learning disability in mathematics involves impairments in the number sense, counting problems, number-fact storage, problems in memorization of arithmetic facts, accuracy of fluid calculation, and mathematical reasoning that involves executive functioning and working memory. Therefore, proficiency in mathematics involves more than computational skills. It also includes a systematic plan toward problem-solving and adequate working memory to complete the task. Good working memory of basic number facts is essential. Typically, a child with impairment in mathematics shows performance similar to that of much younger typically developing children.

Specific learning disability in mathematics is a heterogeneous condition. There may be both intrinsic and extrinsic influences on the acquisition of academic skills in mathematics. The extrinsic factors relate to the complexity of mathematics, poor skill instruction, and lack of mastery of prerequisite math skills. Intrinsic skills relate to general intelligence, executive functioning, quantitative reasoning ability, and visual–spatial ability. Other factors are more attitudinal, such as attitude toward the subject, interest, and sociocultural background.

## History

Hinshelwood (1917b) suggested there are distinctive processes involved in number calculation and proposed separate centers for processing numbers and word reading based on the study of a patient with brain damage. The patient, despite being alexic, retained the ability to read figures rapidly and fluently. Hinshelwood found differential abilities in mental arithmetic among people who are not brain damaged and also claimed that the reverse is true, finding that boys who excelled in reading and other subjects may have difficulty in arithmetic. Hinshelwood acknowledged that others have recognized children who have difficulty in reading figures without corresponding difficulties in reading letters and words. He found that among 12 children with congenital word blindness, only 3 also had difficulty in recognition of figures. Two of his subjects were above average in arithmetic. He wrote (1917a),

> The visual memories of words and figures are deposited in distinct cerebral areas . . . probably close together and possibly contiguous. When defective development was more extensive and thus involved the figure area, then the reading disability included both words and figure.

In the 1930s and 1940s, children with mathematics disorders were found to have associated minimal brain damage or dysfunction. The recognition of minimal brain dysfunction with mathematical problems led to the concept of developmental mathematics disorder. The initial research on mathematics disorder addressed the relationship of visual–spatial skills to problems in numerical computation. Because of issues with visual–spatial skills, the right hemisphere of the brain was thought to be primarily involved. However, the evidence supports the involvement of both hemispheres of the brain in computation and problem-solving tasks, particularly working memory.

## Epidemiology

Math disorder occurs in approximately 3–7% of schoolchildren identified before high school graduation (APA, 2013). This estimate derives from school-aged children of normal intelligence, who do not show adequate attainment in mathematics. An additional 10% are identified as slow math learners, but this varies from year to year in school. Epidemiologic assessment is complicated because achievement in mathematics may depend more on the quality and amount of instruction than is the case for reading. Math achievement is correlated with intelligence, reading achievement, and emotional state (APA, 2013).

## Definition

In DSM-5, impairment in mathematics is a specifier for a neurodevelopmental disorder, specific learning disorder. The specifier includes difficulties in mastering number sense, number facts, fluent calculation, and math reasoning. To meet diagnostic criteria, symptoms must have been unresponsive for at least 6 months of direct remediation interventions. Number sense includes understanding of number sequence (that one number follows in order after another), knowledge of the words for numbers and number symbols, the ability to compare the relative size (smaller or larger) of numbers, and the ability to carry out simple arithmetic calculations.

From a clinical perspective, we can classify presentations depending on the skills and deficits found. One model (Karagiannakis et al., 2014) proposes four subtypes of skills:

*Core number*: Involves numerosity, estimating numbers and quantities, number line ability, managing symbols, and basic counting
*Memory*: Retrieving math facts, performing calculations, and remembering rules and formulae
*Reasoning*: Grasping math concepts, complex math procedures, logical problems, and problem-solving
*Visuospatial*: Geometry, written calculations, and graphs and tables

In the school setting, the major legislation guaranteeing special education services, IDEA (Yell et al., 2006), defines a math disability as one involving mathematics calculation and mathematics problem-solving. Children are evaluated for competency for age in arithmetic and math calculation, solving word problems, and interpreting graphs. They are examined to determine their understanding of money. Concepts of time are taught, as well as how to apply math concepts to solve quantitative math problems. Each state may choose how a *learning disability* is defined based on educational research. School systems are required to screen for learning problems, provide educational intervention for those identified, monitor progress in learning, and make necessary adjustments to the intervention when needed. If a child does not respond to a trial of a specific intervention, evaluation by a multidisciplinary team is conducted to develop an Individualized Educational Plan (IEP). Children with specific learning disability in math are distinguished from those who are low achieving in math. Typically, research on math deficits requires that individuals identified have math achievement scores below the 10th percentile across multiple grade levels, despite interventions. Another category is that of low achieving math students, who consistently score below the 25th percentile on math achievement tests across grades. They may show more typical entry-level math skill and may improve in later grades.

## Assessment

The diagnosis of math disorder is frequently not made until several years after beginning school. Although younger children have learned to count, it is ordinarily not until formal math instruction has begun that the diagnosis is made. The diagnosis may not be made until the third grade, when math problem-solving becomes more complex. Simple counting strategies are no longer successful. Developmental math problems may be recognized in preschool or kindergarten when children have difficulty learning number names, problems counting things out by rote, difficulty remembering number facts, and difficulty understanding quantity and quality relationships. These children find it difficult to print numbers during computation. Moreover, children keeping numbers in a line may have difficulty with word problems. Essentially, there are problems in ordering or sequencing and memory. With impaired memory, problems arise when carrying numbers over and in remembering basic number facts.

Proficiency in solving word problems requires more than computational skills. An inability to solve word problems may result from the child not developing a systematic plan to find solutions. Determining what data are needed to solve a problem requires language ability, basic reading skill, background knowledge to understand the situation proposed, and math computational skills. A careful analysis of the types of errors made is required to help the child.

### Screening

The first step in a diagnostic process in assessing the general student population to identify "at-risk" children (as early as kindergarten) is screening. A positive screen leads to referral to the formal diagnostic process. Common components of screening batteries include assessment of strategic counting, retrieval of basic arithmetic facts, word problems, and numeral recognition (Gersten et al., 2009).

With passage of the original version of IDEA in 1975, specific learning disabilities were recognized as a disability category for special education services. In the law, the operational definition was based on ability–achievement discrepancy (U.S. Office of Education, 1977). Over time, the discrepancy between intellectual functioning and academic achievement model was deemed lacking in validity and replaced by the response to intervention model that is used in DSM-5. The DSM-5 requirement is for early failure to respond to treatment before making the diagnosis. In 2004, the reauthorization of IDEA legislation changed the definition to one based on an inadequate response to research-based interventions (Yell et al., 2006).

Educational testing and psychometric testing are required to diagnose a math disorder. Individually administered intelligence tests along with educational testing are administered to determine overall cognitive capacity and verbal and performance ability. These are followed by standardized educational achievement tests that examine mathematics ability along with reading and spelling ability. Neuropsychological testing is more extensive than psychoeducational assessment, and it is an essential part of specific learning disorder identification because it can provide information on strengths and weaknesses. In early grades (kindergarten and first grade), the diagnosis is focused on basic skills such as core number processing.

This involves symbolic processing skills, language skills, and spatial processing. The diagnosis is made in older children by examining abstract concepts needed in math processing.

## Cognitive Issues: Mathematical Procedures and Mathematical Memory

### Deficit in Counting

Counting is a basic skill in learning arithmetic. Children with math deficits make errors and typically count more slowly. A common error that a first-grade child with an impairment in mathematics makes when "counting on" is to undercount: "6 + 2 = ?." The child may write "6, 7" instead of starting at 6 and counting an additional two numbers. As children with math deficits grow older, they will subtract a larger number from a smaller number. For example, in the problem "73 − 29 = 44," the child makes the mistake of subtracting 3 from 9. Another frequent error is not decreasing the number in the 10s column when borrowing: "64 − 39 = 35." In both adding and subtracting, understanding is lacking about the commutative property of numbers and thus there is a tendency to use repeated addition rather than fact retrieval. Affected children develop these skills much later than their peers.

### Deficits in Number Fact Storage

Storing math facts into memory or retrieving facts is problematic for children with impairment in mathematics—for example, storing number bonds such as "4 + 2 = 6" into memory. Thus, when asked to do simple math, they may calculate answers by counting instead of retrieving the answer from memory directly. They may also have problems in storing information into long-term memory. Unlike dyslexia, in which deficits have been isolated and identified as causal factors involved in the development of an impairment, in mathematics the causes are much more heterogeneous. Alone, none of the processes previously described fully accounts for impairment in mathematics, although all have been implicated as problematic for those struggling with math.

### Deficits in Working Memory

Working memory (short-term memory) is the capacity to store and process information at the same time (Melby-Lervåg & Hulme, 2013). When we calculate, subcomponents of the math problem being solved are held in mind in temporary working memory storage as information processing proceeds. Mastering arithmetic skills involves simple and complex working memory and other executive function processing.

Deficits in working memory are highly associated with problems in arithmetic. They lead to poor performance on complex working memory tasks. These include backward digit span that involves executive function and counting span (Snowling & Hulme, 2015). Nevertheless, these children may be able to carry out simple tasks like their neurotypically functioning peers on simple tests of short-term or phonological memory, unless the task conducted has a numerical aspect.

Deficits in Executive Functioning

In addition to working memory, children with mathematical impairment may also have executive functioning deficits. Executive functions involve the ability to shift psychological set, plan actions, and judge that the actions are reasonable. Thus, these children may have difficulty on executive functioning tests such as the Tool for Real-time Assessment of Information Literacy Skills (TRAILS; in the Delis–Kaplan battery; see Chapter 2) or Wisconsin Card Sorting Test. Other TRAILS tasks require connecting alternating sequences of numbers and letters (e.g., draw a line from 1 to A, 2 to B, etc.) or numbers and colors (e.g., draw a line from 1 to yellow, 1 to pink, 2 to yellow, 2 to pink, etc.). When conducting executive function tests, it is important to clarify if ADHD is a co-occurring diagnosis.

In summary, in mathematics, there are two main domains of competency: computational skills, as demonstrated in paper-and-pencil arithmetic, and problem-solving for word problems. Thus, counting skills, storage to memory and retrieval, problem-solving using working memory, and executive functions are important factors. From a cognitive perspective, mathematics impairment results from several underlying cognitive deficits. Further study is needed by conducting longitudinal follow-up on the outcomes of current intervention strategies.

## Etiology

The underlying basis of impairment in mathematics is less understood than it is for reading impairment. Less is known about the mechanisms involved in mathematical skills and their development, which depend on complex interaction between verbal and nonverbal cognitive systems. In children, there has been considerable interest in determining underlying cognitive deficits that might be characteristic of developmental math disorder. Rourke (1978) suggested that right hemisphere–based visual–spatial skills are essential to the development of normal arithmetic ability. However, this finding has not been supported. Specific learning disability in math is linked to both hemispheres of the brain. From a cognitive perspective, difficulties in mathematics result from several underlying cognitive deficits, including impairment in the approximate number sense system linked to parietal brain areas as well as interacting verbal systems, particularly those involving executive functions such as working memory.

## Neuroimaging Findings

Impairment in mathematics is a neurodevelopmental disorder involving dysfunction in specific brain regions that are linked to math skills. Numerosity, the building block of math skills, involves the visual and auditory association cortices of the brain and the parietal lobe attention system. The attention system involves the intraparietal sulcus within the posterior parietal cortex (Dehaene et al., 2003). This is a brain region specifically involved in the representation and manipulation of numerical quantity (Dehaene et al., 2003). With experience and learning, the intraparietal sulcus builds an amodal, language-independent semantic representation of numerical quantity. Its neural underpinnings depend on bilateral areas of the horizontal intraparietal sulcus. Three parietal circuits have been proposed for number processing. Consistent with the proposal, a specific reduction in gray matter in the left horizontal intraparietal sulcus is reported in a group of adolescents, born prematurely, who had mathematics problems without reading problems compared to a neurotypically developing control group (Isaacs et al., 2001). The difference only applied to those with problems in calculation but not for others studied who had problems in mathematics reasoning.

Children acquire mathematical understanding in a developmental sequence. At first, they rely on procedure-based counting that, when repeated, results in associations used in information retrieval. This is documented in functional imaging studies showing greater activation of the dorsal basal ganglia, which is involved in working memory (Chang et al., 2007). Gradual development continues into second and third grades with information retrieval from long-term memory thus laying down a foundation for increasing complex math skills (Menon, 2016). The brain region associated with complex math is situated in the medial temporal lobe with connections to the hippocampus and the prefrontal cortex. Younger children exhibit greater involvement of the hippocampus and parahippocampal gyrus (De Smedt et al., 2011) compared to adults. The greater activation found in youth may indicate recruitment of resources for memorization (Menon, 2010).

With maturation, there is greater activation in the left posterior parietal cortex and lateral occipital temporal cortex along with lower activation in multiple prefrontal cortex areas as evidence of greater specialization (Menon, 2010). Individuals with impairment in math have reduced activation during math tasks in functional imaging studies involving the intraparietal sulcus. Structural imaging also showed reduced gray matter in the intraparietal sulcus in those with impairment in math and reduced connectivity between parietal and occipitotemporal regions (Rykhlevskaia et al., 2009). A DTI study found evidence of deficient white fiber projection in the superior longitudinal fasciculus (particularly adjacent to the intraparietal sulcus) that connects parietal, temporal, and frontal regions in children with impairment math performance. The authors proposed a "disconnection" or interruption of integration and control of distributed brain processes, suggesting a disconnection syndrome (Kucian et al., 2014).

## Genetics

There are both genetic and environmental influences on the development of skills in mathematics. When heritability of mathematic difficulty was studied in a large sample of children chosen from the bottom 15% of students from teacher ratings of mathematics skills, the heritability of math skills was estimated to be approximately 0.65 (Oliver et al., 2004). The heritability or genetic influence on math skills is consistent across the continuum from high to low math skills. This research emphasizes that although math skills are acquired over time, the stability of math performance is the result of genetic influences. Twin studies reveal high concordance for impairment in mathematics in monozygotic twins if one is affected (Alarcón et al., 1997; Soares et al., 2018). Fifty percent of siblings of individuals with impairment in mathematics also have impairment in mathematics (Shalev et al., 2001). Math ability is thought to be influenced by many genes of small effects across the entire spectrum of ability in GWAS (Docherty et al., 2010). Approximately half of the observed correlation between math and reading ability is due to shared genetic effects (Davis et al., 2014). In a twins study, 60% of the genetic factors that influenced math ability also influenced reading ability, and approximately 95% of the phenotypic correlation between the two is explained by these shared genetic influences (Markowitz et al., 2005).

## Genetic Syndromes

Another approach to understand the relationship of genetics to impairment in mathematics is to examine neurogenetic disorders with associated impairment in mathematics and compare across disorders to determine if there are commonalities in brain dysmorphology linked to mathematics performance profiles.

Several genetic syndromes are associated with increased risk for math problems. Those with fragile X syndrome have both math and reading deficits. Among girls with fragile X syndrome (without an IDD), 75% or more have a math disability by the end of third grade. They score below average in mathematics in kindergarten and first grade. They have impairment in mathematics and poor working memory. Females with fragile X syndrome are accurate when reading numbers and relating math facts, but they show weak understanding of numerical estimations (Mazzocco, 2009; Murphy, 2009).

The frequency of impairment in mathematics in girls with Turner syndrome is similar to that found in girls with fragile X syndrome. Girls with Turner syndrome are age appropriate in number comprehension and processing speed, including single-digit arithmetic. However, a consistent finding in girls with Turner syndrome is that, compared to neurotypically developing students, complex math calculations and numerical estimation are processed at significantly slower speed and with less accuracy. Although girls with Turner syndrome have weak calculation skills, their ability to complete math problems not requiring explicit calculation is similar to that of their peers.

In summary, girls with Turner syndrome have difficulty with math and handwriting despite reading skills above average. Individuals with Turner syndrome have a particular cognitive phenotype associated with problems in visual–spatial tasks that is not limited to the right hemisphere (Mazzocco, 2009).

Children with the 22q11.2 deletion syndrome (22q11.2ds) have considerable impairment in mathematics resulting from impairment in procedural calculation, math word problem-solving, and representing numerical quantities even though math fact retrieval is intact (Dennis et al., 2009). However, their reading is normal. Younger children with this genetic condition (ages 6–10 years) showed similar number sense and calculation skills as neurotypically developing children but weaker math problem-solving. Older children with 22q11.2ds had slower speed in their general number sense and calculations, but accuracy was maintained. Weak counting skills and magnitude comparison have been found in this group of children, suggesting weak visual–spatial processing. Children with myelomeningocele are at greater risk for math difficulties than their unaffected peers. In Williams syndrome, learning assets and deficits varies with developmental age. Abstract representations of quantity are found to be intact in infancy. However, the representations do not show a typical developmental trajectory in the childhood years. Yet in Williams syndrome, preverbal approximate number skills show deficits throughout their lifetime (O'Hearn & Luna, 2009). Math impairments may also occur in fetal alcohol spectrum disorder (FAS). In FAS, deficits in spatial processing may be related to math impairments. Moreover, prenatal alcohol exposure is associated with deficits in mathematics achievement, above and beyond the contribution of general cognitive abilities. Children with fetal alcohol use disorder are at risk for a wide range of difficulties, including cognitive, behavioral, and academic deficits; however, impairment in mathematics has emerged as a specific area of weakness in FAS (Crocker et al., 2015; Howell et al., 2005).

Overall, individual differences in math may relate to genetic variations and features of brain development. In premature children with very low birth weight, a relationship with impairment in math and damage to the left parietal lobe is reported (Isaac et al., 2001). In children and adolescents with 22q11.2ds syndrome, individual differences in mental arithmetic have been correlated with left parietal lobe white matter structure adjacent to the gray matter regions of the intraparietal sulcus, an area commonly linked to math impairment (Barnea-Goraly et al., 2005). In Turner syndrome and in 22q11.2ds, there are similar findings of deficits in spatial attention (Simon et al., 2008).

## Associated Psychiatric Disorders

The coexistence of another condition along with the primary condition under study is considered "co-occurrence." The most prevalent co-occurrence of impairment in mathematics is with impairment in reading; it co-occurs in 30–70% of individuals with math disorder (Kovacs, 2007; Landerl & Moll, 2010; Plomin et al., 2007). The rates tend to be lower when more stringent cutoffs are applied to the definitions of the various disorders (Landerl & Moll, 2010) and also when population samples are studied. Distinguishing impairment in mathematics from co-occurring impairment in mathematics with impairment in reading is based on performance on nonverbal and verbal tests. Students with impairment in reading show more difficulty with phonology; students with both impairment in mathematics and impairment in reading have more difficulty with processing speed and nonverbal reasoning (Cirino et al., 2015). Less research has been done on math impairment co-occurring with ADHD and language impairments. Impairment in mathematics and ADHD may be separate disorders that are independently transmitted in families (Monuteaux et al., 2005). One study examined cognitive profiles between ADHD and impairment in mathematics in children (Iglesias-Sarmiento et al., 2017). Iglesias-Sarmiento et al. found that problems in simultaneous processing were more predictive of impairment in the mathematics group, whereas executive function deficits were predictive in the ADHD group. In a large study involving 476 children with ADHD, there was co-occurrence in 18% (Capano et al., 2008). Moreover, children with language impairment also may have problems with mathematics (Manor et al., 2001), with approximately 25% having co-occurring mathematic impairment. However, specific and primary math impairment does exist without co-occurrence.

It is important to evaluate for both disorders because children with impairment in mathematics are less likely to be referred for additional educational assistance and intervention than students with reading problems. Unfortunately, children identified with both learning challenges perform more poorly across psychosocial and academic measures than children with impairment in mathematics alone.

The differential diagnosis of a developmental math impairment includes ruling out other reasons for poor school achievement. Among these are IDD, borderline intelligence, poor educational experience, and frequent absences from school. It is essential to complete the educational history to establish whether inadequate instruction is a factor, rather than an intrinsic math impairment. Moreover, children with reading impairment and/or language impairment should also be assessed for math disorder.

## Treatment

### Educational Interventions

Specific instructional components may be beneficial for students with impairment in mathematics, including explicit instruction in math skills (counting principles, numerosity, math fact practice, and problem-solving strategies). Controlling task difficulty is best taught in a small group setting or in individual tutorial sessions. In addition, cognitive and meta-cognitive strategies, computer-based interactive lessons, videos, and hands-on projects have been shown to aid math reasoning and performance. Interventions targeting general cognitive skills involved in math, such as working memory or processing speed, have not proved to be effective. However, practice with working memory and speed tasks on computer can advance task performance. These gains transfer to enhance mastery and specific skills in math or reading (Pennington et al., 2019).

When math materials are introduced, they are best presented using concrete materials such as blocks and counting devices. After basic concepts are understood, students are encouraged to automate number facts. This is important because complex computations require speed and accuracy in using basic number facts. Students with impairment in mathematics can be accurate but are very slow in basic computations. Their slow speed at computations can affect their accuracy as they carry out more complex problems.

These core principles of explicit instruction that focus on enhancing skills and corrective feedback are effective in remediating math problems involving word problem-solving (Zheng et al., 2013). Not only those with impairment in math but also all children benefit from explicit math instruction. Those with impairment essentially need more focused instruction that is broken down into smaller steps with continuous review.

fMRI studies have been conducted to determine the effect of a targeted math intervention on brain activity in third-grade students (Iuculano et al., 2015). At baseline, before the intervention, the children showed activation in brain regions on the bilateral distribution network that is linked to math skills. This includes bilateral prefrontal cortex, bilateral insular cortices, bilateral partial cortices, and associated brain regions. Following an 8-week intervention of one-on-one math tutoring (based on the Wise Math program), brain activation was normalized, and the students' performance on arithmetic tasks was maintained when retested.

Gersten et al. (2005) conducted a meta-analysis of the efficacy of the interventions for math impairment. Studies included the evaluation of the effectiveness of well-defined methods with randomized control trials with matching pretest data. The most effective interventions were those that employed explicit instruction on specific math skills and included instruction in general strategy for solving problems, teaching children to give explicit verbal descriptions of the reasoning they used to solve the problems, including sequencing with examples. An overview of interventions is shown in Box 17.2.

Current information on efficiency of treatment has been summarized for impairment in mathematics in a Cochrane review (Furlong et al., 2016) and in a Campbell Collaboration review (Simms et al., 2017). The advantage of using computer-based interactive video programs stressed by both the Cochrane and Campbell reviews is that the pace is set by the child to individualize instruction. Computer software is also available to provide drill and practice in number facts. Graphics and, in particular, animation may facilitate motivation and interest. Frequent follow-up and re-evaluation are essential to maintain progress. Other technologies include computers and tablets with touch screens (Zhang et al., 2015). Clinical presentation is adjusted for the age and

---

### Box 17.2  Interventions for Impairment in Mathematics

1. Teach different mathematics components explicitly (e.g., fact retrieval, procedures, problem-solving) for whole numbers and rational numbers.
2. Teach arithmetic (math facts) in the context of number knowledge principles to support understanding and strategic counting.
3. Provide speeded strategic practice, with immediate corrective feedback on errors, to build long-term associations in memory and encourage automatic retrieval of answers.
4. For procedural computations, explicitly teach the most efficient algorithms as rules, while providing the conceptual basis for why those procedures work. Begin with worked examples, gradually transferring responsibility to the learners, while providing practice with corrective feedback and cumulative review across problem types.
5. For word problem-solving, teach problem types (e.g., combine problems, compare problems), introducing one problem type at a time, but systematically providing cumulative review across all taught problem types and practice in sorting problems into problem types. For each problem type, begin by providing the conceptual basis for the problem type; then explicitly reach the most efficient solution strategy, with worked examples and gradual transfer of work to the learner.
6. Explicitly reach for transfer by explaining the ways in which problems may look novel but still represent the previously taught problem types.
7. Promote self-regulation and independence to encourage generalization throughout the educational process.

*Source:* Fletcher et al. (2019, p. 271).

developmental level of the child, the presence of other co-occurring conditions, and the type of instructional methods used. There may be combined behavioral interventions for co-occurring conditions such as math anxiety.

In summary, the most effective interventions for an impairment in mathematics include explicit instruction on solving specific types of problems and extend over several weeks to several months. General math problem solving generalizes across various math skills unless the skill is part of a more complex math concept. Guidelines for effective interventions for students coping with impairment in math are available from the U.S. Department of Education as a practice guide released through the What Works Clearinghouse. This document provides direction in the identification and treatment of children with math impairment in the educational system.

### Behavioral Interventions

Behavioral-based interventions for math disorders combined with noninvasive transcranial stimulation of brain regions involved in mathematical processing (prefrontal cortex and parietal lobe regions) have shown improvement in typically developing young adults. However, this approach has not shown benefit in people with impairment in mathematics. The standard of care for math impairment is behavioral interventions.

### Math Anxiety

Mathematics anxiety does affect remediation of problems in math (Maloney & Beilock, 2012; Maloney et al., 2015). Math anxiety refers to negative emotions toward math. It may begin early in the school years and impact achievement (Ramirez et al., 2013). If children are anxious about math, they may avoid learning math skills. Moreover, when parents have math anxiety, their children are more likely to develop math anxiety. Their negative attitude toward math by social transmission can be conveyed to children, in contrast to genetic risk. Behavioral interventions to decrease math anxiety are effective in improving the math skills of children with impairment in mathematics through cognitive tutoring and cognitive–behavior therapy. These interventions foster a positive attitude toward math. Cognitive–behavioral intervention with targeted tutoring decreases anxiety, fostering a positive attitude toward math and better performance (Sokolowski & Necka, 2016).

Working memory is especially vulnerable to math anxiety, leading to poorer math achievement (Ramirez et al., 2013). Math anxiety was examined in an fMRI study that showed overactivation in regions of the right amygdala involved in processing negative emotions. There also was reduced activity in the cortical and subcortical networks involved in both math reasoning and emotion regulation. Nevertheless, math anxiety was distinct from trait anxiety (Young et al., 2012).

Cognitive–behavioral treatment for math anxiety targets negative emotions related to math. It recognizes negative thoughts and reframes them. For older students, writing (math journals) about anxiety for 10–15 min before an examination may be beneficial (Emmert, 2015; Ramirez & Beilock, 2011). Finally, because there is evidence for social transmission of math anxiety, it is important to consider math anxiety in parents and teachers that may be conveyed to children (Pennington et al., 2019).

## Impairment in Written Expression

### History

Writing is speech made visible and is thought to have been introduced by the Sumerians in Lower Mesopotamia approximately 5,000 years ago. The earliest known writing systems were based on pictograms that showed a specific image of the object being represented in the real world. The pictogram evolved into the ideogram, which depicted not only the object but also ideas or concepts associated with it. For example, the ancient Egyptian hieroglyphics (sacred carvings) were originally thought to serve this function. Pictograms were stylized and became increasing abstract as they evolved into linguistic symbols. The Sumerian language is said to be logographic; a logogram is a written sign that may stand for a single morpheme (a word form that is the minimal unit needed to convey meaning) or sometimes for a full word. Linguistic symbols assumed a semantic function and came to represent sounds (Temple, 1993).

In the 9th century BC, the Greeks borrowed the earlier symbol systems but found them to be inefficient in representing their language. They introduced symbols taken from the Phoenician system of consonants to represent individual sounds and added vowels to create an alphabetic system (Coe, 1992). Our own writing system owes its remote origins to the Greeks but ultimately is derived from the Roman alphabet. In alphabetic scripts, language is broken down into phonemes—that is, the individual consonants and vowels that make up the sounds of language. In phonetic writing, signs lose all resemblance to the original images of objects and denote only sounds. The Roman alphabet came to England in the 6th century. Stable spelling of words became standardized in the 16th century and was uniformly stabilized in the 17th century in the English language.

J. W. Ogle introduced the term "agraphia" in 1867 to describe a disorder in which writing is severely impaired, in contrast to "aphasia," an adult-acquired language disorder. In 1948, Goldstein studied written and oral expression in adults with brain injury and concluded, as did later investigations, that because writing depended on speech, there must be neural correlates between the two (Fletcher et al., 2019). We now know that there is little cross-communication between them. Developmental and acquired writing disorders show little overlap between them.

### Definition

Written language requires instruction in word acquisition, learning to read words, understanding text (reading comprehension), and written expression (spelling and composition). In DSM-5, impairment in written expression is categorized as a specific learning disorder along with impairment in reading and mathematics. Specific learning disorders in written expression have multiple components, including handwriting, typing, punctuation, spelling, and composition. A meta-analysis of skill writing in children identified that the most clear-cut differences are in spelling, grammar, handwriting, quality of writing, how writing is organized, vocabulary used, and fluency in written sentences (Graham et al., 2017). Written expression involves

## Box 17.3  DSM-5 Criteria for Specific Learning Disorder with Impairment in Written Expression

1. Deficits in specific learning disorders with impairment in written expression:
   a. Spelling accuracy
   b. Grammar and punctuation accuracy
   c. Clarity or organization of written expression
2. Specify current severity:
   a. Mild: Some difficulties in learning skills in one or two academic domains, but mild enough severity that the individual may be able to compensate when provided with appropriate accommodations or support services, especially during the school years.
   b. Moderate: Marked difficulties learning skills in more academic domain(s), so that the individual is unlikely to become proficient without intervals of intensive and specialized teaching during the school years. Some accommodations or supportive services at least part of the day at school, in the workplace, or at home may be needed to complete activities accurately and efficiently.
   c. Severe: Severe difficulties in learning skills, affecting several academic domains, so that the individual is unlikely to learn those skills without ongoing intensive individualized and specialized teaching for most of the school years. Even with an array of appropriate accommodations or services at home, at school, or in the workplace, the individual may not be able to complete all activities efficiently.

*Adapted* from the *Diagnostic and Statistical Manual of Mental Disorders*, fifth edition (Copyright 2013). American Psychiatric Association. pp. 66–67.

most of the same cognitive processes involved (e.g., working memory) in spelling and word-level learning and other specific learning impairments. As children grow older, organization, self-regulation, and oral skills are developed. The DSM-5 criteria are shown in Box 17.3.

Like the other specifiers of specific learning disorder, impairment in written expression requires demonstrable difficulty in learning and using these academic skills. Deficits must have persisted at least 6 months, despite the provision of interventions that target those difficulties. Difficulties with written expression refer to making multiple grammatical or punctuation errors within sentences, using poor paragraph organization, and lack of clarity in the written expression of ideas. DSM-5 specifies problems in "spelling accuracy and/or clarity of organization of written expression."

The levels of the affected academic skills are substantially and quantifiably below those expected for the individual's chronological age and cause significant interference with academic or occupational performance, or with activities of daily living as confirmed by individually administered standardized achievement measures and comprehensive clinical assessment. For individuals aged 17 years or older, a documented history of impairing learning difficulties may be substituted for the standardized assessment.

The IDEA legislation refers to written expression as a category of learning disability. Like DSM-5, IDEA uses the response to intervention model to confirm the diagnosis. Importantly, other authors (Berninger, 2004; Fletcher et al., 2019) separate the skills into written expression involved in the manual act of handwriting and transcription, which is involved in generating text. Writing difficulties are recognized during the school-age years, becoming most apparent when academic demands exceed the affected individual's limited capabilities. Problems in written expression may be identified in timed tests, required reading reports for a tight deadline, or with increasingly heavy academic load in the high school years. In DSM-5, differential diagnosis of impairment in written expression requires that the learning difficulties are not better accounted for by IDD, problems with visual or auditory acuity, other mental or neurologic disorders, psychosocial adversity, lack of proficiency in the language of academic instruction, or inadequate educational instruction.

In keeping with DSM-5, this section uses the term "impairment in written expression" rather than "writing disorder" or "disorder of written expression." Dysgraphia is another term commonly used when referring to children with writing problems. Although often described as synonymous with impairment in written expression, dysgraphia is distinctly different. Dysgraphia is primarily a deficit in motor output (paper-and-pencil skills), whereas impairment in written expression refers to a conceptual weakness in developing, organizing, and expressing ideas in writing. Diagnoses of impairment in written expression or of dysgraphia are made based on their phenotypical features. Examination of spelling, punctuation, grammar, clarity, and writing organization is essential to diagnose impairment written expression. Writing samples of children with disordered writing skills show delay in producing a small amount of content. For those with co-occurring dysgraphia, legibility is poor to indecipherable.

## Epidemiology

The prevalence of impairment in written expression is estimated at 6.9–14.7% (Katusic et al., 2009; Yoshimasu et al., 2011), with the relative risk for impairment in written expression twice as high for boys as for girls. The largest differences between males and females are in handwriting and spelling. The co-occurrence of impairment in reading is approximately 75% among those without reading impairment; 30% have a co-occurring ADHD. These rates are consistent with earlier studies of written composition focusing on the narrative subtext of the test for written language (Hooper et al., 1993). Fletcher et al. (2019) suggest that impairment in written expression affects approximately 10% of school-aged children. The rates for boys and girls vary with ascertainment method. Rates tend to be higher when identified in schools. The male:female ratio is estimated at 1:5 (Hooper et al., 1993). In a twin study, girls scored higher than boys on a writing composite section (Olson et al., 2013).

The risk for writing problems is greater among those with neurodevelopmental disorders. Approximately 50% of children with oral language disorders have impairment in written expression. Children with ADHD and learning disorders are at greater risk. Impairment in written expression is diagnosed in approximately 60% of the combined and inattentive types of ADHD. Any child with working memory deficits and other problems with executive dysfunction is at risk for problems in written expression.

## Etiology

Among the language skills, writing is the last to develop. Writing disorders frequently persist into secondary school for children with developmental language disorder and/or impairment in reading. A writing sample should reveal the child's difficulty in linguistic, motor, and cognitive development. Writing involves the complex integration of several skills, and a variety of developmental dysfunctions present through the child's written output. The study of writing disorders and the writing process has contributed substantially to understanding how a particular child processes information.

Written language includes handwriting, spelling, and syntax. Many aspects of writing dysfunction may exist alone or in combination: illegibility, irregular letter formation, mechanical problems in writing including punctuation and capitalization, poor grammar and sentence structure, misspelling of words, and slow rates of writing to dictation. Early in the development of each skill involved in writing, cognitive effort is required. Optimally, skills involved in motor production, spelling, punctuation, and capitalization (the mechanics of writing) gradually become automatic and require less mental effort as a child matures. Automatic effort is devoted to higher level cognitive skills, such as planning, organization, application of knowledge, and use of varied and emerging vocabulary. For children with impairment in written expression, breakdowns may occur at any and sometimes every stage.

## Transcription and Impaired Written Expression

There is a wide range of "developmentally typical" transcription to letter production and spelling transcription among preschool and primary grade children. In preschool and kindergarten, poor writers are slow to produce letters and write their name. Weak early spelling and reading skills, letter identification, phonologic awareness, and weak oral language predict weak writing skills in later elementary school grades. Children who have difficulty mastering early transcription skills write slowly or, when writing at a reasonable speed, have poor legibility. Vocabulary use in poor spellers is often restricted to words that they can spell. As children move into upper elementary school grades and beyond, new challenges arise. If lower level transcription skills are not mastered, they cannot be applied to more complex written text generation. In addition to transcription, complex written text generation requires the integration of additional cognitive skills.

## Oral Language and Impaired Written Expression

Language is related to writing skills. Writing difficulties are linked to deficits in both expression and comprehension of oral language. Writing by children with specific language impairment differs from that of their unimpaired peers early in the school experience and persists through high school. In preschool and kindergarten, overall, children with language disorders show poorer letter production and have difficulty printing their name. Poor spelling and weak vocabulary contribute to the poor writing skills. In the higher grades, their written narratives are of lower quality and poorly organized with limited vocabulary. Deficits in pragmatic language and higher level language also impact writing skills. Pragmatic language is the social use of language—for example, greeting others and making requests, and adapting conversating to meet the needs of the situation. Higher level language refers to grammatical skills. It includes making and understanding inferences; appropriate use of figurative language; and making cause-and-effect judgments—for example, understanding the extent of the reader's background knowledge and taking it into account in discussion and the use content-specific vocabulary are key to social engagement in conversation.

## Executive Functions

Writing is a complicated process and involves the integration of several cognitive processes to the listener. Executive functions referred to these include planning, problem-solving, monitoring, and making adjustments to the listener's interest as needed. Two elements involved in the writing process are translation of thought into written output and reviewing what is written. Coming up with ideas is the first step when writing a narrative story. The story is then developed to include a plot with characters and a storyline. The narrative is put into an organized whole that flows from beginning to end. Persistence (self-regulation) is needed to complete the task. Successful writers rely on executive functions; children with impairment in written expression struggle to use them.

## Working Memory

Working memory is a key element in written expression. Working memory is defined as the capacity to hold, manipulate, and store information for short time periods. This type of memory is used in problem-solving. Working memory plays an essential role in the writing process. With poor working memory, writing skills that are expected to be automatic continue to require considerable effort. Thus, impairment in writing can persist into adult life.

Children with weak graphomotor skills (poor handwriting) must devote a great effort to accurately produce written language, thereby increasing working memory use to lower level transcription, and limited memory is available to facilitate discourse. The result might be very slow production in writing a legible story; a written passage may be largely illegible. However, if a child's penmanship and spelling have developed normally but their ability to persist with challenging tasks, organize their thoughts, and develop a coordinated plan for written expression is limited, the disorder is primarily an impairment in composition.

## Conceptual Models of Writing

A conceptual framework frequently used to describe the skills involved in writing is the "simple view of writing" (Berninger & Amtmann, 2003) This model addresses the subskills used in a writing task, emphasizing the relationship among those skills. Four categories of skills are (a) transcription, (b) executive function, (c) working memory, and (d) text generation.

As shown in Figure 17.2, the simple view of writing is shown as a triangle with transcription and executive functioning at the base of it. Text generation is at the vertex of the triangle. At the very center of the triangle is working memory because working memory is needed to facilitate each component. For example, a student with impairment in spelling focuses working memory resources on spelling words, leaving less resource memory to keep ideas in mind as they write (Herbert et al., 2019). Distracted by the spelling effort, the child may lose track of the idea being expressed. When transcription becomes automatic, more working memory is available for self-regulation to generate text. This is referenced as the self-regulation strategy development intervention.

## Treatment

Children with disorder of written expression are often not recognized in school. If they can read adequately, they may be overlooked or thought to be poorly motivated in writing. Early diagnosis with explanations to the child's parents and teachers are critical. Impairment in written expression must be taken quite seriously because the stress of output difficulties may be considerable. Appropriate tests should be used to diagnose the impairment, and the child's deficit should be made known to their teachers, not only in the year of diagnosis but also to teachers in subsequent years of schooling.

Once identified, a writing disorder becomes a challenge throughout a child's school career. Generally, these problems do not spontaneously remit with maturation but may, in fact, intensify in secondary school, in which demands for written output continue to increase. Disorder of written expression in adolescents is frequently accompanied by a secondary loss of self-esteem because teachers may not fully appreciate the extent of the problem. The child's writing is constant visual evidence of deficiencies. Because typically intelligent children with writing problems may not have other academic weaknesses, their learning disorder may pass unnoticed or not be taken seriously enough.

The treatment begins with sequential handwriting instruction in school and often tutoring. Specific therapeutic interventions include tasks involving teaching sequencing—for example, the appropriate use of syllables and the use of oral tests and other means to bypass the disability. Compensatory approaches involve the use of note takers for the child, increased time for written tests, provision of copies of long written assignments, and the use of computers.

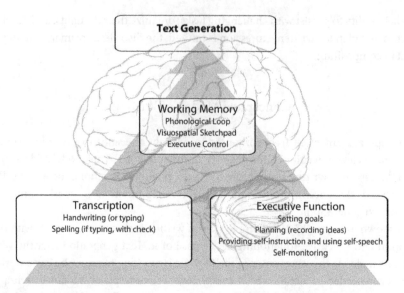

**Figure 17.2** The skills involved in writing, including the subskills that are essential for the writing task and a framework illustrating how those skills are interrelated. The model includes skills in four general categories (from the bottom up): transcription, executive function, working memory, and text generation.
From Hebert et al. (2018); redrawn by Tim Phelps (2021).

Interventions for impairment in written expression should address two principal areas: transcription and composition. Transcription interventions focus on handwriting, spelling, and the use of computer keyboards in writing, whereas composition focuses on generating narrative text. Basic cognitive processes (e.g., working memory) and other executive functions that are shared with other specific learning disorder specifiers are important to consider. Despite ongoing neurological research, distinct neural networks linked to written expression have not been established. Genetic studies do show high heritability. The genetic findings involving written expression overlap with reading-related genetic findings and with reading impairment.

There is ongoing interest in identifying subgroups within the general category of impairment in written expression that are distinct from other language-based disorders. One potential subgroup is handwriting impairment that requires motor control. These studies must consider co-occurring conditions such as ADHD when handwriting may be an issue (Barkley, 2015). Box 17.4 summarizes principles for teaching written expression.

These interventions highlight the importance of concerted instruction in both transcription and text generation in composition (Flower & Hayes, 1980). Meta-analyses of the effectiveness of writing interventions have been conducted to examine interventions in both the elementary school years (Graham et al., 2012) and the adolescent years (Graham & Perrin, 2007). Moreover, meta-analyses have examined the self-regulated strategy development (SRSD) intervention, which appears to be the most effective approach. Other meta-analyses have focused on handwriting and spelling (Santangelo & Graham, 2016) and the use of word processing (Morphy & Graham, 2012).

---

**Box 17.4 Interventions: Teaching Written Expression Learning Disorders**

---

1. Transcription difficulties: Explicitly teach handwriting and spelling with deliberate, regular practice for younger students.
2. Transcription difficulties: Minimize demands for motor output in writing. Use adjuncts such as word processors, keyboards, and spell-checks for older students.
3. Generation problems: Teach written expression in terms style and choice of subject and composition, using self-regulation learning strategies.
4. Permit dictation: Dictation and oral testing as compensatory approaches for older students with impairment in written expression.

---

These meta-analyses show that poor writing skills can be improved with effective treatment. To remediate poor handwriting, there is a popular approach called the Handwriting Without Tears curriculum used by occupational therapists with children. To remediate children with poor handwriting, lower level transcription skills should be focused on until they become automatic. Children should be taught that letter production is essential to broader components of writing. Because working memory constrains the instructional process for students with writing impairment, all components of writing should be taught within the same lesson.

In summary, specific instruction in writing strategies is combined with coaching in self-regulation that addresses the deficits specific to each child. The SRSD intervention is frequently used because of its effectiveness. This model has six stages of implementation: (a) developing and facilitating a student's background knowledge, (b) discussing the writing strategy that is being taught with the student, (c) modeling the strategy for the individual student, (d) assisting the student in memorization of the strategy, (e) supporting the student's use of the strategy during implementation, and (f) independent use of the strategy. The SRSD is applied across various writing situations and implemented until the student has developed mastery of the program's content.

## Special Educational Resources

Children with impairment in written expression may qualify for formal education intervention through federal special education legislation. IDEA requires the development of an IEP when there is a lack of response to targeted interventions over 6 months. A 504 plan requires accommodations and educational support for the interventions. Accommodations provided to a child with impairment in working memory, through an IEP or a 504 plan, include dictation to a scribe when coping with lengthy writing tasks; additional time to complete exams that require writing; and the use of technology such as a computer for typing, speech-to-text dictation software, and writing devices that record teacher instruction. Learning to use technology effectively requires considerable effort but is rewarded by substantial mastery over developmental impairment.

## Further Resources

PBS Parents: http://www.pbs.org/parents/education/math

U.S. Department of Education: *Helping your child learn mathematics*. https://files.eric.ed.gov/fulltext/ED498947.pdf

Zero to Three. *Let's talk about math*. https://www.zerotothree.org/resource/lets-talk-about-math/

## References

Alarcón, M., DeFries, J. C., Light, J. G., & Pennington, B. F. (1997). A twin study of mathematics disability. *Journal of Learning Disabilities, 30*(6), 617–623.

Alexander-Passe, N. (2006). How dyslexic teenagers cope: An investigation of self-esteem, coping and depression. *Dyslexia, 12*(4), 256–275.

Altarac, M., & Saroha, E. (2007). Lifetime prevalence of learning disability among US children. *Pediatrics, 119*(Suppl. 1), S77–S83.

Aman, M. G., & Schroeder, S. R. (1990). Specific learning disorders and mental retardation. In B. Tonge, G. Burrows, & J. Werry (Eds.), *Handbook of Studies on Child Psychiatry* (pp. 209–224). Elsevier.

American Psychiatric Association. (2013). *Diagnostic and statistical manual of mental disorders* (5th ed.). American Psychiatric Publishing.

Bach, S., Richardson, U., Brandeis, D., Martin, E., & Brem, S. (2013). Print-specific multimodal brain activation in kindergarten improves prediction of reading skills in second grade. *NeuroImage, 82*, 605–615.

Barkley, R. A. (Ed.). (2015). *Attention-deficit hyperactivity disorder: A handbook for diagnosis and treatment* (4th ed.). Guilford.

Barnea-Goraly, N., Eliez, S., Menon, V., Bammer, R., & Reiss, A. L. (2005). Arithmetic ability and parietal alterations: A diffusion tensor imaging study in velocardiofacial syndrome. *Cognitive Brain Research, 25*(3), 735–740.

Beauchemin, J., Hutchins, T. L., & Patterson, F. (2008). Mindfulness meditation may lessen anxiety, promote social skills, and improve academic performance among adolescents with learning disabilities. *Complementary Health Practice Review, 13*(1), 34–45.

Berninger, V. W. (2004). Understanding the "graphia" in developmental dysgraphia. In D. Dewey & D. Tupper (Eds.), *Developmental motor disorders: A neuropsychological perspective* (pp. 328–350). Guilford.

Berninger, V. W., & Amtmann, D. (2003). Preventing written expression disabilities through early and continuing assessment and intervention for handwriting and/or spelling problems: Research into practice. In H. L. Swanson, K. R. Harris, & S. Graham (Eds.), *Handbook of learning disabilities* (pp. 345–363). Guilford.

Boets, B., Op de Beeck, H. P., Vandermosten, M., Scott, S. K., Gillebert, C. R., Mantini, D., Bulthe, J., Sunaert, S., Wouters, J., & Ghesquière, P. (2013). Intact but less accessible phonetic representations in adults with dyslexia. *Science, 342*(6163), 1251–1254.

Butterworth, B. (2005). The development of arithmetical abilities. *Journal of Child Psychology and Psychiatry, 46*(1), 3–18.

Capano, L., Minden, D., Chen, S. X., Schachar, R. J., & Ickowicz, A. (2008). Mathematical learning disorder in school-age children with attention-deficit hyperactivity disorder. *Canadian Journal of Psychiatry, 53*(6), 392–399.

Caravolas, M., Hulme, C., & Snowling, M. J. (2001). The foundations of spelling ability: Evidence from a 3-year longitudinal study. *Journal of Memory and Language, 45*(4), 751–774.

Carotenuto, M., Esposito, M., Cortese, S., Laino, D., & Verrotti, A. (2016). Children with developmental dyslexia showed greater sleep disturbances than controls, including problems initiating and maintaining sleep. *Acta Paediatrica, 105*(9), 1079–1082.

Carroll, J. M., Maughan, B., Goodman, R., & Meltzer, H. (2005). Literacy difficulties and psychiatric disorders: Evidence for comorbidity. *Journal of Child Psychology and Psychiatry*, *46*(5), 524–532.

Centers for Disease Control and Prevention. (2016). https://www.psi.org/key-development-partners/the-centers-for-disease-control-and-prevention-cdc/?gclid=Cj0KCQiAtaOtBhCwA RIsAN_x-3Lg1zfRrq7z68JgNIy0baRyQxQJ-3AuwNPAux02VXInS-HQK5EicV4aAucPE ALw_wcB

Chang, C., Crottaz-Herbette, S., & Menon, V. (2007). Temporal dynamics of basal ganglia response and connectivity during verbal working memory. *NeuroImage*, *34*(3), 1253–1269.

Cirino, P. T., Fuchs, L. S., Elias, J. T., Powell, S. R., & Schumacher, R. F. (2015). Cognitive and mathematical profiles for different forms of learning difficulties. *Journal of Learning Disabilities*, *48*(2), 156–175.

Clements, S. D. (1966). *Minimal brain dysfunction in children* (NINDS Monograph No. 3, U.S. Public Health Service Publication No. 1415). U.S. Government Printing Office.

Cobrinik, L. (1974). Unusual reading ability in severely disturbed children. *Journal of Autism and Childhood Schizophrenia*, *4*(2), 163–175.

Coe, M. D. (1992). *Breaking the Maya code*. Thames & Hudson.

Critchley, M. (1970). *The dyslexic child*. Heinemann.

Crocker, N., Riley, E. P., & Mattson, S. N. (2015). Visual–spatial abilities relate to mathematics achievement in children with heavy prenatal alcohol exposure. *Neuropsychology*, *29*(1), 108–116.

Daniel, S. S., Walsh, A. K., Goldston, D. B., Arnold, E. M., Reboussin, B. A., & Wood, F. B. (2006). Suicidality, school dropout, and reading problems among adolescents. *Journal of Learning Disabilities*, *39*(6), 507–514.

Darki, F., Peyrard-Janvid, M., Matsson, H., Kere, J., & Klingberg, T. (2012). Three dyslexia susceptibility genes, *DYX1C1*, *DCDC2*, and *KIAA0319*, affect temporo-parietal white matter structure. *Biological Psychiatry*, *72*(8), 671–676.

Davis, O. S., Band, G., Pirinen, M., Haworth, C. M., Meaburn, E. L., Kovas, Y., Harlaar N., Docherty, S., Hanscombe, K., Trzaskowski, M., Curtis, C. J., Strange, A., Freeman, C., Bellenguez, C., Su, Z., Pearson, R., Vukcevic, D., Langford, C., Deloukas, P., . . . Spencer, C. (2014). The correlation between reading and mathematics ability at age twelve has a substantial genetic component. *Nature Communications*, *5*, 4204.

Dehaene, S., Piazza, M., Pinel, P., & Cohen, L. (2003). Three parietal circuits for number processing. *Cognitive Neuropsychology*, *20*(3–6), 487–506.

Delacato, C. H. (1966). *Neurological organization and reading*. Charles C Thomas.

Denckla, M. B. (2019). *Understanding learning and related disabilities: Inconvenient brains*. Routledge.

Deng, K. G., Zhao, H., & Zuo, P. X. (2019). Association between *KIAA0319* SNPs and risk of dyslexia: A meta-analysis. *Journal of Genetics*, *98*(2), Article 62.

Dennis, M., Berch, D. B., & Mazzocco, M. M. (2009). Mathematical learning disabilities in special populations: Phenotypic variation and cross-disorder comparisons. *Developmental Disabilities Research Reviews*, *15*(1), 80–89.

De Smedt, B., Holloway, I. D., & Ansari, D. (2011). Effects of problem size and arithmetic operation on brain activation during calculation in children with varying levels of arithmetical fluency. *NeuroImage*, *57*(3), 771–781.

Docherty, S. J., Davis, O. S. P., Kovas, Y., Meaburn, E. L., Dale, P. S., Petrill, S. A., Schalkwyk, L., & Plomin, R. (2010). A genome-wide association study identifies multiple loci associated with mathematics ability and disability. *Genes, Brain and Behavior*, *9*(2), 234–247.

Eden, G. F., & Vaidya, C. J. (2008). ADHD and developmental dyslexia: Two pathways leading to impaired learning. *Annals of the New York Academy of Sciences*, *1145*(1), 316–327.

Ehri, L. C. (1997). Learning to read and learning to spell are one and the same, almost. In C. Perfetti, L. Rieben, & M. Fayol (Eds.), *Learning to spell: Research, theory, and practice across languages* (Vol. 13, pp. 237–268). Erlbaum.

Eicher, J. D., Powers, N. R., Miller, L. L., Mueller, K. L., Mascheretti, S., Marino, C., Willcutt, E., DeFries, J., Olson, R., Smith, S., Pennington, B. F., Tomblin, J., Ring, S., & Gruen, J. (2014). Characterization of the *DYX2* locus on chromosome 6p22 with reading disability, language impairment, and IQ. *Human Genetics, 133*(7), 869–881.

Emmert, T. N. (2015). *Examining the effects of mathematics journals on elementary students' mathematics anxiety levels* (Doctoral dissertation, Ohio University).

Farnham-Diggory, S. (1978). *Learning disabilities: A psychological perspective.* Harvard University Press.

Fernald, G. M. (1943). *Remedial techniques in basic school subjects.* McGraw-Hill.

Fletcher, J. M., Lyon, G. R., Fuchs, L. S., & Barnes, M. A. (2019). *Learning disabilities: From identification to intervention.* Guilford.

Flower, L., & Hayes, J. R. (1980). The cognition of discovery: Defining a rhetorical problem. *College Composition and Communication, 31*(1), 21–32.

Francis, D. A., Caruana, N., Hudson, J. L., & McArthur, G. M. (2019). The association between poor reading and internalising problems: A systematic review and meta-analysis. *Clinical Psychology Review, 67,* 45–60.

Frith, U. (1978). Spelling difficulties. *Journal of Child Psychology and Psychiatry, 19,* 279–285.

Frith, U. (1985). Beneath the surface of developmental dyslexia. In K. E. Patterson, J. C. Marshall, & M. Coltheart (Eds.), *Surface dyslexia* (pp. 301–330). Routledge and Kegan-Paul.

Frostig, M. (1969). *Move, grow, learn.* Follet.

Furlong, M., McLoughlin, F., McGilloway, S., Geary, D., & Butterworth, B. (2016). Interventions to improve mathematical performance for children with mathematical learning difficulties (MLD). Cochrane Database of Systematic Reviews, 2016(4), CD012130.

Galaburda, A. M., & Kemper, T. L. (1979). Cytoarchitectonic abnormalities in developmental dyslexia: A case study. *Annals of Neurology, 6*(2), 94–100.

Galaburda, A. M., Sherman, G. F., Rosen, G. D., Aboitiz, F., & Geschwind, N. (1985). Developmental dyslexia: Four consecutive patients with cortical anomalies. *Annals of Neurology, 18*(2), 222–233.

Geary, D. C., Hoard, M. K., Byrd-Craven, J., & DeSoto, M. C. (2004). Strategy choices in simple and complex addition: Contributions of working memory and counting knowledge for children with mathematical disability. *Journal of Experimental Child Psychology, 88*(2), 121–151.

Gersten, R., Beckmann, S., Clarke, B., Foegen, A., Marsh, L., Star, J. R., & Witzel, B. (2009). *Assisting students struggling with mathematics: Response to intervention (RtI) for elementary and middle schools* (NCEE 2009-4060). What Works Clearinghouse.

Gersten, R., Jordan, N. C., & Flojo, J. R. (2005). Early identification and interventions for students with mathematics difficulties. *Journal of Learning Disabilities, 38*(4), 293–304.

Gittelman, R. (1983). Treatment of reading disorders. In M. Rutter (Ed.), *Developmental neuropsychiatry* (pp. 520–541). Guilford.

Gittelman, R., Klein, D. F., & Feingold, I. (1983). Children with reading disorders: II. Effects of methylphenidate in combination with reading remediation. *Journal of Child Psychology and Psychiatry, 24*(2), 193–212.

Göbel, S. M., Watson, S. E., Lervåg, A., & Hulme, C. (2014). Children's arithmetic development: It is number knowledge, not the approximate number sense, that counts. *Psychological Science, 25*(3), 789–798.

Goldberg, T. E., & Rothermel, R. D., Jr. (1984). Hyperlexic children reading. *Brain, 107*(3), 759–785.

Goldston, D. B., Walsh, A., Arnold, E. M., Reboussin, B., Daniel, S. S., Erkanli, A., Nutter, D., Hickman, E., Palmes, G., Snider, E., & Wood, F. B. (2007). Reading problems, psychiatric disorders, and functional impairment from mid- to late adolescence. *Journal of the American Academy of Child & Adolescent Psychiatry, 46*(1), 25–32.

Goswami, U., & Bryant, P. (2016). *Phonological skills and learning to read.* Psychology Press.

Graham, S., Collins, A. A., & Rigby-Wills, H. (2017). Writing characteristics of students with learning disabilities and typically achieving peers: A meta-analysis. *Exceptional Children, 83*(2), 199–218.

Graham, S., McKeown, D., Kiuhara, S., & Harris, K. R. (2012). A meta-analysis of writing instruction for students in the elementary grades. *Journal of Educational Psychology, 104*(4), 879–896.

Graham, S., & Perin, D. (2007). *Writing next-effective strategies to improve writing of adolescents in middle and high schools.* Carnegie Corporation of New York.

Greven, C. U., Rijsdijk, F. V., Asherson, P., & Plomin, R. (2012). A longitudinal twin study on the association between ADHD symptoms and reading. *Journal of Child Psychology and Psychiatry, 53*(3), 234–242.

Grigorenko, E. L., Klin, A., & Volkmar, F. (2003). Annotation: Hyperlexia: Disability or superability? *Journal of Child Psychology and Psychiatry, 44*(8), 1079–1091.

Grafman, J. (Series Ed.). (1992). *Handbook of neuropsychology: Vol. 7. Child neuropsychology* (pp. 187–210). Elsevier.

Haft, S. L., Myers, C. A., & Hoeft, F. (2016). Socio-emotional and cognitive resilience in children with reading disabilities. *Current Opinion in Behavioral Sciences, 10*, 133–141.

Hendren, R. L., Haft, S. L., Black, J. M., White, N. C., & Hoeft, F. (2018). Recognizing psychiatric comorbidity with reading disorders. *Frontiers in Psychiatry, 9*, Article 101.

Hebert, M., Kearns, D. M., Hayes, J. B., Bazis, P., & Cooper, S. (2018). Why children with dyslexia struggle with writing and how to help them. *Language, Speech, and Hearing Services in Schools, 49*(4), 843–863.

Herbert, K. E., Massey-Garrison, A., & Geva, E. (2019). A developmental examination of narrative writing in EL and EL1 school children who are typical readers, poor decoders, or poor comprehenders. *Journal of Learning Disabilities, 53*(1), 36–47.

Hinshelwood, J. (1896). A case of dyslexia: A peculiar form of word-blindness. 1. *Lancet, 148*(3821), 1451–1454.

Hinshelwood, J. (1917a). *Congenital word-blindness.* Lewis.

Hinshelwood, J. (1917b). *Letter; Word and mind-blindness.* Lewis.

Hollingworth, L. S., & Winford, C. A. (1918). *The psychology of special disability in spelling* (No. 88). Teachers College, Columbia University.

Hooper, S. R., Swartz, C. W., Montgomery, J. W., & Reed, M. S. (1993). Prevalence of writing problems across three middle school samples. School Psychology Review, 22(4), 610–622.

Howell, K. K., Lynch, M. E., Platzman, K. A., Smith, G. H., & Coles, C. D. (2005). Prenatal alcohol exposure and ability, academic achievement, and school functioning in adolescence: A longitudinal follow-up. *Journal of Pediatric Psychology, 31*(1), 116–126.

Hulme, C., Bowyer-Crane, C., Carroll, J. M., Duff, F. J., & Snowling, M. J. (2012). The causal role of phoneme awareness and letter-sound knowledge in learning to read: Combining intervention studies with mediation analyses. *Psychological Science, 23*(6), 572–577.

Iglesias-Sarmiento, V., Deaño, M., Alfonso, S., & Conde, Á. (2017). Mathematical learning disabilities and attention deficit and/or hyperactivity disorder: A study of the cognitive processes involved in arithmetic problem solving. *Research in Developmental Disabilities, 61*, 44–54.

Isaacs, E. B., Edmonds, C. J., Lucas, A., & Gadian, D. G. (2001). Calculation difficulties in children of very low birthweight: A neural correlate. *Brain, 124*(9), 1701–1707.

Johnson, W., Bouchard, T. J., Jr., Segal, N. L., & Samuels, J. (2005). General intelligence and reading performance in adults: Is the genetic factor structure the same as for children? *Personality and Individual Differences, 38*(6), 1413–1428.

Karagiannakis, G., Baccaglini-Frank, A., & Papadatos, Y. (2014). Mathematical learning difficulties subtypes classification. *Frontiers in Human Neuroscience, 8*, Article 57.

Katusic, S. K., Colligan, R. C., Weaver, A. L., & Barbaresi, W. J. (2009). The forgotten learning disability: Epidemiology of written-language disorder in a population-based birth cohort (1976–1982), Rochester, Minnesota. *Pediatrics, 123*(5), 1306–1313.

Kelly, D. P., & Natale, M. J. (2020). Neurodevelopmental and executive function and dysfunction. In R. M. Kliegman & J. St. Geme (Eds.), *Nelson textbook of pediatrics* (21st ed.) Elsevier.

Kempe, C., Gustafson, S., & Samuelsson, S. (2011). A longitudinal study of early reading difficulties and subsequent problem behaviors. *Scandinavian Journal of Psychology, 52*(3), 242–250.

Kikuchi, M., Yoshimura, Y., Shitamichi, K., Ueno, S., Hirosawa, T., Munesue, T., Ono, Y., Tsubokawa, T., Haruta, Y., Oi, M., Niida, Y., Remijn, B., Takahashi, T., Suzuki, M., Higashida, H., & Minabe, Y. (2013). A custom magnetoencephalography device reveals brain connectivity and high reading/decoding ability in children with autism. *Scientific Reports, 3,* 1139.

Kirby, P. (2020). Dyslexia debated, then and now: A historical perspective on the dyslexia debate. *Oxford Review of Education, 46*(4), 472–486.

Kirk, S. A., & Bateman, B. (1962). Diagnosis and remediation of learning disabilities. *Exceptional Children, 29*(2), 73–78.

Klassen, R. M., Tze, V. M., & Hannok, W. (2013). Internalizing problems of adults with learning disabilities: A meta-analysis. *Journal of Learning Disabilities, 46*(4), 317–327.

Kucian, K., Ashkenazi, S. S., Hänggi, J., Rotzer, S., Jäncke, L., Martin, E., & von Aster, M. (2014). Developmental dyscalculia: A dysconnection syndrome? *Brain Structure and Function, 219*(5), 1721–1733.

Landerl, K., & Moll, K. (2010). Comorbidity of learning disorders: Prevalence and familial transmission. *Journal of Child Psychology and Psychiatry, 51*(3), 287–294.

Larkin, R. F., & Snowling, M. J. (2008). Comparing phonological skills and spelling abilities in children with reading and language impairments. *International Journal of Language & Communication Disorders, 43*(1), 111–124.

Lonigan, C. J., & Shanahan, T. (2009). *Developing early literacy: Report of the National Early Literacy Panel. Executive summary. A scientific synthesis of early literacy development and implications for intervention.* National Institute for Literacy.

Maloney, E. A., & Beilock, S. L. (2012). Math anxiety: Who has it, why it develops, and how to guard against it. *Trends in Cognitive Sciences, 16*(8), 404–406.

Maloney, E. A., Ramirez, G., Gunderson, E. A., Levine, S. C., & Beilock, S. L. (2015). Intergenerational effects of parents' math anxiety on children's math achievement and anxiety. *Psychological Science, 26*(9), 1480–1488.

Mammarella, I. C., Ghisi, M., Bomba, M., Bottesi, G., Caviola, S., Broggi, F., & Nacinovich, R. (2016). Anxiety and depression in children with nonverbal learning disabilities, reading disabilities, or typical development. *Journal of Learning Disabilities, 49*(2), 130–139.

Manor, O., Shalev, R. S., Joseph, A., & Gross-Tsur, V. (2001). Arithmetic skills in kindergarten children with developmental language disorders. *European Journal of Paediatric Neurology, 5*(2), 71–77.

Markowitz, E. M., Willemsen, G., Trumbetta, S. L., van Beijsterveldt, T. C., & Boomsma, D. I. (2005). The etiology of mathematical and reading (dis) ability covariation in a sample of Dutch twins. *Twin Research and Human Genetics, 8*(6), 585–593.

Mascheretti, S., Trezzi, V., Giorda, R., Boivin, M., Plourde, V., Vitaro, F., Brendgen, M., Dionne, G., & Marino, C. (2017). Complex effects of dyslexia risk factors account for ADHD traits: Evidence from two independent samples. *Journal of Child Psychology and Psychiatry, 58*(1), 75–82.

Maughan, B., Messer, J., Collishaw, S., Pickles, A., Snowling, M., Yule, W., & Rutter, M. (2009). Persistence of literacy problems: Spelling in adolescence and at mid-life. *Journal of Child Psychology and Psychiatry, 50*(8), 893–901.

Maughan, B., Rowe, R., Loeber, R., & Stouthamer-Loeber, M. (2003). Reading problems and depressed mood. *Journal of Abnormal Child Psychology, 31*(2), 219–229.

Maurer, U., Bucher, K., Brem, S., Benz, R., Kranz, F., Schulz, E., van der Mark, S., Steinhausen, H.-C., & Brandeis, D. (2009). Neurophysiology in preschool improves behavioral prediction of reading ability throughout primary school. *Biological Psychiatry, 66*(4), 341–348.

Mazzocco, M. M. (2009). Mathematical learning disability in girls with Turner syndrome: A challenge to defining MLD and its subtypes. *Developmental Disabilities Research Reviews, 15*(1), 35–44.

McArthur, G., Eve, P. M., Jones, K., Banales, E., Kohnen, S., Anandakumar, T., Larsen, L., Marinus, E., Wang, H., & Castles, A. (2012). Phonics training for English-speaking poor readers. *Cochrane Database of Systematic Reviews, 12,* CD009115.

McArthur, G., Sheehan, Y., Badcock, N. A., Francis, D. A., Wang, H. C., Kohnen, S., Banales, E., Anandakumar, T., Marinus, E., & Castles, A. (2018). Phonics training for English-speaking poor readers. *Cochrane Database of Systematic Reviews, 11*(11), CD009115.

McGrath, L. M., Pennington, B. F., Shanahan, M. A., Santerre-Lemmon, L. E., Barnard, H. D., Willcutt, E. G., Defries, J. C., & Olson, R. K. (2011). A multiple deficit model of reading disability and attention-deficit/hyperactivity disorder: Searching for shared cognitive deficits. *Journal of Child Psychology and Psychiatry, 52*(5), 547–557.

Melby-Lervåg, M., & Hulme, C. (2013). Is working memory training effective? A meta-analytic review. *Developmental Psychology, 49*(2), 270–291.

Melby-Lervåg, M., Lyster, S. A. H., & Hulme, C. (2012). Phonological skills and their role in learning to read: A meta-analytic review. *Psychological Bulletin, 138*(2), 322–352.

Menon, V. (2010). Developmental cognitive neuroscience of arithmetic: Implications for learning and education. *Zdm, 42*(6), 515–525.

Menon, V. (2016). A neurodevelopmental perspective on the role of memory systems in children's math learning. In D. Berch, D. Geary, & K. M. Koepke (Eds.), *Development of mathematical cognition: Vol. 2. Neural substrates and genetic influences* (pp. 79–107). Elsevier.

Metsala, J. L., & Siegel, L. S. (1992). Patterns of atypical reading development: Attributes and underlying reading processes. *Handbook of Neuropsychology, 7*, 187–187.

Monuteaux, M. C., Faraone, S. V., Herzig, K., Navsaria, N., & Biederman, J. (2005). ADHD and dyscalculia: Evidence for independent familial transmission. *Journal of Learning Disabilities, 38*(1), 86–93.

Morgan, W. P. (1896). A case of congenital word blindness. *British Medical Journal, 2*(1871), 1378.

Morphy, P., & Graham, S. (2012). Word processing programs and weaker writers/readers: A meta-analysis of research findings. *Reading and Writing, 25*(3), 641–678.

Moura, O., Pereira, M., Alfaiate, C., Fernandes, E., Fernandes, B., Nogueira, S., Moreno, J., & Simões, M. R. (2017). Neurocognitive functioning in children with developmental dyslexia and attention-deficit/hyperactivity disorder: Multiple deficits and diagnostic accuracy. *Journal of Clinical and Experimental Neuropsychology, 39*(3), 296–312.

Murphy, M. M. (2009). A review of mathematical learning disabilities in children with fragile X syndrome. *Developmental Disabilities Research Reviews, 15*(1), 21–27.

Myers, C. A., Vandermosten, M., Farris, E. A., Hancock, R., Gimenez, P., Black, J. M., Casto, B., Drahos, M., Tumber, M., Hendren, R., Hulme, C., & Hoeft, F. (2014). White matter morphometric changes uniquely predict children's reading acquisition. *Psychological Science, 25*(10), 1870–1883.

Nation, K., & Snowling, M. J. (1998). Individual differences in contextual facilitation: Evidence from dyslexia and poor reading comprehension. *Child Development, 69*(4), 996–1011.

National Center for Education Statistics. (2017). https://nces.ed.gov/.

National Center for Education Statistics. (2018). *Children and youth with disabilities.* https://nces.ed.gov/programs/coe/indicator/cgg/students-with-disabilities

Nelson, J. M., & Harwood, H. (2011). Learning disabilities and anxiety: A meta-analysis. *Journal of Learning Disabilities, 44*(1), 3–17.

Nittrouer, S., & Pennington, B. (2010). New approaches to the study of childhood language disorders. *Current Directions in Psychological Science, 19*(5), 308–313.

Norton, E. S., Beach, S. D., & Gabrieli, J. D. (2015). Neurobiology of dyslexia. *Current Opinion in Neurobiology, 30*, 73–78.

Norton, E. S., Black, J. M., Stanley, L. M., Tanaka, H., Gabrieli, J. D., Sawyer, C., & Hoeft, F. (2014). Functional neuroanatomical evidence for the double-deficit hypothesis of developmental dyslexia. *Neuropsychologia, 61*, 235–246.

Nöthem, M. M., Schulte-Koerne, G., Grimm, T., Cichon, S., Vogt, I. R., Müller-Myhsok, B., Propping, P., & Remschmidt, H. (1999). Genetic linkage analysis with dyslexia: Evidence for linkage of spelling disability to chromosome 15. *European child & adolescent psychiatry, 8*(3), 56–59.

Ogle, W. (1867). Aphasia and agraphia. *St. George & Apostles Hospital Report, 2*, 83–122.

O'Hearn, K., & Luna, B. (2009). Mathematical skills in Williams syndrome: Insight into the importance of underlying representations. *Developmental Disabilities Research Reviews*, *15*(1), 11–20.

Oliver, B., Dale, P. S., & Plomin, R. (2004). Verbal and nonverbal predictors of early language problems: An analysis of twins in early childhood back to infancy. *Journal of Child Language*, *31*(3), 609–631.

Olson, R. K., Hulslander, J., Christopher, M., Keenan, J. M., Wadsworth, S. J., Willcutt, E. G., Pennington, B. F., & DeFries, J. C. (2013). Genetic and environmental influences on writing and their relations to language and reading. *Annals of Dyslexia*, *63*(1), 25–43.

Orton, S. T. (1928). Specific reading disability—Strephosymbolia. *Journal of the American Medical Association*, *90*(14), 1095–1099.

Ostrolenk, A., d'Arc, B. F., Jelenic, P., Samson, F., & Mottron, L. (2017). Hyperlexia: Systematic review, neurocognitive modelling, and outcome. *Neuroscience & Biobehavioral Reviews*, *79*, 134–149.

Paracchini, S. (2011). Dissection of genetic associations with language-related traits in population-based cohorts. *Journal of Neurodevelopmental Disorders*, *3*(4), 365–373.

Pennington, B. F. (1991). *Diagnosing learning disabilities*. Guilford.

Pennington, B. F., Johnson, C., & Welsh, M. C. (1987). Unexpected reading precocity in a normal preschooler: Implications for hyperlexia. *Brain and Language*, *30*(1), 165–180.

Pennington, B. F., McGrath, L. M., & Peterson, R. L. (2019). *Diagnosing learning disorders: From science to practice*. Guilford.

Pennington, B. F., & Olson, R. K. (2005). Genetics of dyslexia. In M. J. Snowling & C. Hulme (Eds.), *The science of reading: A handbook* (pp. 453–472). Blackwell.

Peterson, R. L., Boada, R., McGrath, L. M., Willcutt, E. G., Olson, R. K., & Pennington, B. F. (2017). Cognitive prediction of reading, math, and attention: Shared and unique influences. *Journal of Learning Disabilities*, *50*(4), 408–421.

Phillips, A. (1930). Talented imbeciles. *The Psychological Clinic*, *18*(8), 246.

Plomin, R., Kovas, Y., & Haworth, C. M. (2007). Generalist genes: Genetic links between brain, mind, and education. *Mind, Brain, and Education*, *1*(1), 11–19.

Plourde, V., Boivin, M., Brendgen, M., Vitaro, F., & Dionne, G. (2017). Phenotypic and genetic associations between reading and attention-deficit/hyperactivity disorder dimensions in adolescence. *Development and Psychopathology*, *29*(4), 1215–1226.

Ramirez, G., & Beilock, S. L. (2011). Writing about testing worries boosts exam performance in the classroom. *Science*, *331*(6014), 211–213.

Ramirez, G., Gunderson, E. A., Levine, S. C., & Beilock, S. L. (2013). Math anxiety, working memory, and math achievement in early elementary school. *Journal of Cognition and Development*, *14*(2), 187–202.

Ramus, F., & Szenkovits, G. (2008). What phonological deficit? *Quarterly Journal of Experimental Psychology*, *61*(1), 129–141.

Rasinski, T., Samuels, S. J., Hiebert, E., Petscher, Y., & Feller, K. (2011). The relationship between a silent reading fluency instructional protocol on students' reading comprehension and achievement in an urban school setting. *Reading Psychology*, *32*(1), 75–97.

Raskind, W. H., Hsu, L., Berninger, V. W., Thomson, J. B., & Wijsman, E. M. (2000). Familial aggregation of dyslexia phenotypes. *Behavior Genetics*, *30*(5), 385–396.

Richlan, F. (2012). Developmental dyslexia: Dysfunction of a left hemisphere reading network. *Frontiers in Human Neuroscience*, *6*, Article 120.

Richman, L. C., & Kitchell, M. M. (1981). Hyperlexia as a variant of developmental language disorder. *Brain and Language*, *12*, 203–212.

Rivera-Batiz, F. L. (1992). Quantitative literacy and the likelihood of employment among young adults in the United States. *Journal of Human Resources*, *27*, 313–328.

Robinson, H. M. (1972). Visual and auditory modalities related to methods for beginning readers. *Reading Research Quarterly*, *8*, 7–39.

Rose, G. J. (2018). The numerical abilities of anurans and their neural correlates: Insights from neuroethological studies of acoustic communication. *Philosophical Transactions of the Royal Society Series B: Biological Sciences, 373*(1740), 20160512.

Rourke, B. (1978). Reading, spelling and arithmetic disabilities: A neuropsychological analysis. In H. Myklebust (Ed.), *Progress in learning disabilities* (Vol. 4). Grune & Stratton.

Rubenstein, K., Matsushita, M., Berninger, V. W., Raskind, W. H., & Wijsman, E. M. (2011). Genome scan for spelling deficits: Effects of verbal IQ on models of transmission and trait gene localization. *Behavior Genetics, 41*(1), 31–42.

Russell, G., Ryder, D., Norwich, B., & Ford, T. (2015). Behavioural difficulties that co-occur with specific word reading difficulties: A UK population-based cohort study. *Dyslexia, 21*(2), 123–141.

Rykhlevskaia, E., Uddin, L. Q., Kondos, L., & Menon, V. (2009). Neuroanatomical correlates of developmental dyscalculia: Combined evidence from morphometry and tractography. *Frontiers in Human Neuroscience, 3*, Article 51.

Santangelo, T., & Graham, S. (2016). A comprehensive meta-analysis of handwriting instruction. *Educational Psychology Review, 28*(2), 225–265.

Scerri, T. S., & Schulte-Körne, G. (2010). Genetics of developmental dyslexia. *European Child & Adolescent Psychiatry, 19*(3), 179–197.

Schuchardt, K., Fischbach, A., Balke-Melcher, C., & Maehler, C. (2015). The comorbidity of learning difficulties and ADHD symptoms in primary-school-age children. *Zeitschrift fur Kinder-und Jugendpsychiatrie und Psychotherapie, 43*(3), 185–193.

Schulte-Körne, G. (2001). Annotation: Genetics of reading and spelling disorder. *Journal of Child Psychology and Psychiatry and Allied Disciplines, 42*(8), 985–997.

Sexton, C. C., Gelhorn, H. L., Bell, J. A., & Classi, P. M. (2012). The co-occurrence of reading disorder and ADHD: Epidemiology, treatment, psychosocial impact, and economic burden. *Journal of Learning Disabilities, 45*(6), 538–564.

Shalev, R. S., Manor, O., Kerem, B., Ayali, M., Badichi, N., Friedlander, Y., & Gross-Tsur, V. (2001). Developmental dyscalculia is a familial learning disability. *Journal of Learning Disabilities, 34*(1), 59–65.

Shaywitz, B. A., Shaywitz, S. E. (2020). The American experience: Towards a 21st century definition of dyslexia. *Oxford Review of Education, 46*(4), 454–471.

Shaywitz, B. A., Shaywitz, S. E., Blachman, B. A., Pugh, K. R., Fulbright, R. K., Skudlarski, P., Mencl, W., Constable, R., Holahan, J., Marchione, K., Fletcher, J. M., Lyon, G., & Gore, J. (2004). Development of left occipitotemporal systems for skilled reading in children after a phonologically-based intervention. *Biological Psychiatry, 55*(9), 926–933.

Shaywitz, S. E., & Shaywitz, B. A. (2005). Dyslexia (specific reading disability). *Biological Psychiatry, 57*(11), 1301–1309.

Silberberg, N. E., & Silberberg, M. C. (1967). Hyperlexia: Specific word recognition skills in young children. *Exceptional Children, 34*, 41–42.

Silberberg, N. E., & Silberberg, M. C. (1968). Case histories in hyperlexia. *Journal of School Psychology, 7*, 3–7.

Silver, L. B. (1989). Psychological and family problems associated with learning disabilities: Assessment and intervention. *Journal of the American Academy of Child & Adolescent Psychiatry, 28*(3), 319–325.

Simms, V., Gilmore, C., Sloan, S., & McKeaveney, C. (2017). *Interventions to improve mathematics achievement in primary school-aged children: A systematic review.* The Campbell Collaboration.

Simon, T. J., Takarae, Y., DeBoer, T., McDonald-McGinn, D. M., Zackai, E. H., & Ross, J. L. (2008). Overlapping numerical cognition impairments in children with chromosome 22q11.2 deletion or Turner syndromes. *Neuropsychologia, 46*(1), 82–94.

Snowling, M. J, & Hulme, C. (2015). *Rutter's child & adolescent psychiatry* (6th ed.). Wiley.

Snowling, M. J., Hulme, C., & Nation, K. (2020). Defining and understanding dyslexia: Past, present and future. *Oxford Review of Education, 46*(4), 501–513.

Snowling, M. J., & Melby-Lervåg, M. (2016). Oral language deficits in familial dyslexia: A meta-analysis and review. *Psychological Bulletin, 142*(5), 498–545.

Soares, N., Evans, T., & Patel, D. R. (2018). Specific learning disability in mathematics: A comprehensive review. *Translational Pediatrics*, 7(1), 48–62.

Sokolowski, H. M., & Necka, E. A. (2016). Remediating math anxiety through cognitive training: Potential roles for math ability and social context. *Journal of Neuroscience*, 36(5), 1439–1441.

Stevenson, J., Graham, P., Fredman, G., & Mcloughli, V. (1987). A twin study of genetic influences on reading and spelling ability and disability. *Journal of Child Psychology and Psychiatry*, 28(2), 229–247.

Strauss, A. A., & Lehtinen, L. E. (1947). *Psychopathology and education of the brain-injured child.* Grune & Stratton.

Tallal, P., Chase, C., Russell, G., & Schmitt, R. L. (1986). Evaluation of the efficacy of piracetam in treating information processing, reading and writing disorders in dyslexic children. *International Journal of Psychophysiology*, 4(1), 41–52.

Tannock, R., Frijters, J. C., Martinussen, R., White, E. J., Ickowicz, A., Benson, N. J., & Lovett, M. W. (2018). Combined modality intervention for ADHD with comorbid reading disorders: A proof of concept study. *Journal of Learning Disabilities*, 51(1), 55–72.

Tarrasch, R., Berman, Z., & Friedmann, N. (2016). Mindful reading: Mindfulness meditation helps keep readers with dyslexia and ADHD on the lexical track. *Frontiers in Psychology*, 7, Article 578.

Temple, C. (1993). *The brain: An introduction to the psychology of the human brain and behavior.* Penguin.

Therrien, W. J. (2004). Fluency and comprehension gains as a result of repeated reading: A meta-analysis. *Remedial and Special Education*, 25(4), 252–261.

Turkeltaub, P. E., Flowers, D. L., Verbalis, A., Miranda, M., Gareau, L., & Eden, G. F. (2004). The neural basis of hyperlexic reading: An fMRI case study. *Neuron*, 41(1), 11–25.

U.S. Congress. (1975). *Public Law 94-142, Education for All Handicapped Children Act of 1975.* U.S. Government Printing Office.

U.S. Office of Education. (1977). Assistance to states for education of handicapped children: Procedures for evaluating specific learning disabilities. *Federal Register*, 42(250), 65082–65085.

Van der Mark, S., Klaver, P., Bucher, K., Maurer, U., Schulz, E., Brem, S., Martin, E., & Brandeis, D. (2011). The left occipitotemporal system in reading: Disruption of focal fMRI connectivity to left inferior frontal and inferior parietal language areas in children with dyslexia. *NeuroImage*, 54(3), 2426–2436.

Vandermosten, M., Boets, B., Wouters, J., & Ghesquière, P. (2012). A qualitative and quantitative review of diffusion tensor imaging studies in reading and dyslexia. *Neuroscience & Biobehavioral Reviews*, 36(6), 1532–1552.

Wadsworth, S. J., DeFries, J. C., Willcutt, E. G., Pennington, B. F., & Olson, R. K. (2015). The Colorado Longitudinal Twin Study of Reading Difficulties and ADHD: Etiologies of comorbidity and stability. *Twin Research and Human Genetics*, 18(6), 755–761.

Wei, X., Christiano, E., Yu, J., Wagner, M., & Spiker, D. (2015). Reading and math achievement profiles and longitudinal growth trajectories of children with an autism spectrum disorder. *Autism*, 19(2), 200–210.

Welsh, M. C., Pennington, B. F., & Rogers, S. (1987). Word recognition and comprehension skills in hyperlexic children. *Brain and Language*, 32(1), 76–96.

Whitehouse, D., & Harris, J. (1984). Hyperlexia in infantile autism. *Journal of Autism and Developmental Disorders*, 14, 281–289.

Wietecha, L., Williams, D., Shaywitz, S., Shaywitz, B., Hooper, S. R., Wigal, S. B., Dunn, D., & McBurnett, K. (2013). Atomoxetine improved attention in children and adolescents with attention-deficit/hyperactivity disorder and dyslexia in a 16 week, acute, randomized, double-blind trial. *Journal of Child and Adolescent Psychopharmacology*, 23(9), 605–613.

Willcutt, E. G., Betjemann, R. S., McGrath, L. M., Chhabildas, N. A., Olson, R. K., DeFries, J. C., & Pennington, B. F. (2010). Etiology and neuropsychology of comorbidity between RD and ADHD: The case for multiple-deficit models. *Cortex*, 46(10), 1345–1361.

Wilsher, C. R., Bennett, D., Chase, C. H., Conners, C. K., DiIanni, M., Feagans, L., Hanvik, L., Helfgott, E., Koplewicz, H., & Overby, P. (1987). Piracetam and dyslexia: Effects on reading tests. *Journal of Clinical Psychopharmacology, 7*(4), 230–237.

Yell, M. L., Shriner, J. G., & Katsiyannis, A. (2006). Individuals with Disabilities Education Improvement Act of 2004 and IDEA regulations of 2006: Implications for educators, administrators, and teacher trainers. *Focus on Exceptional Children, 39*(1), 1–24.

Yoshimasu, K., Barbaresi, W. J., Colligan, R. C., Killian, J. M., Voigt, R. G., Weaver, A. L., & Katusic, S. K. (2011). Written-language disorder among children with and without ADHD in a population-based birth cohort. *Pediatrics, 128*(3), e605–e612.

Young, C. B., Wu, S. S., & Menon, V. (2012). The neurodevelopmental basis of math anxiety. *Psychological Science, 23*(5), 492–501.

Zhang, M., Trussell, R. P., Gallegos, B., & Asam, R. R. (2015). Using math apps for improving student learning: An exploratory study in an inclusive fourth grade classroom. *TechTrends, 59*(2), 32–39.

Zheng, X., Flynn, L. J., & Swanson, H. L. (2013). Experimental intervention studies on word problem solving and math disabilities: A selective analysis of the literature. *Learning Disability Quarterly, 36*(2), 97–111.

# 18

# Fetal Alcohol Spectrum Disorder

Fetal alcohol spectrum disorder (FASD), a recognized cause of intellectual developmental disorder (IDD) and other neurodevelopmental disorders, often goes undiagnosed. Importantly, alcohol exposure during the prenatal period is preventable. The recommended prevention guideline is that there is no safe amount of alcohol to consume in any trimester of pregnancy (Charness et al., 2016). The manifestations of gestational substance abuse with alcohol are highly correlated with the extent of alcohol use, maternal health, postnatal adversity, and genetic factors (Mela et al., 2019). The most debilitating consequence of prenatal exposure to alcohol is injury to the central nervous system. It is manifest in intellectual, neurological, and behavioral abnormalities.

The lifetime costs for health care, special education, and social services of FASD children are substantial and have been estimated to be in the hundreds of million dollars annually in the United States and Canada (Popova et al., 2011, 2015). These costs take into account growth deficiency, the need to surgically repair structural deficits, the treatment of IDD, and the treatment of learning problems. In the United States, the annual estimated cost of care for all affected individuals ranges from $926 million to $3.2 billion, and it is far higher when adjusted for inflation based on the year of estimation (Greenmyer et al., 2020). IDD alone due to FASD accounts for as much as 11% of the annual cost of all institutionalized residents in the United States and 5% of the cost of all congenital anomalies (Charness et al., 1989; Lupton et al., 2004). Research during the past five decades has established evidence-based education programs for professionals and the public for FASD. These efforts on early recognition, diagnosis, and therapy for disorders along the FASD continuum are leading to improved outcomes (Williams et al., 2015).

This chapter describes the history, epidemiology, diagnosis and classification, clinical features, natural history, etiology (genetics), neuroimaging, associated mental and behavioral disorders, and treatment of FASD.

## History

In 1968, anomalies were observed in 127 French children of alcoholic parents based on effects of alcohol on the developing fetus (Lemoine et al., 1968). Five years later, the pattern of developmental deficits in the offspring of chronic alcoholic mothers was diagnosed as fetal alcohol syndrome (FAS; Jones et al., 1973). Subsequently, it has become apparent that prenatal alcohol exposure is associated with a spectrum of lifelong abnormalities that include physical, cognitive, and behavioral dysfunction. Considerable progress has been made in establishing definitive criteria for diagnosing FASD, which includes FAS, partial fetal alcohol syndrome (PFAS), alcohol-related birth defects (ARBD), alcohol-related neurodevelopmental disorder (ARND), and neurobehavioral disorder with prenatal exposure (ND-PAE) (Hoyme et al., 2016). ND-PAE is a new psychiatric diagnosis included in the appendix of the fifth edition of the *Diagnostic and Statistical Manual of Mental Disorders* (DSM-5; American Psychiatric Association, 2013) the criteria of which require further study. The ND-PAE criteria include prenatal alcohol exposure and central nervous system involvement with impairments in cognition, self-regulation, and adaptive functioning. In contrast to ARBD, ND-PAE may be diagnosed with or without physical dysmorphia associated with alcohol exposure (Hagan et al., 2016). Although ND-PAE is a disorder undergoing further study as a distinct diagnosis, its presentation may be diagnosed under other specific neurodevelopmental disorders (code F88) in DSM-5.

## Epidemiology

Fetal alcohol spectrum disorders are the leading cause of preventable neurodisabilities in the world. The risk for an alcohol-exposed pregnancy in women aged 15–44 years is 7.3% (Green, 2016). Binge drinking by pregnant women is the major concern. Using a conservative approach, the U.S. estimated prevalence for combined FASD among first graders measured in four regional U.S. communities ranged from 1.1% to 5.0% (May et al., 2018). Criteria for diagnosis in these communities were based on the four domains in the FASD continuum: dysmorphic features, physical growth, neurobehavioral development, and prenatal alcohol exposure. The highest rates in the world are reported as 13.5–20.8% in a mixed-race population in South Africa (May et al., 2013). The prevalence of alcohol use during pregnancy in the Aboriginal populations of the United States and Canada has been found to be three or four times higher than that of the general population. The World Health Organization is conducting global studies to determine rates; systematic reviews note that alcohol consumption in pregnancy remains high in many countries. Despite its frequency, FASD often goes unrecognized because many physicians do not systematically inquire about alcohol use and may not recognize the extensive range of the effects of prenatal alcohol exposure.

## Diagnosis and Classification

Diagnostic criteria are based on those developed from a collaboration on FASD prevalence research consortium with modifications drawn from the 1996 Institute of Medicine (now National Academy of Medicine) criteria. Diagnosis is strengthened by documenting the extent of alcohol exposure. Alcohol exposure is defined as six or more drinks for 2 weeks or more during pregnancy and as three or more drinks per drinking event on at least three occasions during pregnancy. In addition, social or legal problems related to alcohol use are factored into the assessment. Although diagnosis is related to binge drinking, lower levels of alcohol also adversely affect brain development. In one prospective study involving 607 children exposed to alcohol during pregnancy, one alcohol drink per day in any trimester was associated with behavioral problems at age 22 years (Day et al., 2013). Prenatal exposure to alcohol is not required when the characteristic dysmorphic facial features are present. The collaboration on the FASD prevalence study included a neurobehavioral component involving cognition and behavior.

Box 18.1 shows the diagnostic criteria for FASD from the Collaboration on Fetal Alcohol Spectrum Disorder Prevalence Study (May et al., 2018). Criteria included dysmorphic facial features, growth deficiency, brain abnormality, cognitive or behavioral impairment, other systemic malformation, and prenatal alcohol exposure. PFAS can

---

**Box 18.1  Diagnostic Criteria for Fetal Alcohol Spectrum Disorder**

## Fetal Alcohol Syndrome (FAS)

For a FAS diagnosis, a child must have (a) a characteristic pattern of minor facial abnormalities including at least two or more of the key features of FAS (palpebral fissures ≤10th percentile, thin vermilion border, or smooth philtrum); (b) evidence of prenatal and/or postnatal growth retardation (height or weight ≤10th percentile); (c) evidence of deficient brain growth (structural brain anomalies or lower occipitofrontal head circumference [OFC] ≤10th percentile); and, when possible, (d) confirmation of maternal alcohol consumption from the mother or a knowledgeable collateral source.

## Partial Fetal Alcohol Syndrome (PFAS)

For a PFAS diagnosis, a child must have (a) evidence of a characteristic pattern of facial abnormalities including two, three, or more of the key features of FAS (above); (b) one or more other characteristics, such as prenatal or postnatal growth retardation (≤10th percentile in height or weight), hypoplastic midface, ocular defects, abnormalities of the fingers, or other physical defects linked to prenatal alcohol exposure; (c) small OFC (≤10th percentile) and/or evidence of a complex pattern of behavioral or cognitive abnormalities inconsistent with developmental level and unexplainable by genetic composition, family background, or environment alone; and, when possible, (d) direct or collateral confirmation of maternal alcohol consumption.

## Alcohol-Related Neurodevelopmental Disorders (ARND)

For an ARND diagnosis, documentation of significant prenatal alcohol exposure is required. The child displays neurological or structural brain abnormalities (e.g., microcephaly) or manifests evidence of a complex and characteristic pattern of behavioral or cognitive abnormalities inconsistent with developmental level as measured by test batteries and are not explained by genetic predisposition, family background, or environment alone.

## Alcohol-Related Birth Defects (ARBD)

For an ARBD diagnosis, criteria include prenatal alcohol exposure, evidence of two or more of the characteristic pattern of facial anomalies, as well as congenital structural defects of varying degree and number but generally normal neurobehavioral performance.

occur without alcohol exposure history when craniofacial features, neurobehavioral impairment and growth deficiency, or abnormal brain development are demonstrated. A diagnosis of ARND requires evidence of alcohol exposure and only cognitive and behavior abnormality. Because criteria are less strict, it makes up a large proportion of cases. The diagnosis of ARBD is less common and includes skeletal or cardiovascular systems.

The diagnostic term neurobehavioral disorder associated with prenatal alcohol exposure is limited in the DSM-5 appendix (Hagan et al., 2016). It is placed in the appendix as a disorder requiring additional study. There are three symptom domains: neurocognition, self-regulation, and adaptive functioning. Currently, there is a lack of consensus on the minimal degree of alcohol exposure at which adverse effects can be demonstrated and the degree of cognitive impairment to make the diagnosis. Moreover, the frequency of impairment in the three symptom domains is being clarified. ND-PAE was included in the May et al. (2019) prevalence survey, and the rates can be estimated from it. When a direct comparison was made among the set of alcohol-related development disorders diagnostic criteria, including the proposed ND-PAE criteria, ND-PAE was correctly identified in 77 of 86 cases (90%; Johnson et al., 2018).

## Clinical Features

More than 80% of children with FAS, the most severe form of FASD, show prenatal and postnatal growth deficiency, microcephaly, infantile irritability, and mild to moderate IDD. Initially, identification of FAS was based on physical stigmata. Subsequently, dysmorphic features were specified in greater detail. The three core facial features established in affected children are short palpebral fissures, thinner upper lip vermillion border, and flattened philtrum (Warren & Foudin, 2001). However, for a diagnosis of FAS, facial stigmata are one of four general areas required for diagnosis. The others are growth impairments, neurocognitive deficits, and history of alcohol exposure. These four characteristics for FAS remain unchanged and are currently used (British Medical Association Board of Science, 2016). For PFAS, facial features and cognitive or behavioral impairment are required. For the other diagnoses, facial features are not required. Cognitive and behavioral features are required for PFAS (Figure 18.1).

Over time, the measurement of these core facial features is increasingly being refined—for example, using three-dimensional photographic tools to measure the details of facial features (Suttie et al., 2013). In addition, there can be additional minor physical anomalies. These include ptosis, epicanthal folds, railroad track ears, forward tilted nostrils, midline flattening, and joint contractures. Gross motor defects occur more frequently when there is moderate to severe alcohol exposure (Lucas et al., 2014). Fine motor skills are also affected, including handwriting skills (Doney et al., 2014).

## Sensory Processing Abnormalities

Prenatal alcohol exposure affects sensory processing. Brain regions involved in taste and odor processing may be affected, leading to impaired odor identification (Bower

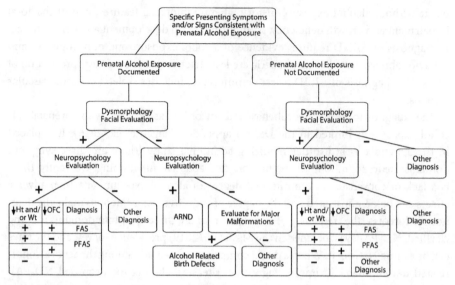

**Figure 18.1**  Decision tree for making FASD diagnoses. At the top of the figure, presented signs and/or symptoms are shown. Fetal alcohol exposure is either documented or not documented. Facial dysmorphology evaluation is examined whether or not alcohol exposure is documented. Neuropsychological evaluation is completed, and categories of FASD are listed separately for documented and not documented alcohol exposure. ARND, alcohol-related neurodevelopmental disorder; FAS, fetal alcohol syndrome; FASD, fetal alcohol spectrum disorder; OFC, occipitofrontal head circumference; PFAS, partial fetal alcohol syndrome.

From Hoyme et al. (2016); redrawn by Tim Phelps (2021).

et al., 2013). In its more severe form, prenatal alcohol can disrupt eye development with microophthalmia, optic nerve hypoplasia, and poor visual acuity (Strömland & Pinazo-Durian, 2002). Hearing, speech, and language problems occur, and difficulty in auditory processing can interfere with the development of reading and writing.

## Cognitive Defects and Social Skills

There is a wide range of cognitive defects. These include IDD; impaired attention, executive dysfunction, and memory; and visual–spatial and visual-motor performance defects. Cognitive defects occur in those with dysmorphic facial features in some but not in all cases. Social skills deficits affect adoptive functioning in school and in the community, and they can lead to legal difficulty.

## Documentation of Prenatal Alcohol Exposure

Alcohol intake is measured based on the quantity of alcohol consumed, standard drinks per drinking day, and frequency of alcohol consumption (daily and number of times per week). The time of alcohol use in gestation should be ascertained. Both human and animal studies have established that drinking three to five drinks or more per occasion defines binge drinking; it is the most detrimental form of alcohol consumption for the fetus. Moreover, it is essential to ask about other substance use (e.g., marijuana and opiates) during pregnancy that may accompany alcohol use. Generally, all this information is collected retrospectively in clinical practice.

## Natural History

Fetal alcohol spectrum disorder is not limited to childhood; the cognitive and behavioral effects and psychosocial problems persist throughout adolescence into adulthood and old age (Wozniak et al., 2019). After puberty, the faces of patients with FAS and PFAS are less distinctive. Affected individuals generally are short and microcephalic; however, their weight tends to reach the adult mean for age. IQ scores widely vary. Maladaptive behaviors throughout life include poor judgment, distractibility, difficulty perceiving social cues, and problems in modulating mood. Adolescents exposed prenatally to alcohol have been shown to rely more on stored, learned, verbal information for daily communication, whereas non-exposed adolescents rely more on abstract thinking and verbal efficacy. Importantly, frequently it is only when there is excessive cognitive load that deficits become apparent. Deficits also include problems with executive functioning (Lange, Probst, et al., 2017; Lange, Rovet, et al., 2017).

## Etiology

Alcohol is a known teratogen that crosses easily through the placenta to the fetus. The fetal liver cannot process alcohol as efficiently as an adult liver because the fetal liver has low activity of the critical catabolic enzyme alcohol dehydrogenase, which metabolizes alcohol (Manriquez et al., 2019). Moreover, the amniotic sac retains alcohol; this compounds toxicity because the fetus swallows the amniotic fluid (Guelinckx et al., 2011). Acetaldehyde, a toxic metabolite of alcohol, interferes with fetal growth and development through its impact on cell differentiation and DNA synthesis. Acetaldehyde also causes dysregulation of the hypothalamic–pituitary–adrenal axis, resulting in an elevation in serum cortisol levels (Keiver et al., 2015).

Ethanol has been shown to have potent effects on neurotransmission in the fetal brain, which is critical for guiding neurogenesis, neuronal migration, and neuronal survival. Specifically, ethanol allosterically enhances $GABA_A$ receptor function, which inhibits neuronal firing. In tandem, ethanol allosterically inhibits NMDA receptor function, an excitatory glutamate receptor, thus further impairing fetal brain neuronal activity (Lotfullina & Khazipov, 2018). Moreover, the NMDA receptor plays a more fundamental role in brain development; it gates the influx $Ca^{2+}$ that drives gene expression, especially genes encoding growth and trophic factors and proteins promoting synaptogenesis. Blocking the NMDA receptors of immature neurons results in the activation of programed cell death or apoptosis (Farber et al., 2010). These effects of ethanol not only account for central nervous system hypoplasia (microencephaly) in FAS but also contribute to facial stigmata because GABA is also a morphogen (Pearl et al., 2007).

## Genetics

Early studies suggested a genetic sensitivity to FASD based on human twin studies. In a study of monozygotic and dizygotic twins, monozygotic twins were 100% concordant for the diagnosis of FASD, whereas dizygotic twins were 64% concordant (Streissguth & Dehaene, 1993), consistent with some genetic risk factors. Nevertheless, the very high concordance in fraternal twins highlights the importance of alcohol exposure alone. Despite such high risk, not all exposure to alcohol results in FASD: Abel (1995) found that only 4.3% of children who had heavy alcohol exposure in utero developed full-blown FAS. However, this does not mean that they were unaffected, and they may be on the fetal alcohol spectrum. Still, other susceptibility factors are likely involved that may determine severity, including genes and environmental factors.

## Genes Involved in Ethanol Metabolism

The major enzyme involved in alcohol metabolism, ethanol, is initially metabolized by alcohol dehydrogenase (ADH) to toxic acetaldehyde, which is then converted to nontoxic acetate. The nontoxic acetaldehyde is converted to acetate by aldehyde dehydrogenase. Some ADH alleles metabolize acetaldehyde more quickly than others. For example, the *ADH1B*3* allele is reported to increase alcohol metabolism, mitigating alcohol effects on attention and behavior problems in adolescents who were exposed to alcohol in utero (Dodge et al., 2014).

Because alcohol-related FASD phenotype is variable, further research is needed to improve diagnosis and to clarify individual risk (Eberhart & Parnell, 2016). Genetic studies demonstrate that the human *L1CAM* gene is important in brain development, and mutations of this gene result in dysgenesis of the corpus callosum, hydrocephalus, and cerebral dysplasia, similar to findings in FASD. Still, not all genotypes are equally sensitive to ethanol. Polymorphisms in genes that are involved in the regulation of the sensitivity of L1 neural cell adhesion molecules to ethanol have been associated with both craniofacial development and brain morphology in humans (Dou et al., 2018).

## Pathophysiological Models of Brain Development

The effects of alcohol on development are largely determined by the dose, pattern of consumption, and timing of prenatal exposure (Wozniak et al., 2019). In studies of mice in gastrulation at the equivalent of 17 days of human gestation, alcohol exposure affects the craniofacial face signature, resulting in small palpebral fissures and lip and philtrum abnormalities. Later alcohol exposure in rodents at the development phase of neurulation, the equivalent of 3 or 4 weeks of human gestation, results in dysmorphic faces similar to that found in 22q11.2 syndrome (Parnell et al., 2018). Even later in gestation, after the completion of organogenesis, there is far less effect of alcohol exposure on craniofacial development. However, brain development is affected by alcohol throughout all three trimesters. Exposure later in gestation may be correlated with behavioral and neurocognitive without craniofacial features in, for example, alcohol-related developmental disorder.

## Neuroimaging

Alcohol produces neurochemical and structural changes throughout the brain (Reynolds et al., 2011). These may not result in gross anatomical change. However, refined imaging frequently reveals subtle structural changes. The three most common brain abnormalities found in FASD neuroimaging studies are small head and brain size (in relation to body size), thinning of corpus callosum, and underdeveloped cerebellum. Moreover, there are abnormalities in overall brain structure, cortical development, white matter microstructure, and functional connectivity. These brain findings affect developmental trajectories and are associated with cognitive and social adaptive deficits. Associated deficits linked to brain imaging abnormalities are found in executive functions, memory, vision, hearing, motor skills, and behavior.

Still, routine radiology reports using conventional magnetic resonance imaging (MRI) typically report neuroimaging findings as nonspecific. Therefore, clinical MRI is not recommended for prenatal alcohol exposure (Wozniak et al., 2019). Quantitative imaging, which is more sensitive, should be used to identify brain regions that are the most susceptible to gestational alcohol exposure. Especially helpful is volumetric assessment with three-dimensional T1-weighted MRI scans. These scans have revealed that white matter volume is disproportionately reduced with alcohol exposure. Moreover, thinning of the corpus callosum, the large white matter tract that connects the two cerebral hemispheres, is frequently reported. Volume reductions have also been reported in the basal ganglia.

In the fetus, white matter may be more sensitive to alcohol-induced brain injury. Diffusion tensor imaging (DTI) in affected children has found microstructural white matter pathology not apparent on clinical MRI (Wozniak et al., 2019). Glial cells, important guides in the structural development of the brain, and myelinated axons seem especially vulnerable to alcohol toxicity. DTI provides quantitative measurements of white matter. Fractional anisotropy and mean diffusivity are measures that can be compared between subjects. DTI allows more sensitive measure of tissue microstructure than standard MRI. Mean diffusivity measured with DTI is a measure of white matter microstructural pathology that is not apparent on clinical MRI. DTI studies of FASD in children and young adults have shown diffusion abnormalities in the corpus callosum. A whole-brain, voxel-based analysis of children and adolescents with FASD showed anisotropy reductions in the splenium of the corpus callosum and right lateral temporal lobe. In one study, 7 of 10 white matter tracts and three of four deep gray matter structures were shown to be abnormal in FASD.

Task-based functional MRI has been used to visualize cognitive processing deficits in FASD and to show that the frontal–parietal connectivity correlates with spatial working memory in affected children and that parietal activity is abnormal during spatial memory processing (Infante et al., 2017; Woods et al., 2015). These brain changes may go undetected until the child reaches an age when cognitive functions are emerging and affect school performance.

The consequences of prenatal alcohol exposure vary widely from mild to disabling brain dysfunction that includes learning and memory, executive functions, social communication, attention, and sensorimotor skills. Childhood depression, anxiety, and other mental health conditions also can be manifestations of primary brain insults or secondary to the neurobehavioral/neurobiological symptoms resulting from alcohol exposure.

## Behavioral Phenotype

The behavioral phenotype for fetal alcohol exposure is characterized by impairments in intellectual functioning, particularly in mathematics, and difficulty understanding cause and effect when generalizing from one situation to another. Inattention, poor concentration, impaired judgment, memory deficits, and problems in abstract reasoning are also characteristic. Behavioral problems include impulsivity, hyperactivity, oppositional behavior, and conduct disorders.

## Associated Mental and Behavioral Disorders

Co-occurring mental and behavioral disorders are a major concern in prenatal alcohol exposure. Individuals with prenatal alcohol exposure evaluated in psychiatric clinics exhibit both internalizing disorders (e.g., depression and anxiety) and externalizing disorders (e.g., attention-deficit/hyperactivity disorder [ADHD] and conduct disorders), along with cognitive and adaptive deficits. FASD is the most common and preventable cause of neurodevelopmental disorders and IDDs in the United States and Europe (O'Leary et al., 2013). A systematic review of 11 studies of co-occurring mental and behavioral disorders with FASD revealed that attention-deficit hyperactivity symptoms occurred in 50% of subjects, a 10-fold increase over the typical population prevalence of 5% (Weyrauch et al., 2017). Oppositional defiant disorder was 5 times more prevalent than expected in the general population, whereas learning disorders were twice the expected rate. IDD, 20 times more common than in the general population, was documented in 23% of the FASD subjects. Psychosis was also found to be 20 times higher. Depression, anxiety disorder, bipolar disorder, and post-traumatic stress disorder were significantly increased over the general population rates. Reactive attachment disorder was 5 times higher than the expected rate. Moreover, there were increased rates of alcohol, tobacco, and other substance abuse beginning in adolescence, together revealing the remarkably high prevalence of co-morbid psychiatric disorders in FASD. These high rates of neurobehavioral disorders are mostly based on studies of FASD cases referred to psychiatric services. Population prevalence rates based on school studies for the same disorders find lower rates (McLennan, 2015).

Rates of epilepsy are also increased in FASD and range from 6% in a retrospective chart review study to as high as 25% in a high-risk international foster care sample

(Boronat et al., 2017; Popova et al., 2016). Sleep problems commonly occur and may compound neurobehavioral problems (McLennan, 2015). In one study using clinical assessment along with polysomnography, 20 of 36 children and adolescents referred to a FASD clinic had sleep disorders—twice the rate in the general population. The most frequent sleep problems were insomnia and parasomnias (sleep arousal disorders). Moreover, 79% showed dysregulation of melatonin secretion with delayed or advanced patterns of melatonin release (Goril et al., 2016). Sleep disturbance may involve central respiratory modulation problems (central apnea), upper airway obstruction, and disrupted circadian rhythms (Hanlon-Dearman et al., 2018). Thus, sleep assessment should be a part of the routine assessment of FASD.

## Treatment

### Prevention

The first issue is prevention of alcohol exposure. There is no clearly established safe dose of alcohol for pregnant women. The Committee on Substance Abuse and the Committee on Children's Disabilities of the American Academy of Pediatrics (2023) recommends that because there is no known safe amount of alcohol consumption during pregnancy, complete abstinence from alcohol for women who are pregnant or who are planning a pregnancy is recommended. The committee recommends a special emphasis on educating the public about the harmful effects of alcohol during pregnancy and identifying children with fetal alcohol exposure early for referral for educational services.

The American Academy of Pediatrics (AAP) and the American College of Obstetrics and Gynecology (ACOG) have active programs to prevent FASD. The AAP medical home program for patients with FASD initiative alerts pediatricians to inform parents about the risk of alcohol use during pregnancy and provides guidelines for routine screening for prenatal alcohol exposure.

ACOG has specific guidelines for preventative counseling and health education for obstetricians and gynecologists. The goal is to empower their members to improve screening and to provide brief intervention and referral to treatment for alcohol use disorders in pregnant women or those planning pregnancy to prevent FASD (Manriquez et al., 2019). This initiative advises members to participate in educational speakers bureaus and to provide educational material for maintenance of board certification in the specialty.

### Management

A comprehensive intervention program begins with parental recognition of the etiology of FASD. Parental counseling should include discussion of the physical and behavioral phenotype and treatment planning. The family should be advised about the need for special educational programs and assisted in behavior management. Family therapy is often required to help family members cope with their child's neurodevelopmental disorder. The impact of the disorder on the family has been poignantly described by Michael Doris (1989) in *The Broken Cord*, his book about raising an adopted son with FAS.

The approach to comprehensive treatment focuses on the individual child. It begins with assessment of cognitive, behavioral, and adaptive deficits in developing comprehensive treatment. In addition to family education and family-focused behavioral interventions, computerized attention training, impulse control management, and special education to address specific social skills development and learning deficits are essential (Coles et al., 2018). In special education, interventions for language disorder, literacy, and mathematics assistance are important (Coles et al., 2009; Petrenko & Alto, 2017).

The most common academic problem is in mathematics for both children and adults with fetal alcohol exposure. Math deficits may involve problems with information processing, visual motor impairments, and executive functioning deficits in planning and working memory. The Math Interactive Learning Experience program is designed to educate parents and teachers about FASD and provides individualized instruction. The program results in significant improvement in math and handwriting skills compared to control groups (Kully-Martens et al., 2018).

A major aspect of treatment is interventions for concurrent psychiatric, emotional, and behavioral problems (Mattson et al., 2019). It is important to assess for age-appropriate communication skills and socialization milestones. Most children with FASD have co-occurring internalizing and externalizing behavioral disorders, higher rates of school disruptions, and legal problems. Those diagnosed with FASD who respond to multimodal treatment interventions have better medical, psychological, and vocational outcomes. Intervention should begin early and continue long term, with modifications in the school environment, social support, parent management strategies, and educational interventions as required. Specialized parent training is needed because traditional parent training is not effective (Mukherjee, 2019).

## Management of Associated Conditions

Medication use for co-occurring conditions should address ADHD, cognitive inflexibility, mood and affect dysregulation, and seizure disorders. Symptomatic medication management must take into account the neurodevelopment features of FASD. For seizures, traditional anti-seizure medications—carbamazepine, oxcarbazepine, and valproic acid—are prescribed. For ADHD, more commonly the inattentive type, patients with FASD are typically treated with stimulants. However, the response to stimulants in FASD is variable compared to other etiologies of ADHD. Nevertheless, a consensus panel on treatment of comorbid ADHD concluded that stimulant medication can improve attention and decrease hyperactivity as part of a carefully developed treatment plan (Young et al., 2016). Although the side effects of stimulants may be similar to those in neurotypically developing children, the side effects in those with FASD can be worse because of their abnormal physiology. Although methylphenidate is the most commonly used medication, atomoxetine can also be effective. Guanfacine and clonidine may be used to address cognitive inflexibility, working memory deficits, and hyperactivity (Calles, 2008). Finally, integrated psychosocial care and medication use is essential. This may require referral to specialty services set up specifically for FASD cases. The Pediatric Medical Home Program provides coordination and continuity of care; it is parent and family focused and provides consistency of care across the life span (Turchi & Smith, 2018).

## Further Resources

Centers for Disease Control and Prevention: https://www.cdc.gov/ncbddd/fasd
FASD United: https://fasdunited.org/
National Institute on Alcohol Abuse and Alcoholism: https://www.niaaa.nih.gov
Substance Abuse and Mental Health Services Administration, FASD Center for Excellence: https://www.fasdcenter.samhsa.gov

## References

Abel, E. L. (1995). An update on incidence of FAS; FAS is not an equal opportunity birth defect. *Neurotoxicology and Teratology, 17,* 437–443.

American Psychiatric Association. (2013). *Diagnostic and statistical manual of mental disorders* (5th ed.) American Psychiatric Publishing.

Boronat, S., Sánchez-Montañez, A., Gómez-Barros, N., Jacas, C., Martinez-Ribot, L., Vazquez, E., & Del Campo, M. (2017). Correlation between morphological MRI findings and specific diagnostic categories in fetal alcohol spectrum disorders. *European Journal of Medical Genetics, 60,* 65–71.

Bower, E., Szajer, J., Mattson, S. N., Riley, E. P., & Murphy, C. (2013). Impaired odor identification in children with histories of heavy prenatal alcohol exposure. *Alcohol, 47,* 275–278.

British Medical Association Board of Science. (2016). *Fetal alcohol spectrum disorders, a guide for healthcare practitioners update.* British Medical Association.

Calles, J. L., Jr. (2008). Use of psychotropic medications in children with developmental disabilities. *Pediatric Clinics of North America, 55,* 1227–1240.

Charness, M. E., Riley, E. P., & Sowell, E. R. (2016). Drinking during pregnancy and the developing brain: Is any amount safe? *Trends in Cognitive Science, 20,* 80–82.

Charness, M. E., Simon, R. P., & Greenberg, D. A. (1989). Ethanol and the nervous system. *New England Journal of Medicine, 321,* 442–454.

Coles, C. D., Kable, J. A., & Taddeo, E. (2009). Math performance and behavior problems in children affected by prenatal alcohol exposure: Intervention and follow-up. *Journal of Developmental and Behavioral Pediatrics, 30,* 7–15.

Coles, C. D., Kable, J. A., Taddeo, E., & Strickland, D. (2018). GoFAR: Improving attention, behavior and adaptive functioning in children with fetal alcohol spectrum disorders: Brief report. *Developmental Neurorehabilitation, 21,* 345–349.

Day, N. L., Helsel, A., Sonon, K., & Goldschmidt, L. (2013). The association between prenatal alcohol exposure and behavior at 22 years of age. *Alcohol: Clinical and Experimental Research, 37,* 1171–1178.

Dodge, N. C., Jacobson, J. L., & Jacobson, S. W. (2014). Protective effects of the alcohol dehydrogenase-ADH1B* 3 allele on attention and behavior problems in adolescents exposed to alcohol during pregnancy. *Neurotoxicology and Teratology, 41,* 43–50.

Doney, R., Lucas, B. R., Jones, T., Howat, P., Sauer, K., & Elliott, E. J. (2014). Fine motor skills in children with prenatal alcohol exposure or fetal alcohol spectrum disorder. *Journal of Developmental and Behavioral Pediatrics, 35,* 598–609.

Doris, M. (1989). *The broken cord.* Harper & Row.

Dou, X., Menkari, C., Mitsuyama, R., Foroud, T., Wetherill, L., Hammond, P., Suttie, M., Chen, X., Chen, S., Charness, M., & Collaborative Initiative on Fetal Alcohol Spectrum Disorders. (2018). L1 coupling to ankyrin and the spectrin–actin cytoskeleton modulates ethanol inhibition of L1 adhesion and ethanol teratogenesis. *FASEB Journal, 32*, 1364–1374.

Eberhart, J. K., & Parnell, S. E. (2016). The genetics of fetal alcohol spectrum disorder. *Alcohol: Clinical and Experimental Research, 40*, 1154–1165.

Farber, N. B., Creeley, C. E., & Olney, J. W. (2010). Alcohol-induced neuroapoptosis in the fetal macaque brain. *Neurobiology of Disease, 40*(1), 200–206.

Goril, S., Zalai, D., Scott, L., & Shapiro, C.M. (2016). Sleep and melatonin secretion abnormalities in children and adolescents with fetal alcohol spectrum disorders. *Sleep Medicine, 23*, 59–64.

Green, P. P. (2016). Vital signs: Alcohol-exposed pregnancies—United States, 2011–2013. *MMWR Morbidity and Mortality Weekly Report, 65*, 91–97.

Greenmyer, J. R., Popova, S., Klug, M. G., & Burd, L. (2020). Fetal alcohol spectrum disorder: A systematic review of the cost of and savings from prevention in the United States and Canada. *Addiction, 115*(3), 409–417.

Guelinckx, I., Devlieger, R., & Vansant, G. (2011). Alcohol during pregnancy and lactation: Recommendations versus real intake. *Archives of Public Health, 68*, 134–142.

Hagan, J. F., Jr., Balachova, T., Bertrand, J., Chasnoff, I., Dang, E., Fernandez-Baca, D., Kable, J., Kosofsky, B., Senturias, Y., Singh, N., Sloane, M., Weitzman, C., Zubler, J., Neurobehavioral Disorder Associated with Prenatal Alcohol Exposure Workgroup, & American Academy of Pediatrics. (2016). Neurobehavioral disorder associated with prenatal alcohol exposure. *Pediatrics, 138*(4), e20151553.

Hanlon-Dearman, A., Chen, M. L., & Olson, H. C. (2018). Understanding and managing sleep disruption in children with fetal alcohol spectrum disorder. *Biochemistry and Cell Biology, 96*, 267–274.

Hoyme, H. E., Kalberg, W. O., Elliott, A. J., Blankenship, J., Buckley, D., Marais, A. S., Manning, M., Robinson, L., Adam, M., Abdul-Rahman, O., Jewett, T., Coles, C., Chambers, C., Jones, K., Adnams, C., Shah, P., Riley, E., Charness, M., Warren, K., & May, P. (2016). Updated clinical guidelines for diagnosing fetal alcohol spectrum disorders. *Pediatrics, 138*(2), e20154256.

Infante, M. A., Moore, E. M., Bischoff-Grethe, A., Tapert, S. F., Mattson, S. N., & Riley, E. P. (2017). Altered functional connectivity during spatial working memory in children with heavy prenatal alcohol exposure. *Alcohol, 64*, 11–21.

Jenssen, B. P., Walley, S. C., Boykan, R., et al; AAP Section on Nicotine and Tobacco Prevention and Treatment, Committee on Substance Use and Prevention. (2023). Protecting Children and Adolescents From Tobacco and Nicotine. *Pediatrics, 151*(5).

Johnson, S., Moyer, C. L., Klug, M. G., & Burd, L. (2018). Comparison of alcohol-related neurodevelopmental disorders and neurodevelopmental disorders associated with prenatal alcohol exposure diagnostic criteria. *Journal of Developmental and Behavioral Pediatrics, 39*, 163–167.

Jones, K., Smith, D., Ulleland, C., & Streissguth, A. (1973). Pattern of malformation in offspring of chronic alcoholic mothers. *Lancet, 301*, 1267–1271.

Keiver, K., Bertram, C. P., Orr, A. P., & Clarren, S. (2015). Salivary cortisol levels are elevated in the afternoon and at bedtime in children with prenatal alcohol exposure. *Alcohol, 49*, 79–87.

Kully-Martens, K., Pei, J., Kable, J., Coles, C. D., Andrew, G., & Rasmussen, C. (2018). Mathematics intervention for children with fetal alcohol spectrum disorder: A replication and extension of the Math Interactive Learning Experience (MILE) program. *Research in Developmental Disabilities, 78*, 55–65.

Lange, S., Probst, C., Gmel, G., Rehm, J., Burd, L., & Popova, S. (2017). Global prevalence of fetal alcohol spectrum disorder among children and youth: A systematic review and meta-analysis. *JAMA Pediatrics, 171*, 948–956.

Lange, S., Rovet, J., Rehm, J., & Popova, S. (2017). Neurodevelopmental profile of fetal alcohol spectrum disorder: A systematic review. *BMC Psychology, 5*, Article 22.

Lemoine, P., Harrousseau, H., Borteryu, J. P., & Menuet, J. C. (1968). Les enfants de parents alcohliques, *Quest Medicale, 21*, 476–482.

Lotfullina, N., & Khazipov, R. (2018). Ethanol and the developing brain: Inhibition of neuronal activity and neuroapoptosis. *The Neuroscientist*, *24*(2), 130–141.

Lucas, B. R., Latimer, J., Pinto, R. Z., Ferreira, M. L., Doney, R., Lau, M., Jones, T., Dries, D., & Elliott, E. J. (2014). Gross motor deficits in children prenatally exposed to alcohol: A meta-analysis. *Pediatrics*, *134*(1), e192–e209.

Lupton, C., Burd, L., & Harwood, R. (2004). Cost of fetal alcohol spectrum disorders. *American Journal of Medical Genetics Part C: Seminars in Medical Genetics*, *127*, 42–50.

Manriquez, M., Starer, J., Parisi, V., Tracy, E., McFadden, T., & Penney, L. (2019). Fetal alcohol spectrum disorder prevention program: SBIRT's role in averting fetal alcohol spectrum disorders. *Birth Defects Research*, *111*, 829–834.

Mattson, S. N., Bernes, G. A., & Doyle, L. R. (2019). Fetal alcohol spectrum disorders: A review of the neurobehavioral deficits associated with prenatal alcohol exposure. *Alcohol: Clinical and Experimental Research*, *43*, 1046–1062.

May, P. A., Blankenship, J., Marais, A. S., Gossage, J. P., Kalberg, W. O., Barnard, R., De Vries, M., Robinson, L., Adnams, C., Buckley, D., Manning, M., Jones, K., Parry, C., Hoyme, H., & Seedat, S. (2013). Approaching the prevalence of the full spectrum of fetal alcohol spectrum disorders in a South African population-based study. *Alcohol: Clinical and Experimental Research*, *37*(5), 818–830.

May, P. A., Chambers, C. D., Kalberg, W. O., Zellner, J., Feldman, H., Buckley, D., & Taras, H. (2018). Prevalence of fetal alcohol spectrum disorders in 4 US communities. *JAMA*, *319*, 474–482.

McLennan, J. D. (2015). Misattributions and potential consequences: The case of child mental health problems and fetal alcohol spectrum disorders. *Canadian Journal of Psychiatry*, *60*, 587–590.

Mela, M., Coons-Harding, K. D., & Anderson, T. (2019). Recent advances in fetal alcohol spectrum disorder for mental health professionals. *Current Opinion in Psychiatry*, *32*, 328–335.

Mukherjee, R. A. (2019). Diagnosis and management of fetal alcohol spectrum disorder. *Current Opinion in Psychiatry*, *32*, 92–96.

O'Leary, C., Leonard, H., Bourke, J., D'Antoine, H., Bartu, A., & Bower, C. (2013). Intellectual disability: Population-based estimates of the proportion attributable to maternal alcohol use disorder during pregnancy. *Developmental Medicine and Child Neurology*, *55*, 271–277.

Parnell, S. E., Riley, E. P., Warren, K. R., Mitchell, K. T., & Charnesse, M. E. (2018). The contributions of Dr. Kathleen K. Sulik to fetal alcohol spectrum disorders research and prevention. *Alcohol*, *69*, 15–24.

Pearl, P. L., Taylor, J. L., Trzcinski, S., & Sokohl, A. (2007). The pediatric neurotransmitter disorders. *Journal of Child Neurology*, *22*(5), 606–616.

Petrenko, C. L., & Alto, M. E. (2017). Interventions in fetal alcohol spectrum disorders: An international perspective. *European Journal of Medical Genetics*, *60*, 79–91.

Popova, S., Lange, S., Burd, L., & Rehm, J. (2015). The economic burden of fetal alcohol spectrum disorder in Canada in 2013. *Alcohol and Alcoholism*, *51*, 367–375.

Popova, S., Lange, S., Shield, K., Mihic, A., Chudley, A., Mukherjee, R., Bekmuradov, D., & Rehm, J. (2016). Comorbidity of fetal alcohol spectrum disorder: A systematic review and meta-analysis. *Lancet*, *387*, 978–987.

Popova, S., Stade, B., Bekmuradov, D., Lange, S., & Rehm, J. (2011). What do we know about the economic impact of fetal alcohol spectrum disorder? A systematic literature review. *Alcohol and Alcoholism*, *46*, 490–497.

Reynolds, J. N., Weinberg, J., Clarren, S., Beaulieu, C., Rasmussen, C., Kobor, M., Dube, M., & Goldowitz, D. (2011). Fetal alcohol spectrum disorders: Gene–environment interactions, predictive biomarkers, and the relationship between structural alterations in the brain and functional outcomes. *Seminars in Pediatric Neurology*, *18*, 49–55.

Streissguth, A. P., & Dehaene, P. (1993). Fetal alcohol syndrome in twins of alcoholic mother: Concordance of diagnosis and IQ. *American Journal of Genetics*, *47*, 857–861.

Strömland, K., & Pinazo-Durán, M. D. (2002). Ophthalmic involvement in the fetal alcohol syndrome: Clinical and animal model studies. *Alcohol and Alcoholism*, *37*, 2–8.

Suttie, M., Foroud, T., Wetherill, L., Jacobson, J. L., Molteno, C. D., Meintjes, E. M., Hoyme, H., Khaole, N., Robinson, L., Riley, E., Jacobson, S. W., & Hammond, P. (2013). Facial dysmorphism across the fetal alcohol spectrum. *Pediatrics, 131*(3), e779–e788.

Turchi, R. M., & Smith, V. C. (2018). The role of integrated care in a medical home for patients with a fetal alcohol spectrum disorder. *Pediatrics, 142*(4), e20182333.

Warren, K. R., & Foudin, L. L. (2001). Alcohol-related birth defects: The past, present, and future. *Alcohol Research & Health, 25*, 153–158.

Weyrauch, D., Schwartz, M., Hart, B., Klug, M. G., & Burd, L. (2017). Comorbid mental disorders in fetal alcohol spectrum disorders: A systematic review. *Journal of Developmental and Behavioral Pediatrics, 38*, 283–291.

Williams, J. F., Smith, V. C., & Committee on Substand Abuse. (2015). Fetal alcohol spectrum disorders. *Pediatrics, 136*(5), e1395–1406.

Woods, K. J., Meintjes, E. M., Molteno, C. D., Jacobson, S. W., & Jacobson, J. L. (2015). Parietal dysfunction during number processing in children with fetal alcohol spectrum disorders. *NeuroImage: Clinical, 8*, 594–605.

Wozniak, J. R., Riley, E. P., & Charness, M. E. (2019). Clinical presentation, diagnosis, and management of fetal alcohol spectrum disorder. *Lancet Neurology, 8*, 760–770.

Young, S., Absoud, M., Blackburn, C., Branney, P., Colley, B., Farrag, E., Fleisher, S., Gregory, G., Gudjonsson, G., Kim, K., O'Malley, K. D., Plant, M., Rodriguez, A., Ozer, S., Takon, I., Woodhouse, E., & Mukherjee, R. (2016). Guidelines for identification and treatment of individuals with attention deficit/hyperactivity disorder and associated fetal alcohol spectrum disorders based upon expert consensus. *BMC Psychiatry, 16*, Article 324.

# 19

# Challenging Behavior

## Aggression and Self-Injury

*Challenging behavior* is a term that collectively refers to self-injury, temper outbursts, and aggressive/destructive behavior. These problem behaviors are a major feature in developmental neuropsychiatric disorders, particularly in severe intellectual developmental disorder (IDD) and autism spectrum disorder (ASD) (Folch et al., 2018; Steenfeldt-Kristensen et al., 2020). Aggression toward others and self-injurious behavior (SIB) are of particular concern for psychiatrists and other health professionals because of their severity, frequency, and resistance to treatment. Aggression/destructive behavior and self-injury have adverse effects on family life and can result in failure of community placement for children and adolescents with neurodevelopmental disorders. Evidence-based behavioral psychological and pharmacological interventions are required along with staff training to implement these treatments. This chapter reviews the epidemiology, classification, differential diagnosis, assessment, predisposing factors, etiologic models, treatment, and medicolegal issues of challenging behavior.

## Epidemiology

Challenging behaviors occur frequently in people with IDD, ASD, and traumatic brain injury. Prevalence rates vary from 5% to 15% in educational, health, and social care services (Dekker et al., 2002). A meta-analysis of total population prevalence of challenging behaviors in individuals with IDD in the United Kingdom found that the lowest functioning had potentially life-threatening problem behaviors, particularly severe self-injury (Emerson et al., 2001). Rates are higher in teenagers and individuals in their 20s, and they are higher in institutional compared to home settings. Those with co-occurring communication problems, sensory impairment, and co-occurring psychiatric disorders are more likely to exhibit severe challenging behaviors. There is increased risk when exposed to crowded, unpredictable environments and in settings in which physical health needs and pain are not recognized or managed properly. Challenging behaviors may be used by the subject to increase sensory stimulation, seek help, or avoid demands (escape behaviors).

Comprehensive population surveys in people with IDD have been conducted in Wales and England. In Wales, 1.2 million individuals receiving IDD services were screened, with interviews conducted with the primary caregivers. The survey identified 4.5/10,000 people with severe challenging behaviors, comprising 10% of the IDD population; disruptive behaviors were the most common form. Moreover, a substantial number had less severe behavior disorders (Lowe et al., 2007). In England, a total population study was carried out in two areas of the country to ascertain rates of challenging behaviors. Like Wales, 10–15% of those with IDD had severe challenging behaviors. Among them, 7% were aggressive, 5% had destructive behaviors, and 4% exhibited self-injury. The majority showed two or more forms of challenging behaviors and two-thirds were male. Nearly half lived at home with their families. Most of those with severe behavior disorders were in the severe range of IDD. In both studies, challenging behaviors were major stressors for families. Those with challenging behaviors were at greater risk of neglect or abuse (Emerson et al., 2001). Treatment of aggressive behaviors is of particular importance because they may lead to reduced services and more restrictive programming (Benson & Brooks, 2008).

Aggressive behaviors are major factors in community placement and create major issues in management. In one study involving more than 3,000 adult men and women receiving services for IDD, the prevalence of aggressive behavior assessed with the Modified Overt Aggression Scale was 52%. Property damage had been caused by 38% of study participants, 24% had SIB, and 10% were sexually aggressive. However, almost all aggressive acts were rated as mild, with verbal aggression being the most common. Nevertheless, in 5%, aggression led to injury of the victim. Physical aggression was most common in those with severe to profound IDD (Crocker et al., 2006).

## Classification

Population-based studies used to access challenging behaviors include the Challenging Behavior Survey (Alborz et al., 1994), Aberrant Behavior Checklist Second Edition (Aman et al., 1985), Behavior Problem Inventory (Lundqvist, 2013), and Behavior Problem Inventory–Short Form (Rojahn et al., 2012a, 2012b). In addition, there is the Criteria for Determining Severe Problem Behavior (CDSPB) rating scale used in Japan that includes elements of the other scales (Inoue, 2019). The CDSPB scale addresses challenging behaviors that are directly harmful (self-biting and head banging) and indirectly harmful (sleep disorders and their behavioral consequences). It covers 11 domains: severe self-injury with or without self-mutilation, severe aggression that injures others (biting, kicking, punching, and hair pulling), stereotyped/restricted behaviors (behaviors that do not respond to intervention), noncompliance, severe property destruction (breaking furniture, punching doors, and tearing one's clothes), sleep disorder that is associated with daytime aggression, severe feeding problems (regurgitation of food and pica), severe problems in elimination (smearing or throwing feces), extreme hyperactivity leading to danger to self or life, unbearable screaming and crying lasting for hours, sustained panic (cannot be calmed), and explosive tantrums linked to trivial environmental change. Behaviors involving food, excretion, sleep patterns, and hyperactivity in the first 3 years of life predict more serious SIB and aggression in later years. As a consequence, early interventions for these behaviors are important.

The term challenging behavior has been introduced into psychiatric classification through the World Health Organization's (WHO) *International Classification of Functioning, Disability, and Health* (ICF; WHO, 2001, 2007). The ICF, unlike the *International Classification of Disease*, addresses how the subject functions in an everyday environment. The youth version, ICF-CY, is used in assessment of children and adolescents. Challenging behaviors, like psychiatric diagnoses, impact social engagement at home, in school, and in community activities. The ICF approach emphasizes not only personal factors but also how social and environmental factors result in problem behaviors in individuals with an IDD.

In the 11th edition of the *International Statistical Classification of Diseases and Related Health Problems* (ICD-11; WHO, 2019), other challenging behaviors are listed under "Symptoms, Signs, or Clinical Findings, Not Elsewhere Classified" and are classified under the MB23 category Symptoms or Signs Involving Appearance and Behavior. Aggressive behavior (MB23.0), disruptive behavior (MB23.8), psychomotor agitation (MS23.M), suicide attempt (MB23.R), suicidal behavior (MS23.S), and other challenging behaviors are coded in this section of ICD-11.

In the fifth edition of the *Diagnostic and Statistical Manual of Mental Disorders* (DSM-5; American Psychiatric Association [APA], 2013), because of its severity, self-injurious behavior is included under the category stereotypical movement disorder with or without self-injury. Diagnostic criteria include repetitive, seemingly driven, and apparently purposeless motor behavior that interferes with social, academic, or other activities and that may lead to self-injury with onset in the developmental period. The behavior is not attributable to the physiological effects of substance abuse or not better explained by another developmental disorder. Among these are hair-pulling disorders (trichotillomania) and obsessive–compulsive disorders with excoriation of skin. Specifiers for stereotypic movement disorder in DSM-5 are with and without self-injurious behavior and association with a known medical or genetic disorder—for example, fetal alcohol syndrome, Lesch–Nyhan syndrome, and other genetic syndromes in which self-injury is a feature. The most common topographies for SIB are head banging and eye gouging. Other challenging behaviors involving self-injury are classified under obsessive–compulsive and related disorders in DSM-5. These are trichotillomania (hair pulling) and excoriation (skin picking) disorder. Other challenging behaviors, such as aggression, are not specifically coded as distinct disorders in DSM-5. Thus, stereotypic movement disorder with self-injurious behavior, trichotillomania (hair pulling), and excoriation (skin picking) disorders are the only challenging behavior categories in DSM-5.

## Differential Diagnosis

The differential diagnosis for stereotypical movement disorder with and without self-injury includes simple stereotypical movements common in infancy and early childhood. ASD, where SIB may be a feature, Tourette syndrome and other tic disorders, obsessive–compulsion and related disorders, and other neurological and medical conditions are among the differential diagnoses. Thus, SIB can be seen as associated features in various disorders. In these disorders, the diagnosis of SIB should not be made unless the self-injury leads to a substantial dysfunction and becomes the focus of treatment. When SIB is diagnosed, any co-occurring mental disorder should be diagnosed as well. Typical types of self-stimulatory behaviors in young children, such as thumb sucking, rocking, and mild head banging, are usually self-limiting and rarely result in tissue damage requiring treatment. Self-stimulatory behaviors associated with blindness in persons not otherwise disabled (so-called blindisms, such as head rocking from side to side or light gazing) usually do not result in dysfunction or in self-injury. Behaviors seen in tic disorder are usually involuntary, nonrhythmic, rapid, exhibited in shorter bursts, and described by the individual as irresistible. Ordinarily, these do not result in self-injury. However, self-injury can be a feature of Tourette syndrome. Factitious disorders are intentional and motivated by the psychological need to assume a sick role and involve deliberate self-harm. In obsessive–compulsive disorders and related disorders, the person feels driven to perform the act in question (which usually is more complex and ritualistic) to prevent or reduce distress; examples are trichotillomania and excoriation disorder. SIB is also associated with some behaviors, such as repetitive hand washing. In people with IDD, obsessions may not be elicited but compulsions may be identified. In Tourette syndrome, these behaviors have been referred to as impulsions rather than compulsions.

In trichotillomania, by definition, the topography of self-injury is limited to hair pulling. The essential feature of trichotillomania is recurrent pulling out of hair resulting in hair loss and failed efforts to voluntarily decrease or stop hair pulling. These hair-pulling cases cause clinically significant distress or impairment in social, occupational, or other areas of functioning. Trichotillomania is not the result of another mental disorder—for example, behavior to change a perceived defect in one's appearance as in body dysmorphic disorder. Hair pulling may occur in any region of the body wherever hair grows—most commonly the scalp, eyebrows, and eyelids. Trichotillomania may occur in brief episodes during the day but also may continue for hours. Efforts may be made to camouflage hair loss (wigs and wearing of scarfs). Distressful symptoms include loss of self-control, shame, and embarrassment. It may be triggered by boredom or anxiety and followed by a sense of relief. Prevalence is 1% or 2% in adolescents and adults, with a female:male ratio of 10:1. Hair pulling commonly has its onset at puberty.

The most essential feature of excoriation (skin picking) disorder is recurrent picking at one's own skin despite repeated attempts to stop. Skin picking leads to significant distress or impairment in social, occupational, or community areas of functioning. Substance abuse or other clinical conditions, such as scabies, are medical causes of skin picking, whereas skin-picking disorder is not better explained by a medical condition or another mental disorder. The most common area picked is the fingernails; however, the face, arms, and hands are picked, including both healthy skin and skin lesions such as pimples.

Self-mutilation (deliberate self-harm) associated with certain psychotic and personality disorders is premeditated, voluntary, intentional, sporadic, and has a meaning for the individual within the context of the underlying severe mental disorder (e.g., it is the result of delusional thinking). Involuntary movements associated with neurological disorders usually follow a typical pattern, and the signs and symptoms of the neurological disorder are present and self-injury usually does not occur.

Stereotypic movement disorder associated with self-injurious behavior needs to be considered phenomenologically as potentially distinct and distinguishable according to its association with other diagnoses. The phenomenology varies considerably among IDD syndromes. For Lesch–Nyhan syndrome, self-biting and self-mutilation of lips and fingers are characteristic, whereas excoriation (skin picking) is associated with Prader–Willi syndrome. The topography (focus and location) of the self-injurious behaviors may be extremely varied from person to person and from one point in time to another in the same person. In some persons with SIB, self-restraining behaviors can be seen, such as holding hands inside shirts or in pockets. When this is prevented, the SIB recurs; this behavior provides evidence for the intention to prevent self-injury.

The psychiatric disorder in children and adolescents that is most associated with SIB is ASD. Stereotypic movements in ASD are, for the most part, distinctive and include echolalia, hand flapping, flipping objects, and lining up objects. Inflexible adherence to routines is common. These rituals, along with deficits in social emotional reciprocity and problems with affect regulation, increase their vulnerability to self-injurious behavior. Children with ASD are approximately six times more likely to self-injure than those with Down syndrome (Richards et al., 2012). In a comparative study, half of the children with an ASD diagnosis self-injured compared to 18% with Down syndrome. Rates of self-injury similar to ASD were found in fragile X syndrome. Among those with ASD, SIB was greatest in those with higher levels of impulsivity and hyperactivity, negative affect, and lower cognitive functioning. Significant impairments in adaptive behavior, communicative language, and social engagement may be present in those with SIB. SIB also occurs in association with psychotic disorders in which self-mutilation is often linked to somatic delusions.

In addition to association with affective disorder and psychosis, SIB is associated with disruptive behavior disorders such as oppositional defiant disorder and conduct disorder. DSM-5 specifiers most often associated with self-injury are Lesch–Nyhan syndrome; Cornelia de Lange syndrome; congenital insensitivity to pain; fragile X syndrome; Rett's syndrome; Tourette disorder; and specific diagnostic etiologies of blindness, such as retrolental fibroplasia. With regard to the consequences of self-injury, chronic tissue damage is present, depending on the topography of the SIB. These may include cuts, scratches, skin infection, bruises, alopecia areata, bite marks, rectal fissures, foreign bodies in bodily orifices and in the gastrointestinal tract, retinal detachment, and abdominal distension (from aerophagia).

## Natural History

There is no typical age or pattern of onset of SIB. The onset may follow a stressful event in a vulnerable person. In nonverbal persons with an IDD, it may be triggered by a painful physical condition, such as middle ear infection in young children. The self-injurious behaviors often peak in adolescence and then gradually decline, but they can also persist for years, especially in persons with severe/profound IDD, ASD, and genetic syndromes with self-injury (Arron et al., 2011). The topography of these behaviors often changes; for example, a person engages in hand biting that may then subside and then head hitting emerges. An individual engaging in a stereotypic behavior usually does not cause in major self-injury (e.g., light head banging and skin picking). However, a stereotypic behavior may progress in its intensity to the point that major self-injury occurs.

The most serious complication is tissue damage. In less severe cases, a chronic skin irritation or calluses from biting, pinching, scratching, or saliva smearing may be present. The more serious complications include blindness (due to retinal detachment following eye gouging or hitting), intestinal obstruction (from pica—swallowing of solid objects), infections, and even death. If these behaviors are extreme and objectionable, there may be psychosocial complications leading to the individual's exclusion from school and community activities. The behavior leads to considerable stress on parents and other family members.

## Predisposing Factors

Various factors have been hypothesized to underlie SIB. Environmental, psychosocial, and biological theories of causation have been proposed (see the section titled "Etiologic Models of Self-Injury"). Mechanisms that have been implicated include dopaminergic receptor supersensitivity, maintenance of physiological homeostasis through reduction of the level of arousal by self-injury, reduction of dysphoria through release of endogenous opioids, escape/avoidance (from aversive situations), and self-stimulation. SIBs do not represent a single homogeneous disorder but, rather, are heterogeneous. Several factors might be involved in their pathogenesis. For instance, a person exhibiting SIB, which was initiated by one mechanism, may learn that SIB results in increased attention from the caregivers. This learned experience might become the factor maintaining the self-injury, especially in nonstimulating institutional environments, in which it is more common. IDD is probably the most important predisposing factor, the risk being higher the more severe the cognitive deficit, especially if it is associated with severe sensory deficits (blindness and deafness), ASD, or lack of response to painful physical illness in a nonverbal person.

## Etiologic Models of Self-Injury

### Isolation Rearing

Nonhuman primates show considerable self-directed behavior, such as scratching and self-grooming, when raised in isolation. Self-directed behavior is typically seen in animals that experience privation or deprivation early in life, especially rearing apart (the deprivation syndrome). Self-directed behaviors include (a) self-clasping—using hands or feet to grasp legs, arms, chest, or head; (b) self-orality involving digit sucking; (c) self-aggression consisting of biting, slapping, or hitting body parts; (d) rocking/swaying back and forth; and (e) saluting, which involves raising a hand to the ipsilateral eye like a salute, occasionally with thumb pressure against the eyeball. These behaviors may be seen in combination, such as self-clasp along with rocking. These behaviors have been noted (a) with fear or frustration, (b) when activities are thwarted or escape is prevented, (c) with apparent environmental dissatisfaction, and (d) when an animal cannot successfully adapt to a new situation. Isolation results in limitations of motor activity, lack of parent and peer contact, impaired learning of social skills, and altered affective state.

These forms of self-stimulation and self-mutilation may be sequelae of isolation during sensitive developmental periods. Animals that received restricted rearing experience were compared with a control group of feral and group-reared animals. At age 5 years, the restriction-reared monkeys showed four times more self-aggression than social aggression; the control monkeys were never observed to be self-aggressive (Anderson & Chamove, 1980). Self-biting occurred in social contexts, such as displacement by a more dominant monkey during social aggression and when startled by sudden movement of others. Self-biting was noted at less than 3 months, frequently in the context of digit sucking. Self-aggression in individually housed, wild-born, stump-tailed macaques has been reported to show decreased in frequency with social pairings (Goosen & Ribbens, 1980). These behaviors are reported in animals raised in captivity as opposed to feral animals transferred to a zoo. These behaviors have been noted in such diverse species as opossums, jackals, hyenas, marmosets, squirrel monkeys, and long-tail monkeys (Meyer-Holzapfel, 1968).

Substantial research has been conducted with rhesus macaques. Rhesus monkeys engage in self-injury approximately 14–25% of the time in captive settings, typically self-biting (Lutz et al., 2003). Self-injury in nonhuman primates is correlated with parental neglect and limitations in social interaction among them (Lutz et al., 2003; Rommeck et al., 2009). Early maternal separation leads to brain abnormality and dysregulation of the serotonin system (Huggins et al., 2012) and hypothalamic–pituitary axis dysfunction (Feng et al., 2011; Shannon et al., 1998). The effects of isolated rearing on self-stimulation and self-injury in humans are reported in children reared in severely deprived and isolated situations in institutionalized settings (Nelson et al., 2014).

The factors related to the development of self-injury after isolation are found more often in the early developmental periods. For example, in one study, two groups of animals were reared under conditions that were identical with respect to physical restriction but differed in terms of the amount of visual stimuli—that is, one group was housed outside and in view of other animals and activities. The visually isolated animals demonstrated greater stereotyped behavior (Mason, 1991). Mason provides two suggestions for the effects of developmental isolation on behavior: (a) the filial response of contact-seeking behavior with the mother to establish attachment, which reduces arousal; and (b) exploratory behavior through social and motor play to increase stimulation or arousal. He suggests that behavior such as a rocking stereotypy may be a self-provision of passive movement stimulation ordinarily received from the parent. Thus, he notes that infant monkeys raised with a mobile surrogate do not show rocking, whereas those raised with a stationary surrogate do rock, indicating the importance of movement stimulation.

The most severe forms of self-injury occur in animals that are the most agitated; self-injury may lead to reduced agitation. This could be a homeostatic mechanism elicited in severely socially deprived environments. Another means of reducing arousal is autogrooming or allogrooming. All grooming between animals leads to reduced arousal. Because an isolated animal has no companion, it may groom itself, resulting in stereotypies and perhaps self-injury. Thus, SIB may be a maladaptive self-soothing strategy. Self-injury may be preceded by autogrooming (Goosen & Ribbens, 1980). SIB also occurs when fighting behavior is prevented. Stereotypy and self-injury might reduce other more aversive stimulation or indicate loss of control in a new and novel situation.

Early experiences can result in behavioral sensitization and predispose for recurrence when there is exposure to a situation analogous to the original one. Children have similar responses, beginning with stereotypies, which may extend to self-injury. The arousal-increasing and arousal-decreasing hypotheses are important, although the evidence for them may be subject to a variety of interpretations. In one study (Wood et al., 2022), 34 of 49 neglected monkeys did not self-injure, suggesting that factors in addition to early neglect are involved, such as peer rejection. Additional research on rearing in social isolation and on early infant stimulation and attachment is needed to better understand the biological factors involved in self-injury. These studies should include the examination of serotonin genotype variation as a genetic risk factor in SIB (Wood et al., 2022).

## The 6-Hydroxydopamine Model

The role of the dopamine system in SIB has been studied by administering the neurotoxin 6-hydroxydopamine (6-OHDA) to neonatal rats during the developmental period, followed by subsequent pharmacological challenge. 6-HODA is selectively accumulated in dopaminergic neurons, where it causes severe oxidative damage, resulting in their selective degeneration. Using this approach, a relationship between dopamine receptor denervation-induced supersensitivity and self-injury has been demonstrated in experimental animals (Breese et al., 1984). Rats were given injections of 6-OHDA at 5 days of age to denervate basal ganglia brain regions of their dopaminergic input, resulting in supersensitive dopamine receptors. Severe self-biting was seen in the lesioned animals when they were challenged as adults with a dopamine agonist (L-dopa or apomorphine); however, untreated adult rats did not show this behavior after being administered dopamine receptor agonists.

Administration of 6-OHDA to immature rats leads to changes in chemoarchitecture of the brains of the 6-OHDA-treated rats in adulthood. The density of D2 receptors is increased or unchanged, whereas that of D1 dopamine receptors is decreased or unchanged in these animals. When a D1 dopamine agonist, SKF 38393, or L-dopa was administered to the 6-OHDA-treated rats, the animals self-injured, in keeping with the sensitization model. The self-injury was blocked by a D1 antagonist, SCH23390, but not by a D2 dopamine antagonist. Overall increased sensitivity of signaling in D1 dopamine receptors is essential for producing SIB in rats lesioned by 6-OHDA in the neonatal period. The lesioned rats also show an increase in striatal serotonin, met-encephalon, substance P, and reduced binding to the μ-opioid receptor. D1 receptor antagonism by olanzapine blocked self-injury in a study of humans who self-injure (Janowsky et al., 2003). Although olanzapine also blocks other dopamine and serotonin receptors, its D1 antagonist action is presumed to account for its effects. Olanzapine also reduces self-injury in neonatal rat models (Moy et al., 2001).

Studies in monkeys that self-injure were carried out by M. Goldstein et al. (1985) to investigate the striatal dopamine regulation of motor activity. Goldstein et al. studied the effects of dopamine agonists on monkeys that for 10–14 years had unilateral denervated nigrostriatal systems. L-Dopa and apomorphine, dopamine agonists, elicited self-biting of the digits of the fingers of the monkeys contralateral to the lesion. This effect was blocked by a D1 dopamine receptor antagonist (SCH 23390) and by fluphenazine, a

D1/D2 antagonist, but it was not blocked by a pure D2 dopamine receptor antagonist. The self-injury was elicited by dopamine receptor agonists, whose effects are predominantly on the D1 receptor, and was blocked by a D1 antagonist, consistent with the D1 dopamine treatment for the self-injury. Ungerstedt (1971) also reported SIB in rats after lesioning the nigrostriatal dopaminergic projection with 6-HODA. The emphasis in all these studies is on injury using developmental models with earlier sensitization and later self-injury. These studies are of considerable importance in animal modeling of self-injury.

## Pemoline Model of Self-Injurious Behavior

Pemoline is a psychostimulant that leads to SIB when chronically administered to rats. Its use leads to behavioral symptoms that are like SIB in humans. Rats given pemoline target specific body areas to SIB, repeatedly injuring them in a stereotypical manner. Moreover, this self-injury is increased if the animals are raised in impoverished environments (Devine, 2019). Pemoline is a long-acting indirect monoamine neurotransmitter agonist. It blocks the reuptake of dopamine, serotonin, and norepinephrine. SIB can be induced by giving a 300 mg/kg dose, which becomes apparent with 48 hr, or following chronic daily treatment with 4–12 doses per day (Devine, 2012). Pemoline causes a 30% depletion in striatal dopamine (Muehlmann & Devine, 2008), thus impairing dopaminergic neurotransmission. Pemoline-induced SIB is blocked by the $N$-methyl-D-aspartate subtype of glutamate receptor antagonist, MK-801 (Muehlmann & Devine, 2008). The suppression of SIB by MK-801 indicates a role for glutamatergic neurotransmission. Finally, SIB caused by pemoline can be modified by manipulations (Devine, 2012). Rats raised in impoverished settings had substantially more tissue injury than those raised in an enriched environment.

## Bay K 8644 Model

Bay K 8644, a calcium channel agonist, causes dystonia and SIB in mice when given soon after weaning (Jinnah et al., 1999). The calcium channel antagonist nifedipine and similar drugs that block dihydropyridine-type calcium channels are caused by the administration of Bay K 8644. The SIB is exacerbated by administering the dopamine indirect agonist amphetamine (Kasim & Jinnah, 2003) and the serotonin uptake inhibitor fluoxetine (Kasim et al., 2002), indicating involvement by the dopaminergic and serotoninergic systems. SIB was also attenuated by co-administration of SCH-23390, the dopamine D1 receptor antagonist that also prevents SIB in the 6-OHDA model in rats. Similarly, D2 dopamine receptor antagonists were ineffective. Moreover, Bay K 8644 worsened self-injury in dopamine D1 receptor null mutant mice that were physically immature (Kasim et al., 2006). Overall, like the 6-OHDA model, the Bay K 8644 model implicates the dopamine and serotonin systems, with behavioral effects medicated by the D1 dopamine receptor.

## Neuromaturational Processes in Development

Neuromaturational and neuroanatomical changes may also be important in the occurrence of stereotypies and SIB. The onset of self-biting during a particular stage of development suggests a relationship to neuromaturational changes. Different regions of the frontal lobe in a rodent are responsible for sucking and chewing (Iriki et al., 1988). Chewing is a developmental acquisition requiring synaptic reorganization that ordinarily takes place around the time teeth erupt. The transition from finger sucking to biting may be a consequence of the maturational acquisition and exercise of chewing. Stimulation of the vestibular system by rocking, spinning, or other forms of body movement has been shown to influence motor development of normal and developmentally delayed children and is a factor in children with abnormalities in this brain region (Clark et al., 1977). From these studies, stereotypy and self-injury might be a way for a person with IDD to provide neurologically based self-stimulation. This stimulation may not only be reinforcing but also necessary for neuronal development.

## Opioid and Non-Opioid Stress-Induced Analgesia

Stress-induced analgesia is an endogenous pain suppression response that takes place during or following exposure to stressful or fearful stimuli and is modified by context. Soldiers in World War II experiencing battle wounds reported little pain, whereas similar injury in a nonthreatening setting was highly painful (Beecher, 1946). These observations led to the understanding that pain is heavily influenced by context (Ford & Finn, 2008). Neurobiologic models of stress-induced analgesia have been studied in both animals and humans. Neurobiologic substrates are important in mediating and modulating endogenous analgesia through the descending inhibitory pain pathway, which is involved in both stress-induced analgesia and regulation of nociceptive signaling of emotionality (Stein, 2016). Recent studies of stress-induced analgesia primarily concern conditional analgesia and distraction-induced analgesia, where key roles for endogenous opioid, monoamines, cannabinoid, γ-aminobutyric acid, and glutamate systems have been identified.

Stress-induced analgesia is an adaptive innate response—essentially a defense response—to immediate danger and an aspect to the flight-or-fight response. Stress-induced anesthesia follows robust and acute stressful stimulation. There is substantial overlap in neural pathways involved in both pain and stress. The endogenous opioid system is a key regulator of the descending pain pathway, with opioid receptors located on astrocytes, microglia, immune cells, and neurons in peripheral tissues (Salemi et al., 2005). Opioid receptors and opioid peptides are found in supraspinal, spinal, and peripheral sites, with key roles in regulating nociceptive signaling and the stress response (Ferdousi & Finn, 2018).

The identification of endogenous opioid peptides with functions similar to morphine opened new avenues for research on pain and pain-related behavior (Snyder, 1977). Three genetically distinct families of opioid peptides have been identified in the central nervous system: endorphin/corticotrophins, enkephalins, and dynorphin/neoendorphins. The localization of their receptors indicates that these peptides play an important role in the control of pain. Increases in opioid peptide production and inhibition in pain responsiveness accompany acutely stressful states, leading to insensitivity to pain—so-called stress-induced analgesia (SIA)—in animals (Butler & Finn, 2009) and humans (Ferdousi & Finn, 2018). These effects are partially reversible with naloxone, an opiate receptor antagonist whose administration has been associated with an increase in threshold for pain (Buchsbaum et al., 1977). The administration of an enkephalinase inhibitor against the enkephalin catabolic enzyme enkephalinase has been shown to potentiate stress-induced analgesia, which is blocked by naloxone. Sensitivity to SIA is influenced by age, gender, and prior experience to stressful stimuli (Butler & Finn, 2009).

The discovery of the opiate receptors also led to investigations into opiate self-administration. Opiate receptors ($\delta$, $\kappa$, and $\mu$) are densely distributed in brain regions associated with SIB in animals, and opiates have been shown to have reinforcing properties for self-stimulation (Ferdousi & Finn, 2018). Animal studies with rhesus monkeys and rats have demonstrated that microinfusions of opioids (methionine enkephalin and morphine) into the ventral tegmentum, substantia nigra, or nucleus accumbens facilitate self-stimulation in a dose-related manner. Animals will bar-press for the delivery of enkephalin, demonstrating its reinforcing properties. The mechanism of inhibition of nociception (experience of pain) involves the activation of receptor subtypes coupled to different intracellular signaling (Millan, 2002). Neurotransmitters that inhibit nociception are endogenous opioids, endocannabinoids, $\gamma$-aminobutyric acid (GABA), glycine, vasopressin, oxytocin, and adenosine. When either naltrexone or naloxone (both opiate receptor antagonists) is administered, the SIA is blocked. Moreover, naloxone increases the aversive response in rats that are exposed to electric shock pain. Systemic or central administration of antagonists for all three opiate receptors attenuates stress-induced analgesia in rats, whereas an enkephalinase inhibitor potentiated the peak effect and duration of stress-induced anesthesia in rats in a naloxone-reversible manner (Butler & Finn, 2009). The antinociceptive effect of opiate receptor activation also may be linked to release of the inhibitory neurotransmitter GABA (Christie et al., 2000).

These findings regarding the opiate system have led to several hypotheses with regard to SIB. First, repeated occurrence of SIB could lead to opioid-mediated stress-induced analgesia that is associated with elevated levels of endogenous opioid peptides which inhibit pain. Second, it is possible that some individuals might engage in SIB as a means of self-administering opioid peptides. These hypotheses have been tested indirectly by administering naloxone or naltrexone in a series of case reports. The authors concluded that the opiate receptor antagonist effects are due to either (a) reducing the pain threshold, therefore intensifying the normally painful effects of SIB, or (b) extinguishing the reinforcing effects of SIB (Christie et al., 2000).

Conflicting results have been reported in studies conducted during the past three decades regarding the effects of opiate receptor antagonists on SIB, including case reports, small case series, and small case–control studies. Trials have been conducted primarily in adults, although there are also studies specific to children. One study involved six male patients, aged 15–31 years, who had IDD and SIB. Naltrexone was administered 50 mg/day (0.6–1.5 mg/kg) for 3 weeks. There was a significant reduction in the severity of SIB in two patients and a trend toward improvement in a third case

(Kars et al., 1990). In a larger double-blind controlled crossover study, naltrexone at 50 mg/day was given to 33 adults with IDD and SIB (Willemsen-Swinkels et al., 1995). On the Aberrant Behavior Checklist and the Clinical Global Impression Scale, naltrexone did not show benefit compared to placebo in this study, and side effects included fatigue, nausea, and sedation. In contrast, in a double-blind controlled study, daily administration of naltrexone to a 12-year-old with ASD led to a drop in self-injury rate to zero for 22 months (Barrett et al., 1989).

Based on the hypothesis that SIB is influenced or maintained by the release of endogenous opioid peptides, a quantitative review of naltrexone use for SIB covering a 20-year period was conducted. The authors identified 27 research articles involving 86 individuals with self-injury. Eighty percent of the subjects were reported to have improved by 47% or more over their baseline rate of SIB. Males were found to respond better than females. No relationship was found between treatment outcome and ASD in this study (Symons et al., 2004).

Support for the endogenous opioid model is also found in preclinical studies of people with SIB. Elevated plasma β-endorphin levels have been reported to predict differential response to treatment with opiate receptor antagonists (Sandman, 2009; Sandman et al., 1997). Similarly, in a study of nonsuicidal people without neurodevelopmental disabilities but exhibiting SIB (e.g., self-cutting and self-burning), the role of endogenous opioids and monoamine neurotransmitters in SIB was examined. Nonsuicidal self-injury is a category designated in the appendix of DSM-5 for further study.

Chronic stress can lead to a blunting of the response to acute stress (Bremner, 2003; Heffernan et al., 2000). Similarly, prenatal stress altered the hypothalamic levels of met-enkephalin in an animal study. In rat pups, the μ-opioid and δ-opiate receptors are downregulated after prenatal stress (Sanchez et al., 1992, 1996). Nonsuicidal SIB is generally followed by improved mood and a decrease in negative affect. Naltrexone has been reported in case reports for successful long-term treatment of SIB in borderline personality disorder (Griengl et al., 2001) and as an adjunct to enhance supportive psychotherapy (Guerdjikova et al., 2014). Buprenorphine, a μ-opiate receptor partial agonist and κ-opiate receptor antagonist, has also been evaluated as a treatment for nonsuicidal SIB. Norelli et al. (2013) described successful treatment of six individuals with SIB with buprenorphine.

## Altered Anatomy and Physiological State

Surgical procedures have resulted in SIB in experimental animals, including lesions in the temporal lobe in macaques (Kluver & Bucy, 1939) and lesions in the spinal cord such as bilateral cervicothoracic dorsal rhizotomy from C5 to T2 (Busbaur, 1974), sciatic nerve section, and transection of the middle of the lateral funiculus (Jones & Barraclough, 1978). A primary consideration is whether the surgery results in the complete elimination of sensory input (anesthesia) or alters input (paresthesia), possibly associated with constant irritation. Taub (Taub, 1977; Taub et al., 1973) found self-injury in sensory deafferented monkeys whose sensory pathways had been disrupted, which suggests sensory isolation as a mechanism for SIB.

Other investigators have studied paresthesia in animals. For example, Innovar (fentanyl citrate/droperidol), a drug causing local irritation, has resulted in SIB in experimental animals. One possible explanation for these stereotypies and SIB is that arousal is increased by local irritation and that stereotypies reduce arousal. Stereotypies and SIB have been frequently observed under conditions of increased arousal, suggesting that (a) neurophysiological arousal causes increased stereotypies and SIB and (b) specific motor activity related to stereotyped and SIB reduces arousal.

## Drug-Induced Changes in Physiological State

In addition to drugs or surgical lesions involving the spinal cord or affecting the peripheral nervous system that lead to SIB, centrally acting drugs that increase stereotypies may lead to SIB in experimental animals. These substances include alcohol, caffeine, methylxanthine, clonidine, pemoline, and amphetamine. Amphetamine administration leads to stereotypies in animals and humans. High-dose pemoline has similar effects to amphetamine on provoking SIB, the effects of which are blocked by the dopamine D2 receptor antagonist haloperidol. Low-dose pemoline administered to adult and weaning rats results in intermittent SIB and stereotypy. However, Mueller et al. (1986) proposed that although they occur together, there are distinctly different mechanisms mediating SIB and stereotypy.

Rats and rabbits that were underfed and then received chronic administration of very high doses of caffeine or theophylline, methylpurine derivatives, eventually developed self-mutilating behavior. Purines such as adenosine are released from cells and influence neuronal activity as presynaptic modulators of neurotransmitter release and as regulators of receptor sensitivity (Kopin, 1981).

Endogenous peptides, such as adrenocorticotropic hormone (ACTH), also may produce stereotypies. Intraventricular administration of ACTH to rats has been shown to produce excessive grooming (Gispen et al., 1976; Jolles et al., 1979); the dopaminergic system has been linked to the effects of ACTH on grooming (Cools et al., 1978). It is suggested that excessive grooming is a response that serves to decrease arousal of the organism following activation of the ACTH system (Delius et al., 1976; Jolles et al., 1979). The response to the particular stimulus continues until the stimulus condition is altered. Once avoidance responding has stabilized, the pituitary–adrenal response to a previously arousing stimulus is attenuated (Hennessey & Levine, 1979). An inhibitory feedback effect on adrenocortical activity is exerted by the execution of species-specific behavior that either removes the external excitatory stimulus (escape, avoidance behavior, etc.) or mitigates the internal state (e.g., arousal stereotypy).

An individual with IDD in an environment that makes excessive demands, creating uncertainty and conflict with no opportunity to escape, will engage in SIB. However, under such conditions, stereotypies may serve as an effective means to reduce the level of arousal. Overall, SIB may represent an extreme form of stereotyped behavior when the individual is stressed and highly aroused. Ordinarily, pain suppresses behavior; however, stress-induced analgesia can occur, leading to a decrease in pain perception in these circumstances.

## Conditions Associated with Self-Injury

### Autism Spectrum Disorder

In the DSM-III (American Psychiatric Association, 1980), "childhood onset pervasive developmental disorder" included SIB among its diagnostic characteristics. Although this condition is no longer included in the classification system, SIB is a major consideration in individuals with ASD (Minshawi et al., 2014). ASD may account for the majority of cases of severe SIB in individuals with co-occurring intellect IDD. There is no specific topography of SIB in this population; head banging, face hitting, self-biting, and other forms of self-injurious behavior are seen.

Bartak and Rutter (1976) compared children with autistic disorder with IQs below 70 above 70 on nonverbal scales. The two groups differed in their pattern of symptoms, although they were similar in meeting diagnostic criteria for an autistic disorder. However, the low IQ and high IQ groups differed substantially in that the lower IQ group had significantly more self-injury and stereotypies.

Based on his neurophysiological studies, Ornitz (1974) suggested that there are problems in sensory modulation and motility in persons with autistic disorder diagnoses. These potential problems in sensory modulation as well as deficits in metacognition and social perception may contribute to self-injury. Complex behavioral interactions require social communication skills that are lacking in persons with ASD and may increase their vulnerability to aggression or self-injury when demands are placed on them. Moreover, persons with ASD show a markedly restricted repertoire of activities and interests that include stereotyped and repetitive movements.

### Lesch–Nyhan Disease

Lesch–Nyhan disease (Lesch & Nyhan, 1964; Nyhan, 1976; see also Harris, 2018) is an inborn error of purine metabolism in which self-injury is a major behavioral manifestation. The full syndrome requires virtual absence of the enzyme. Other syndromes with partial hypoxanthine phosphoribosyltransferase deficiency are associated with gout without the neurological and behavioral symptoms and without self-injury (Harris, 2018).

The onset of self-injury may be as early as 1 year, with eruption of teeth, or rarely as late as the teens. Children demonstrate self-mutilation initially through self-biting, which is intense and causes tissue damage, often leading to amputation of fingers and loss of tissue around the lips (Lesch & Nyhan, 1964; Mizuno & Yugari, 1974). With increasing age, they also may self-mutilate by picking the skin with their fingers. Biting often results in extraction of primary teeth. In type, the self-mutilation behavior is different from that seen in other IDD syndromes with self-injury, in which self-hitting and head banging are the most common presentations. The self-injury occurs although all sensory modalities, including the pain sense, are intact. The SIB often requires that the patient be restrained. Despite their dystonias, when restraints are removed, the child may appear terrified and quickly and accurately place a hand in the mouth. The child may ask for restraints to prevent elbow movement, and when restraints are placed, the child may become relaxed and more good-humored (Nyhan, 1976). The dysarthric speech may result in interpersonal communication problems that cause frustration in social situations. Still, higher functioning children can express themselves and participate in their treatment. Hemiballismic arm movements can also create difficulty because the raised arm is sometimes interpreted as a threatening gesture by others and may be socially reinforced, leading to hitting others.

Understanding the molecular disorder has led to effective drug treatment for those aspects of the disease that are related to uric acid accumulation and subsequent arthritic tophi, renal stones, and neuropathy. However, reduction in uric acid has not influenced the neurological and self-injurious behavior. In fact, some children diagnosed with hypoxanthine-guanine phosphoribosyltransferase deficiency and treated from birth with xanthine oxidase inhibitors for hyperuricemia still have behavioral and neurological symptoms despite never having had high levels of uric acid.

Because it is a condition in which self-injury is a behavioral phenotype uniquely present in all cases, Lesch–Nyhan disease has been investigated as a potential biological model for self-biting. Both anatomical and neurochemical studies have been undertaken in this condition. Brain imaging studies suggest involvement of the presynaptic dopamine system in Lesch–Nyhan disease (Wong et al., 1996). Early studies showing prophylactic effects of L-5 hydroxytryptophan on self-mutilation were not confirmed (Mizuno & Yugari, 1975).

## Cornelia de Lange Syndrome

Self-injury in Cornelia de Lange syndrome includes face hitting, face picking, and lip biting; no one specific pattern has been found, nor is the behavior as intense as that found in Lesch–Nyhan disease (Singh & Pulman, 1979; Srivastava et al., 2021). In a review of 50 cases (aged 5–17 years) using the Children's Yale–Brown Obsessive Compulsive Scale, Aberrant Behavior Checklist, and Vineland Adaptation-Behavior Scales, 45% had some form of self-injury (Srivastava et al., 2021). Typically, self-injury is treated using behavior therapy. However, no specific treatment approach in a series of cases of Cornelia de Lange individuals has been reported. In several cases, onset of SIB is reported to coincide with the eruption of teeth. The relationship of self-injury to tantrums and biological factors related to delayed tooth eruption, chewing behavior, and pain sensitivity requires further evaluation. Furthermore, Greenberg and Coleman (1973) reported low serotonin levels in whole blood in seven of seven males and two of four females ranging in age from 10 to 30 years with the disorder, in contrast to controls; this finding also requires replication. The relationship of serotonin levels and self-injury requires continuing assessment.

## Hereditary Sensory and Autonomic Neuropathies

The hereditary sensory and autonomic neuropathies (HSANs) are inherited disorders with sensory dysfunction with altered pain and temperature perception and depressed reflexes that affect both sexes. Those discussed here are characterized by autosomal recessive inheritance with onset at birth (Axelrod & Gold-von Simson, 2007). People with both congenital insensitivity to pain with anhidrosis (CIPA) and congenital insensitivity without neuropathy (HSAN IV) and Riley–Day syndrome (HSAN III) self-injure. A second congenital insensitivity to pain syndrome also occurs without associated neuropathy (Cox et al., 2006).

## Congenital Insensitivity to Pain

Congenital insensitivity to pain with anhidrosis may occur as an autosomal recessive disorder that is associated with self-mutilation (Pérez-López et al., 2015). In CIPA, the chromosomal location is 1q21–22 and the genes involved are *NTRK1* and *TRKA*. In channelopathy-associated congenital insensitivity to pain without neuropathy, chromosome 2q24.3 and the sodium channel gene *SCN9A* are involved. The self-injury may be accidental and not follow a specific syndrome pattern. The following criteria are required for diagnosis: (a) Pain sensation should be absent from birth, (b) anhidrosis, (c) the entire body should be affected, (d) self-injury, and (e) all other sensory modalities should be intact or minimally impaired with deep tendon reflexes present. IDD is seen in approximately one-third of reported cases. Affected children with a co-occurring behavior disorder may take unnecessary risks that result in self-injury. The sensory insensitivity to pain may lead to self-mutilation, auto-amputation, and corneal scarring. Speech is typically clear. Hypotonia and delay in motor milestones are frequent in early development, but strength normalizes with age. Emotionality, irritability, and hyperactivity are common (Axelrod & Gold-von Simson, 2007) and seen in approximately 50% of cases. Behavior treatment is recommended.

In several studies of patients with congenital insensitivity to pain, endogenous opiates have been strongly implicated. In one study, administration of naloxone dramatically reduced the pain threshold by 67% as measured by the nociceptive flexion reflex (Dehen et al., 1977). Dehen et al. (1986) subsequently reported that spontaneously elevated nociceptive (pain) threshold levels were markedly diminished after naloxone injections in four patients with congenital insensitivity to pain. Although cerebral spinal fluid (CSF) β-endorphin was either not elevated or only slightly elevated in these patients, their clinical response to opioid antagonists suggests a possible treatment in some identified children with this disorder. Another study failed to replicate the antagonist effect of naloxone but noted elevated opioid levels in the CSF (Manfredi et al., 1981). By restoring the pain response with naloxone, accidental self-injury would be expected to be reduced.

Congenital insensitivity, or indifference to pain without neuropathy, has autosomal recessive inheritance. It results from a loss of function mutation in the *SCN9A* gene encoding the voltage-gated sodium channel Nav1.7 and is identified in both humans and a mouse model. A Nav1.7 deletion leads to upregulation of the endogenous opioid system involving met-enkephalin protein in sensory neurons. The opioid antagonist naloxone potentiates peripheral input into the spinal cord and reduces analgesia in both male and female Nav1.7 mutant mice and in a human Nav1.7 null mutant (Nilsen et al., 2009). Thus, Nav1.7 channel blockers may be potentiated by exogenous opioids (Minett et al., 2015). In a human study, there was a dramatic reversal of analgesia with infusion of naloxone.

## Riley–Day Syndrome (Familial Dysautonomia)

Riley–Day syndrome (Riley et al., 1949) or familial dysautonomia is a hereditary autonomic neuropathy. It is an autosomal recessive disorder. The responsible mutant gene, *IKBKAP*, is located at chromosome 9q31 and encodes a scaffolding protein, ELP1 (Rubin & Anderson, 2017). Affected persons are homozygous, with an estimated incidence of 1 per 3,600 live births (Axelrod & Gold-von Simson, 2007). It is almost exclusively found in descendants of Ashkenazi Jews. Patients with Riley–Day syndrome have distinctive physical features that emerge over time and both neurological and physiological abnormalities; the most pertinent to self-injury are those associated with abnormal sensory nerves, nerve fibers, and autonomic nerve plexuses. However, self-mutilation is relatively rare. Taste perception and discrimination are markedly deficient, and pain perception is reduced or absent (Riley et al., 1949). The primary problems are alacrima (absence of tears), gastrointestinal and respiratory dysfunction, and low blood pressure. Studies of Riley–Day syndrome have shown decreases in dopamine β-hydroxylase, the enzyme that converts dopamine to norepinephrine. This is consistent with progressive loss of dopamine neurons that serve as a biomarker (D. Goldstein et al., 2008). This suggests dopamine system involvement in this disease.

## Rett's Syndrome

Rett's syndrome (Rett, 1966) is characterized by hand wringing and hand-to-mouth behavior that may lead to self-injury. The diagnosis of Rett's syndrome is based on a characteristic neurodevelopmental phenotype. The main criteria are shown in Box 19.1 (Neul et al., 2010). There are four main criteria and two exclusion criteria. In its classic presentation, there is apparently normal early psychomotor development in the first 6–12 months, followed by rapid decline with regression in acquired motor skills, loss of spoken language, and purposeful hand use. There is the onset of hand stereotypies, abnormal gait in early life, followed by stabilization as described here.

There is slowing of development beginning in the first 6 months, particularly in motor abilities; hypotonia is present. Developmental delay is insidious at onset, with loss of acquired abilities and onset of characteristic hand wringing and hand-to-mouth movements. These stereotyped behaviors are important diagnostic clues in girls who have lost previously acquired purposeful hand skills. Social withdrawal is accompanied by hyperventilation, clumsy movements, and seizures. The social withdrawal behavior is related to a developing encephalopathy, and the child may be misdiagnosed with ASD. When autistic ASD is considered in girls, Rett's disorder must be ruled out because it is distinct and should not be a specifier for ASD. Over time, there is a plateau in symptomatology with no further loss of skills. Those affected gradually show more social awareness. Seizures are common, as are severe intellectual developmental disorder and gait apraxia/ataxia. In adolescence, motor deterioration continues with decreasing mobility,

---

**Box 19.1 Rhett Syndrome Main Criteria and Exclusion Criteria**

---

Main Criteria
1. Partial or complete loss of acquired purposeful hand skills
2. Partial or complete loss of acquired spoken language
3. Gait abnormalities: Impaired (dyspraxic) or absence of ability
4. Stereotypic hand movements (hand wringing/squeezing, clapping/tapping, mouthing, and washing/rubbing automatisms)

Exclusion Criteria
1. Brain injury secondary to trauma (peri- or postnatally), neurometabolic disease, and severe infections that cause neurological problems
2. Grossly abnormal psychomotor development in first 6 months of life

---

spasticity, scoliosis, muscle wasting, and vasomotor disturbances, whereas social response and eye contact improve (Hagberg et al., 1983, 2002). Differential reinforcement behavioral procedures combined with response interruption techniques have been used to reduce hand-to-mouth behavior. Mutations in the *MECP2* gene located in the X chromosome (x28) account for 95% of typical cases (Ehrhart et al., 2018).

## Tourette Syndrome

Self-injury is an important concern in Tourette syndrome; SIB is underreported in Tourette disorder (Eisenberg et al., 1959; Robertson et al., 1989). Self-destructive behavior in Tourette patients is correlated with obsessionality and hostility on rating scales. Patients with self-injury tend to be at the most severe end of the spectrum. The types of self-injury reported in individuals with Tourette disorder are typically not the same as those encountered with other self-injurious syndromes, such as Lesch–Nyhan disease. The topography of self-injury is more nonspecific and similar to that seen in severe IDD, although Tourette disorder patients are of average intelligence. SIB in individuals with Tourette disorder may stem from obsessions—for example, hitting the head in conjunction with a hand jerk. Other forms of self-injury are more complex and include pulling out teeth and eye poking. Rather than being a tic behavior, the self-injury is heterogeneous and, in some instances, appears compulsive; in others, it may be related to a "directed tic." The topography of self-injury in 30 Tourette disorder patients included head banging, body punching or slapping, head or face punching, hitting the body on hard objects, poking sharp objects into the body, scratching parts of the body, and a variety of other forms (Robertson et al., 1989). Trimble (1992) noted tattooing in some individuals with Tourette disorder and also coprographia. Overall, one-third, or 30 of 90 patients, referred in that study showed SIB.

Self-harm is most common in children and adolescents, rarely beginning in adulthood. It is associated with tic severity, obsessive–compulsive disorder, and attention deficit disorder. Tic severity is the major issue in children, whereas anxiety disorders and other psychiatric disorders are important to address in adults (Szejko et al., 2019). Several studies have focused on lifetime prevalence of self-injury. In one Tourette study, clinical presentations were examined in approximately 300 cases and classified as mild, moderate, and severe. Mild/moderate self-injury was correlated with aggressive compulsions. Severe self-injury correlated with episodic rages and risk-taking behavior. All categories of severity were correlated with severity of tics (Mathews et al., 2004).

## Fragile X Syndrome

Fragile X syndrome has increased rates of challenging behavior. Fragile X syndrome is associated with overactivity, impulsivity, repetitive behavior, and impaired social communication. There is a range of behavioral problems, from difficulties in social communication with strangers to autistic-like behavior, self-injury, and periodic violent outbursts of behavior. Hand flapping was noted in 66% of 50 males, hand biting in 74%, and unusual hand mannerisms in 88% (Hagerman et al., 1986). Most males with fragile X syndrome do not have a pervasive lack of relatedness to caregivers and do not meet criteria for ASD. Males with fragile X syndrome can be happy, likeable, and friendly. Hand flapping, hand biting, perseverative speech, and poor eye contact in a child who is overactive and has an IDD or learning disability suggest the need for an evaluation for fragile X syndrome.

Self-injury is a phenotypic behavior in fragile X syndrome, with a prevalence of 54–58% over the lifetime (Symons et al., 2003), and the prevalence of aggressive behavior has been reported to be 50% (Arron et al., 2011). Hand biting is most common and reported in 26%. Demands and changes in routine are the most common triggers for self-injury. The most common forms of aggressive behavior are hitting (49%) and kicking others (30%) (Hessl et al., 2008). SIB and aggression are persistent over time. In a longitudinal study, there was a 77% persistence in self-injury and 69% persistence in aggression during the 8-year observation period. The baseline level of repetitive behavior predicted persistence of self-injury. Impulsivity predicted persistence of aggression (Crawford et al., 2019). Self-injury also occurs in other genetic syndromes. For example, excoriation (skin picking) is common in Prader–Willi syndrome and Smith–Magenis syndrome (Clarke et al., 2002; Finucane et al., 2001; Whittington & Holland, 2020), and there is a broad topography of SIB that incudes self-hitting and self-biting.

In summary, there is no typical age or pattern of onset of SIB. The onset often follows a stressful environmental event. In nonverbal persons with a severe degree of IDD, it may be triggered by a painful physical condition, such as middle ear infection in young children. SIBs often peak in adolescence and then may gradually decline, but they may also persist for years, especially in persons with severe/profound IDD. The focus of these behaviors often changes; for example, a person may engage in hand biting that may then subside and head hitting may emerge. Quite commonly, an individual engages in a stereotypic behavior that usually does not result in self-injury (e.g., light head banging and skin picking), but at times the stereotypic behavior may progress in its intensity to the point that self-injury results.

## Conditions Associated with Aggressive Behavior

## Mutation in the Structural Gene for Monoamine Oxidase A

A major metabolic pathway involved in the degradation of dietary and neurotransmitter amines utilizes oxidative deamination by the monoamine oxidases (i.e., MAO-A and MAO-B). The genes for these monoamines are located at the p11.3 region of the X chromosome. The *MAOA* gene encodes the key enzyme for the degradation of serotonin and catecholamines (Brunner et al., 1993). Brunner et al. described a nonsense mutation in the *MAOA* gene (RS72554632) in a large Dutch kindred that was significantly linked with a clinical phenotype characterized by borderline IDD and abnormal behavior. There was prominent aggressive and sometimes violent behavior that was triggered by stress. In addition, other forms of antisocial behavior were described, including attempted rape, arson, and exhibitionism. Twenty-four urine specimens in three patients indicated a severe reduction in monoamine metabolites (i.e., metabolites of serotonin and catecholamines). An infant with a second *MAOA* mutation exhibited developmental cognitive deficits and behavioral changes on the autism spectrum (Piton et al., 2014). The child was diagnosed with ASD, attention-deficit/hyperactivity disorder (ADHD), and self-injury. Two of his maternal uncles with the same mutation resulting in reduced *MAOA* activity had severe IDD and a history of aversive treatment in childhood.

Studies of the *MAOA* gene provide evidence that mutations increase the propensity for aggressive, antisocial, and violent behavior. Mouse models of *MAOA* deficiency by gene–environment interactions show similarity to human behavioral phenotypes. Adult *MAOA* knockout mice show high levels of inter-male aggression with elevated serotonin in the brain, especially in the first weeks of life. Aggression in these null mutants is accompanied by deficits in sociability and environmental exploration (Kolla & Bortolato, 2020). A study in humans demonstrated a gene–environment interaction extending the relationship of low *MAOA* activity (*MAOA-L* allele) to more aggressive behavior in response to a perceived loss (McDermott et al., 2009). Congenital *MAOA* deficiency as well as low *MAOA* activity variants are associated with higher risk for antisocial behavior and violence, especially in males with a history of child maltreatment. The interplay between low *MAOA* genetic variants and adversity in early life provides evidence of gene–environment interaction on the pathophysiology of antisocial behavior and aggression (Kolla & Bortolato, 2020). The *MAOA-L* allele has been extensively studied with childhood adversity and mistreatment. This was first reported in 2002 (Caspi et al., 2002; Poulton et al., 2015). Independent meta-analysis has lent some support for the gene–environment interaction, with a modest effect size of 0.18 (Ficks & Waldman, 2014).

Finally, positron emission tomography (PET), magnetic resonance imaging (MRI), and functional MRI studies have examined the role of *MAOA* in aggression and antisocial behavior. A PET study reported that brain *MAOA* levels explained 30% of the variance in trait aggression (Alia-Klein et al., 2008), and *MAOA* density measured with the $[C^{11}]$-harmine as the *MAOA* ligand was lower in the orbitofrontal cortex and ventral striatum in people with antisocial personality with high aggression (Kolla et al., 2015).

A structural MRI study demonstrated decreased surface area of the right amygdala associated with psychopathic traits (Kolla et al., 2017). A functional neuroimaging study revealed *MAOA-L* carriers to have abnormal corticoamygdaloid connectivity (Meyer-Lindenberg et al., 2006).

## Comprehensive Assessment

Self-injurious behavior is multiply determined and requires interdisciplinary assessment. The psychiatrist can function as a primary mental health caregiver or as a core member of an interdisciplinary team, which they lead. In the latter role in the assessment of SIB, the psychiatrist is responsible for diagnosing and for integrating the findings of the interdisciplinary assessment team. In all instances, coordination with nonmedical professionals in the evaluation and treatment of SIB is essential.

The psychiatric assessment requires observations of and interviews with the patient, parent, or guardian and others who are directly involved with the patient's care. The interview with the patient may require augmented and alternative communication devices if the patient is nonverbal. In addition, neurodevelopmental and medical assessment (including syndrome identification), critical review of past psychological tests and cognitive test profiles (the Full Scale IQ score alone is not sufficient because of subtest scatter), request for new tests as needed, psychosocial stressor evaluation (understanding of the social impact of the disability on the parent or guardian and on caregivers), the degree of restrictiveness of treatment needed (e.g., use of restraints), and review of previous treatments (especially behavioral and pharmacological approaches) are included.

In conducting an examination for SIB, the following should be considered. From a neurobiological perspective, SIB is multiply determined and involves maturational factors, current physiological state, past life experience, the social context of the behavior, and whether there is initiation of behavior in novel environmental settings. One must consider a severe form with a seemingly sudden spontaneous onset and a less severe form following stereotypy with regularly repeated injury. The social context must be considered because past social isolation may lead to increased vulnerability for future injury when stressed. In ASD, a deficiency in bonding may enhance vulnerability to self-injury because of lack of responsiveness to social reinforcement. The role of depression and learned helplessness also should be considered in the assessment.

The physiological state of the individual must also be considered. A state of agitation may accompany emotional lability and may be a temperamental factor, an aspect of a mental disorder, or a consequence of environmental variables. Excessive sensory input may result in stereotypies and sometimes can lead to self-injury. Individuals with IDD often have neurological abnormalities involving sensory systems, predisposing them to SIB. Excessive agitation may occur when conditions are perceived by the person as confusing or threatening to themself.

## Diagnostic Formulation

The essential elements to any individual formulation include predisposing, precipitating, perpetuating, and protective factors. Genetic background can be an important predisposing factor. Life circumstances can be precipitating factors. Perpetuating factors include cognition, self-regulation, and lack of family support. Protective factors include temperament, capacity to self-regulate, cognition, and family support. Case formulation follows a neurobehavioral model that includes behavioral history and consideration of biological variables. The formulation begins with a description of the developmental level and listing a current diagnosis, cognition, attachment status, communication skills, associated disabilities (particularly sensory and motor), and environmental contingencies as they relate to self-injury. Aggression and other challenging behaviors should be described in detail. Family environment and psychosocial circumstances are salient. Consideration of co-occurring severe mental illness is particularly important in the case formulation.

## Selection of Treatment

The treatment plan is based on the case formulation and is tailored to the unique aspects of the individual case, taking into account both the behavioral and biological variables from the neurobehavioral model. The approach to treatment is mutimodal and should include individual, family, behavioral (using applied behavior analysis [ABA]), and pharmacological interventions that address the biological variables. Interventions that increase mastery of environmental challenges and enhance positive behaviors by emphasizing communication skills by using augmented communication are important. Behavioral reduction procedures have been reviewed by the National Institutes of Health (NIH, 1991). The NIH consensus statement states that

> behavioral reduction approaches should be selected for their rapid effectiveness only if the exigencies of the clinical situation require such restrictive interventions and only after appropriate review. These interventions should be used only in the context of a comprehensive and individualized behavioral enhancement treatment program.

Careful consideration must be given to the possible biological bases for SIB, its association with organic brain conditions, and how biological factors relate to treatment approaches. Knowledge about the possible biological mechanisms involved in SIB is employed along with other treatment procedures for more effective behavioral management to reduce the considerable cost involved in both initial treatment and generalization of treatment into a home or community setting.

In planning a treatment program dealing with SIB, it is important to consider if there is impairment in reciprocal social interactions and if there is an insecure social attachment. So, an essential component to treatment is the inclusion of a program of functional language communication. Establishing social engagement with the therapist is extremely important because disabled persons with social deficits often do not respond spontaneously. Focused language communication can be needed to initiate social interactions. A lack of social awareness and the failure to establish an attachment relationship are major impediments. The individual with ASD may not seek proximity to their caregivers, and thus social interaction seems unrewarding for them. Lower functioning individuals with ASD, in particular, do not initiate social communication spontaneously or respond to nonverbal cues, such as a frown from an adult or other gestures that ordinarily serve as a signal to end an inappropriate activity. Thus, addressing impairments in communication and imaginative skills is a critical element in program planning. The stereotypies that these children exhibit may be used as reinforcers in working with the children—for example, using hand flapping as a reinforcer as part of the treatment. Ongoing involvement in treatment by family members, caregivers, and staff members is vital. The same approach to treatment must be consistently applied across treatment settings.

Regarding behavioral interventions, a high-quality non-aversive behavioral intervention should include the following components: (a) a systematic functional analysis or assessment followed by a multicomponent treatment intervention based on the results of the analysis, (b) a focus on building functionally equivalent skills to replace the problem behaviors, and (c) altering living environments to promote lifestyle changes that minimize problem behaviors. Treatment must be individualized to recognize individual differences in emotional responsiveness (Woodcock & Blackwell, 2020). In some instances, mindfulness may be incorporated into the treatment package (Singh et al., 2019). Finally, supportive psychotherapy and mindfulness approaches are needed to assist parents and caregivers to mitigate the stress in caring for the patient (Singh et al., 2019). Regular follow-up and case review are essential to monitor the emergence of social attachment and self-regulation, the appropriateness of behavioral interventions, and the effectiveness of pharmacological treatments.

## Treatment Planning

The risk for challenging behavior increases with the severity of IDD, concurrent ASD, deficits in communication, sensory impairments, and recognition of challenging behavior in genetic syndromes such as Lesch–Nyhan syndrome and Cornelia de Lange syndrome. In planning a treatment program dealing with challenging behaviors, especially self-injury, it is important to consider the impairments in reciprocal social interactions and the extent of development of social attachment. An essential component in treatment is communication and, for the more severely cognitively impaired, the establishment of a program of functional language communication. Establishing social attention is extremely important because disabled persons with social deficits often do not respond spontaneously to language communication or initiate social interaction. Their lack of social awareness and the failure to establish secure attachment are major factors in choosing therapeutic strategies. For example, an individual with ASD may not show attachment by seeking proximity of the caretaker, and social interactions can be unrewarding to them. Their impairments in communication and imaginative skills are critical elements to consider in program planning. Lower functioning individuals with ASD do not initiate social communication spontaneously or respond to nonverbal cues such as a frown from an adult or other gestures that ordinarily serve as a signal to end an activity. Stereotypies in children with ASD can be used as reinforcers in working with these children. Involvement of family members, caregivers, and staff members in treatment is vital so that the same approach is consistently applied across school, home, and community settings.

In treatment planning, the personal characteristics of the patient are taken into consideration in formulating interventions for challenging behaviors, especially when using behavioral interventions. In addition, the relationship between the type of injury, its severity, and the trajectory of SIB and other challenging behaviors must be assessed. Comorbid medical conditions, severity of IDD, and the presence of ASD are risk factors to consider for challenging behaviors (Oliver et al., 2017). An example of a medical risk factor is a unrecognized pain—for example, an otitis media that leads to SIB. ASD is a personal characteristic associated with higher levels of anxiety and stereotypical behavior associated with SIB (Cervantes & Matson, 2015). A study involving 152 children with ASD found that the severity of the symptoms correlated with the degree of SIB (Rattaz et al., 2015).

Stereotypical behaviors predict SIB regardless of the co-occurrence of ASD. In one study, the cumulative 1-year incidence of SIB associated with stereotypy was nearly 5% (Davies & Oliver, 2016). The onset of SIB was predicted by the presence of repetitive behaviors, and onset of aggression was predicted by the presence of impulsivity (Barnard-Brak et al., 2015). Importantly, SIB is a behavioral phenotype in certain genetic disorders. In addition, there is a relationship between sleep disorders, SIB, and anxiety (Williams et al., 2015). For example, anxiety is related to some aspects of repetitive behaviors in fragile X syndrome (Oakes et al., 2016). There is also the issue of the relationship of internal physiologic state to SIB and aggression. Because higher cortisol levels have been reported in children with ASD who engage in SIB (Lydon et al., 2015), pain can provoke or exacerbate SIB in vulnerable individuals.

## Parental Interventions

The most successful parent interventions combine behavioral approaches with other strategies. Parent–child interactional therapy (PCIT), initially developed for neurotypically developing children, is applicable for those with neurodevelopmental disorders. It focuses on helping parents interact with their children utilizing attachment theory and social learning theory (Zlomke & Jeter, 2020). A review of the literature examined applications of PCIT to ASD and ADHD in 18 published studies over a period of 16 years using parent–child ratings and reported significant improvement in challenging behaviors.

Parents whose children have neurodevelopmental disorders, especially parents with children exhibiting challenging behaviors, have high levels of stress, anxiety, and depression. The anxiety that they experience must be reduced to allow them to fully engage in parent–child training sessions. Several psychoeducational approaches combine teaching and sharing information about the disability as well as teaching stress reduction strategies. Mindfulness-based stress reduction has a strong evidence base. Mindfulness, combined with positive behavioral support, has also led to reduction in parental stress and improvements in children's challenging behaviors (Singh et al., 2019). A randomized trial of 243 mothers compared a mindfulness-based stress reduction approach to a positive psychology intervention after 6 months of treatment (Dykens et al., 2014). Both treatments showed benefits with regard to sleep, well-being, parental stress, depression, and anxiety; however, the mindfulness group showed more rapid improvements.

## Cognitive and Self-Regulatory Interventions

Behavioral models that use operant approaches focus on antecedent/behavior/consequences strategies in the behavioral analyses. These approaches rely on noncognitive procedural (nondeclarative) memory and reinforce more adaptive behavior. In contrast, cognitive and self-regulatory behavioral interventions rely on cognitive engagement with the person. These approaches emphasize developing greater self-awareness and encourage the patient to make choices consistent with their cognitive level of functioning to facilitate social engagement and social communication. For example, teaching sign language to nonverbal children with IDD facilitates choice and may reduce challenging behavior through encouraging communication of interests and needs. Providing a means to communicate a specific need reduces challenging behaviors (Neely et al., 2018). For example, a nonverbal child was taught the sign for the word "go" when he became restless, and then he was allowed to actively roam around the room. He was less disruptive after learning this one sign. Similarly, when eating, he was taught the sign for the word "more." This made him more manageable at mealtime, helping him self-regulate because he could eat as much food as he wanted.

When introducing cognitive/self-regulation approaches, it is important to consider personal characteristics. This approach addresses the underpinnings of challenging behaviors in the particular patient. For example, preservation of sameness is characteristic of ASD. Disruption of behavioral routines may result in panic, leading to challenging behaviors. These behaviors are precipitated when transitions are required to move on to other activities. Recognition of preservation of sameness is a trigger for challenging behavior in ASD. Personal problems coping with anger are also emotional triggers for challenging behavior. Treatment of emotional dysregulation includes teaching the child skills in emotion recognition. Staff training focuses on promoting self-management in individuals with IDD. Overall, it is important to assess individualized cognitive and emotional processing. Parental mindfulness-based behavior support may have beneficial effects in management of the child's challenging behavior. Mindfulness training and yoga have been reported to benefit children with ADHD whose intelligence is in the typical range (Huguet et al., 2019).In contrast, the use of mindfulness in children with ASD and those with IDD is limited by the extent of their cognitive capacity to cope with and adapt to environmental tasks. There is greater benefit in managing challenging behavior using mindfulness in individuals with higher intellectual functioning (Woodcock & Blackwell, 2020).

## Digital Technology Assisted Interventions

Digital technologies are now available to facilitate cognitive skill training and emotion regulation interventions for patients with challenging behaviors. Digital technology includes the use of mobile phones, tablets, and computers. This includes, for example, the use of functional communication applications such as Go Talk Now, which was found to be useful in ASD for teaching self-monitoring of behavior (Muharib et al., 2019). Telehealth delivery is now being used for function-based behavioral treatment transfer to generalize treatment from controlled clinic and hospital settings to noncontrolled home environments.

## Psychotropic Medications: Mental Disorders with Challenging Behaviors

Mental disorders may precipitate challenging behavior in people with neurodevelopmental disorders. Recognition, assessment, and treatment of the comorbid mental disorders are essential to effectively treat people with challenging behavior. Historically, psychotropic drugs have been used almost exclusively and, unfortunately, excessively in some institutional settings to control challenging behaviors. This excessive use led to a class action lawsuit to ensure comprehensive treatment and not medication alone for behavioral control. Currently, behavioral and other psychosocial interventions have largely replaced stand-alone medication management of challenging behavior. Because of past excessive drug use, psychotropic medications are now typically prescribed for diagnosable mental disorders or as adjunctive treatment when established psychosocial interventions fail to reduce or terminate challenging behavior. A meta-analysis of 14 studies that included 912 participants found that the neuroleptic drugs risperidone and aripiprazole reduced challenging behaviors during the largely short-term treatment periods ($p = .001$). Weight gain and elevated prolactin levels were the most significant side effects with these two drugs. However, the quality of the studies was "typically low" (McQuire et al., 2015). As noted, most studies of psychotropic drug treatment of challenging behaviors in neuropsychiatric disorders are short term; long-term follow-up is needed to determine whether the treatment effects persist and what side effects emerge.

Risperidone and aripiprazole are the medications most frequently prescribed for challenging behaviors. Both medications are approved for behavior problems in ASD. In a large study, risperidone was effective and well-tolerated for reducing tantrums, aggression, or SIB in children with ASD (McCracken et al., 2002). In addition, olanzapine also was found to be effective in treating challenging behaviors (SIBs, aggression, and destructive/disruptive behavior). Weight gain and sedation are the most common side effects for all three medications (Janowsky et al., 2003).

Dopamine D1 receptor antagonists cause substantial reductions in SIB in the 6-OHDA rodent model of SIB (Moy et al., 2001). In this model, olanzapine, an atypical antipsychotic drug that also is a dopamine D1 receptor antagonist, was also found to reduce SIB. In addition to olanzapine's effects on dopamine D1 and D2 receptors, serotoninergic neurotransmission may play a role in its effects (Bymaster et al., 1999).

This was suggested when mianserin, a selective 5-HT$_{2C}$ receptor antagonist, blocked SIB in the rodent model (Kostrzewa, 1995).

SIB with self-mutilation is the behavioral phenotype in Lesch–Nyhan disease. Ecopipam, a selective dopamine D1 receptor antagonist, has been examined in a double-blind, placebo-controlled crossover trial in patients with Lesch–Nyhan disease to reduce SIB because the dopamine D1 receptor appeared to be etiologically involved in the 6-HODA rat model of SIB. The topographies of self-injury in this disorder include self-biting, self-hitting, head banging, and other injurious activities. Impulsivity and aggression are also characteristic in Lesch–Nyhan disease. Although the ecopipam study was terminated because of unanticipated side effects, including sedation and dystonia in some subjects likely due to high initial doses, the drug appeared to reduce self-injury in most patients who could continue the trial. In an open label extension lasting 1 year, one subject showed virtually complete cessation of SIB with no significant side effects (Khasnavis et al., 2016).

## The Role of Electroconvulsive Treatment for Intractable Self-Injurious Behavior

Intractable cases of SIB present with high intensity and high rates of such severe self-injury that protective equipment (helmets, arm restraints, face shields, neck pillows, and sports padding) is required to prevent self-harm and self-mutilation. Intractable cases may also require constant caregiver supervision to prevent SIB throughout waking hours, which results in limited participation in school or recreational activities. Because of the severity of this behavior, involved adolescents are separated from family members in treatment facilities for substantial periods of time.

Functional behavioral assessment finds no operant reinforcement strategy for intervention in these treatment-resistant cases. They are considered to be in a category referred to as "behavior-maintained by internal reinforcement" (Kahng et al., 2002) and require continuous restraint to avoid severe self-harm. When SIB is not responsive to psychosocial, behavioral, or psychopharmacologic interventions or their combined use, the diagnosis may be agitated catatonia. The first line of treatment for catatonia is benzodiazepine, typically lorazepam (Mazzone et al., 2014). In refractory patients, SIB may persist despite trials of multiple psychopharmacological medications, given singularly or in combination, along with long-term unsuccessful behavioral interventions (Wachtel et al., 2018).

Electroconvulsive therapy (ECT) can be an efficacious treatment for self-injury associated with agitated catatonia. Catatonia is recognized as the syndrome most responsive to treatment with ECT (Fink, 2013). The recognition of self-injury in ASD potentially as a form of catatonia has resulted in ECT treatment in treatment-resistant cases. This is entirely different than the controversial use of contingent electric shock as a response-reduction behavioral intervention. Although reduction in self-injury using contingent electric shock was reported in the 1960s, the use of painful punishment procedures such as contingent electric shock has been largely abandoned for treating challenging behavior. This procedure has been abused, resulting in litigation (Duker & Seys, 1996).

In DSM-5, catatonia is recognized as occurring in the context of several psychiatric disorders. Catatonia is not recognized as a separate diagnosis in DSM-5 but may co-occur in neurodevelopmental disorders and psychotic, bipolar, depressive, and other disorders. Catatonia is defined by marked psychomotor disturbance that may involve decreased motor activity (mutism), decreased social engagement, or excessive and peculiar motor activity. The presentation ranges from marked unresponsiveness to marked agitation with stereotypy. Careful supervision is needed to prevent self-harm or harm to others with catatonia. It is defined by the presence of three or more psycho-motor features listed in the DSM-5 criteria. Catatonia is recognized as a co-occurring psychiatric syndrome with motor (agitation), vocal (mutism, negativism, and echo-lalia), and behavioral/motor (catalepsy, waxy flexibility, posturing, mannerisms, echo-praxia, stereotypy, and grimacing) symptoms.

The Bush–Francis Catatonia Rating Scale that is used in clinical research lists 23 symptoms of catatonia (Bush et al., 1996). Affective illness and psychosis are most frequently associated with catatonia (Fink & Taylor, 2006). Among the neurodevelopmental disorders, catatonia is most commonly associated with ASD. Large studies from Sweden, the United Kingdom, and the United States have identified catatonia as a specifier for ASD, occurring in 15–20% of cases. Two of the studies fo-cused on catatonic psychomotor retardation, emphasizing passivity, lack of motivation, and slow movement in a population-based study in the United Kingdom (Wing & Shah, 2000). A Swedish population-based study with 13- to 22-year follow-up of 120 cases of ASD diagnosed in childhood with re-evaluation at ages 17–40 years found that 50% of catatonic cases self-injured (Billstedt et al., 2005). U.S. studies identifying catatonia have been based on chart reviews (Ghaziuddin et al., 2012).

Bates and Smeltzer (1982) first reported a substantial reduction of head injury in a 25-year-old man in response to ECT. In a 2008 case report, the relationship of SIB to catatonia was proposed in an 18-year-old girl with classic catatonia (mutism, stupor, grimacing, and food refusal), with the SIB leading to trauma and retinal detachment; ECT completely resolved her catatonic symptoms, with healing of her eye (Wachtel et al., 2008). Subsequent single-case reports have documented response to ECT in individuals with SIB and ASD. Response to ECT treatment of agitated catatonia in ASD is summarized in a review of 22 individuals (16 males and 6 females, ranging in age from 8 to 26 years) with ASD with catatonia (Wachtel, 2019). Catatonia was diagnosed using DSM-5 criteria. The patients were treated with a combination of lorazepam and ECT. Thirteen of the 22 subjects were continued on maintenance ECT at the end for the study period. ECT was beneficial in reducing agitated catatonic symptoms and alleviating treatment-resistant SIB. The ECT in these cases followed a standard pro-tocol with propofol or methohexital anesthesia, muscle relaxation with succinylcho-line, and bitemporal application. Initially, the course of treatment was 3 weekly sessions until there was symptom relief, which was followed by continued maintenance ECT as indicated.

Studies have shown resolution of cortisol and thyroid functional abnormalities after repeated ECT treatments. This normalization is consistent with the proposed neuro-endocrine mechanism (Shorter & Fink, 2010). Additional research in animal models supports an increase in hippocampal neurogenesis with ECT. There was an increase in brain cells after induced seizures (Madsen et al., 2000; Öngür & Heckers, 2004). ECT has also been shown to be beneficial for catatonia in youth with SIB but without ASD in single-case reports with co-occurring bipolar disorder, major depression, and psychotic depression.

Ethical considerations have been raised about ECT use in children younger than age 18 years, particularly those diagnosed with IDD, who can neither consent nor assent to the procedure. This issue has been addressed by Robertson et al. (2013). When ECT is performed in youth with neurodevelopmental disorders, consent can be provided by the parent after a detailed disclosure of the safety and efficacy of ECT for intractable treatment-resistant SIB in people with ASD. Educational videotapes of prior successful treatments are shown to parents, and a discussion is held with parents whose children have received successful ECT treatment.

In summary, ECT may be indicated when there is intractable, treatment-resistant, repetitive SIB in ASD. Catatonia is conceptualized within the spectrum of DSM-5 as diagnosable agitated catatonia. In carefully selected cases, ECT has been shown to be efficacious, allowing previously medically and psychosocially incapacitated children to return to home, school, and community settings without further SIB. There is ongoing research to further refine the diagnosis of catatonia in ASD to optimize the use of ECT in individuals with treatment refractory SIB.

## Applied Behavior Analysis/Functional Behavioral Assessment

Behavioral analytic research on challenging behaviors concerns the use of functional assessment procedures governing behavior. ABA employs objective measurements of behavior along with systematic examination of environmental factors. ABA interventions are an important element in a comprehensive, problem-focused treatment plan. The application of comprehensive intensive behavioral interventions for ASD typically involves 20–40 hours per week of programming (Reichow, 2012). Challenging behaviors such as aggression and SIB are addressed through such problem-focused treatment approaches. These interventions are time-limited and typically initiated in outpatient settings (Doehring et al., 2014; Hagopian & Gregory, 2016).

A functional behavioral assessment considers the function of the behavior. A functional assessment uses noncognitive operant reinforcement interventions. The function of behavior refers to what initiates and maintains a behavior. The function of challenging behaviors may be, for example, to gain attention from others or to escape from demanding tasks (referred to as escape behavior). The analysis of the function of the behavior experimentally simulates real-world situations in which the behavior may take place. In these simulated settings, antecedents and consequences for problem behavior are manipulated to measure their effects on behavior. The functional analysis methodology utilizes a series of test and control situations for the assessment of problem behavior for clinical research and clinical practice.

The operant functional behavioral situations examined are (a) access to attention, (b) escape from instructional demands, and (c) access to preferred items and reinforcement when none of these maintain behavior. In a review of 981 functional analysis data sets from more than 30 years, Beavers et al. (2013) found that approximately three-fourths of the challenging behavior cases were controlled by social conditions: attention or escape from the demands and access to preferred items. In contrast, for 16–20% of the cases, the problem behaviors occurred independent of these social variables; that is, they were automatically reinforced. In these instances, neurobiological processes, especially behavioral phenotypes in neurogenetic syndromes such as Lesch–Nyhan syndrome and Cornelia de Lange syndrome, were involved. Problem behaviors that were automatically reinforced included SIB and pica. Finally, in this review, a function could not be ascertained in 6% (Hagopian et al., 2013, 2015). Thus, in 20–25% of the cases, the challenging behaviors were not socially mediated.

The term automatic reinforcement is used by behavioral psychologists for these nonresponsive, non-socially mediated cases because the behavior is considered to produce its own reinforcement. Behavioral psychologists have proposed subtypes of automatic self-injurious behavior and examined the subtypes by applying the criteria to hospitalized cases. Examination of data sets of automatically reinforced SIB led to the identification of the following subtypes (Hagopian et al., 2015):

> Subtype 1: SIB is highest when the person is left alone with no interactions and is lowest in a play condition (41% of the cases).
> Subtype 2: SIB is high and variable across all functional assessment situations (38% of the cases).
> Subtype 3: SIB is automatically reinforced with high levels of self-restraint (20% of the cases).

Subtype 1 proved more responsive to behavioral interventions than Subtypes 2 and 3, whereas the other two subtypes were more resistant. None of the Subtype 2 cases reached criteria for reinforcement-based treatment and could not be treated without restraint. In nonhospitalized cases, these results were replicated for Subtypes 1 and 2. Importantly, operant behavioral approaches exclusively consider observed behavior without clarifying co-occurring psychiatric disorders, patient characteristics such as emotional lability, or behavioral phenotype of genetic syndromes.

## Medicolegal Issues

Medicolegal issues are essential considerations in the treatment of SIB. Informed consent by the parent or legal guardian is required for the initiation and implementation of the treatment plan, as well as for making major changes in the plan. State guidelines are of particular importance in monitoring the use of psychotropic drugs. The use of aversive interventions remains controversial; empirical, ethical, and legal considerations restrict their use.

## Conclusion

Challenging behaviors, especially SIB, occur most often in persons with severe IDD. One should consider if SIB is a learned response, the result of deviant development in a neurogenetic disorder, or an ethologically derived pattern of behavior elicited in stressful circumstances.

Environmental experiences during sensitive periods of development have been implicated in SIB in animals. Isolation, particularly from social contact with mothers or peers, results in subsequent impairment in social skills. Isolation is one of the best documented examples of an environmental etiology occurring during a sensitive period.

SIB follows increased arousal, leading to frustration and rage. Some forms of SIB involve exaggerations of the grooming mechanisms, whereas others avert fighting behavior. SIB has been specifically associated with ASD and with several types of IDD. With regard to brain mechanisms, catecholamine, indoleamines, and opioid neurotransmitter systems have been implicated. In animal models, psychotropic drugs such as amphetamine and pemoline, acting through dopaminergic receptors and intranigral muscimol activating $GABA_A$ receptors, elicit stereotypy and SIB. These effects are antagonized by D1 dopamine receptor antagonists.

6-HODA lesion of the nigrostriatal dopaminergic pathway early in development or sensory deafferentation are lesion models of SIB in experimental animals. Stress-induced analgesia may be a factor in eliciting or maintaining self-injury. Whether subjects self-stimulate to facilitate sensory input or to cause the release of endogenous opioids is an open question because the issue of whether stress-induced analgesia is a secondary consequence of the behavior remains unresolved.

In formulating treatment for patients, each of these mechanisms should be considered in conjunction with cognitive assessment, capacity for self-regulation, behavioral phenotype of a neurogenetic syndrome, and the psychiatric diagnosis. The final treatment plan is derived from integrating the findings from a comprehensive interdisciplinary assessment.

# References

Alborz, A., Bromley, J., Emerson, E., Kiernan, C., & Qureshi, H. (1994). *Challenging behaviour survey: Individual schedule.* Hester Adrian Research Centre, University of Manchester.

Alia-Klein, N., Goldstein, R. Z., Kriplani, A., Logan, J., Tomasi, D., Williams, B., Telang, F., Shumay, E., Biegon, A., Craig, I., Henn, F., Wang, G., Volkow, N., & Fowler, J. (2008). Brain monoamine oxidase A activity predicts trait aggression. *Journal of Neuroscience, 28*(19), 5099–5104.

Aman, M. G., Singh, N. N., Stewart, A. W., & Field, C. J. (1985). The Aberrant Behavior Checklist: A behavior rating scale for the assessment of treatment effects. *American Journal of Mental Deficiency, 89,* 485–491.

American Psychiatric Association. (1980). *Diagnostic and statistical manual of mental disorders* (3rd ed.).

American Psychiatric Association. (2013). *Diagnostic and statistical manual of mental disorders* (5th ed.). American Psychiatric Publishing.

Anderson, J. R., & Chamove, A. S. (1980). Self-aggression and social aggression in laboratory-reared macaques. *Journal of Abnormal Psychology, 89*(4), 539–550.

Arron, K., Oliver, C., Moss, J., Berg, K., & Burbidge, C. (2011). The prevalence and phenomenology of self-injurious and aggressive behaviour in genetic syndromes. *Journal of Intellectual Disability Research, 55*(2), 109–120.

Axelrod, F. B., & Gold-von Simson, G. (2007). Hereditary sensory and autonomic neuropathies: Types II, III, and IV. *Orphanet Journal of Rare Diseases, 2*(1), Article 39.

Barnard-Brak, L., Rojahn, J., Richman, D. M., Chesnut, S. R., & Wei, T. (2015). Stereotyped behaviors predicting self-injurious behavior in individuals with intellectual disabilities. *Research in Developmental Disabilities, 36*, 419–427.

Barrett, R. P., Feinstein, C., & Hole, W. T. (1989). Effects of naloxone and naltrexone on self-injury: A double-blind, placebo-controlled analysis. *American Journal of Mental Retardation, 93*(6), 644–651.

Bartak, L., & Rutter, M. (1976). Differences between mentally retarded and normally intelligent autistic children. *Journal of Autism and Childhood Schizophrenia, 6*, 109–120.

Bates, W. J., & Smeltzer, D. J. (1982). Electroconvulsive treatment of psychotic self-injurious behavior in a patient with severe mental retardation. *American Journal of Psychiatry, 139*(10), 1355–1356.

Beavers, G. A., Iwata, B. A., & Lerman, D. C. (2013). Thirty years of research on the functional analysis of problem behavior. *Journal of Applied Behavior Analysis, 46*(1), 1–21.

Beecher, H. K. (1946). Pain in men wounded in battle. *Annals of Surgery, 123*(1), 96–105.

Benson, B. A., & Brooks, W. T. (2008). Aggressive challenging behaviour and intellectual disability. *Current Opinion in Psychiatry, 21*(5), 454–458.

Billstedt, E., Gillberg, I. C., & Gillberg, C. (2005). Autism after adolescence: Population-based 13- to 22-year follow-up study of 120 individuals with autism diagnosed in childhood. *Journal of Autism and Developmental Disorders, 35*(3), 351–360.

Breese, G. R., Baumeister, A. A., McCown, T. J., Emerick, G., Frye, G. D., Crotty, K., & Mueller, R. A. (1984). Behavioral differences between neonatal and adult 6-hydroxy-dopamine-treated rats to dopamine agonists: Relevance to neurological symptoms in clinical syndromes with reduced brain dopamine. *Journal of Pharmacology and Experimental Therapeutics, 231*, 343–354.

Bremner, J. D. (2003). Long-term effects of childhood abuse on brain and neurobiology. *Child and Adolescent Psychiatric Clinics of North America, 12*(2), 271–292.

Brunner, H. G., Nelen, M. R., van Zandvoort, P., Abeling, N. G., van Gennip, A. H., Wolters, E. C., Kuiper, M., Ropers, E. C., & van Oost, B. A. (1993). X-linked borderline mental retardation with prominent behavioral disturbance: Phenotype, genetic localization, and evidence for disturbed monoamine metabolism. *American Journal of Human Genetics, 52*(6), 1032–1039.

Buchsbaum, M. S., Davis, G. C., & Bunney, W. E. (1977). Naloxone alters pain perception and somatosensory evoked potentials in normal subjects. *Nature, 270*(5638), 620–622.

Busbaur, A. I. (1974). Effects of central lesion on disorders produced by dorsal rhizotomy in rats. *Experimental Neurology, 42*, 490–501.

Bush, G., Fink, M., Petrides, G., Dowling, F., & Francis, A. (1996). Catatonia: I. Rating scale and standardized examination. *Acta Psychiatrica Scandinavica, 93*(2), 129–136.

Butler, R. K., & Finn, D. P. (2009). Stress-induced analgesia. *Progress in Neurobiology, 88*(3), 184–202.

Bymaster, F., Perry, K. W., Nelson, D. L., Wong, D. T., Rasmussen, K., Moore, N. A., & Calligaro, D. O. (1999). Olanzapine: A basic science update. *British Journal of Psychiatry, 174*(Suppl. 37), 36–40.

Caspi, A., McClay, J., Moffitt, T. E., Mill, J., Martin, J., Craig, I. W., Taylor, A., & Poulton, R.(2002). Role of genotype in the cycle of violence in maltreated children. *Science, 297*(5582), 851–854.

Cervantes, P. E., & Matson, J. L. (2015). Comorbid symptomology in adults with autism spectrum disorder and intellectual disability. *Journal of Autism and Developmental Disorders, 45*(12), 3961–3970.

Christie, M. J., Connor, M., Vaughan, C. W., Ingram, S. L., & Bagley, E. E. (2000). Cellular actions of opioids and other analgesics: Implications for synergism in pain relief. *Clinical and Experimental Pharmacology and Physiology, 27*(7), 520–523.

Clark, D. L., Kreutzberg, J. R., & Chee, F. K. W. (1977). Vestibular stimulation influence on motor development in infants. *Science, 196*, 1228–1229.

Clarke, D. J., Boer, H., Whittington, J., Holland, A., Butler, J., & Webb, T. (2002). Prader–Willi syndrome, compulsive and ritualistic behaviours: The first population-based survey. *British Journal of Psychiatry, 180*(4), 358–362.

Cools, A. R., Wiegant, U. M., & Gispen, W. H. (1978). Distinct dopaminergic systems in ACTH induced grooming. *European Journal of Pharmacology, 50,* 265–268.

Cox, J. J., Reimann, F., Nicholas, A. K., Thornton, G., Roberts, E., Springell, K., Karbani, G., Jafri, H., Mannan, J., Raashid, Y., Al-Gazali, L., Hamamy, H., Valente, E., Gorman, S., Williams, R., McHale, D., Wood, J., Gribble, F., & Woods, C. (2006). An SCN9A channelopathy causes congenital inability to experience pain. *Nature, 444*(7121), 894–898.

Crawford, H., Karakatsani, E., Singla, G., & Oliver, C. (2019). The persistence of self-injurious and aggressive behavior in males with fragile X syndrome over 8 years: A longitudinal study of prevalence and predictive risk markers. *Journal of Autism and Developmental Disorders, 49*(7), 2913–2922.

Crocker, A. G., Mercier, C., Lachapelle, Y., Brunet, A., Morin, D., & Roy, M. E. (2006). Prevalence and types of aggressive behaviour among adults with intellectual disabilities. *Journal of Intellectual Disability Research, 50*(9), 652–661.

Davies, L. E., & Oliver, C. (2016). Self-injury, aggression and destruction in children with severe intellectual disability: Incidence, persistence and novel, predictive behavioural risk markers. *Research in Developmental Disabilities, 49,* 291–301.

Dehen, H., Amsallem, B., Colas-Linhart, N., & Cambier, J. (1986). Cerebrospinal fluid beta-endorphin in congenital insensitivity to pain. *Revue Neurologique, 142*(5), 541–544.

Dehen, H., Willer, J. C., Boureau, F., & Cambier, J. (1977). Congenital insensitivity to pain, and endogenous morphine-like substances. *Lancet, 310*(8032), 293–294.

Dekker, M. C., Koot, H. M., Ende, J. V. D., & Verhulst, F. C. (2002). Emotional and behavioral problems in children and adolescents with and without intellectual disability. *Journal of Child Psychology and Psychiatry, 43*(8), 1087–1098.

Delius, J. D., Craig, B., & Chaudoir, C. (1976). Adrenocorticotropic hormone: Glucose displacement activities in pigeon. *Zeitschrift fur Tierpsychologie, 40,* 183–193.

Devine, D. P. (2012). The pemoline model of self-injurious behaviour. *Psychiatric Disorders: Methods and Protocols,* 155–163.

Devine, D. P. (2019). The pemoline model of self-injurious behavior: An update. *Psychiatric Disorders: Methods and Protocols,* 95–103.

Doehring, P., Reichow, B., Palka, T., Phillips, C., & Hagopian, L. (2014). Behavioral approaches to managing severe problem behaviors in children with autism spectrum and related developmental disorders: A descriptive analysis. *Child and Adolescent Psychiatric Clinics, 23*(1), 25–40.

Duker, P. C., & Seys, D. M. (1996). Long-term use of electrical aversion treatment with self-injurious behavior. *Research in Developmental Disabilities, 17*(4), 293–301.

Dykens, E. M., Fisher, M. H., Taylor, J. L., Lambert, W., & Miodrag, N. (2014). Reducing distress in mothers of children with autism and other disabilities: A randomized trial. *Pediatrics, 134*(2), e454–e463.

Ehrhart, F., Sangani, N. B., & Curfs, L. M. (2018). Current developments in the genetics of Rett and Rett-like syndrome. *Current Opinion in Psychiatry, 31*(2), 103–108.

Eisenberg, L., Ascher, E., & Kanner, L. (1959). A clinical study of Gilles de la Tourette's disease (maladie des tics) in children. *American Journal of Psychiatry, 115,* 715–723.

Emerson, E., Kiernan, C., Alborz, A., Reeves, D., Mason, H., Swarbrick, R., Mason, L., & Hatton, C. (2001). The prevalence of challenging behaviors: A total population study. *Research in Developmental Disabilities, 22*(1), 77–93.

Feng, X., Wang, L., Yang, S., Qin, D., Wang, J., Li, C., Lv, L., Ma, Y., & Hu, X. (2011). Maternal separation produces lasting changes in cortisol and behavior in rhesus monkeys. *Proceedings of the National Academy of Sciences of the USA, 108*(34), 14312–14317.

Ferdousi, M., & Finn, D. P. (2018). Stress-induced modulation of pain: Role of the endogenous opioid system. Progress in *Brain Research, 239,* 121–177.

Ficks, C. A., & Waldman, I. D. (2014). Candidate genes for aggression and antisocial behavior: A meta-analysis of association studies of the 5HTTLPR and MAOA-uVNTR. *Behavior Genetics*, 44(5), 427–444.

Fink, M. (2013). Rediscovering catatonia: The biography of a treatable syndrome. *Acta Psychiatrica Scandinavica*, 127, 1–47.

Fink, M., & Taylor, M. A. (2006). *Catatonia: A clinician's guide to diagnosis and treatment*. Cambridge University Press.

Finucane, B., Haines Dirrigl, K., & Simon, E. W. (2001). Characterization of self-injurious behaviors in children and adults with Smith–Magenis syndrome. *American Journal of Mental Retardation*, 106(1), 52–58.

Folch, A., Cortés, M. J., Salvador-Carulla, L., Vicens, P., Irazábal, M., Muñoz, S., Rovira, L., Orejuela, C., Haro, J., Vilella, E., & Martínez-Leal, R. (2018). Risk factors and topographies for self-injurious behaviour in a sample of adults with intellectual developmental disorders. *Journal of Intellectual Disability Research*, 62(12), 1018–1029.

Ford, G. K., & Finn, D. P. (2008). Clinical correlates of stress-induced analgesia: Evidence from pharmacological studies. *Pain*, 140(1), 3–7.

Ghaziuddin, N., Dhossche, D., & Marcotte, K. (2012). Retrospective chart review of catatonia in child and adolescent psychiatric patients. *Acta Psychiatrica Scandinavica*, 125(1), 33–38.

Gispen, W. H., Wiegant, M. M., Grevan, H. M., & De Wied, D. (1976). The induction of excessive grooming in the rat by intraventricular application of peptides derived from ACTH: Structure-activity studies. *Life Sciences*, 17, 645–652.

Goldstein, D. S., Holmes, C., & Axelrod, F. B. (2008). Plasma catechols in familial dysautonomia: A long-term follow-up study. *Neurochemical Research*, 33(9), 1889–1893.

Goldstein, M., Anderson, L. T., Reuben, R., & Dancis, J. (1985). Self-mutilation in Lesch–Nyhan disease is caused by dopaminergic denervation. *Lancet*, 1, 338–339.

Goosen, C., & Ribbens, L. G. (1980). Autoaggression and tactile communication in pairs of adult stumptailed macaques. *Behaviour*, 73(3–4), 155–174.

Greenberg, A., & Coleman, M. (1973). Depressed whole blood serotonin levels associated with behavioral abnormalities in the de Lange syndrome. *Pediatrics*, 52(5), 720–724.

Griengl, H., Sendera, A., & Dantendorfer, K. (2001). Naltrexone as a treatment of self-injurious behavior—A case report. *Acta Psychiatrica Scandinavica*, 103(3), 234–236.

Guerdjikova, A. I., Gwizdowski, I. S., McElroy, S. L., McCullumsmith, C., & Suppes, P. (2014). Treating nonsuicidal self-injury. *Current Treatment Options in Psychiatry*, 1(4), 325–334.

Hagberg, B., Aicardi, J., Dias, K., & Ramos, O. (1983). A progressive syndrome of autism, dementia, ataxia, and loss of purposeful hand use in girls: Rett's syndrome: Report of 35 cases. *Annals of Neurology*, 14(4), 471–479.

Hagberg, B., Hanefeld, F., Percy, A., & Skjeldal, O. L. A. (2002). An update on clinically applicable diagnostic criteria in Rett syndrome: Comments to Rett Syndrome Clinical Criteria Consensus Panel Satellite to European Paediatric Neurology Society meeting, Baden Baden, Germany, 11 September 2001. *European Journal of Paediatric Neurology*, 6(5), 293–297.

Hagerman, R. J., Jackson, A. W., Levitas, A., Rimland, B., & Braden, M. (1986). An analysis of autism in fifty males with fragile X syndrome. *American Journal of Medical Genetics*, 23, 359–374.

Hagopian, L. P., & Gregory, M. K. (2016). Behavior analytic approaches to problem behavior in intellectual disabilities. *Current Opinion in Psychiatry*, 29(2), 126–132.

Hagopian, L. P., Rooker, G. W., Jessel, J., & DeLeon, I. G. (2013). Initial functional analysis outcomes and modifications in pursuit of differentiation: A summary of 176 inpatient cases. *Journal of Applied Behavior Analysis*, 46(1), 88–100.

Hagopian, L. P., Rooker, G. W., & Zarcone, J. R. (2015). Delineating subtypes of self-injurious behavior maintained by automatic reinforcement. *Journal of Applied Behavior Analysis*, 48(3), 523–543.

Harris, J. C. (2018). Lesch–Nyhan syndrome and its variants: Examining the behavioral and neurocognitive phenotype. *Current Opinion in Psychiatry*, 31(2), 96–102.

Heffernan, K., Cloitre, M., Tardiff, K., Marzuk, P. M., Portera, L., & Leon, A. C. (2000). Childhood trauma as a correlate of lifetime opiate use in psychiatric patients. *Addictive Behaviors, 25*(5), 797–803.

Hennessey, J. W., & Levine, S. (1979). Stress, arousal, and the pituitary adrenal system: A psychoendocrine hypothesis. Progress in *Psychobiology* and *Physiological Psychology, 8*, 133–178.

Hessl, D., Tassone, F., Cordeiro, L., Koldewyn, K., McCormick, C., Green, C., Wegelin, J., Yuhas, J., & Hagerman, R. J. (2008). Brief report: Aggression and stereotypic behavior in males with fragile X syndrome—Moderating secondary genes in a "single gene" disorder. *Journal of Autism and Developmental Disorders, 38*(1), 184–189.

Huggins, K. N., Mathews, T. A., Locke, J. L., Szeliga, K. T., Friedman, D. P., Bennett, A. J., & Jones, S. R. (2012). Effects of early life stress on drinking and serotonin system activity in rhesus macaques: 5-Hydroxyindoleacetic acid in cerebrospinal fluid predicts brain tissue levels. *Alcohol, 46*(4), 371–376.

Huguet, A., Eguren, J. I., Miguel-Ruiz, D., Vallés, X. V., & Alda, J. A. (2019). Deficient emotional self-regulation in children with attention deficit hyperactivity disorder: Mindfulness as a useful treatment modality. *Journal of Developmental and Behavioral Pediatrics, 40*(6), 425–431.

Inoue, M. (2019). Assessments and interventions to address challenging behavior in individuals with intellectual disability and autism spectrum disorder in Japan: A consolidated review. *Yonago Acta Medica, 62*(2), 169–181.

Iriki, A., Shuicki, N., & Nakamura, Y. (1988). Feeding behavior in mammals: Corticobulbar projection is reorganized during conversion from sucking to chewing. *Developmental Brain Research, 44*, 189–196.

Janowsky, D. S., Barnhill, L. J., & Davis, J. M. (2003). Olanzapine for self-injurious, aggressive, and disruptive behaviors in intellectually disabled adults: A retrospective, open-label, naturalistic trial. *Journal of Clinical Psychiatry, 64*(10), 1258–1265.

Jinnah, H. A., Yitta, S., Drew, T., Kim, B. S., Visser, J. E., & Rothstein, J. D. (1999). Calcium channel activation and self-biting in mice. *Proceedings of the National Academy of Sciences, 96*(26), 15228–15232.

Jolles, J., Rompa-Barendregt, I., & Gispen, W. H. (1979). ACTH-induced excessive grooming in the rat: The influence of environmental and motivational factors. *Hormones and Behavior, 12*, 60–72.

Jones, I. H., & Barraclough, B. M. (1978). Auto-mutilation in animals and its relevance to self-injury in man. *Acta Psychiatrica Scandinavica, 58*, 40–47.

Kahng, S., Iwata, B. A., & Lewin, A. B. (2002). Behavioral treatment of self-injury, 1964 to 2000. *American Journal of Mental Retardation, 107*(3), 212–221.

Kars, H., Broekema, W., Glaudemans-van Gelderen, I., Verhoeven, W. M. A., & Van Ree, J. M. (1990). Naltrexone attenuates self-injurious behavior in mentally retarded subjects. *Biological Psychiatry, 27*(7), 741–746.

Kasim, S., Blake, B. L., Fan, X., Chartoff, E., Egami, K., Breese, G. R., . . . Jinnah, H. A. (2006). The role of dopamine receptors in the neurobehavioral syndrome provoked by activation of L-type calcium channels in rodents. *Developmental Neuroscience, 28*(6), 505–517.

Kasim, S., Egami, K., & Jinnah, H. A. (2002). Self-biting induced by activation of L-type calcium channels in mice: Serotonergic influences. *Developmental Neuroscience, 24*(4), 322–327.

Kasim, S., & Jinnah, H. A. (2003). Self-biting induced by activation of L-type calcium channels in mice: Dopaminergic influences. *Developmental Neuroscience, 25*(1), 20–25.

Khasnavis, T., Torres, R. J., Sommerfeld, B., Puig, J. G., Chipkin, R., & Jinnah, H. A. (2016). A double-blind, placebo-controlled, crossover trial of the selective dopamine D1 receptor antagonist ecopipam in patients with Lesch–Nyhan disease. *Molecular Genetics and Metabolism, 118*(3), 160–166.

Kluver, H., & Bucy, A. S. (1939). Preliminary analysis of functions of the temporal lobe in monkeys. *Archives of Neurology and Psychiatry, 42*, 978–1000.

Kolla, N. J., & Bortolato, M. (2020). The role of monoamine oxidase A in the neurobiology of aggressive, antisocial, and violent behavior: A tale of mice and men. *Progress in Neurobiology, 194,* 101875

Kolla, N. J., Matthews, B., Wilson, A. A., Houle, S., Bagby, R. M., Links, P., . . . Meyer, J. H. (2015). Lower monoamine oxidase-A total distribution volume in impulsive and violent male offenders with antisocial personality disorder and high psychopathic traits: An [(11)C] harmine positron emission tomography study. *Neuropsychopharmacology, 40*(11), 2596–2603.

Kolla, N. J., Patel, R., Meyer, J. H., & Chakravarty, M. M. (2017). Association of monoamine oxidase-A genetic variants and amygdala morphology in violent offenders with antisocial personality disorder and high psychopathic traits. *Scientific Reports, 7*(1), 1–13.

Kopin, I. J. (1981). Neurotransmitters and the Lesch–Nyhan syndrome. *New England Journal of Medicine, 305,* 1148–1150.

Kostrzewa, R. M. (1995). Dopamine receptor supersensitivity. *Neuroscience and Biobehavioral Reviews, 19*(1), 1–17.

Lesch, M., & Nyhan, W. L. (1964). A familial disorder of uric acid metabolism and central nervous system function. *American Journal of Medicine, 36,* 561–570.

Lowe, K., Allen, D., Jones, E., Brophy, S., Moore, K., & James, W. (2007). Challenging behaviours: Prevalence and topographies. *Journal of Intellectual Disability Research, 51*(8), 625–636.

Lundqvist, L. O. (2013). Prevalence and risk markers of behavior problems among adults with intellectual disabilities: A total population study in Örebro County, Sweden. *Research in Developmental Disabilities, 34*(4), 1346–1356.

Lutz, C., Well, A., & Novak, M. (2003). Stereotypic and self-injurious behavior in rhesus macaques: A survey and retrospective analysis of environment and early experience. *American Journal of Primatology, 60*(1), 1–15.

Lydon, S., Healy, O., Roche, M., Henry, R., Mulhern, T., & Hughes, B. M. (2015). Salivary cortisol levels and challenging behavior in children with autism spectrum disorder. *Research in Autism Spectrum Disorders, 10,* 78–92.

Madsen, T. M., Treschow, A., Bengzon, J., Bolwig, T. G., Lindvall, O., & Tingström, A. (2000). Increased neurogenesis in a model of electroconvulsive therapy. *Biological Psychiatry, 47*(12), 1043–1049.

Manfredi, M., Bini, G., Cruccu, G., Accornero, N., Berardelli, A., & Medolago, L. (1981). Congenital absence of pain. *Archives of Neurology, 38*(8), 507–511.

Mason, G. J. (1991). Stereotypies: A critical review. *Animal Behaviour, 41*(6), 1015–1037.

Mathews, C. A., Waller, J., Glidden, D., Lowe, T. L., Herrera, L. D., Budman, C. L., Erenberg, G., Naarden, A., Bruun, R., Freimer, N., & Reus, V. I. (2004). Self injurious behaviour in Tourette syndrome: Correlates with impulsivity and impulse control. *Journal of Neurology, Neurosurgery, and Psychiatry, 75*(8), 1149–1155.

Mazzone, L., Postorino, V., Valeri, G., & Vicari, S. (2014). Catatonia in patients with autism: Prevalence and management. *CNS Drugs, 28*(3), 205–215.

McCracken, J. T., McGough, J., Shah, B., Cronin, P., Hong, D., Aman, M. G., Arnold, L., Lindsay, R., Nash, P., Hollway, J., McDougle, C. J., Posey, D., Swiezy, N., Kohn, A., Scahill, L., Martin, A., Koenig, K., Volkmar, F., Carroll, D., Lancor, A., . . . Research Units on Pediatric Psychopharmacology Autism Network. (2002). Risperidone in children with autism and serious behavioral problems. *New England Journal of Medicine, 347*(5), 314–321.

McDermott, R., Tingley, D., Cowden, J., Frazzetto, G., & Johnson, D. D. (2009). Monoamine oxidase A gene (MAOA) predicts behavioral aggression following provocation. *Proceedings of the National Academy of Sciences of the USA, 106*(7), 2118–2123.

McQuire, C., Hassiotis, A., Harrison, B., & Pilling, S. (2015). Pharmacological interventions for challenging behaviour in children with intellectual disabilities: A systematic review and meta-analysis. *BMC Psychiatry, 15*(1), Article 303.

Meyer-Holzapfel, M. (1968). Abnormal behavior in zoo animals. In M. Fox (Ed.), *Abnormal behavior in animals* (pp. 476–503). Saunders.

Meyer-Lindenberg, A., Buckholtz, J. W., Kolachana, B., Hariri, A. R., Pezawas, L., Blasi, G., Wabnitz, A., Honea, R., Verchinski, B., Callicott, J., Egan, M., Mattay, V., & Weinberger, D. (2006). Neural mechanisms of genetic risk for impulsivity and violence in humans. *Proceedings of the National Academy of Sciences of the USA, 103*(16), 6269–6274.

Millan, M. J. (2002). Descending control of pain. *Progress in Neurobiology, 66*(6), 355–474.

Minett, M. S., Pereira, V., Sikandar, S., Matsuyama, A., Lolignier, S., Kanellopoulos, A. H., Mancini, F., Iannetti, G., Bogdanov, Y., Santana-Varela, S., Millet, Q., Baskozos, G., MacAllister, R., Cox, J., Zhao, J., & Wood, J., (2015). Endogenous opioids contribute to insensitivity to pain in humans and mice lacking sodium channel Nav1.7. *Nature Communications, 6*, 8967.

Minshawi, N. F., Hurwitz, S., Fodstad, J. C., Biebl, S., Morriss, D. H., & McDougle, C. J. (2014). The association between self-injurious behaviors and autism spectrum disorders. *Psychology Research and Behavior Management, 7*, 125–136.

Mizuno, T., & Yugari, Y. (1975). Prophylactic effect of L-5 hydroxytryptophan on self-mutilation in the Lesch–Nyhan syndrome. *Neuropuediatrie, 6*, 13–23.

Mizuno, T. I., & Yugari, Y. (1974). Self-mutilation in Lesch–Nyhan syndrome. *Lancet, 303*(7860), 761.

Moy, S. S., Knapp, D. J., & Breese, G. R. (2001). Effect of olanzapine on functional responses from sensitized D 1-dopamine receptors in rats with neonatal dopamine loss. *Neuropsychopharmacology, 25*(2), 224–233.

Muehlmann, A. M., Brown, B. D., & Devine, D. P. (2008). Pemoline (2-amino-5-phenyl-1, 3-oxazol-4-one)-induced self-injurious behavior: A rodent model of pharmacotherapeutic efficacy. *Journal of Pharmacology and Experimental Therapeutics, 324*(1), 214–223.

Muharib, R., Correa, V. I., Wood, C. L., & Haughney, K. L. (2019). Effects of functional communication training using GoTalk Now iPad application on challenging behavior of children with autism spectrum disorder. *Journal of Special Education Technology, 34*(2), 71–79.

National Institute for Health and Care Excellence. (2019). *Challenging behaviour and learning disabilities: Prevention and interventions for people with learning disabilities whose behaviour challenges.* http://www.nice.org.uk/guidance/ng11

National Institutes of Health. (1991, September). *Consensus Development Conference on the Treatment of Destructive Behaviors in Persons with Developmental Disabilities* (NIH Publication No. 91–2410). U.S. Department of Health and Human Services, Public Health Service.

Neely, L., Garcia, E., Bankston, B., & Green, A. (2018). Generalization and maintenance of functional communication training for individuals with developmental disabilities: A systematic and quality review. *Research in Developmental Disabilities, 79*, 116–129.

Nelson, C. A., Fox, N. A., & Zeanah, C. H. (2014). *Romania's abandoned children: Deprivation, brain development, and the struggle for recovery.* Harvard University Press.

Neul, J. L., Kaufmann, W. E., Glaze, D. G., Christodoulou, J., Clarke, A. J., Bahi-Buisson, N., Leonard, H., Bailey, M., Schanen, N., Zappella, M., Renieri, A., Huppke, P., Percy, A., & RettSearch Consortium. (2010). Rett syndrome: Revised diagnostic criteria and nomenclature. *Annals of Neurology, 68*(6), 944–950.

Nilsen, K. B., Nicholas, A. K., Woods, C. G., Mellgren, S. I., Nebuchennykh, M., & Aasly, J. (2009). Two novel SCN9A mutations causing insensitivity to pain. *Pain, 143*(1–2), 155–158.

Norelli, L. J., Smith, H. S., Sher, L., & Blackwood, T. A. (2013). Buprenorphine in the treatment of non-suicidal self-injury: A case series and discussion of the literature. *International Journal of Adolescent Medicine and Health, 25*(3), 323–330.

Nyhan, W. L. (1976). Behavior in the Lesch–Nyhan syndrome. *Journal of Autism and Childhood Schizophrenia, 6*(3), 235–252.

Oakes, A., Thurman, A. J., McDuffie, A., Bullard, L. M., Hagerman, R. J., & Abbeduto, L. (2016). Characterising repetitive behaviours in young boys with fragile X syndrome. *Journal of Intellectual Disability Research, 60*(1), 54–67.

Oliver, C., Licence, L., & Richards, C. (2017). Self-injurious behaviour in people with intellectual disability and autism spectrum disorder. *Current Opinion in Psychiatry, 30*(2), 97–101.

Öngür, D., & Heckers, S. (2004). A role for glia in the action of electroconvulsive therapy. *Harvard Review of Psychiatry, 12*(5), 253–262.

Ornitz, E. M. (1974). The modulation of sensory input and motor output in autistic children. *Journal of Autism and Childhood Schizophrenia, 4*, 197–215.

Pérez-López, L. M., Cabrera-González, M., Gutiérrez-de la Iglesia, D., Ricart, S., & Knörr-Giménez, G. (2015). Update review and clinical presentation in congenital insensitivity to pain and anhidrosis. *Case Reports in Pediatrics*, 2015, 589852.

Piton, A., Poquet, H., Redin, C., Masurel, A., Lauer, J., Muller, J., Thevenon, J., Herenger, Y., Chancenotte, S., Bonnet, M., Pinoit, J. M., Huet, F., Thauvin-Robinet, C., Jaeger, A.-S., Le Gras, S., Jost, B., Gerard, B., Peoch, K., Launay, J.-M., . . . Mandel, J.-L. (2014). 20 ans apres: A second mutation in MAOA identified by targeted high-throughput sequencing in a family with altered behavior and cognition. *European Journal of Human Genetics, 22*(6), 776–783

Poulton, R., Moffitt, T. E., & Silva, P. A. (2015). The Dunedin Multidisciplinary Health and Development Study: Overview of the first 40 years, with an eye to the future. *Social Psychiatry and Psychiatric Epidemiology, 50*(5), 679–693.

Rattaz, C., Michelon, C., & Baghdadli, A. (2015). Symptom severity as a risk factor for self-injurious behaviours in adolescents with autism spectrum disorders. *Journal of Intellectual Disability Research, 59*(8), 730–741.

Reichow, B. (2012). Overview of meta-analyses on early intensive behavioral intervention for young children with autism spectrum disorders. *Journal of Autism and Developmental Disorders, 42*(4), 512–520.

Rett, A. (1966). Uber ein Eigenartiges hirnatrophisches Syndrome bei Hyperammonamie in Kindsalter. *Wiener Medizinishe Wochenschrift, 116*, 723–726.

Richards, C., Oliver, C., Nelson, L., & Moss, J. (2012). Self-injurious behaviour in individuals with autism spectrum disorder and intellectual disability. *Journal of Intellectual Disability Research, 56*(5), 476–489.

Riley, C. M., Day, R. L., Greeley, D. M., & Langford, W. S. (1949). Central autonomic dysfunction with defective lacrimation. *Pediatrics, 3*, 468–478.

Robertson, M., Rey, J. M., & Walter, G. (2013). Ethical and consent aspects. In N. Ghaziuddin & G. Walter (Eds.), *Electroconvulsive therapy in children and adolescents* (pp. 56–75). Oxford University Press.

Robertson, M. M., Trimble, M. R., & Lees, A. L. (1989). Self-injurious behaviour and the Gilles de la Tourette syndrome: A clinical study and review of the literature. *Psychological Medicine, 19*, 611–625.

Rojahn, J., Rowe, E. W., Sharber, A. C., Hastings, R., Matson, J. L., Didden, R., Kroes, D., & Dumont, E. L. M. (2012a). The Behavior Problems Inventory–Short Form for individuals with intellectual disabilities: Part I. Development and provisional clinical reference data. *Journal of Intellectual Disability Research, 56*(5), 527–545.

Rojahn, J., Rowe, E. W., Sharber, A. C., Hastings, R., Matson, J. L., Didden, R., Kroes, D., & Dumont, E. L. M. (2012b). The Behavior Problems Inventory–Short Form for individuals with intellectual disabilities: Part II. Reliability and validity. *Journal of Intellectual Disability Research, 56*(5), 546–565.

Rommeck, I., Anderson, K., Heagerty, A., Cameron, A., & McCowan, B. (2009). Risk factors and remediation of self-injurious and self-abuse behavior in rhesus macaques. *Journal of Applied Animal Welfare Science, 12*(1), 61–72.

Rubin, B. Y., & Anderson, S. L. (2017). *IKBKAP/ELP1* gene mutations: Mechanisms of familial dysautonomia and gene-targeting therapies. *The Application of Clinical Genetics, 10*, 95–103.

Salemi, S., Aeschlimann, A., Reisch, N., Jüngel, A., Gay, R. E., Heppner, F. L., Michel, B., Gay, S., & Sprott, H. (2005). Detection of kappa and delta opioid receptors in skin—Outside the nervous system. *Biochemical and Biophysical Research Communications, 338*(2), 1012–1017.

Sanchez, M. D., Milanes, M. V., Fuente, T., & Laorden, M. L. (1992). Prenatal stress alters the hypothalamic levels of methionine–enkephalin in pup rats. *Neuropeptides, 23*(2), 131–135.

Sanchez, M. D., Milanés, M. V., Pazos, A., Diaz, A., & Laorden, M. L. (1996). Autoradiographic evidence of μ-opioid receptors down-regulation after prenatal stress in offspring rat brain. *Developmental Brain Research, 94*(1), 14–21.

Sandman, C. A. (2009). Efficacy of opioid antagonists in attentuating self-injurious behavior. In R. Dean, E. Bilsky, & S. Negus (Eds.), *Opiate receptors and antagonists* (pp. 457–472). Humana Press.

Sandman, C. A., Hetrick, W., Taylor, D. V., & Chicz-DeMet, A. (1997). Dissociation of POMC peptides after self-injury predicts responses to centrally acting opiate blockers. *American Journal of Mental Retardation, 102*(2), 182–199.

Shannon, C., Champoux, M., & Suomi, S. J. (1998). Rearing condition and plasma cortisol in rhesus monkey infants. *American Journal of Primatology, 46*(4), 311–321.

Shorter, E., & Fink, M. (2010). *Endocrine psychiatry: Solving the riddle of melancholia.* Oxford University Press.

Singh, N. N., Lancioni, G. E., Karazsia, B. T., Myers, R. E., Hwang, Y. S., & Anālayo, B. (2019). Effects of mindfulness-based positive behavior support (MBPBS) training are equally beneficial for mothers and their children with autism spectrum disorder or with intellectual disabilities. *Frontiers in Psychology, 10,* Article 385.

Singh, N. N., & Pulman, R. M. (1979). Self injury in the de Lange syndrome. *Journal of Mental Deficiency Research, 23,* 79–84.

Snyder, S. H. (1977). Opiate receptors in the brain. *New England Journal of Medicine, 296,* 266–271.

Srivastava, S., Clark, B., Landy-Schmitt, C., Offermann, E. A., Kline, A. D., Wilkinson, S. T., & Grados, M. A. (2021). Repetitive and self-injurious behaviors in children with Cornelia de Lange syndrome. *Journal of Autism and Developmental Disorders, 51*(5), 1748–1758.

Steenfeldt-Kristensen, C., Jones, C. A., & Richards, C. (2020). The prevalence of self-injurious behaviour in autism: A meta-analytic study. *Journal of Autism and Developmental* Disorders, *50*(11), 3857–3873.

Stein, C. (2016). Opioid receptors. *Annual Review of Medicine, 67,* 433–451.

Symons, F. J., Clark, R. D., Hatton, D. D., Skinner, M., & Bailey, D. B., Jr. (2003). Self-injurious behavior in young boys with fragile X syndrome. *American Journal of Medical Genetics Part A, 118*(2), 115–121.

Symons, F. J., Thompson, A., & Rodriguez, M. C. (2004). Self-injurious behavior and the efficacy of naltrexone treatment: A quantitative synthesis. *Mental Retardation and Developmental Disabilities Research Reviews, 10*(3), 193–200.

Szejko, N., Jakubczyk, A., & Janik, P. (2019). Prevalence and clinical correlates of self-harm behaviours in Gilles de la Tourette syndrome. *Frontiers in Psychiatry, 10,* Article 638.

Taub, E. (1977). Movement in nonhuman primates deprived of somatosensory feedback. Exercise and *Sports Sciences Reviews, 4,* 335–376.

Taub, E., Perrella, P. N., & Barro, G. (1973). Behavioral development following forelimb deafferentation on the day of birth in monkeys with and without blinding. *Science, 181,* 959–960.

Trimble, M. (1992). Gilles de Ia Tourette syndrome [Paper presentation]. Annual Meeting of the American Psychiatric Association, Washington, DC.

Wachtel, L. E. (2019). Treatment of catatonia in autism spectrum disorders. *Acta Psychiatrica Scandinavica, 139*(1), 46–55.

Wachtel, L. E., Shorter, E., & Fink, M. (2018). Electroconvulsive therapy for self-injurious behaviour in autism spectrum disorders: Recognizing catatonia is key. *Current Opinion in Psychiatry, 31*(2), 116–122.

Whittington, J., & Holland, A. (2020). Developing an understanding of skin picking in people with Prader–Willi syndrome: A structured literature review and re-analysis of existing data. *Neuroscience & Biobehavioral Reviews, 112,* 48–61.

Willemsen-Swinkels, S. H., Buitelaar, J. K., Nijhof, G. J., & van Engeland, H. (1995). Failure of naltrexone hydrochloride to reduce self-injurious and autistic behavior in mentally retarded adults: Double-blind placebo-controlled studies. *Archives of General Psychiatry, 52*(9), 766–773.

Williams, S., Leader, G., Mannion, A., & Chen, J. (2015). An investigation of anxiety in children and adolescents with autism spectrum disorder. *Research in Autism Spectrum Disorders, 10,* 30–40.

Wing, L., & Shah, A. (2000). Catatonia in autistic spectrum disorders. *British Journal of Psychiatry*, *176*(4), 357–362.

Wong, D. F., Harris, J. C., Naidu, S., Yokoi, F., Marenco, S., Dannals, R. F., Ravert, H., Yaster, M., Evans, A., Rousset, O., Bryan, R. N., Gjedde, A., Kuhar, M., & Breese, G. (1996). Dopamine transporters are markedly reduced in Lesch–Nyhan disease in vivo. *Proceedings of the National Academy of Sciences of the USA, 93*(11), 5539–5543.

Wood, E. K., Kruger, R., Day, J. P., Day, S. M., Hunter, J. N., Neville, L., Lindell, S., Barr, C., Schwandt, M., Goldman, D., Suomi, S., Harris, J., & Higley, J. (2022). A nonhuman primate model of human non-suicidal self-injury: Serotonin transporter genotype-mediated typologies. Neuropsychopharmacology, *47*(6), 1256–1262.

Woodcock, K. A., & Blackwell, S. (2020). Psychological treatment strategies for challenging behaviours in neurodevelopmental disorders: What lies beyond a purely behavioural approach?. *Current Opinion in Psychiatry, 33*(2), 92–109.

World Health Organization. (2001). *International classification of functioning, disability, and health.*

World Health Organization. (2007). *International classification of functioning, disability, and health for children and youth.*

World Health Organization. (2019). *International statistical classification of diseases and related health problems* (11th ed.).

Ungerstedt, U. (1971). Postsynaptic supersensitivity after 6-hydroxydopamine induced degeneration of the nigro-striatal dopamine system. *Acta Psychiatrica Scandinavica, 367*(suppl.), 69–93.

Zlomke, K. R., & Jeter, K. (2020). Comparative effectiveness of parent–child interaction therapy for children with and without autism spectrum disorder. *Journal of Autism and Developmental Disorders, 50*(6), 2041–2052.

# Index